# SLEEP DEPRIVATION

# LUNG BIOLOGY IN HEALTH AND DISEASE

*Executive Editor*

**Claude Lenfant**

*Former Director, National Heart, Lung, and Blood Institute*
*National Institutes of Health*
*Bethesda, Maryland*

**ADDITIONAL VOLUMES IN PREPARATION**

*The opinions expressed in these volumes do not necessarily represent the views of the National Institutes of Health.*

# SLEEP DEPRIVATION

## Clinical Issues, Pharmacology, and Sleep Loss Effects

### Clete A. Kushida
*Stanford University*
*Stanford, California*

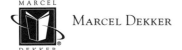

MARCEL DEKKER

NEW YORK

**Library of Congress Cataloging-in-Publication Data**
A catalog record for this book is available from the Library of Congress.

**ISBN: 0-8247-2094-6**

Marcel Dekker, 270 Madison Avenue, New York, NY 10016

**Distribution Center**
Marcel Dekker, Cimarron Road, Monticello, New York 12701, U.S.A.

Current printing (last digit):

10  9  8  7  6  5  4  3  2  1

PRINTED IN THE UNITED STATES OF AMERICA

# Introduction

The second half of the past century was a time of remarkable scientific expansion and knowledge explosion. Biology and health fields were the beneficiaries of many genuine observations and discoveries and, as a result, the health of individuals and the public as a whole improved markedly. The area of sleep and sleep disorders illustrates the advances in knowledge that occurred.

Sleep is a topic that has long been addressed by writers—but much more frequently by poets than by researchers. As an example, in the beginning of the nineteenth century, Samuel Taylor Coleridge gave us this verse:

> Oh, Sleep! It is a gentle thing,
> Beloved from pole to pole

Unquestionably, during the last few decades the study of sleep and its biology in health and disease has moved to the forefront of research, and it has revealed a wealth of observations. At the same time, it has attracted the interest of many investigators with expertise in diverse basic disciplines and clinical areas.

The association of sleep disorders with other clinical fields such as cardiology, neurology, mood and attention disorders, and pneumology is well recognized. Sleep deprivation is a medical issue, but also a social one. As a consequence, we have seen a number of societal and regulatory changes to ensure that appropriate sleep time is available.

This series of monographs, *Lung Biology in Health and Disease*, includes a number of volumes on sleep, the first one having been published in 1984. Seven of these volumes have been exclusively about one or another aspect of sleep, and others, on different subjects, included components related to sleep. However, *lack* of sleep did not achieve stardom in this series until Dr. Clete Kushida from the world-famous Stanford Sleep Disorders Clinic and Research Center accepted the invitation to edit this volume on *Sleep Deprivation: Clinical Issues, Pharmacology, and Sleep Loss Effects*.

This volume and its companion on *Sleep Deprivation: Basic Science, Physiology, and Behavior* are true landmarks in the area of sleep biology and medicine. Dr. Kushida enrolled contributors who have pioneered exploration of the field, and I am grateful to them all for the opportunity to introduce this volume to the readership.

**Claude Lenfant, M.D.**
Bethesda, Maryland

# Preface

"That we are not much sicker and much madder than we are
is due exclusively to that most blessed and blessing
of all natural graces, sleep."

—Aldous Huxley

"Be alert. The world needs more lerts."

I remember this prominent sticker posted on the office door of Dr. Mary Carskadon, when she was at Stanford University. Since her office was next to the entrance of the Sleep Research Laboratory where I conducted undergraduate sleep research, this was the first item I saw when I entered and exited the lab. Needless to say, these words became forever stamped on my mind and, in a modern society in which increased work and family commitments threaten sleep, these are undoubtedly words to live by.

The field of sleep research is experiencing an enviable period of growth since the discovery of REM sleep in 1953. Yet there are still fundamental questions in our field that remain unanswered; many of these questions are within the realm of sleep loss and sleep deprivation. Fortunately, there are many talented investigators who have assumed the responsibility of answering some of these questions, and we look forward to their important breakthroughs.

This work is a direct outcome of the vision and efforts of Dr. Claude Lenfant at the National Heart, Lung and Blood Institute. This monograph could not exist without the outstanding contributions of the talented group of international authors; their diligent work is greatly appreciated. I am deeply indebted to the renowned and true pioneers of our field, Drs. William C. Dement and Allan Reschtschaffen, who provided both direct and indirect supportive expertise for this project. In all of my endeavors, I can always count on my parents, Samiko and Hiroshi Kushida, to assist me; this monograph was no exception.

Lastly, the major theme of this work is that sleep deprivation has profound repercussions on the well-being of the individual and society. It is my sincere hope that the reader becomes proactive and participates in our field's crusade to eliminate sleep loss. The following goals may serve to guide the reader in this crusade:

- To strive to eliminate personal sleep debt, and to encourage others to do the same.
- To prevent those who are sleep deprived from operating motor vehicles or hazardous machinery, or otherwise placing themselves or others in unsafe situations.
- To advise those who are persistently sleepy to seek medical opinion.
- To educate the public on the importance of sleep, and to advocate social change in educational and professional situations where sleep deprivation is currently the norm.

**Clete A. Kushida**
Stanford, California

# Contributors

**Christine Acebo**
E. P. Bradley Hospital/Brown Medical School, East Providence, Rhode Island, U.S.A.

**Lamia Afifi**
Cairo University Medical School Hospitals, Cairo, Egypt

**Thomas J. Balkin**
Walter Reed Army Institute of Research, Silver Spring, Maryland, U.S.A.

**Gregory Belenky**
Walter Reed Army Institute of Research, Silver Spring, Maryland, U.S.A.

**Selim R. Benbadis**
University of South Florida and Tampa General Hospital, Tampa, Florida, U.S.A.

**Michael H. Bonnet**
Dayton Department of Veterans Affairs Medical Center, Wright State University, Kettering Medical Center, and the Wallace Kettering Neuroscience Institute, Dayton, Ohio, U.S.A.

**Amber (Tietzel) Brooks**
Flinders University, Adelaide, South Australia, Australia

**J. Lynn Caldwell**
San Antonio, Texas, U.S.A.

**John A. Caldwell**
San Antonio, Texas, U.S.A.

**Eugenia E. Calle**
American Cancer Society, Atlanta, Georgia, U.S.A.

**Mary A. Carskadon**
Brown Medical School and E. P. Bradley Hospital,
East Providence, Rhode Island, U.S.A.

**Meagan Daley**
Université Laval, Québec, Canada

**Dawn Daniel**
Stanford University, Stanford, California, U.S.A.

**Ritu Davé**
Kaiser Permanente, Stockton Medical Center, Stockton, California, U.S.A.

**William C. Dement**
Stanford University, Stanford, California, U.S.A.

**David F. Dinges**
University of Pennsylvania School of Medicine, Philadelphia, Pennsylvania, U.S.A.

**Jillian Dorrian**
University of Pennsylvania School of Medicine, Philadelphia, Pennsylvania, U.S.A.

**Pingfu Feng**
Case Western Reserve University and Wade Park VA Medical Center,
Cleveland, Ohio, U.S.A.

**David J. C. Flower**
Alertness Solutions, Cupertino, California, U.S.A.

**Fabio Garcia-Garcia**
Washington State University, Pullman, Washington, U.S.A.

**Erika Gaylor**
Stanford University, Stanford, California, U.S.A.

**Kevin B. Gregory**
Alertness Solutions, Cupertino, California, U.S.A.

**Christian Guilleminault**
Stanford University, Stanford, California, U.S.A.

**W. Edward Jung**
Alertness Solutions, Cupertino, California, U.S.A.

**Thomas S. Kilduff**
SRI International, Menlo Park, California, U.S.A.

**Jacqueline D. Kloss**
Drexel University, Philadelphia, Pennsylvania, U.S.A.

**James M. Krueger**
Washington State University, Pullman, Washington, U.S.A.

**Daniel F. Kripke**
University of California–San Diego, La Jolla, California, U.S.A.

**Clete A. Kushida**
Stanford University, Stanford, California, U.S.A.

**Leon Lack**
Flinders University, Adelaide, South Australia, Australia

**Mélanie LeBlanc**
Université Laval, Québec, Canada

**Matthias K. Lee**
Virginia Mason Sleep Disorders Center, Seattle, Washington, U.S.A.

**Rachel Manber**
Stanford University, Stanford, California, U.S.A.

**Matthew R. Marler**
University of California–San Diego, La Jolla, California, U.S.A.

**Merrill M. Mitler**
National Institute of Neurological Disorders and Stroke,
Bethesda, Maryland, U.S.A.

**Charles M. Morin**
Université Laval, Québec, Canada

**Ferenc Obal, Jr.**
University of Szeged, Szeged, Hungary

**Heather N. Odle-Dusseau**
Clemson University, Clemson, South Carolina, U.S.A.

**Judith A. Owens**
Rhode Island Hospital, Providence, Rhode Island, U.S.A.

**Markku Partinen**
University of Helsinki, Espoo, Finland

**Pierre Philip**
Clinique du Sommeil Chu Bordeaux, Bordeaux, France

**June J. Pilcher**
Clemson University, Clemson, South Carolina, U.S.A.

**Craig J. Pritzlaff**
Southern Methodist University, Dallas, Texas, U.S.A.

**Allan Rechtschaffen**
Chicago, Illinois, U.S.A.

**Thomas P. Reilly**
Liverpool John Moores University, Liverpool, England

**Timothy Roehrs**
Henry Ford Hospital, Sleep Disorders and Research Center, and Wayne State University, School of Medicine, Detroit, Michigan, U.S.A.

**Naomi L. Rogers**
University of Pennsylvania School of Medicine, Philadelphia, Pennsylvania, U.S.A.

**Mark R. Rosekind**
Alertness Solutions, Cupertino, California, U.S.A.

**Thomas Roth**
Henry Ford Hospital, Sleep Disorders and Research Center, and Wayne State University, School of Medicine, Detroit, Michigan, U.S.A.

**Daniel W. Shuman**
Southern Methodist University, Dallas, Texas, U.S.A.

**Alexander McCall Smith**
University of Edinburgh, Edinburgh, Scotland

**Roger S. Smith**
Stanford University, Stanford, California, U.S.A.

**Riccardo Stoohs**
Dortmund Sleep Disorders Center, Dortmund, Germany

**Jacques Taillard**
Clinique du Sommeil Chu Bordeaux, Bordeaux, France

**Akira Terao**
SRI International, Menlo Park, California, U.S.A.

**James K. Walsh**
St. John's Mercy Medical Center, St. Luke's Hospital, and Saint Louis University, St. Louis, Missouri, U.S.A.

**Nancy J. Wesensten**
Walter Reed Army Institute of Research, Silver Spring, Maryland, U.S.A.

**Amy R. Wolfson**
College of the Holy Cross, Worcester, Massachusetts, U.S.A.

**Kin Yuen**
Stanford University, Stanford, California, U.S.A.

# Contents

## EVALUATION OF SLEEP LOSS

## CRITICAL THEORETICAL AND PRACTICAL ISSUES

# 1

# Questionnaires and Rating Scales

**SELIM R. BENBADIS**

University of South Florida and Tampa General Hospital,
Tampa, Florida, U.S.A.

## I.  Introduction

Sleep disorders are common, and are generally underdiagnosed. The two major complaints related to sleep are insomnia ("I can't sleep") and excessive daytime sleepiness (EDS, "I can't stay awake"). EDS is a relatively nonspecific symptom. It can be the end result of any factor that causes sleep disruption, and it can be caused by "primary" or "intrinsic" sleep disorders. Insomnia of any cause can result in sleep deprivation and subsequent EDS. The most common cause of EDS *in the general population* is self-imposed sleep deprivation, or "insufficient sleep syndrome." By contrast, the most common causes of EDS seen *in a sleep center* are primary (intrinsic) disorders of EDS. The American Academy of Sleep Medicine (AASM, formerly the American Sleep Disorders Association) classification of sleep disorders includes over 80 diagnoses that are associated with EDS, but the majority of patients evaluated at sleep centers have sleep apnea, narcolepsy, idiopathic hypersomnia, or periodic limb movements of sleep.

EDS, of any cause, is common. The exact prevalence is difficult to determine, since sleepiness is not an all-or-none phenomenon, but it can be estimated. Using a subjective scale, the Epworth Sleepiness Scale (ESS), about 26% of normal subjects score >10 and about 2.5% score >15 (1). Using an objective method, the MSLT, about 32% of subjects score in the severely sleepy range (2). In addition to being common, EDS is a significant public health problem, as it is responsible for a significant proportion of motor vehicle and industrial accidents.

This chapter will review the questionnaires and rating scales available for the evaluation of sleep deprivation and EDS. Other questionnaires used for sleep disorders but not directly related to EDS (e.g., sleep disorders questionnaires, questionnaires for specific symptoms, restless legs, cataplexy) will not be reviewed.

## II.  General Features of Questionnaires and Rating Scales

Questionnaires and rating scales are by nature subjective. Subjects are asked questions, which they answer according to how they perceive their symptoms. Thus, administering questionnaires and rating scales is best viewed as an extension and systematic version of "regular" history taking. Their value, in general, is that they add standardization and formal and quantitative grading of symptoms. Their major weakness is precisely in their definition: they are by nature subjective, and an important question is how they relate to *objective* measures of sleepiness.

Questionnaires and rating scales for sleepiness can be divided into two broad categories: those that estimate short-term, or moment-to-moment fluctuations, and those that assess more long-term (steady-state, permanent) states. The former is typified by the Stanford Sleepiness Scale (SSS), and is best suited for evaluation of sleepiness/alertness throughout the circadian cycle. The latter are typified by the ESS, and are best suited for the evaluation of sleep disorders.

## III.  Available Questionnaires and Rating Scales

### A.  Visual Analog Scales

A visual analog scale can be used for sleepiness, and is similar to what is commonly used in the assessment of pain. It typically uses a horizontal line (e.g., 10 cm), on which subjects can draw a vertical mark indicating their degree of alertness or sleepiness. In theory this provides a continuous measure, rather than a discrete integer. This is probably overly simplistic to measure a multidimensional and complex phenomenon like sleepiness. It does not add much to simple history taking, and is overall rarely used (3,4).

### B.  Stanford Sleepiness Scale

The Stanford Sleepiness Scale (SSS) (5) was the most commonly used scale for sleepiness prior to the ESS. It seems to reliably quantify sleepiness in healthy persons (5,6), but its usefulness in sleep disorders is less certain. The SSS consists of seven descriptive phrases that describe the subject's state (see Fig. 1), of which subjects must choose the *one* that best describes how they feel at the time. Thus,

The subject is to choose the statement that best describes his/her state.

1    Feeling active and vital, alert, wide awake

2    Functioning at high level, but not at peak, able to concentrate

3    Relaxed, awake, not at full alertness, responsive

4    A little foggy, not at peak, let down

5    Fogginess, beginning to lose interest in remaining awake, slowed down

6    Sleepiness, prefer to be lying down, fighting sleep, woozy

7    Almost in reverie, sleep onset soon, lost struggle to remain awake

**Figure 1**    The Stanford Sleepiness Scale. (From Ref. 5.)

the SSS is the prototype of a scale that refers to a degree of sleepiness at a *particular point in time*. It is therefore best suited to evaluate *short-term* changes, e.g., moment-to-moment fluctuations of an individual throughout the circadian rhythm (7), rather than a comparison among multiple subjects.

### C.  Karolinska Sleepiness Scale

The Karolinska Sleepiness Scale (8) is comparable to the SSS. The choice here is among nine descriptive statements (phrases that describe the subject's state). Here the statements specifically refer to how the patient felt in the previous 10 min.

### D.  Sleep-Wake Activity Inventory

The Sleep-Wake Activity Inventory (SWAI) (9) was scientifically and rigorously developed, using a stepwise regression analysis with the mean sleep latency. As a result, it is a multidimensional measure, and is quite extensive, with 59 items in the questionnaire. The factors tested include EDS, but also other related factors, termed psychic distress, social desirability, energy level, ability to relax, and nocturnal sleep. This scale appears to be sensitive to different levels of sleepiness, and also seems to reliably reflect improvements associated with treatment (9). Despite being published in 1993, the SWAI has not been widely used in clinical practice, most likely because it is more complex and lengthy than the ESS. It may be better suited for clinical research protocols. It does appear to reliably distinguish normal alertness from pathological sleepiness (10).

### E.  Functional Outcomes of Sleep Questionnaire

The Functional Outcomes of Sleep Questionnaire (FOSQ) was proposed in 1997 (11). Its objective was to assess the functional outcome related to EDS, i.e., patients' actual ability to function in daily life along multiple dimensions, including physical, mental, and social functioning. Specifically, the FOSQ comprises a total of 30 items, grouped in five "factors": activity level, vigilance, intimacy/sexuality, general productivity, and social. It takes about 15 min to complete. Like the SWAI, the FOSQ has not been widely used in clinical practice, most likely because of its complexity and length, and is probably better suited for clinical research. There are other questionnaires (e.g., SAQLI [Sleep Apnea Quality of Life Inventory], QWB-SA [Quality of Well-Being-Sleep Apnea]) that are designed to assess quality-of-life in patients with specific sleep disorders.

### F.   Epworth Sleepiness Scale

The Epworth Sleepiness Scale (ESS) was described in 1991 (12), and has rapidly supplanted other similar scales. It is easy to administer, and is currently (by far) the most widely used subjective scale (13–19), including important clinical trials for narcolepsy (20–23). It is an eight-item questionnaire where each question is answered with a score from 0 (would never doze) to 3 (high chance of dozing), thus yielding a total between 0 (minimum) and 24 (maximum sleepiness). Questions inquire of the tendency to fall asleep during the following circumstances: (a) sitting and reading, (b) watching television, (c) sitting inactive in a public place, (d) as a passenger in a car for 1 hr without a break, (e) lying down in the afternoon, (f) sitting and talking to someone, (g) sitting quietly after lunch, and (h) in a car while stopped for a few minutes in traffic (Fig. 2).

Because of its conciseness, the ESS easily fits on a single $8 \times 11$ sheet of paper, and takes less than 3 min for patients or families to complete. Its items are short, simple, easily understandable even by poorly educated patients, and it yields a simple number (from 0 to 24). Unlike the SSS, which refers to a state at a particular time of the day or night, the ESS refers to a general state, and is more suited to evaluate disease versus health. For those reasons, it is currently and by far the most used sleepiness scale, both in clinical practice and in research.

### G.   Other Questionnaires and Scales

Other (less specific) scales have also been used as part of the evaluation of EDS. The basic Nordic Sleep Questionnaire (24) is a quantitative measure of subjective sleep *complaints* not limited to sleepiness. It focuses on events that happen (during sleep or wakefulness), and grades them on a five-point scale from 1 (never) to 5 (almost every day/night). Thus it is best suited for "events" but not for sleepiness as such. The Sleep Disorders Questionnaire (SDQ) (25) was extracted from another comprehensive questionnaire, the Sleep Questionnaire and Assessment of Wakefulness (SQAW) of Stanford, but is more geared for the diagnosis of specific sleep disorders (e.g., sleep apnea, narcolepsy) than for the evaluation and quantification of EDS.

How likely are you to doze off or fall asleep in the following situations, in contrast to feeling just tired? This refers to your usual way of life in recent times. Even if you have not done some of these things recently, try to work out how they would have affected you.

Use the following scale to choose the most appropriate number for each situation:

0: would *never* doze
1: *slight* chance of dozing
2: *moderate* chance of dozing
3: *high* chance of dozing

**Activity**　　　　　　　　　　　　　　　　　　　　　　**Chance of Dozing**

Sitting and Reading　　　　　　　　　　　　　　　　　　　_____

Watching TV　　　　　　　　　　　　　　　　　　　　　_____

Sitting inactive in a public place (meeting, theater, etc.)　　_____

As a passenger in a car for 1 hour without a break　　　　_____

Lying down in the afternoon when circumstances permit　　_____

Sitting and talking to someone　　　　　　　　　　　　　_____

Sitting quietly after lunch without alcohol　　　　　　　　_____

In a car, while stopped for a few minutes in traffic　　　　_____

**Total**　　　　　　　　　　　　　　　　　　　　　　　_____

**Figure 2**　The Epworth Sleepiness Scale. Each question is answered with a number from 0 (not at all likely to fall asleep) to 3 (very likely to fall asleep). This yields a total of 0 (minimum) to 24 (maximum), and scores above 10 are thought to warrant investigation.

## IV.　The Relationship Between Subjective (Questionnaires) and Objective Measures of EDS

It is important for clinicians and researchers alike to know whether they should rely on objective or subjective measures of sleepiness, or both, and how the two types of measures relate to each other. Since sleep latency on the MSLT is considered the "gold standard" for objective measure and grading of sleepiness, studies have used this as the objective gold standard. However, not all subjective scales have been studied. Several investigators have reported weak or no association between sleep latency and subjective scales such as the Stanford Sleepiness Scale (26–29). The SWAI, or more specifically its EDS subscale, appears to reliably predict sleep latencies on the MSLT, as evaluated with a regression analysis ($r = 0.386$). The nocturnal sleep subscale of the SWAI was also somewhat predictive of the sleep latency, but much less ($r = 0.033$) (9).

By far the best-studied subjective scale in regard to its relationship to (objective) sleep latency is the ESS. In a series (30) of 102 consecutive patients evaluated for EDS, there was no significant association between ESS score and mean sleep latency. There was no difference in mean ESS score among three groups defined by mean sleep latency as normal (>10 min), moderate (5–10 min), or severe (<5 min) sleepiness. Results of a receiver operating characteristic analysis were no better than random guessing, i.e., the Epworth scale could not reliably distinguish patients with abnormal and normal sleep latency. No Epworth score could adequately discriminate a sleep latency less than or equal to 10. There was no Epworth value where both the sensitivity and specificity were high. Finally, the ESS score could not distinguish abnormal from normal sleep latency. There was (as expected) a gradual increase in median ESS score with increase in sleep latency severity, but with a wide variability of ESS score within each sleep latency level. In another study of a comparable clinical population (31), there was a statistically significant but only moderate correlation of -0.37 ($p = 0.004$). In another series of 522 drug-free narcoleptics (21), there was a statistically significant but weak correlation ($r = -0.27$, $p < .001$) between ESS scores and sleep latency. In the original description of the ESS, Johns (12) reported a correlation of -0.514 ($p < .01$). However, this was based on a smaller sample skewed toward very sleepy patients (11 with narcolepsy, 14 with idiopathic hypersomnia, and 2 with sleep apnea), with "concentrated" values for both Epworth score and sleep latency.

While correlation may not be the optimal measure of the usefulness of the Epworth scale for discrimination or prediction (32), there also appears to be no *categorical* association between ESS score and sleep latency (30,33,34). Thus, although the ESS may be predictive of other variables such as general health status (16) or respiratory disturbance index (12), most of the evidence suggests that its association with sleep latency is tenuous. Similar results emerge from studies comparing ESS with the other (newer) objective measure of EDS, the maintenance of wakefulness test (MWT). In a large narcolepsy sample, the correlation between ESS and MWT was weak ($r = -0.29$, $p < .001$) (35).

The lack of association, or weak correlation, between subjective scales and objective measures suggests that subjective and objective measures evaluate different aspects of sleepiness. This is the prevailing view (15,30,31,35,36), and it is supported by the association between the ESS, nocturnal sleep latency (on polysomnogram), and respiratory disturbance index (12).

## V.  Sleepiness and Its Borderland

Several symptoms are commonly encountered in medicine, that are possibly related to sleepiness. Various terms for these symptoms include *fatigue, tiredness, lack of energy*, and *"asthenia"* (a very widely used term in Europe). While sleepiness is in theory distinct in that it is a tendency to truly fall asleep, differentiating these much less specific symptoms from true sleepiness in clinical practice can be challenging. This issue is epitomized by the controversial association between vague syndromes like "fibromyalgia" and "chronic fatigue" and sleep disturbances (37,38). Most of the evidence suggests that vague fatigue-type symptoms are not caused by intrinsic (primary) sleep disorders (39,40). However, there is also evidence that many patients use these terms interchangeably, so the prevalence of sleep disorders in patients who report "fatigue"-type symptoms is relatively high (38). In fact, patients with well-documented sleep apnea may use vague terms *more often* than accurate ones like sleepiness (38), suggesting that such symptoms should often be evaluated in the same way as "sleepiness." This important finding, together with the notorious underdiagnosis of disorders of excessive sleepiness, suggests that the classic dichotomy between sleepiness and fatigue may be impractical and obsolete (40). Therefore, a reasonable approach is to have a low threshold of using a sleepiness scale (e.g., ESS) in patients who report less specific symptoms such as *fatigue, tiredness, lack of energy,* or *"asthenia."*

## References

1. Benbadis SR, Perry MC, Sunstad LS, Wolgamuth BR. Prevalence of daytime sleepiness in a population of drivers. Neurology 1999; 52:209–210.
2. Bonnet MH, Arand DL. We are chronically sleep deprived. Sleep 1995; 18:908–911.
3. Yoon IY, Jeong DU, Kwon KB, Kang SB, Song BG. Bright light exposure at night and light attenuation in the morning improve adaptation of night shift workers. Sleep 2002; 25:351–356.
4. Takahashi M, Arito H. Maintenance of alertness and performance by a brief nap after lunch under prior sleep deficit. Sleep 2000; 23:813–819.
5. Hoddes E, Zarcone V, Smythe H, Phillips R, Dement WC. Quantification of sleepiness: a new approach. Psychophysiology 1973; 10:431–436.
6. Herscovitch J, Broughton R. Sensitivity of the Stanford Sleepiness Scale to the effects of cumulative partial sleep deprivation and recovery over sleeping. Sleep 1981; 4:83–92.
7. Danker-Hopfe H, Kraemer S, Dorn H, Schmidt A, Ehlert I, Herrmann WM. Time-of-day variations in different measures of sleepiness (MSLT, pupillography, and SSS) and their interrelations. Psychophysiology 2001; 38:828–835.
8. Akerstedt T, Gillberg M. Subjective and objective sleepiness in the active individual. Int J Neurosci 1990; 52:29–37.
9. Rosenthal L, Roehr TA, Roth T. The sleep-wake activity inventory: a self-report measure of daytime sleepiness. Biol Psychiatry 1993; 34:810–820.
10. Johnson EO, Breslau N, Roth T, Roehr T, Rosenthal L. Psychometric evaluation of daytime sleepiness and nocturnal sleep onset scales in a representative community. Biol Psychol 1999; 45:764–770.
11. Weaver TE, Laizner AM, Evans LK, Maislin G, Chugh DK, Lyon K, Smith PL, Schwartz AR, Redline S, Pack AI, Dinges DF. An instrument to measure functional status outcomes for disorders of excessive sleepiness. Sleep 1997; 20:835–843.

12.  Johns MW. A new method of measuring sleepiness: the Epworth Sleepiness Scale. Sleep 1991; 14:540–545.
13.  Maycock G. Sleepiness and driving: the experience of UK car drivers. J Sleep Res 1996; 5:229–237.
14.  Hardinge FM, Pitson DJ, Stradling JR. Use of Epworth Sleepiness Scale to demonstrate response to treatment with nasal continuous airway pressure in patients with obstructive sleep apnoea. Respir Med 1995; 89:617–620.
15.  Johns MW. Sleepiness in different situations measured by the Epworth Sleepiness Scale. Sleep 1994; 17:703–710.
16.  Briones B, Adams N, Strauss M, Rosenberg C, Whalen C, Carskadon M, Roebuck T, Winters M, Redline S. Relationship between sleepiness and general health status. Sleep 1996; 19:583–588.
17.  Bassetti C, Aldrich MS, Chervin RD, Quint D. Sleep apnea in patients with transient ischemic attack and stroke: a prospective study of 59 patients. Neurology 1996; 47:1167–1173.
18.  Melamed S, Oksenberg A. Excessive daytime sleepiness and risk of occupational injuries in non-shift daytime workers. Sleep 2002; 25:315–322.
19.  Arnulf I, Konofal E, Merino-Andreu M, Houeto JL, Mesnage V, Welter ML, Lacomblez L, Golmard JL, Derenne JP, Agid Y. Parkinson's disease and sleepiness: an integral part of PD. Neurology 2002; 58:1019–1024.
20.  Fry J. A new alternative in the pharmacological management of somnolence: a phase III study of modafinil in narcolepsy. Ann Neurol 1998; 43:88–97.
21.  Sangal RB, Sangal JM, Belisle C. MWT and ESS measure different abilities in 41 patients with snoring and daytime sleepiness. Sleep Res 1997; 26:493.
22.  Broughton RJ, Fleming JA, George CF, Hill JD, Kryger MH, Moldofsky H, Montplaisir JY, Morehouse RL, Moscovitch A, Murphy WF. Randomized, double-blind, placebo-controlled crossover trial of modafinil in the treatment of excessive daytime sleepiness in narcolepsy. Neurology 1997; 49:444–451.
23.  Anonymous. A randomized, double blind, placebo-controlled multicenter trial comparing the effects of three doses of orally administered sodium oxybate with placebo for the treatment of narcolepsy. Sleep 2002; 25:42–49.
24.  Partinen M, Gislason T. The basic Nordic Sleep Questionnaire (BNSQ): a quantitated measure of subjective sleep complaints. J Sleep Res 1995; 4(S1):150–155.
25.  Douglass AB, Bornstein R, Nino-Murcia G, Keenan S, Miles L, Zarcone VP Jr, Guilleminault C, Dement WC. The Sleep Disorders Questionnaire. I. Creation and multivariate structure of SDQ. Sleep 1994; 17:160–167.
26.  Seidel WF, Balls S, Cohen S, Patterson N, Yost D, Dement WC. Daytime alertness in relation to mood, performance and nocturnal sleep in chronic insomniacs and non-complaining sleepers. Sleep 1984; 7:230–238.
27.  Pressman MR, Fry JM. Relationship of autonomic nervous system activity to daytime sleepiness and prior sleep. Sleep 1989; 12:239–245.
28.  Hoch CC, Reynolds CF, Jennings R, Monk TH, Buysse DJ, Machen MA, Kupfer D. Daytime sleepiness and performance among healthy 80 and 20 year olds. Neurobiology of aging 1991; 13:353–356.
29.  Harnish MJ, Chard SR, Orr WC. Relationship between measures of objective and subjective sleepiness. Sleep Res 1996; 25:492.
30.  Benbadis SR, Mascha E, Perry MC, Wolgamuth BR, Smolley LA, Dinner DS.. Association between Epworth Sleepiness Scale and MSLT in a clinical population. Ann Intern Med 1999; 130:289–292.

31. Chervin R, Aldrich MS, Pickett R, Guilleminault C. Comparison of the results of Epworth Sleepiness Scale and multiple sleep latency test. J Psychosom Res 1997; 42:145–155.

32. Greenland S, Schlesselman JJ, Criqui MH. The fallacy of employing standardized regression coefficients and correlations as measures of effect. Am J Epidemiol 1986; 123:203–208.

33. Smolley LA, Ivey C, Farkas M, Faucette E, Murphy S. Epworth Sleepiness Scale is useful for monitoring daytime sleepiness. Sleep Res 1993; 22:389.

34. Sander AM, Mohan KK, Axelrod BN, Nahhas A, Kapen S. The Epworth Sleepiness Scale: an unworthy adversary to clinical interview. Sleep Res 1996; 25:355

35. Sangal RB, Mitler MM, Sangal JM. Subjective sleepiness ratings (Epworth Sleepiness Scale) do not reflect the same parameter of sleepiness as objective sleepiness (maintenance of wakefulness test) in patients with narcolepsy. Clin Neurophysiol 1999; 110:2131–2135.

36. Sangal RB, Mitler MM, Sangal JM and US modafinil in narcolepsy multicenter study group. MSLT, MWT and ESS: indices of sleepiness in 522 drug-free patients with narcolepsy. Sleep Res 1997; 26:492.

37. Moldofsky H. Fibromyalgia, sleep disorder and chronic fatigue syndrome. Ciba Found Symp 1993; 173:262–271.

38. Le Bon O, Hoffmann G, Murphy J, De Meirleir K, Cluydts R, Pelc I. How significant are primary sleep disorders and sleepiness in the chronic fatigue syndrome? Sleep Res Online 2000; 3:43–48.

39. Lichstein KL, Means MK, Noe SL, Aguillard RN. Fatigue and sleep disorders. Behav Res Ther 1997; 35:733–740.

40. Chervin RD. Sleepiness, fatigue, tiredness, and lack of energy in obstructive sleep apnea. Chest 2000; 118:372–379.

# 2

# Multiple Sleep Latency Test

**LAMIA AFIFI**

Cairo University Medical School Hospitals, Cairo, Egypt

**CLETE A. KUSHIDA**

Stanford University, Stanford, California, U.S.A.

**MARY A. CARSKADON**

Brown Medical School and E. P. Bradley Hospital,
East Providence, Rhode Island, U.S.A.

## I.  Introduction

Excessive daytime sleeepiness (EDS) leads to impaired performance, diminished intellectual capacity, and is a major cause of accidents and other catastrophes (1). Thus, quantification of EDS is an important procedure, as positive findings willl require a thorough search and treatment of the cause or causes. The method of measurement, however, must be reliable and reproducible so that its results are respected in experimental and clinical settings.

A number of methods can be used to measure sleepiness (see also Chapters 1, 3, and 4) or its consequences. Introspective measures, requiring self-assessment of internal state, have been used for decades. One of the first to be designed and validated specifically to measure sleepiness was the Stanford Sleepiness Scale (SSS), developed by Hoddes and colleagues (2). The SSS was carefully constructed as a seven-point rating scale of equal-appearing intervals from wide awake to devastatingly sleepy, and validated against sleep deprivation. Though it is a well-validated measure for assessing sleepiness in controls, patients with chronic sleepiness appear to lose the ability to assess their internal level of sleepiness accurately (3). Another approach to measuring sleepiness is exemplified by the Epworth Sleepiness Scale, introduced by Johns (4). This scale is commonly used by sleep specialists and evaluates *behavior* not internal state. Thus, the patient is asked to rate the likelihood of falling asleep in eight specific real-life situations. The score ranges from 0 to 24, and a score of 10 or more usually warrants further investigation (5). Performance tasks have also been used to mark the consequences of sleep loss or correlates of excessive sleepiness. Though tasks that are long, repetitious, self-paced, and simple were once thought best to assess the effect of sleepiness, more recent work with brief high-signal-load tasks, such as the psychomotor vigilance task (PVT) of Dinges and colleagues, show a significant sensitivity to sleepiness resulting from sleep deprivation or sleep restriction (6).

The technique most commonly used for objective evaluation of daytime sleepiness is the Multiple Sleep Latency Test (MSLT). It is composed of a series of naps during which subjects are asked not to resist sleep. The speed of falling asleep on tests across time is the chief outcome of the MSLT, which has achieved widespread acceptance because of its simple, intuitive approach to sleepiness. Hence, the greater levels of sleepiness are indicated by more rapid sleep onsets. Furthermore, the MSLT provides several opportunities to test for sleep-onset rapid-eye-movement (REM) episodes, the primary diagnostic sign of narcolepsy.

The MSLT was developed by Mary A. Carskadon and William C. Dement (7) in the Stanford University laboratory of Dr. Dement during the early 1970s. The impetus for developing the MSLT arose from both clinical and experimental needs. In terms of clinical needs, the assessment of excessive sleepiness in narcolepsy and other hypersomnias relied principally upon self-report and, often, a single daytime nap in which the amount and distribution of sleep were evaluated. The difficulty of relying on a single nap, in particular, arose owing to a significant number of false-negative appraisals and the perceived need for repeated assessments. Experimental studies also suffered from the lack of a specific objective metric for evaluating sleepiness. Thus, simultaneous with the clinical need arose the need to understand sleepiness and the regulation of sleep across 24 hr in some meaningful and objective manner. One approach was the 90-min day, in which a 30-min "night" was provided every 90 min.

In the 1960s, the Mayo Clinic group had used pupillometry (8) as an objective measure of sleepiness; however, this technique did not achieve widespread use owing to its limitation by ocular or autonomic lesions, dependence on the patient's cooperation, and difficulties in data interpretation. In the early 1970s, the Stanford group, perceiving the difficulties associated with pupillometry, began by first developing the Stanford Sleepiness Scale and later developing the MSLT. The MSLT arose directly from the results of the 90-min day experiments (9). Most important was the identification during the 90-min day study that the amount of the 30-min night filled with sleep, which was nearly 100%, correlated to the speed of falling asleep, varied across the 24 hr, and was associated with the temporal distribution of sleep and feelings of sleepiness. During the same era, the study of sleep deprivation was of growing scientific interest. The work of the Walter Reed group and the San Diego Naval Research Lab, as well as international efforts, were poised to carry the understanding of sleep deprivation and its impact to the next level. These experiments utilized measures of performance and a variety of self-report measures to evaluate the response of subjects to various sleep deprivation and sleep restriction paradigms. Others have gone on to identify other performance parameters that may be relative to sleep deprivation; however, the key behavioral outcome, that is, sleepiness or sleep tendency, remained a secondary focus and was not always well discriminated.

Thus, in the mid-1970s, the Stanford group devised the MSLT and tested its usefulness, first in a study of sleep deprivation of the prototypical experimental psychology research subject, the "normal" college student. The timing of the MSLT was based on several considerations including:

> The need for a repeated measure of sleep within a day for clinical evaluations.
>
> The need for a test that could be done at intervals providing for other measures during experimental assessment of sleep deprivation.
>
> The reluctance to place assessments at intervals of 90 min which, at the time, were thought to possibly be overshadowed by an ultradian rhythmic process.

The 20-min length of each test was determined based on:

> The needs of experimental and clinical protocols.
>
> The notion that a reversal of sleep states, i.e., REM sleep onset (important for clinical assessments), should be evident within 20 min.
>
> The need for experimental studies in which, for individuals who demonstrate no sleepiness, the task would not be excessively long and boring.

The Stanford group has consistently referred to the MSLT as a measure of sleep tendency from which sleepiness can be inferred (10). This 20-min test, at 2-hr intervals, was first performed with six college students over the course of a 6-day protocol that included 2 baseline days, a 60-hr sleep deprivation, and 2 recovery days. Between the MSLTs, participants were engaged in performance testing and made introspective appraisals (SSS) of their alertness at frequent intervals. The participants in this initial validation study were kept on a fixed-sleep schedule for the week before the study, based on their stated usual sleep pattern and sleep need. Thus, two of the participants were on a schedule permitting 9 and 7 hr of sleep each. The first lesson learned from this initial study was that the fear of boredom from an overlong test was not realized. Indeed, of all the MSLT evaluations that occurred in this study, only one participant remained awake for the entire 20-min test. The baseline data collected were the first to show a now common pattern on the MSLT, with longer sleep latencies mornings and evenings as compared to midday. The validation with prolonged wakefulness showed a clear decline in sleep latency across the waking period that was well related to both subjective appraisals and performance test results (11). Recovery from the sleep deprivation period included 2 nights of sleep on the participants' nominal schedules, and the most remarkable finding from this initial study was the unexpected pattern of sleep latencies on the first recovery day. To wit, the sleep latencies were significantly shorter than baseline during the first test in the morning and then achieved baseline levels in the afternoon. After a second night of sleep, recovery values were indistinguishable from the baseline levels.

This experiment provided sufficient evidence for the Dement group to continue to use the Multiple Sleep Latency Test in both experimental and clinical settings with great success, particularly in the clinical domain (12–15). Subsequent experimental studies have provided data to confirm the validity and sensitivity of the MSLT to varying levels of sleep deprivation and sleep extension. The evaluations of MSLT tests under conditions of total sleep deprivation have been performed in a number of age groups. As mentioned earlier, the initial assessment was done in college-aged participants. The Stanford group has also performed sleep deprivation studies with the MSLT in adolescents and the elderly, and other groups have examined sleep deprivation with this measure in other ages using the MSLT test—really to gauge the physiological process of sleep loss in humans. Finally, the physiological sleepiness measured by the MSLT cannot be reliably assessed by most subjects (16). For example, recent evidence found no correlation between the subjective Epworth Sleepiness Scale and the objective MSLT, suggesting subjective and objective methods may assess different aspects of sleepiness (17). This discrepancy may also relate to the ways in which such measures detect state versus trait characteristics. On the other hand, a number of groups have shown that with chronic partial sleep loss, for example, introspective sleep assessments show a far different pattern from the MSLT (18) or performance (19).

## II.  Procedure of the MSLT

The MSLT technique is well standardized (20). An overnight polysomnogram is carried out the night before the MSLT to examine both the quality and quantity of the night's sleep, which influence the MSLT results. For example, the MSLT may be influenced by sleep for up to 7 nights before the test (18); thus it is ideal that subjects complete sleep diary forms or otherwise have their sleep assessed (e.g., actigraphy) for 1–2 weeks before the MSLT. A sleep diary generally includes information on bedtime, wakeup time, napping, and the use of drugs. Subjects should also stop any medication that might affect sleep latency (e.g., sedatives, hypnotics, antihistamines) or REM latency (e.g., tricyclic antidepressants) 2 weeks before the study. A urine drug screen on the morning of the MSLT is helpful in identifying patients in whom drug effects are suspected. Subjects should be prohibited from taking caffeine and alcohol the day of the study; however, acute withdrawal from high doses of caffeine may affect test results.

The MSLT is routinely performed at 2-hr intervals, beginning 1.5–3 hr after awakening from nocturnal sleep, and consists of 4–6 naps. Subjects should be in bed 5 min before the scheduled start of the test, to allow for calibrations of the recorded parameters and to establish a standard lead-in into the test. This is an important step as different levels of activity before the nap affect the sleep latency (21). Between the naps, the subject should remain out of bed and technicians should check that the subject is not sleeping. The naps should be carried out in a sleep-inducing environment; thus, the rooms must be dark and quiet and the temperature adjusted to a comfortable level. The subject is instructed to try to sleep and not to resist sleeping, with the same instructions given for each nap. Bedroom lights are then turned off, signaling the start of the test, from which sleep latency is calculated. The test is ended after 20 min if there has been no sleep, or after 15 min from the beginning of sleep (20), though in experimental studies, an SLT is often terminated at unequivocal sleep onset.

The recording montage includes the standard Rechtschaffen and Kales (22) technique; central electroencephalogram (EEG), horizontal electrooculogram (EOG), and chin electromyogram (EMG) electrodes. Strongly recommended additions to this montage are occipital EEG, vertical EOG, and electrocardiogram (ECG) electrodes. In clinical studies of patients known to snore, measures of respiratory flow and respiratory sounds may be helpful to identify occasions when snoring affects the sleep onset (23).

## III.  MSLT Results

For each nap, sleep onset latency and sleep stages are recorded according to standard criteria (22). The criteria used for sleep onset are also somewhat variable, with some preferring to score sleep onset by the first 30-sec epoch of sleep, while others require three 30-sec epochs to determine sleep onset. Standard guidelines recommend defining sleep latency as the first single 30-sec epoch of sleep (24). The MSLT can sometimes be difficult to interpret, and different raters may vary in their findings of whether a patient has sleep-onset REM periods, but less so for the sleep-onset latency (25). For experimental studies, the latter score is the most common measure. Whether to use a value indicating the full day's score, such as daily mean or median, or to examine each SLT value individually depends up the goal of the study.

The underlying assumption of the MSLT is that lower scores indicate greater sleepiness and vice versa. A common rubric holds that a daily average score of less than 5 min indicates a pathological level of daytime sleepiness. This level is associated with impaired performance in patients and in sleep-deprived normal subjects (26). Scores of adult normal controls usually range from 10 to 20 min (27). Scores between 5 and 10 min indicate moderate sleepiness, and may or may not be associated with pathological conditions (23).

Abnormal sleep-onset REM periods, which occur within 15 min of sleep onset, are of major importance in the diagnosis of narcolepsy. Other causes of sleep-onset REM periods, such as sleep deprivation or other sleep disorders (e.g., obstructive sleep apnea), must be excluded (28).

## IV.  Applications of the MSLT

Using the MSLT as an objective laboratory assessment of the clinical symptom of sleepiness, as well as abnormal sleep structure, has greatly facilitated the diagnosis, differentiation, and treatment of various disorders of excessive daytime somnolence (EDS). A brief review of its applications is described below.

### A.  Sleep Deprivation

The MSLT has been utilized in many studies to examine the effects of sleep deprivation on daytime sleepiness. As described earlier, Carskadon and Dement (11) performed the first MSLT study to test the effects of two nights of sleep loss in six young subjects. The scores fell to about 1 min at 0600 on the first night of sleep loss and remained at similarly low values throughout the sleep loss period. After one night of recovery sleep the scores remained significantly below baseline levels, which were not achieved until after the second recovery night.

The effects of various time-in-bed (TIB) conditions on daytime sleepiness and total sleep time (during a 24-hr enforced bedtime) were investigated by Rosenthal et al. (29). Thirty-two subjects were randomly assigned to spend 8, 6, 4, or 0 hr in bed, followed the next day by a standard MSLT. The sleep latencies were shorter for those subjects in the 0-hr condition when compared to the other three conditions. Also, the sleep latencies of those subjects in the 4- and 6-hr conditions were comparable to, but different from, those of subjects in the 8- and 0-hr TIB conditions.

Another study, by Devoto et al. (30), evaluated the effects of different amounts of sleep and SWS restriction on the ensuing daytime sleepiness. Six men, after one adaptation night and an initial 8-hr baseline night, were allowed to sleep 5, 4, 3, 2, and 1 hr with a 1-week interval between conditions. The following day, four sleep-onset MSLT trials were carried out. Results indicated a linear increase in the propensity to sleep as a function of the increase in sleep restrictions.

Howard and colleagues (31) suggested a reform of residents' work and duty hours based on a study that assessed the levels of physiological and subjective sleepiness in 11 anesthesia residents in three conditions: (1) during a normal (baseline) work schedule, (2) after an in-hospital 24-hr on-call period, and (3) after a period of extended sleep. MSLT scores were shorter in the baseline (6.7 min) and postcall (4.9 min) conditions, compared with the extended-sleep condition (12 min), and there was no significant difference between the baseline and postcall conditions. Residents' daytime sleepiness on the MSLT in both baseline and postcall conditions was near or below levels associated with clinical sleep disorders, and residents were subjectively inaccurate determining EEG-defined sleep onset.

The effect of sleep deprivation on different age groups has also been tested using the MSLT. Sleep loss in young adolescents was assessed by examining the effects of one night's sleep loss in 12 subjects whose ages ranged from 11.7 to 14.6 years. MSLTs showed a marked reduction of sleep-onset latency from 0530 throughout the day of sleep loss. In contrast to the subjective measures, sleep latency test scores did not recover to basal levels until the afternoon of the first recovery day. In general, the sleep loss response of young adolescents showed no marked differences as from published reports of sleep loss in older subjects (32). Another study, by Carskadon and Dement (26), assessed sleepiness in 10 elderly volunteers, aged 61–77 years, before, during, and after 38 hrs of sleep loss. Reported subjective sleepiness increased and latency to sleep onset on the MSLT declined. All measures returned to basal values after a night of sleep. With this exception, the response was similar to that reported in younger volunteers, although shorter-lived. Direct comparison of sleep deprivation in healthy 80-year-olds and 20-year-olds was carried out in a study by Brendel et al. (33). The protocol consisted of three nights of baseline sleep, one night of total sleep deprivation, and two nights of recovery sleep. Daytime sleepiness was measured by five naps on the days following the third and sixth nights. Surprisingly, young subjects had shorter daytime sleep latencies than the old, suggesting a greater unmet sleep need in the former group. This finding suggests that acute total sleep loss is a more disruptive procedure for the young than for the old.

Chronic partial sleep restriction is a topic of current interest and one that was examined two decades ago by Carskadon and Dement (18). During a week of restriction to 5 hr of sleep a night, 10 college-aged adults manifested an accumulating decrease of sleep latency scores that did not plateau. A more recent chronic sleep restriction study (34) showed a .95 correlation of performance measures with the Carskadon and Dement MSLT scores. These studies provided important support for the concept of sleep deficits that continue to grow as sleep reduction is prolonged. A more recent interpretation implicates "excess wake" as the primary factor rather than sleep deficit (35).

Another interesting question that was examined using MSLT was the effect of deprivation of specific sleep stages. Because slow-wave sleep (SWS) has been theorized to be an intense form of NREM sleep, Walsh et al. (36) examined in 12 healthy adult volunteers the effects of marked SWS deprivation (SWD) for two nights versus a controlled sleep disruption (CD) condition in which minutes of SWS were preserved and a no sleep disruption (ND) condition. Results showed that two nights of SWD did not cause greater daytime sleepiness on the MSLT than did CD, although sleepiness in both conditions was increased compared to the ND condition. Thus, selective deprivation of SWS does not appear to produce greater decrements in alertness; however, a larger sample may be required to fully assess this phenomenon. Another study, by Glovinsky et al. (37), studied the effects of selective sleep-stage restriction, measuring sleep tendency with a "modified" MSLT before and after two nights of awakenings from either REM or stage 2 sleep in 16 normal young adults. During the modified MSLT, subjects were allowed up to 25 min to fall asleep, and only 2 consecutive min of any stage of sleep before being awakened. In addition, sleep latency was defined as the time from lights out to the first epoch of two consecutive 30-sec epochs of any stage of sleep, and a value of 25 min was assigned to a nap if no sleep occurred. REM sleep and stage 2 awakenings produced comparable levels of sleepiness during subsequent daytime MSLTs.

Nykamp and colleagues (38) reported a contradictory finding from a study of sleeping subjects awakened each time they entered stage REM sleep and yoked control subjects who were awakened concomitantly with the REM-deprived subjects when not in stage REM sleep. The yoked control subjects manifested significantly lower MSLT scores on deprivation days owing to decreased total sleep time. Also, the REM-deprived subjects did not demonstrate any changes in MSLT scores compared to baseline nights. These investigators concluded that the REM-deprivation procedure antagonized the effects of sleep loss on daytime sleepiness, resulting in increased alertness for REM-deprived subjects compared to yoked control subjects. The mechanism by which REM deprivation would exert such an alerting effect is unknown.

### B.  Sleep Fragmentation

The effect of sleep fragmentation on daytime sleepiness was studied by Levine et al. (39), who combined sleep deprivation with sleep fragmentation in an experiment where 40 subjects were deprived of sleep for one night, then randomly assigned to one of five conditions: at 8:30 A.M. they were given 100 min of natural sleep; sleep with arousals 1/5 min, 1/3 min, 1/1 min; or no sleep. After the recovery nap, sleep latencies were evaluated at 12:00 P.M., 2:00 P.M., 4:00 P.M., and 6:00 P.M. Mean sleep latencies increased linearly as the rate of arousal during the recuperative nap decreased. Although the natural sleep provided recuperation relative to no sleep or fragmented sleep, it did not restore daytime sleepiness to the screening level. Roehrs et al. (40) carried out another sleep fragmentation study without sleep deprivation. Thirty-six subjects were studied in an experimental model of sleep fragmentation in whom sleep was disrupted on two nights by presenting tones that produced brief electroencephalographic (EEG) arousals (without shortening sleep time). Daytime function was assessed the following day with the MSLT and a divided attention performance test. These investigators found that sleep fragmentation produced significant disruption of nocturnal sleep and reduced daytime alertness.

### C.  Sleep Extension (See Also Chaps. 25 and 28)

Studies of adults extending sleep beyond an average of 7.5 hr at night have produced contradictory findings. While Roehrs and colleagues (41) found that sleep extension reduced MSLT scores significantly, Harrison and Horne (42) found that extended sleep produced no improvements to self-rated mood or subjective sleepiness. In fact, MSLT scores during extended sleep in the latter study showed small (about 1 min) reductions. These investigators suggested that their findings provided little support to the view of chronic sleep deprivation in the average 7.5-hr sleeper. On the other hand, Carskadon and Dement have shown substantial differences in daily MSLT scores in several age groups as a function of sleep times that are shorter or longer than thought to be "usual" sleep need or that extended sleep with a daytime nap (1,43).

### D. Narcolepsy

Sleepiness is a primary symptom of narcolepsy, often preceding the onset of the other well-known symptoms of the disease, namely cataplexy, sleep paralysis, and hypnagogic hallucinations (44). Evaluation of the MSLT of narcoleptic patients has demonstrated a short sleep latency (<5 min) and multiple sleep-onset REM periods (SOREMPs). The more specific finding in the MSLT of narcoleptic patients is more than 2 SOREMPs, shown to reach a specificity of 99% by Amira et al. (45), which further increased to 99.2% if 3 SOREMPs were recorded (46). On the other hand, more than one SOREMP can occur in nonnarcoleptic patients, such as those with sleep apnea, sleep deprivation, depression, periodic limb movements, circadian rhythm disruption, or withdrawal from REM-suppressing medications (5,47). Thus, the findings of the MSLT, which is always performed for suspected narcoleptic patients, must be interpreted in view of the clinical history and nocturnal PSG.

### E. Diagnosis of Various Disorders of EDS

The differential diagnosis of EDS includes narcolepsy, sleep apnea syndrome, sleep deprivation, periodic limb movement disorder, idiopathic central nervous system (CNS) hypersomnia, psychiatric diseases and use of sedating medications (48). Attempts to reach a differential diagnosis using the MSLT have been made by several groups. For example, Reynolds et al. (49) and Zorick et al. (50) carried out the MSLT for groups of patients with various disorders of EDS. They found that the patients with narcolepsy or sleep apnea had the shortest sleep latency (<5 min), while patients with psychiatric disorders showed the longest latency (>10 min), reaching values similar to those of normals. Patients with idiopathic CNS hypersomnia, periodic limb movement disorder, or insufficient sleep occupied a middle position (5-10 min). REM latency was significantly shorter in narcolepsy than in apnea, and more than 70% of the naps were SOREMP-positive in narcolepsy and less than 20% in the other disorders. A nonstandard MSLT measure, sleep percentage, was gradually reduced from a mean of 52.5% to a mean of 39.8% during the day in depressives, paralleling improvement in mood and energy levels. In contrast, sleep percentages increased and sleep latencies decreased during the day in patients with narcolepsy or sleep apnea.

In a study by Van den Hoed et al. (23), 100 sleep-apnea-free patients with EDS due to other disorders underwent the MSLT and nocturnal PSG. When the results were compared to the established diagnosis in an attempt to verify the MSLT's ability to classify patients, mean sleep latency alone correctly classified 82% of narcoleptics. In addition, the MSLT mean sleep latency value and the sleep latency on the nocturnal PSG were able to objectively differentiate between different groups with EDS.

In a more selective study, Kayumov et al. (51) studied 22 patients with depression/anxiety and 47 nondepressed patients with sleep apnea using the PSG, MSLT, and Maintenance of Wakefulness Test (MWT). They found that depressed patients with more disturbed nocturnal sleep paradoxically showed greater daytime alertness. Of course, these parallel findings may indicate an underlying factor that inhibits sleep at night and in the daytime. In contrast, the more disturbed nocturnal sleep was in the sleep apnea patients, the lower (sleepier) their scores on the MSLT. These findings illustrate the value of the MSLT as a clinical tool in the differential diagnosis for complaints of EDS.

### F.  Insomnia

A rather different clinical application of the MSLT is the assessment of patients with insomnia. One might expect that, as in the sleep-deprived individuals, patients with insomnia would have a short sleep latency on the MSLT; however, in a study by Siedel and Dement (52), only 7% of insomniacs were in the pathological range on MSLT (< 5 min), while 17% were in the "gray area" (5–10 min), and 41% had scores >15 min. These data suggest that insomniacs are a heterogeneous population and that many respond abnormally to restricted nocturnal sleep.

Bonnet and Arand (53) performed a study in which sleep recordings from 10 insomniacs were used as a template for disrupting similar sleep in a group of matched normal sleepers for seven nights. They wished to determine if specific electroencephalographic (EEG) sleep patterns were responsible for the secondary insomnia symptoms reported by the insomniacs, and MSLT was used as an outcome measure. Insomniacs had increased sleep latencies on the MSLT, while normals showed decreased latencies following the sleep manipulation. Both groups complained of decreased vigor. These investigators concluded that the secondary symptoms reported by patients with primary insomnia are probably not related to their poor sleep per se, but occur secondary to CNS hyperarousal.

The previous studies led to the hypothesis that the insomnia patients may be suffering from a state of chronic activation that disturbs night sleep but protects against or prevents EDS from occurring in the morning. Conversely, such patients may be naturally "short sleepers" whose sleep need may be fulfilled with relatively short sleep at night.

### G.   Effect of Treatment

Different lines of treatment for sleep disorders associated with EDS, such as continuous positive airway pressure or airway surgery, were evaluated using the MSLT. In comparing pre- and posttreatment symptoms, a subject may perceive an improvement of awareness as very substantial, whereas the MSLT may reveal that the vulnerability remains. Hence, objective assessment of the response is offered by the MSLT (16,54). The alerting effect of caffeine has been proven by its ability to increase the sleep latency on the MSLT of normal sleep-deprived subjects (55).

Hypnotic drug efficacy depends not only on its action on improving the quality of nocturnal sleep, but also on the diurnal effects of the drug. The ideal sleeping pill would increase the amount and consolidation of nocturnal sleep, which should improve waking alertness or at least should not further compromise it. Carskadon and colleagues (56) compared two groups of insomniacs treated with a short-acting (e.g., triazolam) and a long-acting (e.g., flurazepam) benzodiazepine and found that the flurazepam group had a shorter sleep latency on the MSLT with the drug than on baseline, while the triazolam group had a longer sleep latency with treatment. These findings were attributed to a carryover of sedating effects of the long-acting compounds, and improvement of daytime alertness with short-acting compounds due to improved nocturnal sleep. In another study, sleep deprivation was combined with midazolam or a placebo drug. It was found that both groups had similar latencies on the MSLT with partial sleep deprivation, and the placebo group had a shorter latency with complete sleep deprivation, suggesting that bedtime midazolam does not affect alertness the following day (57).

The MSLT has also been used for assessment of other types of compounds that may affect diurnal somnolence. Antihistamines, for example, are commonly associated with subjective sleepiness. Roehrs et al. (58) showed that certain types of antihistamines increase sleepiness, with the MSLT used as the objective measure, while other types do not.

These studies underscore the potential of the MSLT as a valuable tool for assessing many types of compounds, not only for those in which the primary action is sleep-inducing. The assessment of various drug regimens using a sensitive measure of diurnal somnolence may aid in the determination of appropriate treatment strategies while minimizing sleepiness-inducing side effects (1).

## V. Summary and Conclusions

The MSLT is the most common method of objectively measuring daytime sleepiness in sleep laboratories. This test has been standardized into a form that reliably measures sleepiness in various populations. The MSLT has been used to evaluate levels of sleepiness: (1) in conditions of sleep deprivation, reduction, fragmentation, and extension; (2) in suspected narcoleptic patients; (3) in patients with various disorders of excessive daytime sleepiness; (4) in patients with insomnia; and (5) in the posttreatment condition of patients with sleep disorders associated with daytime sleepiness. Further work is needed to compare subjective measures of sleepiness and newer performance measures with the MSLT.

## References

1. Carskadon MA, Dement WC. Daytime sleepiness; quantification of a behavioural state. Neurosci Biobehav Rev 1987; 11(3):307–317.
2. Hoddes E, Dement WC, Zarcone V. The development and use of the Stanford Sleepiness Scale (SSS). Psychophysiology 1972; 1:150–157.

3. Herscovitch J, Broughton R. Sensitivity of the Stanford Sleepiness Scale to the effects of cumulative sleep deprivation and recovery oversleeping. Sleep 1981; 4: 83–92.

4. Johns MW. A new method of sleepiness: the Epworth Sleepiness Scale. Sleep 1991; 14:540–545.

5. Benbadis S. Daytime sleepiness: when is it normal? When to refer?. Cleveland Clinic J Med 1998 November/December: 543–549.

6. Dinges DF. Probing the limits of functional capability: the effects of sleep loss on short-duration tasks. In: Broughton RJ, Ogilvie R, eds. Sleep, Arousal and Performance. Cambridge; MA: Birkhauser-Boston, 1992:176–188.

7. Carskadon MA, Dement WC. Sleep tendency; an objective measure of sleep loss. Sleep Res 1977; 6:200.

8. Yoss RE, Moyer NJ, Ogle KN. The pupillogram and narcolepsy; a method to measure decreased levels of wakefulness. Neurology 1969; 19:921–928.

9. Carskadon M, Dement W. Sleep studies on a 90–min day. EEG Clin Neurophysiol 1975; 39:145–155.

10. Carskadon MA, Dement WC. The multiple sleep latency test: what does it measure? Sleep 1982; 5:S67–S72.

11. Carskadon, MA, Dement WC. Effects of total sleep loss on sleep tendency. Percept Mot Skills 1979; 48(2):495–506.

12. Richardson GS, Carskadon MA, Flagg W, et al. Excessive daytime sleepiness in man: multiple sleep latency measurement in narcoleptic and control subjects. Electroencephalog Clin Neurophysiol 1978; 45:621–627.

13. Carskadon MA, Harvey K, Dement WC. Sleep loss in young adolescents. Sleep1981; 4(3):299–312.

14. Carskadon MA, Dement WC. Multiple sleep latency tests during the constant routine. Sleep1992; 15(5):396–399.

15. Chervin RD, Kraemer HC, Guilleminault C. Correlates of sleep latency on the multiple sleep latency test in a clinical population. Electroencephalog Clinical Neurophysiol 1995; 95:147–153.

16. Zorick F, Roehrs T, Conway W, Fujita S, Wittig R, Roth T. Effects of uvulopalatopharyngoplasty on the daytime sleepiness associated with sleep apnea syndrome. Bull Eur Physiopathol Respir 1983; 19: 600–603.

17. Benbadis SR, Mascha E, Perry MC, Wolgamuth BR, Smolley LA, Dinner DS. Association between the Epworth Sleepiness Scale and the multiple sleep latency test in a clinical population. Ann Intern Med 1999; 130(4): 289–292 .

18. Carskadon MA, Dement WC. Cumulative effects of sleep restriction on daytime sleepiness. Psychophysiology 1981; 18: 107–113.

19. Dorrian J, Lamond N, Holmes AL, Burgess HJ, Roach GD, Fletcher A., Dawson D. The ability to self-monitor performance during a week of simulated night shifts. Sleep 2003; 26(7):871–877.

20. Carskadon MA, Dement WC, Mitler MM, Roth T, Westbrook PR, Keenan S. Guidelines of the Multiple Sleep Latency Test (MSLT): a standard measure of sleepiness. Sleep 1986; 9(4):519–524.

21. Bonnet MH, Arand DL. Sleepiness as measured by modified multiple sleep latency testing varies as a function of preceding activity. Sleep 1998; 21:477–483.

22. Rechtschaffen A, Kales A. A Manual of Standardised Terminology, Techniques and Scoring System for Sleep Stages of Human Subjects. Los Angeles, UCLA Brain Information Service/Brain Research Institute, 1968.

23. Van den Hoed J, Kraemer H, Guilleminault C, Zarcone P, Laughton EM, Dement WC, Mitler MM. Disorders of excessive daytime somnolence: polygraphic and clinical data for 100 patients. Sleep 1981; 4:23–27.

24. Benbadis SR, Perry M, Wolgamuth BR, Mendelson WB, Dinner DS. The multiple sleep latency test: comparison of sleep onset criteria. Sleep 1996; 8: 632–636.

25. Benbadis SR, Qu Y, Warnes H, Dinner D, Perry M, Piedmonte M. Interrator reliability of the multiple sleep latency test. Electroencephalogr Clin Neurophysiol 1995; 95:302–304.

26. Carskadon MA, Dement WC. Sleep loss in elderly volunteers. Sleep 1985; 83(3):207–221.

27. Richardson GS, Carskadon MA, Orav EJ, Dement WC. Circadian variation of sleep tendency in elderly and young adult subjects. Sleep 1982; 5 (suppl):82–94.

28. Mitler MM, Van den Hoed J, Carskadon MA, Richardson G, Park R, Guilleminault C, Dement WC. REM sleep episodes during the Multiple Sleep Latency Test in narcoleptic patients. Electroencephalogr Clin Neurophysiol 1979; 46:479–481.

29. Rosenthal L, Roehrs TA, Rosen A, Roth T. Level of sleepiness and total sleep time following various time in bed conditions. Sleep 1993; 16(3):226–232.

30. Devoto A, Lucidi F, Violani C, Bertini M. Effects of different sleep reductions on daytime sleepiness. Sleep 1999; 22(3):336–343.

31. Howard SK, Gaba DM, Rosekind MR, Zarcone VP. The risks and implications of excessive daytime sleepiness in resident physicians. Acad Med 2002; 77(10):1019–1025.

32. Carskadon MA, Harvey K, Dement W. Sleep loss in young adolescents. Sleep 1981; 4(3):299–312.

33. Brendel DH, Reynolds CF 3rd, Jennings JR, Hoch CC, Monk TH, Berman SR, Hall FT, Buysse DJ, Kupfer DJ. Sleep stage physiology, mood, and vigilance responses to total sleep deprivation in healthy 80–year-olds and 20–year-olds. Psychophysiology 1990; 27(6):677–85.

34. Dinges DF, Pack F, Williams K, Gillen KA, Powell JW, Ott GE, Aptowicz C, Pack AI. Cumulative sleepiness, mood disturbance, and psychomotor vigilance performance decrements during a week of sleep restricted to 4–5 hours per night. Sleep 1997; 20(4):267–277.

35. Van Dongen HP, Maislin G, Mullington JM, Dinges DF. The cumulative cost of additional wakefulness: dose-response effects on neurobehavioral functions and sleep physiology from chronic sleep restriction and total sleep deprivation. Sleep 2003; 26(2):117–126.

36. Walsh JK, Hartman PG, Schweitzer PK. Slow-wave sleep deprivation and waking function. J Sleep Res 1994; 3(1): 16–25.

37. Glovinsky PB, Spielman AJ, Carroll P, Weinstein L, Ellman SJ. Sleepiness and REM sleep recurrence: the effects of stage 2 and REM sleep awakenings. Psychophysiology 1990; 27(5):552–559.

38. Nykamp K, Rosenthal L, Folkerts M, Roehrs T, Guido P, Roth T. The effects of REM sleep deprivation on the level of sleepiness/alertness. Sleep 1998; 21(6):609–614.

39. Levine B, Roehrs T, Stepanski E, Zorick F, Roth T. Fragmenting sleep diminishes its recuperative value. Sleep 1987; 10(6):590–599.

40. Roehrs T, Merlotti L, Petrucelli N, Stepanski E, Roth T. Experimental sleep fragmentation. Sleep 1994; 17(5):438–443.

41. Roehrs T, Shore E, Papineau K, Rosenthal L, Roth T. A two-week sleep extension in sleepy normals. Sleep 1996; 19(7):576–582.

42. Harrison Y, Horne JA. Long-term extension to sleep—are we really chronically sleep deprived? Psychophysiology 1996; 33(1):22–30.

43. Carskadon MA. Determinants of Daytime Sleepiness: Adolescent Development, Extended and Restricted Nocturnal Sleep. Ph.D. dissertation, Stanford University, Stanford, CA, 1979.

44. Dement WC, Carsadon MA, Guilleminault C, Zarcone V. Narcolepsy. Diagnosis and treatment. Prim Care 1976; 3(4): 609–623.

45. Amira SA, Johnson TS, Logowitz NB. Diagnosis of narcolepsy using the Multiple Sleep Latency Test: analysis of current laboratory criteria. Sleep 1985; 8(4):325–331.

46. Aldrich MS, Chervin RD, Malow BA. Value of the Multiple Sleep Latency Test (MSLT) for the diagnosis of narcolepsy. Sleep 1997; 20(8):620–629.

47. Kader G. Narcolepsy. Presented at the first Cairo Symposium for Sleep Disorders, 1998.

48. Parkes JD. Daytime sleepiness. Br Med J 1993; 306:772–775.

49. Reynolds CF, Coble PA, Kupfer DJ, Holzer BC. Application of multiple sleep latency test in disorders of excessive sleepiness. Electroencephalogr Clin Neurophysiol 1982; 53(4):443–452.

50. Zorick F, Roehrs T, Koshorek G, Sicklesteel J, Hartse K, Wittig R, Roth T. Patterns of sleepiness in various disorders of excessive daytime somnolence. Sleep 1982; 5(suppl):165–174.

51. Kayumov L, Rotenberg V, Buttoo K, Auch C, Pandi-Perumal SR, Shapiro CM. Interrelationships between nocturnal sleep, daytime alertness, and sleepiness: two types of alertness proposed. J Neuropsychiatry Clin Neurosci 2000; 12(1):86–90.

52. Seidel WF, Dement WC. Sleepiness in insomnia; evaluation and treatment. Sleep 1982; 5(suppl):182–190.

53. Bonnet MH, Arand DL. The consequences of a week of insomnia. Sleep1996; 19(6):453–461.

54. Wittig R, Zorick F, Conway W, Ward J, Roth T. Normalization of the MSLT after six weeks of CPAP for sleep apnea syndrome. Presented at the first annual meeting of the Association of Professional Sleep Societies, Columbus, OH, 1986.

55. Lumley M, Roehrs T, Asker D. Ethanol and caffeine effects on daytime sleepiness/alertness. Sleep 1987; 10:306–312.

56. Carskadon MA, Seidel F, Greenblatt DJ, Dement WC. Daytime carry-over effects of triazolam and flurazepam in elderly insomniacs. Sleep 1982; 5:361–371.

57. Borbely AA, Balderer G, Trachsel L, Tobler I. Effect of midazolam and sleep deprivation on day-time sleep propensity. Arzneimittelforschung 1985; 35(11):1696–1699.

58. Roehrs T, Tietz E, Zorick F, Roth T. Daytime sleepiness and antihistamines. Sleep 1984; 7:137–141.

# 3

# Maintenance of Wakefulness Test

**MERRILL M. MITLER**

**National Institute of Neurological Disorders and Stroke,
Bethesda, Maryland, U.S.A.**

## I.  Measurement of the Symptom of Sleepiness

In clinical, industrial, and research settings, the symptom of sleepiness can manifest as a complaint about feeling too sleepy to function or about falling asleep inappropriately. This complaint may be voiced by an individual or by another party such
as a spouse, employer, or teacher. Such sleepiness can represent a serious, potentially life-threatening condition that affects not only the individual but also the individual's family, co-workers, and society in general. In these cases, it is often
desirable to have reliable, objective, and physiologically based measurements of
sleepiness. Until the mid-1980s, clinical EEG examination and the Multiple Sleep
Latency Test (MSLT) were the two testing options most often ordered.

### A.  Physiological Sleepiness Versus Manifest Sleepiness

The Maintenance of Wakefulness Test (MWT) was developed as an alternative,
physiologically based test of sleepiness (1). The test was designed for use with
patients whose sleepiness during the day might adversely affect performance or
safety. Reasoning on the basis of face validity, a person who has little difficulty
with falling asleep inappropriately should be able to stay awake in a quiet, sedentary situation such as during MWT trials. Beyond the procedure's face validity,
there are other rationales for the use of the MWT, as discussed below.

The MWT involves instruction to remain awake while sitting in a comfortable position in a partially reclining chair or propped-up in bed (1). A similar protocol for assessing the ability to maintain wakefulness, the Repeated Test of Sustained Wakefulness (RTSW), was developed by Hartse et al. (2) and involves instruction to remain awake while lying in bed. The RTSW seems to produce data similar to the MWT. Both the MWT and the RTSW are outgrowths of the MSLT and can be thought of as measures of *manifest* sleepiness, as opposed to *physiological* sleepiness. The MWT and RTSW quantify the tendency for sleep to occur while trying to stay awake in comfortable, sleep-permissive circumstances. As is discussed elsewhere in this volume, the Multiple Sleep Latency Test (MSLT) is considered a measure of *physiological* sleepiness. The MSLT quantifies the tendency to fall asleep while trying to do so in comfortable, sleep-permissive circumstances. As such, the MSLT can be regarded as an estimator of the greatest possible tendency to fall asleep at the nap times studied. Since the MWT instructs subjects to stay awake, one might predict that, all other factors being equal, sleep latencies on the MWT would be longer than on the MSLT (3). However, studies have not always supported this prediction (4,5).

### Effect of Measurement Conditions

It seems clear from our everyday experience as well as from scientific literature that conditions such as ongoing activity, posture, and environmental distractions can affect the likelihood of a person's falling asleep. A recent study by Bonnet and Arand (3) quantitatively estimated the relative contribution of the instruction and posture. They assessed sleep latency in healthy controls in the following conditions: lay down and sleep (MSLT); lay down and stay awake; sit up and sleep; sit up and stay awake (MWT); and sit in a chair in front of a computer and stay awake. Average sleep latencies were: lay-sleep—11.1 min; sit-sleep—17.7 min; lay-awake—21.7 min; sit-awake—29.0 min; computer—30.1 min. Correlations between conditions declined as subjects sat up. All differences were significant except the sit-awake and computer conditions. The authors concluded that the MWT differed from the MSLT because motivation and posture are additive factors that favor falling asleep on MSLT naps more than on the MWT trials. They further suggested that MSLT and MWT data may not correlate because the MWT data reflect the combined effects of the sleep and arousal systems while the MSLT measures only sleepiness. However, as will be demonstrated, this conceptualization, that the MWT is simply an MSLT with additive factors that prolong sleep latency, is not consistent with several MWT findings.

We now examine MWT operating characteristics in detail. The MWT protocol was devised to, and on the face of things seems to, measure the ability to sustain wakefulness. As Bonnet and Arand have shown, motivation and posture are important factors that can reduce the tendency to fall asleep and reciprocally, although not linearly, increase the ability to maintain wakefulness. The ability to stay awake can, of course, also be influenced by factors including, but not limited to, amount of prior sleep, pharmacological status, central nervous system status, and time of day. Considerations of conditions such as prior sleep and medical status are important, but are straightforward and common—usually involving pretest standardization, documentation, and grouping of data with those of comparable subjects. Time of day deserves additional discussion. A large number of studies and normative data exist for physiologically based metrics of daytime sleepiness. If it is necessary to assess sleepiness during the night, choices of validated tools are generally limited to performance tests. While physiologically based metrics readily detect nighttime drops in alertness in normal and sleep-deprived volunteers, guidelines as to what degree of sleepiness is *pathological* during the night have not been established. It is *normal* to be very sleepy at 4:00 A.M.

### Effect of Testing Protocol

Under some conditions, feelings of sleepiness may be great and protocols that must be run when subjects are extremely sleepy encounter the problem of "floor effects." For example, physiological sleepiness may be so great because of a drug effect that sleep latencies are too short to be above statistical noise. In these circumstances, it is difficult to detect subjects with abnormal sleepiness or to detect the effect of any remedial intervention.

### MSLT Versus MWT

The MSLT can be conceptualized as a standardized protocol adapted from early studies on the effects of experimentally dividing the normal nighttime sleep period into multiple opportunities for sleep distributed throughout the 24-hr day (e.g., 1 hr for sleep offered every 3 hr or 30 min for sleep every 90 min) (6–8). The most extreme forms of this type of "two thirds wake, one third sleep" protocol are the ultra-short-cycle studies of Lavie and colleagues that have used cycles as brief as 20 min (13 min of wakefulness and 7 min of sleep) (9–11). The MWT, in turn, can be conceptualized as an outgrowth of the MSLT with altered instructions and body position. Some studies have shown that the MSLT and MWT produce similar data when detecting remedial interventions. The multicenter study of modafinil in patients with narcolepsy was able to detect therapeutic effects of comparable size with both the MSLT and MWT (12). However, other studies suggest that the MSLT and the MWT correlate only weakly and may measure fundamentally different abilities (4,5). Discordancy between the MSLT and the MWT may be partly understood, as Bonnet and Arand suggest, in terms of the additive effects of instruction and posture. However, the instruction and posture are not simply additive, subject by subject. One cannot expect a perfect correlation between lower MSLT scores and higher MWT scores. For example, consider the following hypothetical average MSLT scores on five subjects (9–13) and the following average MWT scores on the same five subjects (19–23). The numbers of the second set were obtained by adding 3 (for the effect of sitting as opposed to lying down) and 7 (for the effect of instruction to stay awake as opposed to go to sleep) to each number in the first set. In these hypothetical data sets, the correlation between the two measures is 1.0. Such a strong correlation between the MSLT and the MWT has not been reported in the literature. An example that better fits with the literature is one in which some random method is used to add posture and instruction numbers to MSLT scores, such that an average increase is obtained.

Figure 1 presents a scatter plot of the results of MSLTs and MWTs done on each of 258 patients evaluated by Sangal and colleagues in Troy, Michigan for the complaint of excessive sleepiness. While the correlation, 0.41, between the two tests is statistically significant, much discordancy remains. Less than 17% of the variability is explained by the linear relationship between the two tests. These data demonstrate that patients with the symptom of excessive somnolence may be discordant on the two tests. There are patients who have low sleep latency on MSLT and high sleep latency on MWT (lower right quadrant) and others who have high sleep latency on MSLT and low sleep latency on MWT (upper left quadrant). The narrow ellipse denotes the range (2.0–20.0 min) in MSLT scores for those 76 patients who were able to remain awake on all MWT trials. A factor analysis suggested that two factors, alertness and sleepiness, account for 91% of all variance (Fig. 1).

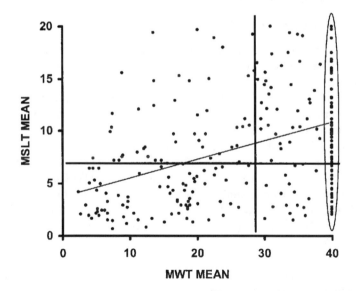

**Figure 1**   Scatter plot of MSLT and MWT scores (redrawn from the data of Sangal et al. [5]). An MSLT and an MWT were administered on the same day to 258 consecutive patients whose clinical presentation required evaluation for excessive sleepiness. The horizontal and vertical lines represent the midpoint in the MSLT and the MWT distributions, respectively. The correlation between MSLT and MWT sleep latencies is 0.41 (note the trend line arising from point MWT = 2.4, MSLT = 4.1). The narrow ellipse denotes the range (2.0–20.0 min) in MSLT scores for those 76 patients who were able to remain awake on all MWT trials.

Another potential explanation for differences between the MSLT and the MWT is that the MWT, because of its instructions to remain awake, adds a nonlinear motivational factor that is not present with the MSLT. The MWT often reveals improvement in treated patients who continue to be physiologically sleepy. Thus, the MWT is sometimes considered to be a way of extending the sensitivity range of the MSLT (13). Reasoning that an MWT is simply an MSLT plus a motivational component (even a nonlinear component) falters, however, because it assumes that motivational factors are not present in the MSLT. Such an assumption with respect to the MSLT is not justified.

## B. Motivational Factors

In a testing situation, a rational, self aware, honest individual who is a good historian and has no agenda other than complying with the testing protocols presents no problem. In clinical practice, such individuals are relatively uncommon.

### Reasons for Objective Testing

With increasing frequency, assessment of sleepiness is being done for regulatory and judicial purposes. In such situations, objective and repeatable testing is usually necessary. The incentives for a subject to show a high or a low degree of sleepiness should not be ignored in objective physiologically based testing.

### Perceived Gains and Losses of Subject

Within the objective testing situation, there may be incentives for a sleepy person to appear less sleepy (e.g., to preserve driving privileges) or an alert person to appear more sleepy (e.g., to obtain prescription stimulants). Therefore, it is important to consider instructions to the patient and the tasks to be performed as they pertain to patient motivations as well as to test instructions.

### Faking Possibilities

Most experienced sleep specialists have encountered patients who seemed to be trying to fake results on the MSLT. Some try to fake short sleep latency and even sleep-onset REM periods, possibly to secure a diagnosis of narcolepsy and prescription stimulants. Others struggle to remain awake to avoid appearing excessively sleepy. Less frequent, but possible, are individuals who try to fake results on an MWT by ignoring instructions to remain awake or use extraordinary methods to avoid sleep. Proper testing procedures can obviate some of these problems. However, selecting an objective, physiologically based test that is aligned with the purposes at hand can simplify problems with divergence between instructions and incentives, thereby reducing the problem of faking. If one is interested in how quickly a person falls asleep when told to do so, then faking problems are minimal with a properly administered MSLT. In properly screened and prepared subjects, it is hard to imagine faking low sleep latencies on the MSLT. If one is interested in how well a person can resist falling asleep in quiet, sedentary conditions, then an MWT is a good choice of tests. In properly screened and prepared subjects, it is hard for a subject to fake alertness on the MWT.

## II.  MWT Protocols

Polysomnographic procedures used to conduct the MWT are similar to those used for the MSLT (1,14). The major difference is the instruction given to the test subject. The person being tested is placed in a seated or propped-up position and told *to attempt to remain awake*. The MWT assesses an individual's capability to not be overwhelmed by sleepiness. If the wakefulness system fails, sleepiness becomes manifest. This laboratory situation parallels circumstances in which sleep onset occurs inadvertently while a person is passive and sedentary in a nonstimulating environment. In the MWT there is no task other than to remain awake. During the MWT, an individual is monitored for electroencephalographic sleep onset during 4–6 sessions, scheduled at 2-hr intervals commencing 2-hr after awakening from the previous night's sleep. Studies comparing MWT and MSLT sleep latencies find, as expected, that subjects take longer to fall asleep when instructed to remain awake than when told not to resist sleep.

### A.   Rationale for 40-, 30-, and 20-Min Trials

There are several MWT variants with respect to trial duration. This variation stems from the fact that the MWT can be adapted to a variety of situations depending on the degree of sleepiness and motivational characteristics of the population to be studied. As examples, with extremely somnolent subjects such as patients with narcolepsy, a shorter trial duration, say 20 min, can be used with minimal ceiling effects. In individuals who are only moderately sleepy (say, MSLT sleep latencies in the 6–10 min range), as opposed to extremely sleepy (say, MSLT sleep latencies in the 0–5 min range), MWT trial durations of 30 min or 40 min are needed to reduce problems with ceiling effects (15–17).

### B.   Instructions to Subject

In the MWT the subject is instructed to stay awake, remain in a sitting position, and not use extraordinary methods to comply, such as face slapping, singing, etc. The rules for trial termination and the activities that are permitted after trial termination are not explained to the subject. Unless dictated by the overall project underway, the subject is permitted to use the usual amount of caffeine.

### C.   Setting

The setting of the MWT is the sleep laboratory room. The subject may be seated in a reclining easy chair or propped-up in bed with pillows or a bolster. The room lights are dimmed to the levels at which nocturnal polysomnography is performed.

### D. Termination of Each MWT Trial

Several methods of terminating an MWT trial can be chosen depending on the subject population and the purposes of the test. It is true that such protocol variability can limit comparability of data from study to study. However, variability within a particular subject population can actually be reduced by the judicious selection of MWT protocol parameters so that ceiling effects are minimized and incentives to comply with instructions are optimized. Possible trial termination rules include the following:

1. Let each trial last the maximum time (e.g., 20, 30, or 40 min) regardless of whether or not the subject falls asleep.
2. Awaken the subject after sleep onset and remove him/her from the testing situation until the next trial.
3. Awaken the subject and enforce wakefulness while keeping him/her in the testing situation.

Rules for termination of each MWT trial can also be adjusted to the testing purpose and to the incentives for the actual subject population under study to comply with instructions. With populations in which motivation to stay awake is judged to be low, trials can be terminated after sleep onset. Moreover, activities permitted after trial termination can also be restricted to reduce incentives to exit the MWT trials. In all cases, subjects are to remain in the laboratory and not engage in strenuously physical activity. Below is an example protocol that was developed for a research project on the effects of nasal CPAP in patients with sleep apnea (National Heart Lung and Blood Institute Grant 1 UO1 HL68060-01A1 "Apnea Positive Pressure Long-Term Efficacy Study," William C. Dement, PI). The choice of trial duration and trial termination were selected for this research application and the reasons for those decisions are discussed.

#### Protocol for the Maintenance of Wakefulness Test

The maintenance of wakefulness test (MWT) is a daytime polysomnographic procedure that addresses the symptom of excessive sleepiness by measuring the subject's ability to remain awake during soporific circumstances. The MWT will follow nighttime polysomnography. For each MWT trial, the subject is instructed to remain awake while sitting comfortably in bed in a darkened bedroom. The subject will be seated up in bed with the support of a bolster pillow ("bedrest"). Polysomnographic procedures and scoring are conducted as in the MSLT.

It is recognized that various MWT trial durations and rules for termination of trials have been used depending on the setting. Choices among these variations allow the MWT to be adapted to a variety of settings and needs. For example, if there are concerns about sleep accumulation during trials or about sleep inertia after trials, termination occurs at some defined point shortly after sleep onset. Making adjustments with respect to the activities that are permitted after trial termination can adapt the MWT to various presumed levels of subject motivation to succeed in remaining awake. If a subject in a clinical setting risks losing driving privileges by performing poorly on the MWT, one may suppose that the subject's motivation is high. However, a research subject for whom failure to remain awake has no personal consequences may not try hard to remain awake and may look forward to social contacts and other activities after early termination of an MWT trial.

*MWT trial duration:*
MWT trial duration will be 20 min. The rationales for this decision are that the 20-minute trial MWT has been used in both clinical and research settings and has been validated against longer MWT trials. Moreover, pilot data showed that an MWT with 20-minute trials statistically distinguishes subjects on active CPAP from subjects on sham CPAP.

*Rules for trial termination:*
MWT trials will be terminated after no less than six 30-second epochs of continuous sleep.

If there is no sleep episode lasting six epochs, the trial is terminated after 20 min. Once a trial is terminated, the room lights are turned on, the subject is asked to open his/her eyes, stay seated in bed, and remain awake until the 20 min scheduled for the trial have elapsed. The reasons for these termination rules are that by requiring a full 3 min of sleep, the termination rules will minimize the chances of an MWT trial being prematurely terminated because the technologist incorrectly misread waking EEG as asleep. Termination shortly after sleep onset also minimizes the chances of subjects being awakened from an MWT trial and then being confronted with neurocognitive testing within the next few minutes. These termination rules also compensate for low motivational levels since, in this research protocol, failure to remain awake has few negative consequences for the subject. The trial termination rules will increase motivation by giving subjects negative feedback if they fail to stay awake. Yet, subjects will not be rewarded with naps (as would be the case with uniform 20-min trials) or with social contact after early failures to stay awake (as would be the case with allowing the subject to get out of bed after falling asleep).

*Specific procedures:*
1.   Four 20-minute trials are to be run at 1000, 1200, 1400 and 1600 hr
2.   Subjects to be seated in bed, propped up using a bolster pillow with arms (reading pillow)
3.   Room lights will be dimmed so that no more than 0.10–0.13 lux is present at the subject's eye level
4.   Subjects will be instructed to remain awake without using extraordinary measures (e.g., vocalizing, face slapping)
5.   The PSG will be monitored continuously during each trial
6.   A trial will be ended after 20 min or after six consecutive 30-second epochs of any stage of sleep, whichever occurs first
7.   If a trial is terminated before 20 min, the technologist will turn on the room lights, ask the subject to keep his/her eyes open, and remain awake. The tech-

nologist will continue to monitor the PSG and awaken the subject as soon as any further sleep is detected.

8. The subject will get out of bed only after the 20 min have elapsed.

### E. Limitations

With the growing interest in sleepiness and public safety, demand for tests to assess sleepiness has increased. Indeed, the Federal Aviation Administration recognizes the MWT as a means to determine whether noncommercial pilots can be licensed after treatment for sleep apnea (18). Validation for this use of MWT has not been done. It is not known whether failures on MWT trials predict unsafe vehicle operation. While the MWT has proven useful in identifying patients who have worrisome difficulty maintaining alertness on the job and for evaluating treatment effects in patients with narcolepsy and sleep-related breathing disorders, the MWT should not be used as the sole determinant for any clinical, administrative, or judicial decision. It should also be noted that MSLT and MWT do not correlate well in patients complaining of excessive sleepiness (5). Many patients who will fall asleep rapidly when not resisting sleep can remain awake on MWT trials. Paradoxically, there are also patients who fall asleep more quickly when trying to stay awake on the MWT than when trying to fall asleep on the MSLT (see Fig. 1). Underlying neurophysiological mechanisms for maintaining alertness may be distinct from those that regulate and coordinate sleep.

### III. Interpretation of MWT Results

The MWT does have some face validity in that one expects a person who has no difficulty with falling asleep inappropriately in daily life to be able to stay awake on MWT trials. However, caution is advised. No physiologically based test, including the MWT, has been shown to be a valid predictor of operator errors on the highway or in the workplace. Furthermore, the motivational factors present during an MWT done for, say, reinstatement of a driver's license may be too strong. In fact, these factors may lead to overestimation of alertness while driving. For example, such an MWT may overestimate that level of alertness the patient experiences when driving home after the test. For reasons such as the foregoing, results for the MWT should not be considered in isolation of the clinical and/or experimental conditions under which they were obtained. Interpretation of results should reflect intrasubject factors such as presence of a sleep disorder, prior sleep history, time of day, and drug history. Also important are normative values in relation to MWT results.

#### A. Normal Values and Variation

Normative data using 40-min trials terminated after sleep onset have been published with extrapolations to estimate results if 20- and 30-min trials had been used. Figure 2 is a frequency histogram and Table 1 is a summary of parameters for normative MWT data gathered in the international, multisite cooperative

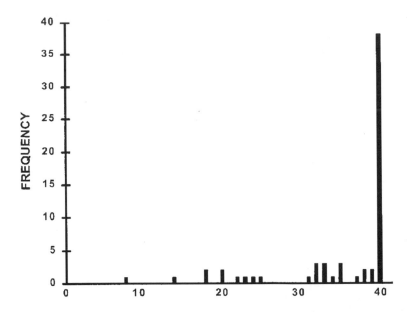

**Figure 2** Normative MWT data. Average sleep latencies over four 40-min long MWT trials were calculated for each of 64 healthy volunteers and plotted in frequency histogram format. (See text and Ref. 11 for details.)

study (14,19). In this study, 64 healthy subjects (27 males and 37 females) were evaluated. Subjects adhered to uniform procedural conditions including a nighttime polysomnographic recording, designed to rule out clinically significant leg movement and respiratory abnormalities, and daytime polysomnographic montage, illuminance level (0.10–0.13 lux at eye level), seating position (propped-up to 45–90° degrees by a reading pillow with arm rests), room temperature (22°C), meal timing (breakfast at least 1 hr before the first MWT trial). Subjects were instructed as follows: "Please sit still and remain awake for as long as possible. Look ahead of you, and do not look directly at the lights." Subjects were not allowed to use extraordinary measures such as slapping the face or singing.

Table 1 presents a summary of some commonly used parametric data. The entire database has been made available on the Internet (http://post.queensu.ca/~listserv/wwwarch/sleep-1.html). Interested parties may download the entire data set and are free to perform other types of data reductions as desired.

## B. Determining Whether Pathology Is Present

The problem of defining abnormal performance on tests such as the MWT has no universal solution. The normative MWT sleep latencies form a skewed distribution that is truncated at 40 min (Fig. 2) with most subjects able to maintain wake-

**Table 1**  Maintenance of Wakefulness Test (MWT) Sleep Latency Norms

| | | | | |
|---|---|---|---|---|
| N = 64 | | | | |
| Sex: 27 Males; 37 females | | | | |
| Age: 47.8 ± 11.4 years | | | | |

**MWT-40 (Trial duration of 40 minutes)**

| | | | | |
|---|---|---|---|---|
| Trial time | 10:00:00 A.M. | 12:00:00 P.M. | 2:00:00 P.M. | 4:00:00 P.M. |
| Trial mean (min) | 36.27 | 33.95 | 34.25 | 36.49 |
| S.D. | 9.16 | 12.03 | 11.48 | 8.79 |
| | **OVER ALL 40-MIN TRIALS:** | | | |
| **Average SL** | 35.24 | **Average No. of Failures** | | 0.81 |
| **S.D.** | 7.93 | **S.D.** | | 1.25 |
| **10th percentile** | 20.00 | | | |

**MWT-30 (Projected by limiting sleep latency to 30)**

| | | | | |
|---|---|---|---|---|
| Trial time | 10:00:00 A.M. | 12:00:00 P.M. | 2:00:00 P.M. | 4:00:00 P.M. |
| Trial mean (min) | 27.92 | 26.12 | 26.39 | 28.16 |
| S.D. | 5.98 | 8.12 | 7.58 | 5.73 |
| | **OVER ALL 30-MIN TRIALS (Projected):** | | | |
| **Average SL** | 28.24 | **Average No. of Failures** | | 0.69 |
| **S.D.** | 4.57 | **S.D.** | | 1.14 |
| **10th percentile** | 21.50 | | | |

**MWT-20 (Projected by limiting sleep latency to 20)**

| | | | | |
|---|---|---|---|---|
| Trial time | 10:00:00 A.M. | 12:00:00 P.M. | 2:00:00 P.M. | 4:00:00 P.M. |
| Trial mean (min) | 19.08 | 18.09 | 18.39 | 19.20 |
| S.D. | 3.06 | 4.37 | 3.90 | 3.20 |
| | **OVER ALL 20-MIN TRIALS (Projected):** | | | |
| **Average SL** | 18.69 | **Average No. of Failures** | | 0.56 |
| **S.D.** | 2.63 | **S.D.** | | 1.02 |
| **10th percentile** | 14.00 | | | |

Summary statistics for normative MWT data. For 64 healthy volunteers, the average sleep laten-cies for four 40-min trials are presented as well as the average across the four-trial MWT. Results for 30-min and 20-min trial durations have been estimated by truncation. (See text and Ref. 11 for details.)

fulness on each trial, but with a few subjects failing to maintain wakefulness after as little as 10 min. Because of the skew in the normative data, the use of a pathol-ogy definition based on the standard deviation of the normative data is problem-atic. Some investigators have suggested using a percentile cutoff, calling abnormal, average MWT scores below, say, the 10th percentile (see Table 1). Others suggest that pathology should be defined by the number of trials in which a subject failed to maintain wakefulness. According to Table 1, the average num-ber of failures to remain awake over four 40-min trials is less than 1 (0.81 ± 1.25).

As stated previously, the MWT should be considered as one index from a set of indices for a subject or patient. Furthermore, the reason for doing an MWT evaluation is important. If the subject or patient is being evaluated as part of a fitness-for-duty examination in connection with a safety-sensitive job, the range of acceptable performance might be narrowed. If the subject or patient is being evaluated to determine whether an experimental intervention has improved ability to remain awake, then the focus may be shifted from average sleep latency to a metric reflective of change from baseline.

### C.  Detecting Effect of Therapeutic Intervention

The MWT and the RTSW have been shown to be sensitive to pharmacological interventions aimed at reducing sleepiness (20–22).

In this connection, the issue of intersubject variability is important when considering sleepiness and change in sleepiness. We can measure, by any of several methods, an increase in sleepiness in a before-and-after experimental manipulation such as a night with no sleep. It sometimes happens that the initial sleepiness value for one person exceeds the final value for another. Thus, change in sleepiness does not speak directly to the question of the presence or absence of pathological sleepiness. To address the question of abnormal sleepiness outside the time interval evaluated in the multicenter normative study (Fig. 2 and Table 1), it is necessary to refer to other normative data for MWT-like tests. For example, data on the ability to sustain wakefulness during the night in healthy volunteers are becoming available in connection with baseline and/or placebo conditions evaluated during studies of the remedial effects of napping and caffeine on functioning during simulated shiftwork (20,23–26). A thorough comparison of the physiological methods for assessing sleepiness and alertness has been presented elsewhere (27).

### D.  Patients with Safety-Sensitive Jobs

The MWT is often done for patients with safety-sensitive jobs such as airline pilots. The testing may be in the course of a clinical evaluation or in the course of a fitness-for-duty evaluation mandated by an employer or regulatory agency. As stated earlier, no physiologically based test, including the MWT, has been shown to be a valid predictor of operator errors on the highway or in the workplace. Therefore, it is not justified to use the MWT as a stand-alone tool in determining fitness for duty. That having been said, poor performance on the MWT should not be ignored by decision makers when evaluating patients with safety-sensitive jobs. No cutoff points with respect to average sleep latency or number of failed MWT trials are suggested here. However, it is wise to consider several MWT parameters (e.g., average sleep latency, number of failed trials, etc.) as part of a comprehensive evaluation. It may also be useful to establish, with the participation of relevant stakeholders, guidelines for pass/fail ranges.

## Acknowledgments

Dr. Mitler was supported by research grant number NS37571 and GCRC grant number RR00833 while he conducted the research discussed in this chapter while at the Scripps Research Institute; he is now at the National Institute of Neurological Disorders and Stroke (NINDS). The author wishes to thank Dr. Michael Bonnet for his careful evaluation. Thanks are due Janet Molsberry for her help in manuscript preparation.

## References

1. Mitler MM, Gujavarty KS, Browman CP. Maintenance of wakefulness test: a polysomnographic technique for evaluation treatment efficacy in patients with excessive somnolence. Electroencephalogr Clin Neurophysiol 1982; 53:658–661.

2. Hartse KM, Roth T, Zorick FJ. Daytime sleepiness and daytime wakefulness: the effect of instruction. Sleep 1982; 5:s107–s118.

3. Bonnet MH, Arand DL. Arousal components which differentiate the MWT from the MSLT. Sleep 2001; 24:441–447.

4. Sangal RB, Thomas L, Mitler MM. Disorders of excessive sleepiness: treatment improves ability to stay awake but does not reduce sleepiness. Chest 1992; 102:699–703.

5. Sangal RB, Thomas L, Mitler MM. Maintenance of wakefulness test and Multiple Sleep Latency Test: measurement of different abilities in patients with sleep disorders [see comments]. Chest 1992; 101:898–902.

6. Weitzman ED, Nogeire C, Perlow M, et al. Effects of a prolonged 3–hour sleep-wake cycle on sleep stages, plasma cortisol, growth hormone and body temperature in man. J Clin Endocrinol & Metab 1974; 38:1018–1030.

7. Carskadon MA, Dement WC. Sleep studies on a 90–minute day. Electroencephalogr Clin Neurophysiol 1975; 39:145–55.

8. Mitler MM, Gujavarty KS, Sampson MG, Browman CP. Multiple daytime nap approaches to evaluating the sleepy patient. Sleep 1982; 5:s119–s127.

9. Lavie P, Scherson A. Ultrashort sleep-waking schedule. I. Evidence of ultradian rhythmicity in "sleepability." Electroencephalogr Clin Neurophysiol 1981; 52:163–174.

10. Lavie P, Zomer J. Ultrashort sleep-waking schedule. II. Relationship between ultradian rhythms in sleepability and the REM-NONREM cycles and effects of the circadian phase. Electroencephalogr and Clin Neurophysiol 1984; 57:35–42.

11. Lavie P. Ultrashort sleep-waking schedule. III. Gates and "forbidden zones" for sleep. Electroencephalogr Clin Neurophysiol 1986; 63:414–425.

12. U.S. Modafinil in Narcolepsy Multicenter Study Group. Randomized trial of modafinil for the treatment of pathological somnolence in narcolepsy. Ann Neurol 1998; 43:88–97.

13. Mitler MM, Miller JC. Methods of testing for sleepiness [corrected] [published erratum appears in Behav Med 1996 Spring;22(1):following table of contents]. Behavioral Medicine 1996; 21:171–83.

14. Doghramji K, Mitler MM, Sangal RB, et al. A normative study of the maintenance of wakefulness test (MWT). Electroencephalogr Clin Neurophysiol 1997; 103:554–562.

15.  Ionescu D, Driver HS, Heon E, Flanagan J, Shapiro CM. Sleep and daytime sleepiness in retinitis pigmentosa patients. J Sleep Res 2001; 10:329–335.
16.  Timms RM, Shaforenko R, Hajdukovic RM, Mitler MM. Sleep apnea syndrome: quantitative studies of nighttime measures and daytime alertness. Sleep Res 1985; 14:222.
17.  Poceta JS, Timms RM, Jeong DU, Ho SL, Erman MK, Mitler MM. Maintenance of wakefulness test in obstructive sleep apnea syndrome [see comments]. Chest 1992; 101:893–897.
18.  Department of Transportation. Sleep Apnea Evaluation Specifications. Federal Aviation Administration Specification Letter, Oct 6, 1992.
19.  Mitler MM, Doghramji K, Shapiro C. The Maintenance of Wakefulness Test: normative data by age. J Psychosom Res 2000; 49:363–365.
20.  Sugerman JL, Walsh JK. Physiological sleep tendency and ability to maintain alertness at night. Sleep 1989; 12:106–112.
21.  Mitler MM, Hajdukovic R, Erman M, Koziol JA. Narcolepsy. J Clin Neurophysiol 1990; 7:93–118.
22.  U.S. Modafinil in Narcolepsy Multicenter Study Group. Randomized trial of modafinil as a treatment for the excessive daytime somnolence of narcolepsy. Neurology 2000; 54:1166–1175.
23.  Walsh J, Schweitzer P, Sugarman J, Muehlbach M. Transient insomnia associated with a three-hour phase advance of sleep time and treatment with zolpidem. J Clin Psychopharmacol 1990; 10:184–189.
24.  Walsh JK, Muehlbach MJ, Humm TM, Dickins QS, Sugerman JL, Schweitzer PK. Effect of caffeine on physiological sleep tendency and ability to sustain wakefulness at night. Psychopharmacology (Berl) 1990; 101:271–273.
25.  Walsh JK, Humm T, Muehlbach MJ, Sugerman JL, Schweitzer PK. Sedative effects of ethanol at night. J Stud Alcohol 1991; 52:597–600.
26.  Walsh JK, Schweitzer PK, Anch AM, Muehlbach MJ, Jenkins NA, Dickins QS. Sleepiness/alertness on a simulated night shift following sleep at home with triazolam. Sleep 1991; 14:140–146.
27.  Mitler MM, Carskadon MA, Hirshkowitz M. Evaluating sleepiness. In: Kryger MH, Roth T, Dement WC, eds. Principles and Practice of Sleep Medicine. Philadelphia: WB Saunders, 2000:1251–1257.

# 4

## Psychomotor Vigilance Performance: Neurocognitive Assay Sensitive to Sleep Loss

JILLIAN DORRIAN, NAOMI L. ROGERS, AND DAVID F. DINGES

University of Pennsylvania School of Medicine, Philadelphia, Pennsylvania, U.S.A.

## I.  Overview

It is well established that sleep deprivation, both acute total and chronic partial sleep restriction, results in significant impairment of neurobehavioral functioning. To quantify the magnitude of such changes, as well as to track the temporal profile in neurobehavioral degradation as sleep loss accumulates, a wide array of neurocognitive assays have been used. However, many of these tests are not well suited for assessment of performance across multiple sleep-wake cycles owing to significant inter- and intrasubject variability. To provide an accurate and useful measure of performance during sleep loss, and the expression of waking neurobehavioral integrity as it changes dynamically over time, neurocognitive assessments must validly and reliably reflect fundamental aspects of waking functions that are altered by sleep deprivation. Since such neurobehavioral assays will need to be administered to persons of different aptitudes and repeatedly over time, they should be devoid of substantial intersubject and intrasubject (e.g., learning) variability. Such assays should also provide meaningful outcome variables that can be easily interpreted relative to neurobiological and cognitive constructs. In this chapter we review one neurobehavioral assay that has met these criteria—the psychomotor vigilance task (PVT).

## II.  Sleep Deprivation and Neurocognitive Performance

It has long been established that sleep deprivation degrades aspects of waking neurobehavioral capability (reviewed in Refs. 1–4). In humans, numerous tests have been designed to capture specific elements of waking cognitive functions. The resulting neurocognitive performance measures provide an index of the degree of functional impairment present in an individual, and they have been used to answer both applied and theoretical questions about the nature of neurobehavioral capability in healthy people deprived of sleep.

Decades of research on human sleep deprivation have resulted in the view that the extent to which a given cognitive task reveals changes during sleep deprivation depends upon such task parameters as duration (5–7), complexity (8,9), response rate (10), and interest (5,8,11,12). As such, findings regarding the type and magnitude of performance impairment during sleep deprivation are, to a large extent, contingent as much on these task parameters as on any particular type of cognitive test. In recent years, a focus on the effects of sleep loss on specific brain regions—especially the prefrontal cortex (PFC)—has resulted in use of tasks that are thought to uniquely activate this substrate.

A wide variety of tests have been used in sleep deprivation experiments ranging from simple tests of reaction time (e.g., Refs. 1,2,13) to complex tasks of higher-order cognitive capacity and PFC function (e.g., Refs. 9,14,15). The diversity of performance tests available for use in performance testing leads to a fundamental question: *What are the criteria for an effective neurocognitive assay under conditions of sleep deprivation, where "effective" means theoretically meaningful, empirically sensitive, and practically useful?*

### A.  Stimulus-Response Approach

Since the first published experimental study of sleep deprivation and human cognitive performance in 1896 (13), investigators have employed a plethora of performance tests to measure the effects of sleep loss on neurobehavioral functioning. One common testing approach is the "stimulus-response" (S-R) method. This typically involves repeated presentation of visual or auditory stimuli, requiring a timely response from the experimental subject. Behavioral alertness is a core feature of the S-R approach as applied to the study of sleep deprivation. Examples of S-R tasks range from the attention-rich demands of simple reaction time tasks to sustained-attention vigilance tasks (as used in Ref. 2 and Ref. 16, respectively). S-R tasks predicated on sustaining attention over time have been used since the earliest studies of human sleep deprivation and performance (2,13). Several fundamental observations were made during these investigations, with experimenters describing phenomena that we now refer to as *microsleeps, hypnagogic reverie, lapsing, circadian* variation in performance, and increased depth of *recovery sleep* (2,3,13). Thus, the effects of sleep deprivation on the neurobiology of focused attention appear to be at the heart of the sensitivity of S-R tasks to sleep deprivation (3). The mechanisms of attention have also recently been recognized to be a fundamental component of higher-order cognitive tasks subserved by the prefrontal cortex.

## B.   Executive Function Approach

In recent years, the effects of sleep loss have been increasingly evaluated using neurocognitive tests that focus on complex cognitive functions, particularly tests putatively subserved by the prefrontal cortex. Horne and colleagues, in particular, have championed the view that sleep loss uniquely affects PFC. Deficits on tasks subserved by PFC have been observed following sleep deprivation; examples include verbal fluency, creative thinking, nonverbal planning (15), confidence judgment (metamemory), temporal memory (14), response inhibition, verb-to-noun word generation (14,15) and word fluency (17,18). These findings have contributed to a frontal lobe hypothesis, which contends that sleep deprivation acts primarily in the frontal lobe, to produce frontal cortex dysfunction, reversible by recovery sleep (19).

A PFC-related function that has received particular study in the scientific literature is working memory. Imaging studies have indicated that performance on working memory tasks is reliant on dopamine receptors in the dorsolateral pre-frontal cortex (20,21). It has been argued that working memory is dependent on a central executive attention system (22,23), and that constructs of executive attention and working memory are closely related (24), if not isomorphic (25). Importantly, performance on working memory tasks is predictive of performance on a range of other tasks of cognitive tests (25). Indeed working memory and its underlying executive attention are likely to be fundamental to performance on virtually any neurocognitive task. Put simply, without the basic ability to hold or sustain attention, it is impossible to perform any task in a goal-directed manner (3). Stable sustained attention is therefore a necessary, but not sufficient, criterion for normal cognitive functioning.

## III.   Criteria for a Neurocognitive Assay Sensitive to Sleep Deprivation

Proposed criteria for a sensitive behavioral assay for studying the temporally dynamic features of sleep deprivation are summarized in Table 1. Ideally, a neurocognitive assay for measuring the effects of sleep loss during waking performance should reflect an aspect of cognition that is: (1) basic to or essential for many expressions of performance, and (2) sensitive to the homeostatic drive for sleep in interaction with the endogenous circadian pacemaker. The ability to sustain attention on a task meets this first criterion because it is a basic feature of nearly all cognitive performance tests, including tests that have proven to be sensitive to sleep deprivation [i.e., from tests of vigilance (16) to creative thinking (15)]. A second criterion for an effective neurobehavioral assay of human sleep depriva-

**Table 1**   Criteria for a Neurocognitive Assay for Assessing the Effects of Sleep Deprivation

| Criteria | Explanation/examples |
| --- | --- |
| Reflects a fundamental aspect of waking neurocognitive functions | Measures the ability to use attention or working memory over time |
| | Capitalizes on brain structures subserving basic cognitive functions |
| Suitable for repeated administration | Has a minimal learning curve |
| | Underlying psychometric properties do not change with repeated testing |
| Easily performed with no aptitude effects | Yields consistent results among a wide range of subject populations |
| | Can be taught quickly |
| | Can be used in laboratory experiments, simulator scenarios, and field situations |
| Task duration relatively brief | Prevents extraneous factors (e.g., lack of interest) from altering performance |
| | Easily integrated into experimental protocols involving repeated measurements |
| | Does not result in greatly augmented subject burden |
| High signal load | Provides a large number of behavioral samples in a brief period of time |
| Reliability | Challenges the subject to maintain cognitive output |
| | Provides test-retest stability |
| | Reflects trait-like inter-individual differences |
| Validity | Convergent validity—sensitive to many forms of sleep deprivation |
| | Ecological validity—sensitive to performance used in everyday functioning |
| | Theoretical validity—reflects changes consistent with theorized functions of sleep |
| Can be interpreted in a meaningful way | Yields metrics that can be translated to "real world" performance |
| | Yields metrics that can be related to sleep/wake physiology |

tion is that the cognitive task should be easy to learn and perform (i.e., minimal intersubject variability in performance due to aptitude, and easily implemented in experimental protocols). This maximizes its utility across a larger segment of the population.

Since a large proportion of experiments investigating human performance during sleep deprivation involve repeated measures designs to properly evaluate temporally dynamic changes in neurocognitive functions over time, a performance task should ideally have a minimal learning curve to prevent masking effects from skill acquisition (26). It is important to note that exposing subjects to a period of training prior to sleep deprivation may reduce learning, but it rarely completely eliminates learning during the experimental testing period, even if subjects reach asymptotic performance levels during training (26). Furthermore, repeated testing should not change the underlying psychometric properties of the test. For example, novelty is an important aspect of several tasks purported to measure PFC function, such as the Haylings Sentence Completion Task (27). Such tests are not suitable for multiple administrations during a study of sleep deprivation (i.e., within-subjects designs) as the task properties are significantly altered.

Other criteria for a neurobehavioral assay of the cognitive effects of sleep deprivation include task duration and signal load (i.e., stimulus rate). Tasks that are very long with low signal rates can induce excessive levels of task-related fatigue, boredom, and reduced motivation, which can contaminate sleep deprivation effects. To avoid this problem, a cognitive task assay during sleep deprivation should require a relatively large number of responses in a short time period. The high signal load allows the experimenter to sample a greater amount of behavior involving sustained cognitive output, and avoid the criticism commonly leveled at low signal load tasks, that the subject falls asleep because he/she is in a passive state.

Finally, a cognitive performance assay used repeatedly during sleep deprivation should have high test-retest reliability; it should be demonstrated to be sensitive to a large proportion of the performance phenomena associated with sleep loss; and it should have the capacity to reflect aspects of "real world" performance (i.e., ecological validity).

## IV. Psychomotor Vigilance Task (PVT) as a Neurocognitive Assay for Sleep Loss

With all of the above criteria in mind, the psychomotor vigilance task (PVT) was developed as a neurocognitive assay for tracking the temporally dynamic changes induced by interaction of the homeostatic drive for sleep and endogenous circadian pacemaker. Its focus is on measurement of the ability to sustain attention and respond in a timely manner to salient signals (28). With a combination of PFC executive attention and traditional stimulus-response testing, the PVT involves a simple (as opposed to choice) reaction time (RT) test—the avoidance of choice RT was deliberate to minimize continued learning and strategy shifts that can occur even in four-choice RT tasks. The PVT requires responses to a small, bright-red-light stimulus (LED-digital counter) by pressing a response button as soon as the stimulus appears, which stops the stimulus counter and displays the RT in milliseconds for a 1-sec period. The subject is instructed to press the button as soon as each stimulus appears, to keep the reaction time as low as possible, but not to press the button too soon [which yields a false start (FS) warning on the display]. Simple to perform, the PVT has only very minor learning effects

(29–31) on the order of a 1–3-trial learning curve (32) [which contrasts dramatically with the 30- to 60-trial learning curve of other supposedly simple learning tasks such as the digit symbol substitution task (33)]. The PVT interstimulus interval varies randomly from 2 sec to 10 sec, and the task duration is typically 10 min, which yields approximately 90 RTs per trial (i.e., a relatively high signal load). The sensitivity of the PVT can be increased by using longer task durations (e.g., 20 min), which can be useful when studying mild to moderate levels of sleepiness or in the assessment of interventions purporting to reduce sleepiness [e.g., various pharmacological agents, naps, work-rest schedules (34)].

### A. PVT Reliability

Reliability statistics have been calculated for the PVT using data from $n = 9$ subjects who were allowed an 8-hr sleep opportunity per night (i.e., the control group) as part of a larger chronic partial sleep deprivation protocol (35). PVT performance was assessed throughout the waking portion of each day. Test-retest statistics were obtained using daily performance averages (from tests taken at 09:30, 11:25, 13:20, and 15:15) on a baseline day and 5 consecutive experimental days. Intraclass correlation coefficients (ICC) measure the proportion of the variance explained by between-subject differences, as opposed to within-subject error. The ICC indicated maximal reliability for the number of PVT lapses (ICC $= 0.888$, $p <.0001$) and median response times (ICC $= 0.826$, $p <.0001$), falling into the standardized "almost perfect" range for a measurement assay (as discussed in Ref. 36).

### B. PVT Validity

The PVT was designed to be sensitive to sleep deprivation (experimental, occupational, and clinical) induced in many different ways (i.e., through sleep fragmentation, acute prolonged waking, chronic partial sleep restriction, etc.). Research has repeatedly shown this to be the case (Table 2) and demonstrated that the PVT captures the neurocognitive effects of sleep loss on wake state stability as reflected in sustained attention. Furthermore, the PVT is without the confounds induced by extraneous intersubject (e.g., aptitude) and intrasubject (e.g., learning) sources of variance that plague most other cognitive tasks. In fact, there is considerable evidence that the PVT meets all of the criteria in Table 1. Use of the PVT to reflect neurocognitive performance changes that are consistent with theorized functions of sleep (i.e., theoretical validity) and to demonstrate sensitivity to many forms of sleep deprivation (i.e., convergent validity) will be considered in the following sections of this chapter. In particular, evidence will be reviewed on the extent to which PVT performance reveals: (1) behavioral lapses, variability, and state instability; (2) circadian and homeostatic variation; (3) the effects of chronic partial sleep deprivation; (4) the benefits of interventions for the neurobehavioral effects of sleep loss; and (5) individual differences in vulnerability to sleep loss. Further, interpretation of PVT data will be considered, with partic-

**Table 2**  Summary of Published Literature on PVT Sensitivity to Sleep Deprivation

| Context | References |
| --- | --- |
| Interaction of homeostatic sleep drive and endogenous circadian pacemaker | Dinges & Kribbs, 1991 (3); Wyatt et al., 1997 (59); Rogers et al., 2002 (106); Graw et al., 2004 (127) |
| Total sleep deprivation | Dinges et al., 1994 (105); Kribbs & Dinges, 1994 (32); Jewett et al., 1999 (30); Konowal et al., 1999 (94); Atzram et al., 2001 (95); Doran et al., 2001 (44); Van Dongen et al., 2003 (68) |
| Chronic sleep restriction (cumulative partial sleep deprivation) | Dinges et al., 1997 (29); Rowland, 1997 (107); Kuo et al., 1998 (108); Johnson et al., 1998 (109); Jewett et al., 1999 (30); Balkin et al., 2000 (110); Drake et al., 2001 (71); Van Dongen et al., 2003 (35); Van Dongen et al., 2003 (68); Belenky et al., 2003 (70) |
| Prophylactic naps in sleep-deprived subjects | Dinges et al., 1987 (77); Rosekind et al., 1994 (31) |
| Caffeine in sleep-deprived subjects | Wright et al., 1997 (84); Dinges et al., 2000 (76); Van Dongen et al., 2001 (78); Wyatt et al., 2004 (124) |
| Body posture changes in sleep-deprived subjects | Caldwell et al., 2003 (111) |
| Sleepiness in the elderly | Pack et al., 1997 (116); Maislin et al., 2001 (117) |
| Slow eyelid closures of the kind experienced by drowsy drivers | Dinges et al., 1998 (112); Mallis et al., 1999 (113); Price et al., 2003 (96) |
| Simulated night shift work in laboratory | Hughes et al., 2001 (114); Lamond et al, 2003 (115); Caldwell et al., 2003 (130); Lamond et al., 2004 (128) |
| Jet lag and simulated night flights in transoceanic pilots | Rosekind et al., 1994 (31); Neri et al., 2002 (118); Russo et al., 2004 (126) |
| Astronauts during space missions | Dijk et al., 2001 (119) |
| On-call demands of medical house staff | Geer et al., 1995 (120); Smith-Coggins et al., 1997 (121); Howard et al., 2003 (125) |
| Intra- and intersubject variability | Doran et al., 2001 (44); Van Dongen et al., 2003 (68) |
| Excessive sleepiness from untreated sleep apnea (OSA), and residual sleepiness in OSA patients treated with nCPAP | Kribbs et al., 1993 (89); Kribbs & Dinges, 1994 (32); Chugh et al., 1998 (87); Dinges et al., 1998 (88); Powell et al., 1999 (102); Dinges & Weaver, 2003 (34) |
| Effects of modafinil on residual sleepiness in OSA patients treated with nCPAP | Dinges & Weaver, 2003 (34) |
| Effects of bright light | Phipps-Nelson et al., 2003 (129) |
| Sleep history and apnea severity in commercial truck drivers | Pack et al., 2002 (122) |
| Effects of alcohol | Powell et al., 1999 (102); Powell et al., 2001 (101) |
| Sedating effects of melatonin | Graw et al., 2001 (123) |

ular reference to drowsy driving, in order to establish that the PVT is sensitive to types of performance used in everyday functioning (i.e., ecological validity), and that PVT metrics can be meaningfully translated in "real world" terms. To set the validity of the PVT as a neurocognitive measure of sleep deprivation, we first review theoretical perspectives on the cognitive effects of sleep loss.

## V. Theories of How Sleep Loss Affects Cognitive Functions

There have been many descriptive hypotheses, but remarkably few theories to explain the cognitive effects of sleep deprivation. Early investigators assumed that because remaining awake for 3 or 4 days was so difficult, the ability to perform neurobehavioral tasks (ranging from finger tapping to IQ tests) should be lost when healthy, motivated persons were deprived of sleep (44). Although the seminal experiment by Patrick and Gilbert (13) reported that 90 hr of continuous wakefulness caused both motor and cognitive deficits in three adults, these findings were not replicated in early-twentieth-century experiments (reviewed in Ref. 2 and 44). Between 1923 and 1934, Nathaniel Kleitman published a series of reports on sleep deprivation ("experimental insomnia") that were intended to clarify the literature (1,2). Kleitman, and a few associates, remained awake between 60 hr and 114 hr but were unable to provide conclusive evidence that sleep loss eliminated the ability to perform specific motor or cognitive functions, because subjects could often transiently perform at baseline levels even after days without sleep. This ultimately led some investigators to assert that the neurocognitive effects of sleep deprivation were primarily to reduce motivation to perform and not cognitive lesions (reviewed in Ref. 3). In subsequent years, refinements were made in experimental measures, cognitive tasks, and statistical analyses, which resulted in less extreme theoretical perspectives on the neurocognitive effects of sleep loss—fewer investigators felt the evidence supported either cognitive lesion hypotheses or motivation hypotheses. Rather, these perspectives were replaced by theories based on evidence that suggested sleep deprivation induced increasing cognitive variability (and hence unpredictability) in specific human neurobehavioral functions.

### A. Response Blocks and the Lapse Hypothesis

The history of cognitive performance testing in human sleep deprivation is marked by several theoretical approaches. As described earlier, early investigators (e.g., Refs. 2,13) initially adopted a functional lesion framework. The possibility that sleep loss left no specific cognitive lesion, but markedly affected variability or stability of responding took decades to establish. The bias that sleep loss must produce cognitive lesions to have functional significance affected test design and, importantly, interpretation of experimental results. A particularly clear example of the latter can be found in Kleitman's (2) exhaustive review of sleep deprivation experiments up to 1963. In describing a seminal experiment by Warren and Clarke (37), who studied four subjects during 48–65 hr of wakefulness, Kleitman stated, "The results were largely negative, as were our own by the same technique" (2, p. 225). However, a reading of the original published report by Warren and Clarke (37) reveals that their results were far from negative (3). Rather, their work, inspired by Bills' research on "mental fatigue" (38–40), laid the foundation for a new theoretical framework. Notably, Bills was not studying the effects of sleep deprivation, but rather, minute-by-minute changes in the performance of non-sleep-deprived subjects. Bills observed an increase in "blocks," defined as "a pause in responses equivalent to the time of two or more average responses" (39, p. 231), with time-on-task. Warren and Clarke (37) applied Bills' block-recording system, and found that while subjects were capable of baseline performance levels while fatigued, they demonstrated increasing numbers of these performance "blocks" as sleep loss progressed. They noted that sleep loss did not produce complete destruction of the aspects of cognitive function they measured, but instead resulted in moment-to-moment performance variability. More than a decade later, Bjerner (41) showed that "blocks" were accompanied by distinct changes in brain activity (EEG) and eye movements (EOG), although he argued these were not "microsleeps." A decade after that observation, in the 1950s, investigators at Walter Reed Army Research Institute (43) hypothesized that the unevenness of performance in sleep-deprived subjects was due to "lapses" [another word for "blocks" (3)], caused by "microsleeps" in EEG and EOG changes.

For approximately two decades, the "lapse hypothesis" was the dominant theoretical explanation for the effects of sleep loss on cognitive performance. In their seminal monograph, Williams, Lubin, and Goodnow (43) reported that performance lapses on experimenter-paced RT tasks increased with increasing hours of wakefulness, and that while poorest performance worsened, subjects were still able to perform at almost optimum levels between lapse periods. Thus, the longer subjects remained awake, the more variable their performance became. Importantly, this was observed regardless of the type (simple vs. choice) or duration (10 vs. 30 min) of RT task, and whether or not subjects were provided with performance feedback.

### PVT Performance Reveals Lapses

Psychomotor vigilance task performance is exquisitely sensitive to lapses as classically defined by Bills (39), Warren and Clarke (37), Bjerner (41), and Williams et al. (43). Figure 1 displays consecutive individual reaction times during a 10-min PVT task from a single subject at 12, 36, 60, and 84 hr of wakefulness during an 88-hr total sleep deprivation protocol (44). After 12 hr of wakefulness, responses were maintained at a fast and consistent level. In contrast, much longer responses become evident in PVT trials undertaken as time awake increased. The lapses (conventionally defined at RT $\geq$ 500 msec) demonstrated not only

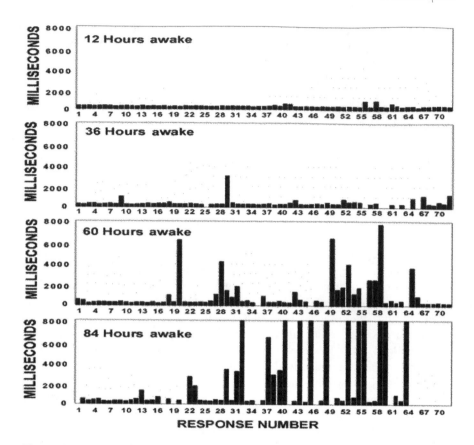

**Figure 1** Individual PVT reaction times (msec) for a representative subject undergoing 88 hr (3.67 days) of total sleep deprivation. Reaction times are from the 10-min visual PVT test bouts at 20:00 on each day of deprivation at 12, 36, 60, and 84 hr of sustained wakefulness. Reaction times after presentation of each stimulus are represented by black bars. Blank spaces between reaction times represent false starts (errors of commission). Reaction times > 500 msec are termed performance lapses, or lapses in attention. After 12 hr of wakefulness, reaction times were comparable across the test bout, with no false starts. At 36 hr of wakefulness, there were occasional lapses in attention (RT > 500 msec), with some false starts near the end of the test bout. After 60 hr awake the frequency of performance lapses was increased a few minutes into the performance bout. At 84 hr of sustained wakefulness, there were significantly more lapses of attention, with RTs > 8000 msec, and a greater incidence of false starts. (From Ref. 44.)

increased frequency as hours awake increased, but they also increased in duration, and in variability (from RT to RT). These data clearly indicate that lapsing, which refers to a failure to respond in a timely manner to a stimulus one is expecting, is an easily recognized occurrence in the performance of sleep-deprived subjects. Lapsing has been consistently recorded in studies of sleep deprivation and performance (e.g., Refs. 13,43–45), making it a primary outcome when using the PVT to assess sleepiness.

## VI.    Beyond the Lapse Hypothesis

The lapse hypothesis marked a significant, conceptually consolidating advance in theoretical approaches to the effects of sleep deprivation on cognitive performance. However, as a largely descriptive explanation of performance during sleep loss, the lapse hypothesis never rose to the level of a theory (i.e., no conceptual basis for lapsing was proffered). It also quickly became clear that the lapse hypothesis failed to account for several aspects of cognitive impairment commonly seen in sleep-deprived individuals. In a series of articles, Kjellberg (46–48) concluded that lapsing was not an adequate explanation for performance impairment during sleep loss. He suggested that lapses were not discrete periods of lowered arousal, but rather that sleep loss lowered arousal, which, after reaching a certain threshold level, resulted in a performance lapse. He concluded therefore that sleep loss resulted in changes to other aspects of performance. Indeed, at least three phenomena are beyond the explanatory scope of the lapse hypothesis. These include optimum response shifts, time-on-task effects, and the increase in errors of commission (false responses) during extended wakefulness (for thorough reviews on this topic the reader is directed to Refs. 3,46–49).

### A.    Response Slowing

The lapse hypothesis explicitly predicted that responses between lapses would be normal, which has not proven to be the case (3,5). In addition to performance lapses, Kjellberg (47) noted a slowing of reaction times that was independent of lapsing. Response slowing, a phenomenon recognized by Williams and colleagues (43), has been experimentally demonstrated using 10-min simple reaction time tasks. For example, Lisper and Kjellberg (50) demonstrated that the fastest 25% of reaction times on an auditory RT task were impaired during 24 hr of sleep deprivation. Similarly, during 54 hr of sustained wakefulness, Dinges and Powell (6) observed a clear decline in what they termed the "optimum response" domain (fastest 10% RTs) on both 10-min visual and 10-min auditory sustained attention tasks. Psychomotor vigilance task performance has also been found to show similar adverse effects of sleep loss on the fastest RTs (33). [The sensitivity of such brief sustained vigilance tasks to sleep loss also showed that Wilkinson's (8) claim in the 1960s that only long-duration (e.g., 40–60 min) vigilance tasks would be sensitive to sleep loss, was incorrect.]

### *Time-on-Task Decrements*

A second observation that cannot be explained by the lapse hypothesis is the well-documented time-on-task decrement (5,6,32,44), which refers to systematic deterioration in performance as a function of increasing duration of a cognitive task. Kleitman referred to this effect as a loss of endurance (2). In an experiment using a color-naming task, he observed that during sleep deprivation, significant slowing of response time and increases in errors could be seen as the task duration was extended from 1 to 12 min (103). He observed that during sleep deprivation most abilities could be maximally utilized by a "new effort" but that "the effect of increased effort disappeared when the test became one of endurance" (103, p. 150).

PVT performance in sleepy individuals frequently shows the effects of time-on-task on lapse rates at any severity of experimental sleep deprivation (e.g., see Fig. 1). Sleep deprivation can markedly worsen this "fatigue" effect in PVT performance, regardless of whether the elevated sleep pressure is experimentally induced (5), or through sleep disorders such as the obstructive sleep apnea syndrome (32). Thus, cognitive performance becomes more variable with both time awake *and* time-on-task (44).

Furthermore, it appears that time-on-task effects are not limited to immediate observable deterioration across single trials. A sleep deprivation experiment involving repeated PVT performance assessments revealed a "cost" associated with completing a longer-duration PVT trial. That is, extending the time-on-task (duration) of the PVT affected performance during subsequent trials. Figure 2 (data from Ref. 51) displays the performance of subjects who completed either a 10-min PVT (lower-workload group) or 20-min PVT (higher-workload group) every 2 hr during 40 hr of continuous wakefulness. Results from the *first* 10 min of the 20-min PVT group were compared to the results from the 10-min PVT group. Figure 2 illustrates a separation in PVT performance scores for the two groups after approximately 22 hr awake (i.e., from 08:00 to 12:00 and 16:00 to 20:00), indicating greater impairment in the high-workload group (i.e., 20-min PVT). Thus, higher cumulative workload further increased PVT deficits as sleep deprivation progressed. This suggests that there is a neurobiological cost to performing the PVT that becomes more evident as sleep loss progresses. It also suggests that in addition to factors such as time awake and time-on-task, prior workload should be accounted for when considering an individual's impairment level during sleep loss.

### Errors of Commission

A third limitation of the lapse hypothesis involved its inability to account for errors of commission, which involve responses when no stimulus is present (44). Studies have demonstrated a higher incidence of errors of commission with increasing hours of wakefulness (42,44). Importantly, errors of commission show the same profile of circadian-modulated increases across days of total sleep deprivation that is seen for errors of omission (i.e., lapses) (44). Such errors occur as premature responses during PVT performance, and are represented by blank spaces in between RT bars in Figure 1. After 12 hr of sustained

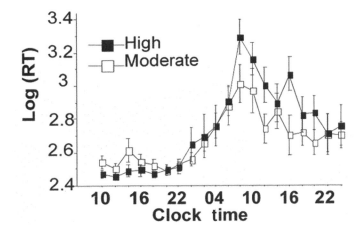

**Figure 2** Mean PVT reaction times (log msec ± sem) across 40 hr of total sleep deprivation. Data from the first 10 min of a 20-min visual PVT performance bout—high workload—are represented by the closed squares; data from the entire duration of a 10-min visual PVT performance bout—low workload—are represented by the open squares. The reaction time data (log transformed) were compared between the two groups using a mixed-model (workload by time awake) ANOVA. Reaction times during the first 10 min of the high-workload performance tests were significantly higher than those in the low-workload performance tests ($F_{9, 456} = 19.87$, $p < .001$). In addition, a decrease in reaction times across the 40 hr of wakefulness was evident in both workload groups ($F_{9, 456} = 2.17$, $p < 0.003$). (From Doran et al., 2000.)

wakefulness this subject experienced no false starts in a single 10-min PVT trial, compared to seven premature responses after 36 hr, five after 60 hr, and 15 after 60 hr. Of note, a time-on-task effect is also evident, with a greater number of false starts occurring later during each trial—a profile similar to that found for lapses.

### State Instability

As described above, both errors of omission involving performance lapses (i.e., failing to respond in a timely manner to a stimulus that is present) and errors of commission involving false starts (i.e., responding when no stimulus is present) have been experimentally demonstrated to increase during sleep deprivation (42,44). Figure 3 shows the profiles of each of these two types of cognitive errors in PVT performance across an 88-hr period of continuous wakefulness, relative to a control condition involving a 2-hr sleep opportunity every 12 hr across the vigil (44). The ability to engage in behavior to compensate for the effects of sleep loss has been observed by numerous investigators (2,13,52). We have suggested that the concomitant increase in errors of commission reflects an increased compensatory effort (albeit inefficient) in reaction to the effects of sleep loss (44). If

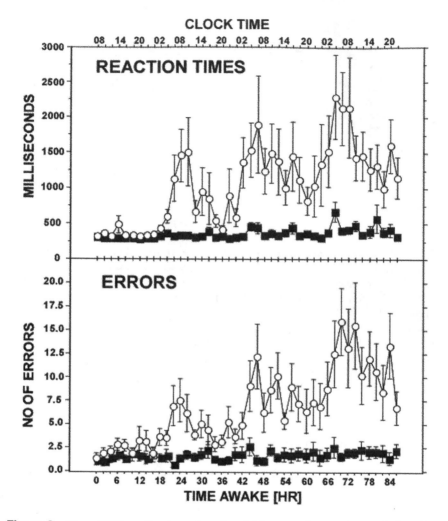

**Figure 3** Mean PVT reaction times (msec) and false starts (errors of commission) during 88 hr of total sleep deprivation and 88 hours of sleep deprivation with two 2-hour nap opportunities each day. Subjects in the total sleep deprivation (TSD) group (*n* = 13) are represented by the open circles. Subjects in the 88-hr sleep deprivation plus two 2-hr nap opportunities (NAP) group (*n* = 15) are represented by the closed squares. Nap opportunity periods were at 02:45-04:45 and 14:45-16:45 each day. The top panel illustrates mean reaction times (± s.e.m.) for each test bout across the experimental protocol. Subjects in the NAP group demonstrated little variation in reaction times across the experimental period, while subjects in the TSD group experienced significant impairment in performance, reflected in the increasing reaction times as time awake increased, with circadian variation in performance capability evident. The bottom panel illustrates mean number of errors (± s.e.m.) per test bout across the experimental protocol. A similar pattern of performance degradation in this variable was evident for both the NAP and TSD groups. (From Ref. 44.)

this hypothesis is correct, increasing motivation and effort to perform well during sleep deprivation may actually have the unintended consequence of producing additional errors of another type.

To explain the neurocognitive effects of sleep loss, what we term the *state instability* hypothesis (44) was developed after observing: (1) the emergence of both errors of omission and errors of commission during sleep loss; (2) their covariation over time in a manner consistent with the interaction of the homeostatic drive for sleep and endogenous circadian pacemaker (33); and (3) their increase with time-on-task. According to this hypothesis, an individual performing under the stress of an elevated homeostatic sleep drive may be overcome by sleepiness to the point of falling asleep uncontrollably while performing, which in turn leads to compensatory effort to resist the rapid and brief intrusions of sleep. Consequently, the state instability means that at any given moment in time the cognitive performance of the individual is unpredictable, and a product of interactive, competing neurobiological systems (connections, receptors, molecules) mediating sleep initiation and wake maintenance. In this conceptualization, the neurocognitive effects of sleep loss are but one manifestation of the broader neurobehavioral consequences of both sleep initiation and wake maintenance neurobiology co-occurring, with inadequate reciprocal inhibition between them. Theoretically, the state instability concept suggests that there are multiple, parallel neurobiological mechanisms by which waking and sleep states can interact. This is consistent with the fact that there are a growing number of candidate molecules that could be involved in the co-occurrence of sleep and waking (53).

A focus of both the state instability and the lapse hypothesis is the use of sustained attention tasks as sensitive assays of cognitive performance variability during sleep deprivation. The difference between the two viewpoints is in the explanation for the variability. The lapse hypothesis contends that performance during sleep deprivation is essentially "normal" until it becomes disrupted by lapses (brief periods of low arousal) (43). In contrast, according to the state instability hypothesis (51), performance variability is produced by the influence of homeostatically controlled sleep initiating mechanisms on the endogenous capacity to maintain alertness, and therefore utilize executive attention (prefrontal cortex). With its relatively high signal rate (input) and utilization of millisecond changes in response time (output), the PVT is designed to be maximally sensitive to state stability-instability during cognitive performance.

## VII. Sensitivity of PVT Performance to Neurobiological Causes of Elevated Sleep Drive

The theoretical and practical utility of any putative cognitive test of the effects of sleep deprivation must be grounded in its demonstrated sensitivity to known neurobiological sources of elevated sleep drive. The following sections review the sensitivity of the PVT to such factors.

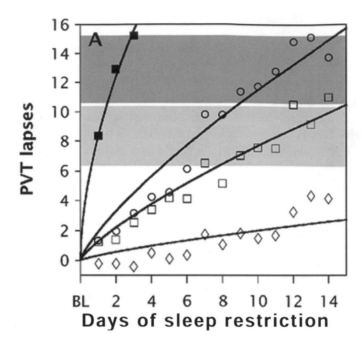

**Figure 4** PVT performance responses to varying doses of daily sleep. Mean PVT lapses per day (07:30–23:30), measured at 2-hr intervals, expressed relative to baseline (BL), in subjects randomized to an 8-hr ($n = 9$; open diamond), 6-hr ($n = 13$; open square), or 4-hr ($n = 13$; open circle) sleep opportunity per day for 14 consecutive days or 0-hr ($n = 13$; closed square) sleep condition across 3 days. The curves represent statistical non-linear model-based best-fitting profiles of the PVT performance response to sleep loss. The mean (± s.e.m.) ranges of neurobehavioral functions for 1 and 2 days of total sleep deprivation (0 hr sleep) are illustrated by the light and dark bands, respectively, allowing comparison of the 3-day total sleep deprivation condition and the 14-day chronic sleep restriction conditions. (From Ref. 35.)

### A.  Cognitive Performance Relative to the Two-Process Model of Sleep-Wake Regulation

Changes in performance capability during continuous wakefulness can be conceptualized as a two-process interaction (33), derived from the two-process model of sleep regulation (54). Specifically, sleepiness and performance are influenced by the homeostatic sleep drive (producing monotonic increases in impairment) and by circadian rhythmicity (near 24-hr cycles) (33,58). Daily circadian modulation of neurocognitive performance has been consistently noted since the first studies of sleep deprivation and human performance (2,13).

The interaction between endogenous circadian rhythmicity and homeostatic sleep drive results in a pattern in neurobehavioral functioning such that cognitive performance capability increases across the diurnal portion of each day (despite increasing time awake), and decreases across the night, reaching a nadir in the first 8 hr of the morning. A less marked and at times ephemeral midafternoon dip in performance has also been reported (55), referred to as the postprandial, or postlunch, dip (56,57). It is consistent with much scientific literature on the endogenous tendency for increased sleep propensity and napping at this time of day (104). Further, with increasing time awake, the escalating drive for sleep amplifies the circadian performance rhythm such that over successive days the level of impairment at the nadir of the rhythm becomes incrementally greater (42,57).

As noted earlier, an effective assay of the cognitive impact of sleep loss should be sensitive to the homeostatic drive for sleep in interaction with the endogenous circadian pacemaker (33,58). From Figure 3, it is evident that the PVT fulfills this requirement, with performance during 88 hr of sleep deprivation demonstrating both a monotonic component to impairment, which increases with increasing time awake, and a rhythmic oscillation in performance, which fluctuates in daily cycles.

Task sensitivity to homeostatic and circadian drives can be even more manifestly illustrated under constant routine conditions. Constant routine protocols allow investigators to study circadian rhythms without masking effects from factors such as sleep, physical activity, meals, light exposure, and social contact that will affect circadian phase markers. Subjects remain awake for longer than 24 hr (often several days), with fixed posture, ambient temperature (approximately 24°C), and lighting (typically <50 lux). Physical activity, meals and social contact are also kept constant (for a review of constant routine procedures, see Ref. 58). Van Dongen and Dinges (33) observed homeostatic and circadian modulations in subjective sleepiness and core body temperature during a 36-hr constant routine protocol ($n = 5$), which were closely reflected by the fastest 10% of PVT RTs. Similarly, a study by Wyatt and colleagues (59) demonstrated the interaction of homeostatic and circadian processes in the modulation of PVT performance. Thus, the psychomotor vigilance task appears to reflect the temporal dynamics of the two endogenous neurobiological systems (process S and process C) controlling daily wakefulness.

### B. Chronic Partial Sleep Deprivation

Chronic partial sleep deprivation has been defined as "preventing subjects from obtaining their usual amount of sleep within a 24-hour period" (60, p. 221). A wide range of partial sleep deprivation paradigms have been conducted, including selective deprivation of particular sleep stages (61–63), gradual sleep reduction over time (64), fixed-duration, reduced sleep opportunities in continuous (65) and distributed schedules (65), and situations where the time in bed is specifically reduced relative to the individual subject's habitual time in bed (29). The time span of these protocols has ranged from 24 hr (66) to 8 months (64).

Long-term investigations of partial sleep deprivation (from 21 days to 8 months) have not found consistent evidence of impairment (26,64,66,67). Such conflicting results are likely due to inadequacy of measurement outcomes and the lack of appropriate laboratory controls for timing and duration of sleep periods (68). In contrast, more tightly controlled, laboratory-based studies of chronic partial sleep deprivation, using more sensitive cognitive performance outcomes, have found clear evidence of performance impairment (29,35,65,69–71). Importantly, findings indicate that the effects of partial sleep deprivation are cumulative, such that performance and alertness become progressively worse across days of sleep restriction (35,70).

The PVT has been a primary performance assay for demonstrating the cumulative neurocognitive effects from chronic partial sleep deprivation (35,70). For example, in the two largest laboratory-controlled dose-response experiments conducted to date on the neurobehavioral effects of chronic sleep restriction, cumulative increases were evident in the average number of PVT lapses per 24 hr across days of sleep restricted to 3, 4, 5, and 6 hr per night (35,70). Moreover, daily PVT lapse rates increased at a more rapid rate in the reduced sleep conditions. Figure 4 displays the results from the first of these studies, in which subjects were restricted to 4, 6, or 8-hr time in bed for sleep for 14 consecutive days (35). The results were compared to 88 hr of total sleep deprivation. Figure 4 illustrates the dose-response relationship between sleep opportunity and the degree of impairment in PVT performance. Interestingly, this cumulative impairment was found to be almost linear for lapse rates. Further, subjects randomized to the 4- and 6-hr sleep restriction conditions reached levels of impairment equivalent to those of subjects undergoing 1–2 nights of total sleep deprivation.

In an earlier experiment, cumulative increases in PVT lapses across 7 days of sleep restricted to approximately 5 hr per night (29) were shown to be strongly related ($r = -0.95$) to sleep onset latency as assessed by the Multiple Sleep Latency Test (MSLT) in a nearly identical protocol (72). It appears that PVT performance lapse frequency and the well-validated physiological measure of sleep propensity may reflect the same basic process of escalating sleep pressure with sleep loss.

### C.   Interventions to Reduce Sleepiness

Interventions such as naps and caffeine to counteract the neurobehavioral effects of sleep loss and sleepiness in healthy adults have been found to improve PVT performance (73–77). The PVT has been successfully used to track the effects of napping in laboratory (77) and operational (31) settings. The use of naps in the laboratory to augment the performance of sleep-deprived subjects is illustrated in the control condition of Figure 3, which shows that PVT errors of omission and commission during 88 hr of sleep deprivation are substantially reduced by 2-hour naps taken every 12 hr.

There is evidence of performance benefits from combining naps and caffeine consumption during sleep loss (79,80). Although these studies did not use the PVT, performance on the PVT has been found to be sensitive to sleep inertia, which refers to feelings of grogginess and severe cognitive impairment after awakening from deep sleep. A potential reason for the advantage of combining naps and caffeine in sleep-restricted subjects has been demonstrated in a study by Van Dongen and colleagues (78), which revealed that sustained low-dose caffeine intake significantly reduced the effects of sleep inertia on PVT performance at awakening from naps during prolonged partial sleep deprivation.

Exposure to bright light during periods of sleep loss has also been used to attenuate performance degradation (e.g., Refs. 81–83). A modified version of the PVT has been used to assess the effects of countermeasure strategies involving combinations of bright light and caffeine (84) during 45.5 hr of total sleep deprivation. PVT performance was sensitive to differences between treatment groups, with best performance achieved by the bright-light/caffeine group, followed by the dim-light/caffeine group, with worse performance in the two groups who received placebo. Thus, it appears that in addition to showing the effects of sleep deprivation in healthy adults, PVT performance is sensitive to the alertness-promoting effects of bright light, naps, and caffeine in sleepy subjects.

### D. Obstructive Sleep Apnea Syndrome

Psychomotor vigilance task performance has also been shown to be sensitive to reduced behavioral alertness associated with obstructive sleep apnea syndrome (OSAS), and the efficacy of interventions for OSAS. Performance of patients with OSAS is impaired on tasks that rely on the ability to sustain attention (85,86). As a measure of behavioral alertness, PVT performance has been demonstrated to be a sensitive method for assessing the attentional capability of patients with OSAS (32,87,88). Kribbs and colleagues (89) found that PVT performance and sleepiness, measured by the MSLT, both reflected the benefits of CPAP use (reduction in respiratory events during sleep). Similarly, the PVT has been used to demonstrate the positive effects of modafinil (a wake-promoting compound) on the capacity to sustain attention in a group of OSAS patients (34).

### VIII. PVT Sensitivity to Other Factors Relevant to Sleepiness and Sedation

The PVT has also proven to be sensitive to other factors associated with neurobehavioral vulnerability to sleep loss and its consequences. The following sections review a few of the more salient ones.

### A. Interindividual Differences in Response to Sleep Loss

An important phenomenon that has been demonstrated using PVT performance results is that increasing time awake (sleep deprivation) in healthy adults is associated with increasing between-subject differences in PVT performance (3,44,68). This can be seen in the 88-hour total sleep deprivation protocol (44) shown in Figure 3, as evidenced by increasing error bars across time. Figure 5 displays PVT reaction time means plotted against standard deviations for 13 subjects from that experiment (44). Linear regression lines were fit for each individual. The different lengths of the regression lines in Figure 5 indicate that the magnitude of impairment differs between individuals. Interindividual differences in susceptibility to the impairing effects of sleep deprivation are an important area of interest, receiving increasing attention. In one of the only systematic studies on the topic to date, Van Dongen and colleagues (68) investigated PVT lapses in the same individuals who underwent 36-hr periods of total sleep deprivation on two separate occasions. Results revealed that interindividual differences accounted for 78.9% of the variance in PVT lapses performance, demonstrating reliable trait-like differences in vulnerability to sleep deprivation as measured using PVT performance (i.e., stable differential vulnerability to the cognitive effects of sleep deprivation).

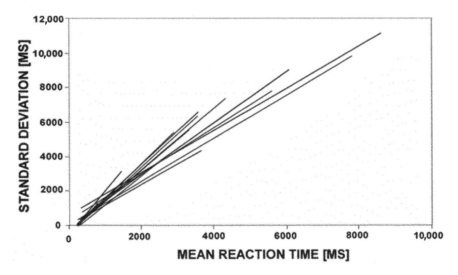

**Figure 5**   Least-square regression lines fit for the linear relationship between mean and standard deviation of PVT reaction times (msec). Data are from $n = 13$ subjects undergoing 88 hr (3.67 days) of total sleep deprivation. This figure illustrates that while all subjects experienced a decline in neurobehavioral performance on the PVT, as illustrated by increased reaction times when responding to the visual stimuli, there is a significant degree of interindividual variability in the magnitude of neurobehavioral impairment, evident by the differing lengths of the lines fit to the data. (From Ref. 44.)

## B. PVT and "Real World" Performance: Drowsy Driving

When interpreting results of laboratory-based cognitive tests, it must be remembered that they are not absolute indicators of "real world" performance. Although a given cognitive task may track the direction of changes in functioning as sleep deprivation increases, such tasks often do not permit a direct extrapolation to estimates of ability to perform everyday tasks. The PVT has some advantages in this regard, because it taps the ability to sustain attention and respond quickly to salient signals—features of a great many real-world tasks. In this sense it has high ecological validity, especially for tasks that require paying attention and responding in a timely manner (e.g., operating any transportation vehicle; monitoring radar, x-ray, and surveillance equipment; etc.).

Motor vehicle operation is a task performed by the vast majority of adults. It is heavily dependent on the ability to sustain attention and respond quickly, and it can have serious medical and economic consequences if not performed reliably. Transport accident data suggest that after controlling for traffic density, there are two main determinants of motor accident frequency: time of day and time spent driving (90). Specifically, accident frequency increases with time spent driving (i.e., time-on-task), and it is temporally distributed in a bimodal fashion. When adjustments are made for exposure (i.e., the number of motor vehicles on the road), crashes cluster disproportionately between 00:00 and 07:00, with a secondary peak around 15:00 (91–93). If inability to sustain attention were a major contributor to such accidents, it would be expected that a similar distribution would be found for prolonged performance lapses on the PVT. Indeed, this is the case. A study investigating PVT lapses greater than 30 sec, which are evidence of severe drowsiness attacks while attempting to perform, found that these attacks had a distribution similar to that of roadway crashes (see Fig. 6), with peaks of occurrence at 07:00 and at 16:00 and increasing prevalence with time-on-task (94).

From data described earlier (92,94), it is apparent that PVT lapses can be considered a temporal indicator of vulnerability to hypovigilance and sleepiness attacks of the kind that can occur during drowsy driving. Furthermore, PVT sensitivity allows a more fine-grained analysis of the circumstances leading up to a 30-sec sleep attack (95). Figure 7 displays PVT reaction times in the 6 min leading up to the first uncontrolled sleep attack in two experiments. A clear increase in reaction times (i.e., lengthening of lapse durations) prior to a 30-sec sleep attack is evident (95). These results suggest that such severe sleep attacks are not simply periods of nonresponding that punctuate normal alert performance; rather, a period of escalating impairment is evident during the min leading up to a 30-sec lapse. Not only is there temporal evidence that PVT lapses may be indicative of sleep attacks, but there is extensive evidence of a close correlation between PVT lapses and percent of time in slow eyelid closures while driving (96–98). The risks posed by increasing periods of slow eyelid closures while driving are obvious.

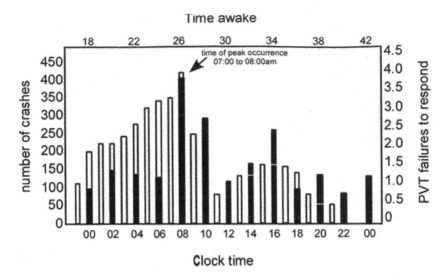

**Figure 6**  Frequency histogram for time of day of motor vehicle crashes and fall-asleep attacks on the PVT. The open bars represent the 60-min frequency of 4333 crashes in which the driver was judged to be asleep but not intoxicated across the 24-hr day; and the solid bars represent fall-asleep attacks (failure to respond for 30 sec on the PVT) in *n* = 14 subjects, measured at 120-min intervals across 42 hr of total sleep deprivation. Both the fatigue-related crashes and fall-asleep attacks follow an equivalent temporal profile across the day, with occurrences increasing across the nocturnal period, and peaking between 07:00 and 08:00. (Adapted from Refs. 92 and 94.)

### C.  Quantifying Impairment: PVT Performance and Alcohol

Attempts have been made to assess the magnitude of performance decrement during sleep loss using positive controls with widely accepted and quantified levels of impairment. Since the impairing effects of alcohol intoxication are readily recognized via public policy and legal regulation, studies have been conducted comparing the effects of sleep deprivation and alcohol.

Experimental comparisons between the performance effects of alcohol intoxication and sleep deprivation have found quantitative and qualitative similarities for numerous performance parameters including unpredictable tracking (9,99), vigilance (100), and response latency in a logical reasoning task (9). These studies have suggested that after 17–18 hr of sleep deprivation, performance is equivalent to (or greater than) that of a person with a blood alcohol concentration (BAC) of 0.05% (the legal driving limit in Australia) (100), and that after 20–25 hr awake, performance impairment is equivalent to (or greater than) a BAC of 0.10% (the legal driving limit in many states in the United States) (9).

Similar results have been found for PVT performance. Powell and colleagues (101) measured PVT performance after acute (1 night without sleep) or

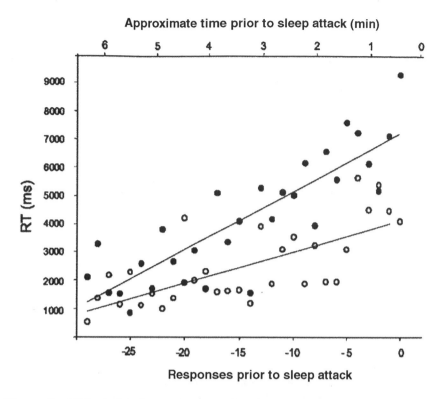

**Figure 7** PVT reaction times prior to the first uncontrolled sleep attack during total sleep deprivation. Fourteen subjects completed 42 hr of total sleep deprivation and completed a 20-min PVT every 2 hr (represented by the closed circles); 19 subjects completed 88 hr of total sleep deprivation and completed a 10-min PVT every 2 hr (represented by the open circles). The number of test bouts (up to 30) prior to an uncontrolled sleep attack (failure to respond for 30 sec on the PVT) is represented on the bottom abscissa, with time prior to the sleep attack (up to 6 min) represented on the top abscissa. In both subject groups a progressive decline in performance on the visual PVT was evident within minutes of an uncontrolled sleep attack on console. This study also demonstrated an increase in subjective sleepiness (measured using the Stanford Sleepiness Scale) in the test bouts prior to the one in which the first sleep attack occurred. Taken together, these findings suggest that even a very sleepy subject cannot fall asleep while performing computerized tasks without some levels of awareness. (From Ref. 95.)

partial (2 hr less sleep per night for 1 week) sleep loss compared to alcohol intoxication (mean concentration = 0.089 g/dL). They found that performance impairment on the PVT was not significantly different in the alcohol and sleep deprivation intervention groups, and the magnitude of impairment was similar. They also compared healthy subjects given alcohol with patients with untreated obstructive sleep apnea on measures of psychomotor vigilance performance

(102). Those with sleep-disordered breathing had worse RT performance than subjects with blood alcohol concentrations of 0.057% or greater.

Such research suggests that while the PVT is extremely sensitive to sleep deprivation, this does not negate its relevance to "real world" performance risks. That is to say, PVT impairment from sleep loss may be an indicator of "real world" task decrement to a degree that may be considered of operational (and legal) concern.

## IX.  Summary and Conclusions

Accurate assessment of neurobehavioral performance capability during sleep deprivation protocols requires cognitive performance assays to be: (a) indicative of a fundamental aspect of waking cognitive function; (b) easily performed; (c) minimally affected by aptitude and learning; (d) as brief as possible; (e) valid and reliable; (f) sensitive; and (g) able to provide meaningful outcome variables that can be easily interpreted. In this chapter we have reviewed the evidence that the psychomotor vigilance task meets these requirements.

The PVT was developed as a neurocognitive test of behavioral alertness to track temporally dynamic changes induced by interaction of the homeostatic drive for sleep and endogenous circadian pacemaker, focusing on assessing ability to sustain attention and respond in a timely manner to salient signals. Repeated administration (every 2 hr during waking periods) of the PVT to subjects allowed 8 hr sleep per night for 5 nights demonstrated the reliability of performance on this task across experimental days. Intraclass correlation coefficients indicated maximal reliability for both number of PVT performance lapses and median response times.

The PVT has been tested under a number of conditions recognized to induce neurocognitive deficits due to sleep loss, including total sleep deprivation, chronic partial sleep deprivation, and sleep fragmentation. Irrespective of the mode of sleep loss, results of extensive experiments on PVT performance have demonstrated that the task is capable of capturing the effects of sleep loss on stability of sustained attention, and that it can reliably reveal the accumulation of cumulative state instability in chronic sleep loss. As an assay of the neurocognitive effects of sleep loss, the PVT has also been used to assess the effectiveness of countermeasures to sleep loss (e.g., naps, caffeine, modafinil). The PVT has also been used to quantify daytime functioning levels in patients with OSAS, in relation to drowsy driving and in alcohol intoxication protocols.

Taken together these studies illustrate the efficacy and sensitivity of the PVT in the assessment of neurocognitive performance in a number of experimental, clinical, and operational paradigms. Because of its high degree of reliability, validity, lack of dependence on aptitude, and ability to be repeatedly administered, the PVT can be used to quantify the effects of sleep loss, and other manipulations, on neurobehavioral capability across a number of days. Studies have suggested that PVT performance has relevance to "real world" risks, such as drowsy driving and alcohol impairment.

## Acknowledgments

The substantive evaluation on which this chapter was based was supported by NIH grant NR04281; Air Force Office of Scientific Research grant F49620-00-1-0266; NASA Cooperative Agreement NCC 9–58 with the National Space Biomedical Research Institute and the Institute for Experimental Psychiatry Research Foundation.

## References

1. Kleitman N. Deprivation of sleep. In: Kleitman N, ed. Sleep and Wakefulness, 1939:215–229.
2. Kleitman N. Deprivation of sleep. In: Kleitman N, ed. Sleep and Wakefulness, 1963:215–229.
3. Dinges DF, Kribbs NB. Performing while sleepy: effects of experimentally-induced sleepiness. In: Monk TH, ed. Sleep, Sleepiness and Performance: J Wiley, New York: 1991:97–128.
4. Harrison Y, Horne JA. The impact of sleep deprivation on decision making: a review. J Exp Psychol: Appl 2000; 6:236–249.
5. Dinges DF, Powell JW. Sleepiness is more than lapsing. Sleep Res 1988; 17:84.
6. Dinges DF, Powell JW. Sleepiness impairs optimum response capability. Sleep Res 1989; 18:366.
7. Findley LJ, Suratt PM, Dinges DF. Time-on-task decrements in "steer clear" performance of patients with sleep apnea and narcolepsy. Sleep 1999; 22:804–809.
8. Wilkinson RT. Effects of up to 60 hours sleep deprivation on different types of work. Ergonomics 1964; 7:175–186.
9. Lamond N, Dawson D. Quantifying the performance impairment associated with fatigue. J Sleep Res 1999; 8:255–262.
10. Williams HL, Lubin A. Speeded addition and sleep loss. J Exp Psychol 1967; 73:313–317.
11. Johnson LC. Sleep deprivation and performance. In: Webb WB, ed. Biological Rhythms, Sleep and Performance. New York: Wiley, 1982.
12. Bohlin G. Monotonous stimulation, sleep onset and habituation of the orienting reaction. Electroencephalogr & Clin Neurophysiol. 1971; 31:593–601.
13. Patrick GT, Gilbert JA. On the effects of loss of sleep. Psychol Rev 1896; 3:469–483.
14. Harrison Y, Horne JA, Rothwell A. Prefrontal neuropsychological effects of sleep deprivation in young adults—a model for healthy aging? Sleep 2000; 23:1067–1073.
15. Horne JA. Sleep loss and "divergent" thinking ability. Sleep 1988; 11:528–536.
16. Glenville M, Broughton R, Wing AM, Wilkinson RT. Effects of sleep deprivation on short duration performance measures compared to the Wilkinson auditory vigilance task. Sleep 1978; 1:169–176.

17. Harrison Y, Horne JA. Sleep deprivation affects speech. Sleep. 1997; 20:871–877.
18. Harrison Y, Horne JA. Sleep loss impairs short and novel language tasks having a prefrontal focus. J of Sleep Res. 1998; 7:95–100.
19. Horne JA. Human sleep, sleep loss and behaviour: implications for the prefrontal cortex and psychiatric disorder. Br J of Psychiatry 1993; 162:413–419.
20. Abi-Dargham A, Mawlawi O, Lombardo I, Gil R, Martinez D, Huang Y, Hwang DR, Keilp J, Kochan L, Van Heertum R, Gorman JM, Laruelle M. Prefrontal dopamine D1 receptors and working memory in schizophrenia. J of Neurosci. 2002; 22:3708–3719.
21. Cools R, Clark L, Owen AM, Robbins TW. Defining the neural mechanisms of probabilistic reversal learning using event-related functional magnetic resonance imaging. J Neurosci. 2002; 22:4563–4567.
22. Baddeley A. Working memory. Science 1992; 255:556–559.
23. Baddeley AD. Is working memory still working? Am Psychol 2001; 56:851–864.
24. Kane MJ, Bleckley MK, Conway ARA, Engle RW. A controlled-attention view of working-memory capacity. J of Exp Psychol: Gen 2001; 130:169–183.
25. Engle RW. Working memory capacity as executive attention. Curr Directi Psychol Sci 2002; 11:19–23.
26. Horne JA, Wilkinson S. Chronic sleep reduction: daytime vigilance performance and EEG measures of sleepiness, with particular reference to "practice" effects. Psychophysiology 1985; 22:69–78.
27. Burgess P, Shallice T. Response suppression, initiation and strategy use following frontal lobe lesions. Neuropsychologia 1996; 34:263–272.
28. Dinges DF, Powell JW. Microcomputer analyses of performance on a portable, simple visual RT task during sustained operations. Behav Res Metho Instrum Comput 1985; 17:652–655.
29. Dinges DF, Pack F, Williams K, Gillen KA, Powell JW, Ott GE, Aptowicz C, Pack AI. Cumulative sleepiness, mood disturbance, and psychomotor vigilance performance decrements during a week of sleep restricted to 4–5 hours per night. Sleep 1997; 20:267–277.
30. Jewett ME, Dijk DJ, Kronauer RE, Dinges DF. Dose-response relationship between sleep duration and human psychomotor vigilance and subjective alertness. Sleep 1999; 22:171–179.
31. Rosekind MR, Graeber RC, Dinges DF, Connell LJ, Rountree MS, Spinweber CL, Gillen KA. Crew factors in flight operations. IX. Effects of planned cockpit rest on crew performance and alertness in long-haul operations. Technical Memorandum. 108839. 1994.
32. Kribbs NB, Dinges DF. Vigilance decrement and sleepiness. In: Harsh JR Ogilvie RD, eds. Sleep Onset Mechanisms. Washington, DC: American Psychological Association, 1994:113–125.
33. Van Dongen HPA, Dinges DF. Circadian rhythms in fatigue, alertness and performance. In: Kryger MH, Roth T, Dement WC, eds. Principles and Practice of Sleep Medicine. Philadelphia: WB Saunders, Company 2000:391–399.
34. Dinges DF, Weaver T. Effects of modafinil on sustained attention performance and quality of life in OSA patients with residual sleepiness while being treated with nCPAP. Sleep Med. 2003; 4:393–402.
35. Van Dongen HPA, Maislin G, Mullington JM, Dinges DF. The cumulative cost of additional wakefulness: dose-response effects on neurobehavioral functions and

sleep physiology from chronic sleep restriction and total sleep deprivation. Sleep 2003; 26:117–126.

36. Landis JR, Koch GG. The measurement of observer agreement for categorical data. Biometrics 1977; 33:159–174.

37. Warren N, Clarke B. Blocking in mental and motor tasks during a 65–hour vigil. J Exp Psychol 1937; 21:97–105.

38. Bills AG. Fatigue in mental work. Physiol Rev 1937; 17:436–453.

39. Bills AG. Blocking: a new principle in mental fatigue. Am J Psychol 1931; 43:230–245.

40. Bills AG. Some additional principles of mental fatigue. Psychol Bull 1934; 31:671.

41. Bjerner B. Alpha depression and lowered pulse rate during delayed actions in a serial reaction test: a study of sleep deprivation. Aviat Space Environ Med 1949; 6:233–235.

42. Lubin A. Performance under sleep loss and fatigue. In: Kety SS, Evarts EV, Williams HL, eds. Sleep and Altered States of Consciousness. Vol. XLV. New York: Williams & Wilkins, 1967:507–513.

43. Williams HL, Lubin A, Goodnow JJ. Impaired performance with acute sleep loss. Psychol Monogra Gen Appl 1959; 73:1–25.

44. Doran SM, Van Dongen HP, Dinges DF. Sustained attention performance during sleep deprivation: evidence of state instability. Archi Ital Biol: Neurosci 2001; 139:253–267.

45. Broadbent DE. Noise, paced performance and vigilance tasks. Br J of Psychol 1953; 44:295–303.

46. Kjellberg A. Sleep deprivation and some aspects of performance. I. Problems of arousal changes. Waking and Sleeping. Vol. 1, 1977:139–143.

47. Kjellberg A. Sleep deprivation and some aspects of performance. II. Lapses and other attentional effects. Waking and Sleeping. Vol. 1, 1977:145–148.

48. Kjellberg A. Sleep deprivation and some aspects of performance. III. Motivation, comment and conclusions. Waking and Sleeping. Vol. 1, 1977:149–153.

49. Dinges DF. Probing the limits of functional capability: the effects of sleep loss on short-duration tasks. In: Broughton RJ, Ogilivie RD, eds. Sleep, Arousal and Performance. Boston: Birkhauser, 1992.

50. Lisper HO, Kjellberg A. Effects of 24–hour sleep deprivation on rate of decrement in a 10–minute auditory reaction time task. J of Exp Psychol 1972; 96:287–290.

51. Doran SM, Van Dongen HPA, Powell JW, Mallis MM, Konowal NM, Dinges DF. Effects of cumulative workload on vigilance decrement during total sleep deprivation. Sleep 2000; 23:A240–A241.

52. Horne JA, Pettitt AN. High incentive effects on vigilance performance during 72 hours of total sleep deprivation. Acta Psychol (Amst) 1985; 58:123–139.

53. Mignot E, Taheri S, Nishino S. Sleeping with the hypothalamus: emerging therapeutic targets for sleep disorders. Nature Neurosci. 2002; 5:1071–1075.

54. Borbély AA. A two process model of sleep regulation. Hum Neurobiol 1982; 1:195–204.

55. Lavie P. Ultrashort sleep-waking schedule. III. "Gates" and "forbidden zones" for sleep. Electroencephalogr Clin Neurophysiol 1986; 63:414–425.

56. Carrier J, Monk T. Effects of sleep and circadian rhythms on performance. In: Turek FW, Zee PC, eds. Regulation of Sleep and Circadian Rhythms. New York: Marcel Dekker, 1999:527–566.

57. Babkoff H, Caspy T, Mikulincer M. Subjective sleepiness ratings: the effects of sleep deprivation, circadian rhythmicity and cognitive performance. Sleep 1991; 14:534–539.

58.  Czeisler CA, Khalsa SBS. The human circadian timing system and sleep-wake regulation. In: Kryger MH, Roth T, Dement WC, eds. Principles and Practice of Sleep Medicine. Philadelphia: WB Saunders, 2000:353–376.
59.  Wyatt JK, Dijk DJ, Ronda JM, Jewett ME, Powell JW, Dinges DF, Czeisler CA. Interaction of circadian- and sleep/wake homeostatic-processes modulate psychomotor vigilance test (PVT) performance. Sleep Res 1997; 26:759.
60.  Webb WB. Partial and differential sleep deprivation. In: Kales A, ed. Sleep Physiology and Pathology: A Symposium. Philadelphia: JB Lippincott, 1969:221–231.
61.  Ferrara M, De Gennaro L, Bertini M. The effects of slow-wave sleep (SWS) deprivation and time of night on behavioral performance upon awakening. Physiol Behav 1999; 68:55–61.
62.  Ferrara M, De Gennaro L, Casagrande M, Bertini M. Selective slow-wave sleep deprivation and time-of-night effects on cognitive performance upon awakening. Psychophysiology 2000; 37:440–446.
63.  Walsh JK, Hartman PG, Schweitzer PK. Slow-wave sleep deprivation and waking function. J Sleep Res 1994; 3:16–25.
64.  Friedmann J, Globus G, Huntley A, Mullaney D, Naitoh P, Johnson L. Performance and mood during and after gradual sleep reduction. Psychophysiology 1977; 14:245–250.
65.  Hartley LR. A comparison of continuous and distributed sleep schedules. Q J Exp Psychol 1974; 26:8–14.
66.  Webb WB, Agnew HW Jr. The effects of a chronic limitation of sleep length. Psychophysiology 1974; 11:265–274.
67.  Blagrove M, Alexander C, Horne JA. The effects of chronic sleep reduction on the performance of cognitive tasks sensitive to sleep deprivation. Appl Cogn Psychol 1995; 9:21–40.
68.  Van Dongen HPA, Rogers NL, Dinges DF. Understanding sleep debt: theoretical and empirical issues. Sleep Biolo Rhythms 2003; 1:4–12.
69.  Tilley AJ, Wilkinson RT. The effects of a restricted sleep regime on the composition of sleep and on performance. Psychophysiology 1984; 21:406–412.
70.  Belenky G, Wesensten NJ, Thorne DR, Thomas ML, Sing HC, Redmond DP, Russo MB, Balkin TJ. Patterns of performance degradation and restoration during sleep restriction and subsequent recovery: a sleep-dose response study. J Sleep Res 2003; 12:1–12.
71.  Drake CL, Roehrs TA, Burduvali E, Bonahoom A, Rosekind M, Roth T. Effects of rapid versus slow accumulation of eight hours of sleep loss. Psychophysiology. 2001; 38:979–987.
72.  Carskadon MA, Dement WC. Cumulative effects of sleep restriction on daytime sleepiness. Psychophysiology 1981; 18:107–113.
73.  Hayashi M, Watanabe M, Hori T. The effects of a 20 min nap in the mid-afternoon on mood, performance and EEG activity. Clin Neurophysiol 1999; 110:272–279.
74.  Sallinen M, Harma M, Akerstedt T, Rosa R, Lillqvist O. Promoting alertness with a short nap during a night shift. J of Sleep Res 1998; 7:240–247.
75.  Lagarde D, Batejat D, Sicard B, Trocherie S, Chassard D, Enslen M, Chauffard F. Slow-release caffeine: a new response to the effects of a limited sleep deprivation. Sleep 2000; 23:651–661.

76. Dinges DF, Doran SM, Mullington J, Van Dongen HP, Price N, Samuel S, Carlin MM, Powell JW. Neurobehavioral effects of 66 hr of sustained low-dose caffeine during 88 hr of total sleep deprivation. Sleep 2000; 23:A20–A21.

77. Dinges DF, Orne MT, Whitehouse WG, Orne EC. Temporal placement of a nap for alertness: contributions of circadian phase and prior wakefulness. Sleep 1987; 10:313–329.

78. Van Dongen HPA, Price NJ, Mullington JM, Szuba MP, Kapoor SC, Dinges DF. Caffeine eliminates psychomotor vigilance deficits from sleep inertia. Sleep 2001; 24:813–819.

79. Bonnet MH, Arand DL. Impact of naps and caffeine on extended nocturnal performance. Physiol Behav 1994; 56:103–109.

80. Bonnet MH, Arand DL. The use of prophylactic naps and caffeine to maintain performance during a continuous operation. Ergonomics 1994; 37:1009–1020.

81. Martin SK, Eastman CI. Medium-intensity light produces circadian rhythm adaptation to simulated night-shift work. Sleep 1998; 21:154–165.

82. Bougrine S, Mollard R, Ignazi G, Coblentz A. Days off and bright light: effects on adaptation to night work. Int J Indus Ergonom 1998; 21:187–198.

83. Campbell SS, Dawson D. Enhancement of nighttime alertness and performance with bright ambient light. Physiol Behav 1990; 48:317–320.

84. Wright KP, Jr., Badia P, Myers BL, Plenzler SC. Combination of bright light and caffeine as a countermeasure for impaired alertness and performance during extended sleep deprivation. J Sleep Res 1997; 6:26–35.

85. Findlay, L., Suratt, P., Dinges, D.F.: Time-on-task decrements in "steer clear" performance of patients with sleep apnea and narcolepsy. Sleep 1999; 22(6):804–80.

86. Bedard MA, Montplaisir J, Richer F, Malo J. Nocturnal hypoxemia as a determinant of vigilance impairment in sleep apnea syndrome. Chest 1991; 100:367–370.

87. Chugh DK, Weaver TE, Dinges DF. Psychomotor vigilance performance in sleep apnea compared patients presenting with snoring without apnea. Sleep 1998; 21:491.

88. Dinges DF, Maislin G, Staley B, Pack F, Woodle C, Pack AI. Sleepiness and neurobehavioral functioning in relation to sleep apnea severity in a cohort of commercial motor vehicleoperations. Sleep 1998; 21:199.

89. Kribbs NB, Pack AI, Kline LR, Getsy JE, Schuett JS, Henry JN, Maislin G, Dinges DF. Effects of one night without nasal CPAP treatment on sleep and sleepiness in patients with obstructive sleep apnea. Am Revi Respir Dis 1993; 147:1162–1168.

90. Folkard S. Black times: temporal determinants of transport safety. Accident Anal Prevent. 1997; 29:417–430.

91. Mitler MM, Carskadon MA, Czeisler CA, Dement WC, Dinges DF, Graeber RC. Catastrophes, sleep, and public policy: consensus report. Sleep 1988; 11:100–109.

92. Pack AI, Pack AM, Rodgman E, Cucchiara A, Dinges DF, Schwab CW. Characteristics of crashes attributed to the driver having fallen asleep. Accident Anal Prevent 1995; 27:769–775.

93. Horne JA, Reyner LA. Sleep related vehicle accidents. Bri Med J 1995; 310:565–567.

94. Konowal NM, Van Dongen HPA, Powell JW, Mallis MM, Dinges DF. Determinants of microsleeps during experimental sleep deprivation. Sleep 1999; 22:S328–S329.

95. Atzram M, Chow C, Price NJ, Rogers NL, Van Dongen HP, Dinges DF. Can sleep attacks occur without feeling sleepy? Sleep 2001; 24:A428–A429.

96.  Price NJ, Maislin G, Powell JW, Ecker AJ, Szuba MP, Mallis MM, Dinges DF. Unobtrusive detection of drowsiness-induced PVT lapses using infrared retinal reflectance of slow eyelid closures. Sleep 2003; 26:A177.

97.  Dinges DF, Mallis MM, Maislin G, Powell JW. Evaluation of techniques for ocular measurement as an index of fatigue and the basis for alertness management. Final report for the U.S. Department of Transportation, National Highway Traffic Safety Administration. NHTSA Report No. HS 808 762. 1998.

98.  Mallis MM, Maislin G, Konowal N, Byrne V, Bierman D, Davis R, Grace R, Dinges DF. Biobehavioral responses to drowsy driving alarms and alerting stimuli. Final report to develop, test and evaluate a drowsy driver detection and warning system for commercial motor vehicle drivers sponsored by the National Highway Traffic Safety Administration, Federal Highway Administration, Office of Motor Carriers. 1999.

99.  Dawson D, Reid K. Fatigue, alcohol and performance impairment. Nature 1997; 388:235.

100.  Williamson MA, Feyer A. Moderate sleep deprivation produces impairments in cognitive and motor performance equivalent to legally prescribed levels of alcohol intoxication. Occup Environ Medi 2000; 57:649–655.

101.  Powell NB, Schechtman KB, Riley RW, Li K, Troell R, Guilleminault C. The road to danger: the comparative risks of driving while sleepy. Laryngoscope 2001; 111:887–893.

102.  Powell NB, Riley RW, Schechtman KB, Blumen MB, Dinges DF, Guilleminault C. A comparative model: reaction time performance in sleep-disordered breathing versus alcohol-impaired controls. Laryngoscope 1999; 109:1648–1654.

103.  Lee MAM, Kleitman N. Studies on the physiology of sleep. II. Attempts to demonstrate functional changes in the nervous system during experimental insomnia. Am J Physiol 1923; 67: 141–152.

104.  Dinges DF, Broughton RJ: The significance of napping: a synthesis. In: Dinges DF, Broughton RJ, eds. Sleep and Alertness: Chronobiological, Behavioral and Medical Aspects of Napping. New York: Raven Press, 1989: 299–308.

105.  Dinges DF, Douglas SD, Zaugg L, Campbell DE, McMann JM, Whitehouse WG, Orne, EC, Kapoor SC, Icaza E, Orne MT. Leukocytosis and natural killer cell function parallel neurobehavioral fatigue induced by 64 hours of sleep deprivation. J Clin Investig 1994; 93:1930–1939.

106.  Rogers NL, Van Dongen HPA, Powell I JW, Carlin MM, Szuba MP, Maislin G, Dinges DF. Neurobehavioral functioning during chronic sleep restriction at an adverse circadian phase. Sleep 2002; 25S:A126–A127.

107.  Rowland L, Thorne D, Balkin T, Sing H, Wesensten N, Redmond D, Johnson D, Anderson, A, Cephus R, Hall S, Thomas M, Powell JW, Dinges DF, Belenky G. The effects of four different sleep-wake cycles on psychomotor vigilance. Sleep Research 1997; 26:627.

108.  Kuo A, Carlin MM, Powell JW, Dinges DF. Chronic restriction of sleep to 4 hours per night for 14 nights changes performance linearly but not subjective sleepiness. Sleep 1998; 21S:169.

109.  Johnson D, Thorne D, Rowland L, Balkin T, Sing H, Thomas M, Wesensten N, Redmond D, Russo M, Welsh A, Aladdin R, Cephus R, Hall S, Powell J, Dinges D, Belenky G. The effects of partial sleep deprivation on psychomotor vigilance. Sleep 1998; 21S:137.

110. Balkin T, Thorne D, Sing H, Thomas M, Redmond D, Wesensten N, Williams J, Hall S, Belenky G. Effects of Sleep Schedules on Commercial Motor Vehicle Driver Performance. FMCSA Report No. DOT-MC-00-133, May, 2000.

111. Caldwell JA, Prazinko B, Caldwell JL. Body posture affects electronencephalographic activity and psychomotor vigilance task performance in sleep-deprived subjects. Clin Neurophysiol 2003; 114(1):23–31.

112. Dinges DF, Mallis M, Maislin G, Powell JW. Evaluation of techniques for ocular measurement as an index of fatigue and the basis for alertness management. Final report for the U.S. Department of Transportation, National Highway Traffic Safety Administration, 1998.

113. Mallis MM, Maislin G, Powell JW, Konowal NM, Dinges DF. Perclos predicts both PVT lapse frequency and cumulative lapse duration. Sleep 1999; 22S1:S149.

114. Hughes RJ, Van Dongen HPA, Dinges DF, Rogers NL, Wright KP, Edgar DM, Czeisler, CA. Modafinil improves alertness and performance during simulated night work. Sleep 2001; 24S:A200.

115. Lamond N, Dorrian J, Roach GD, McCulloch K, Holmes AL, Burgess HJ, Fletcher A, Dawson D. The impact of a week of simulated night work on sleep, circadian phase and performance. Occup Environ Med 2003; 60:1–9.

116. Pack AI, Dinges DF, Gehrman PR, Pack FM, Maislin G. Sleepiness in the elderly, role of sleep apnea: A case-control approach. Sleep Res 1997; 26:453.

117. Maislin G, Pack AI, Samuel S, Dinges DF. Objectively measured sleep behaviors and vigilance in community residing elderly with and without complaints of daytime sleepiness. Sleep 2001; 24S:A224.

118. Neri DF, Oyung RL, Colletti LM, Mallis MM, Tam PY, Dinges DF. Controlled breaks as a fatigue countermeasure on the flight deck. Aviation, Space, Environ Med 2002; 73(6):1–11.

119. Dijk DJ, Neri DF, Wyatt JK, Ronda JM, Riel E, Ritz-De Cecco A, Hughes RJ, Elliott AR, Prisk GK, West JB, Czeisler CA. Sleep, performance, circadian rhythms, and light-dark cycles during two space shuttle flights. Am J Physiol Regul Integr Comp Physiol 2001; 281(5):R1657–1664.

120. Geer RT, Jobes DR, Gilfor J, Traber KB, Dinges D. Reduced psychomotor vigilance in anesthesia residents after 24-hr on call. Anesthesiol 1995; 83(S3A):A1008.

121. Smith-Coggins R, Rosekind MR, Buccino KR, Dinges DF, Moser RP: Rotating shiftwork schedules: Can we enhance physician adaptation to night shifts? Academic Emerg Med 1997; 4:951–961.

122. Pack AI, et al. A study of prevalence of sleep apnea among commercial truck drivers. Final report on contract DTFH61-93-R-00088, 2002.

123. Graw P, Werth E, Kräuchi K, Gutzwiller F, Cajochen Co, Wirz-Justice A. Early morning melatonin administration impairs psychomotor vililance. Behavioral Brain Research 2001; 121:167–172.

124. Wyatt JK, Cajochen C, Ritz-De Cecco A, Czeisler CA, Dik DJ. Low-dose repeated caffeine administration for circadian-phase-dependent performance degradation during extended wakefulness. Sleep 2004; 27(3):374–381.

125. Howard SK, Gaba DM, Smith BE, Weinger MB, Herndon C, Keshavacharya S, Rosekind MR. Simulation study of rested versus sleep-deprived anesthesiologists. Anesthesiol 2003; 98:1345–1355.

126. Russo MB, Sing H, Santiago S, et al. Visual neglect: Occurrence and patterns in pilots in a simulated overnight flight. Aviation, Space, Environ Med 2004; 75(4):323–332.

127. Graw P, Krauchi K, Knoblauch V, et al. Circadian and wake-dependent modulation of fastest and slowest reaction times during the psychomotor vigilance task. Physiol and Behav 2004; 80(5):695–701.

128. Lamond N, Dorrain J, Burgess HJ, et al. Adaptation of performance during a week of simulated night work. Ergonomics 2004; 47(2):154–165.

129. Phipps-Nelson J, Redman JR, Dijk DJ, et al. Daytime exposure to bright light, as compared to dim light, decreases sleepiness and improves psychomotor vigilance performance. Sleep 2003; 26(6):695–700.

130. Caldwell JL, Prazinko BF, Rowe T, et al. Improving daytime sleep with temazepam as a countermeasure for shift lag. Aviation, Space, & Environ Med 2003; 74(2):153–163.

# 5

## Major Sleep Disorders

**CHRISTIAN GUILLEMINAULT AND DAWN DANIEL**

Stanford University, Stanford, California, U.S.A.

## I. Introduction

Sleep disorders have been subdivided into disorders of initiating and maintaining sleep and disorders of excessive daytime sleepiness (1); however, this distinction is fairly arbitrary. For instance, DSM-IV (2) requires the diagnosis of chronic insomnia, a disorder of initiating and maintaining sleep, to be associated with daytime consequences. Most sleep disorders involve some degree of sleep deprivation, which impacts daytime alertness, cognitive function, and quality of life. To induce sleep deprivation, a sleep disorder must increase the normal rate of arousals and awakenings during sleep.

## II. Arousals, Awakenings, and Autonomic Nervous System Activation

The definition of what constitutes a normal awakening from sleep is not well characterized. Although the normative amount is unknown, it appears to vary with age. A significant amount of data from studies of young adults and small groups of subjects, collected with polysomnography, has been published. Awakenings and arousals were defined based on electroencephalographic (EEG) recordings using central leads (3). However, Pivik (4) demonstrated that investigating brain activity using multiple EEG leads will show different views of sleep

71

onset. Sleep offset will probably show similar patterns. Our understanding of arousals and awakenings in this context is thus limited.

EEG arousals have been defined with visual markers. However, the discriminative ability of the human eye of an expert is limited. It has been shown that an event must be a minimum of 3 sec to be visually detected (5). A 2002 study showed that for such short segments, beta EEG bursts are recognized but alpha bursts are not (6). The number of short EEG arousals necessary to induce sleep deprivation is unknown at this time.

Some investigators tried to define "awakenings" behaviorally by analyzing continuous video recordings. Comparisons of EEG recordings and behavioral analyses showed that brief arousals are not detected with the latter approach. Martin et al. (7) tried to exclude the use of EEG recordings and instead used changes in heart rate to detect arousals. Their rationale was that a change in the state of alertness is associated with a change in autonomic nervous system (ANS) activity with an overall increase in parasympathetic activity and a secondary decrease in heart rate during sleep. Arousals and awakenings are associated with an increase in sympathetic activity and changes in heart rate. Unfortunately, heart rate is highly variable during both wakefulness and sleep (8). The state of alertness is not the only factor that affects heart rate. Changes in heart rate are directly related to stroke volume and cardiac output.

Moruzzi (9) already clearly dissociated "activation" from "arousal." Stimulation from the sensory terminals leads to monosynaptic and more often polysynaptic reflexes. These polysynaptic reflexes relay in subcortical structures. Depending on the intensity of stimulation, the degree of neuronal recruitment, and so forth, the number of brain structures involved will vary. Stimulation may affect the thalamus, basal forebrain, and a newly recognized loop called the corticothalamocortical loop (10).

However, activation of the central nervous system (CNS) does not equate with EEG arousals or awakenings. CNS activation implies that integrative neurons were activated and sent information to descending pathways, the nucleus tractus solitarius, and sympathetic controlling cells. An ANS modulation is always associated with an efferent response. CNS activation may lead to an arousal, an awakening, or an important ANS activity change, but activation may be limited to a polysynaptic reflex response with ANS change and no EEG arousal (6).

Therefore, using ANS output such as heart rate will lead to a much higher arousal count than what would be seen with a cortical EEG recording. When the many autonomic regulations of NREM and REM sleep are considered, one may again be dubious about the usage of peripheral markers of ANS as indicators of arousals and awakenings (6). One would have to filter the ANS response to use it as an effective marker. Individual differences in ANS responses exist and would probably complicate the matter further. Thus, the term "ANS arousal" is a misnomer and should not be used until further investigations are performed. The term "ANS activation" is currently the only valid one.

### III. Major Sleep Disorders, Arousals, and Consequent Sleep Deprivation

#### A. Periodic Limb Movement Disorder

Periodic limb movement disorder (PLMD), originally described by Symonds as "nocturnal myoclonus" (11), was questioned as being an epileptic equivalent. Lugaresi et al. (12) demonstrated that it was not epileptic in nature and found a close association between it and restless legs syndrome. Guilleminault et al. (13) showed that it may be associated with insomnia, nocturnal sleep disruption, and daytime fatigue. Further studies have shown that periodic limb movements can vary greatly in severity.

As a basic phenomenon, periodic limb movements typically involve a repetitive extension of the big toes that has a 20–40-sec rhythm. It was equated to a Babinski sign (14). It may be associated with the equivalent of a Babinski maneuver and may even involve the upper part of the body. The etiology of PLMD is unknown, and it is unknown whether all types of periodic limb movements have the same cause. Repetitive jerks may lead to repetitive short arousals, and, depending on the time during the night, may lead to prolonged awakenings. The increasing length of the awakenings is related to the decrease in homeostatic pressure (15) when the arousal occurs after 3–4 hr of sleep. These awakenings are compounded by the frustration of being awakened again with progressive development of confounding fear of sleep and nocturnal awakening with secondary conditioning and apprehension. It was demonstrated that many of the leg movements that cause an autonomic activation (indicated by an increase in heart rate) do not induce EEG arousals. The number of periodic limb movements associated with arousals appears to be the important variable for evidence of daytime complaints. These complaints are similar to the ones seen with sleep deprivation. But great variability of complaints is seen from patient to patient with similar frequencies of arousals.

#### B. Restless Legs Syndrome

Restless legs syndrome (RLS) (16) is a dysesthesia that presents an important circadian relationship. It is a sensation, often difficult for patients to describe clearly, equated to "water running under the skin" or "a snake crawling on muscles" that forces the patients to move their limbs. It is usually bilateral and predominantly in the lower limbs, despite the fact that it can occur in both arms and legs. In its principal presentation, it is associated with a normal neurological evaluation, including normal deep tendon reflexes, sensory evaluation, nerve conduction, and electromyogram. It is prominent in the early evening and during the first part of the sleep period and often decreases in the morning. Several members of the same family of different generations are frequently affected, but sporadic cases are also seen (17).

It can be seen alone or in association with periodic limb movements (12). When associated, RLS will be prominent during the first part of the night (18) while periodic limb movements are noted throughout the night. The dysesthesia forces the patients to get up and move. The sleep deprivation varies in severity from difficulty with falling asleep at bedtime due to the abnormal sensations but with no further sleep disruption to several episodes of nocturnal awakenings leading to important sleep deprivation and daytime consequences of sleepiness, fatigue, irritability, depression, and cognitive dysfunction. In very severe cases, suicidal ideation has been seen. The relationship between the degree of nocturnal disturbances and degree of daytime consequences is based on complaints and subjective reports. Very little is documented with objective testing.

Patients with iron deficiency are reported to have greater risk of RLS, and iron supplements may help the syndrome. In most cases, iron and ferritin are normal and iron treatment is ineffective. However, some type of dysfunction of iron usage has been hypothesized, but the supportive evidence is limited (19,20).

Treatment will call upon dopamine agonists, opioid medications, a benzo-diazepine (clonazepam) that increases total sleep time, and drugs most commonly used as antiepileptic medication, such as gabapentin or equivalent. Dopamine agonists are the most effective and reduce the sleep deprivation and the patients' complaints. But not all patients respond to dopamine agonists and methadone has been prescribed in the most refractory cases (21).

## C.  Sleep-Disordered Breathing Syndromes

Objective evaluations of the consequences of the sleep fragmentation are few in number. Most of them have been performed through studies of sleep-disordered breathing (SDB) syndromes: upper airway resistance syndrome (UARS) and obstructive sleep apnea syndrome (OSAS) (22). SDB is associated with repetitive sleep-related occlusion of the airway, mostly at the level of the oropharynx. Reopening of the airway and air exchange is commonly associated with arousal and awakenings. These patients experience significant sleep deprivation from spending more than 50% of their nocturnal sleep with an awake EEG. The day-time consequences are significant and include daytime fatigue, sleepiness, involuntary napping, lapses leading to industrial and driving accidents, and decreased memory and cognitive functioning. Investigations using the Multiple Sleep Latency Test (MSLT) (23) and cognitive testing have confirmed the important impact of this disabling disorder. However, correlations between the number of complete (apnea) and partial (hypopnea) occlusions of the upper airway during sleep and MSLT (or an equivalent test called the Maintenance of Wakefulness Test [MWT]) have been poor (24–27). More studies need to be performed to determine whether it is the cumulative effect of arousals and awakenings associated with SDB that leads to individual differences in daytime consequences.

The upper airway resistance syndrome (UARS) (28) does not lead to complete collapse of the upper airway, but to increased respiratory effort and often nasal flow limitation without a drop in oxygen saturation below 94%. But the abnormal breathing leads to important change in sleep EEG (29). Short EEG arousals may be present but the use of a computerized technique of EEG analysis, spectral analysis on 2–4-sec windows of the EEG, indicates that there is a large overall increase in alpha EEG frequency during the night. The alpha power (amount of alpha frequencies during a given time window compared to other EEG frequencies) is much higher than age- and gender-matched controls (30). Thus, in this syndrome, there are not only visually recognizable EEG arousals and behavioral awakenings that leads to sleep deprivation, but also a change in the underlying EEG frequency distribution. This pattern is not visually recognizable but it impacts the sleep quality and the individual's behavior the following day (29,30).

How to quantify the sleep deprivation related to this very specific change is not determined and UARS is a model of a problem seen with several sleep disorders related to an insomnia complaint, such as fibromyalgia (31). Interestingly, UARS patients frequently emphasize the nocturnal sleep disruption. They complain of poor nocturnal sleep and may develop a secondary apprehension to sleep and a typical insomnia pattern (i.e., difficulty falling asleep, disrupted nocturnal sleep, and early morning awakening) (32). The nocturnal disruption conditions the patient to poor sleep and leads to secondary anxiety at bedtime. The sleep deprivation will lead more to complaints of fatigue, irritability, and decreases in intellectual functioning, than to daytime sleepiness (32,33).

The MSLT has been performed in patients with UARS, and abnormal results have been reported, but the test is often borderline normal, equating well with the complaint of fatigue. No systematic study of cognitive function has been performed in UARS patients, and investigation of mental lapses using tests such as the psychomotor vigilance task (PVT), a reaction-time test, is also lacking. But reevaluation of subjects treated with nasal CPAP demonstrated that sleep efficiency and MSLT scores improve (28).

The sleep disruption associated with SDB thus has an impact on daytime activities. But the impact seems variable in patients with similar severity of disease based on the amount of abnormal breathing or decreases in oxygen saturation. It also seems to be variable with relation to the type of SDB. As visual scoring is often difficult, no valid study on the cumulative amount of sleep loss or the distribution of the sleep loss throughout the night has been conducted on OSAS patients. There are very few studies using EEG spectral analyses, and only one comparing OSAS and UARS subjects (30). The notion that sleep deprivation occurs during sleep with OSAS was well demonstrated in the 1980s (25,26) but no investigations on the degree of the sleep deprivation associated with OSAS have been conducted.

### D. Narcolepsy

Narcolepsy is, by now, a well-described syndrome with daytime sleepiness, the need to take short naps that are usually refreshing, and the very frequent association with auxiliary symptoms, particularly cataplexy (34). This latter symptom is pathognomonic of narcolepsy but sleep paralysis and hypnopompic and hypnagogic hallucinations are not. It is an abrupt weakness, which may be complete, leading to a fall, or partial, limited to head/neck drop, knee buckling, or arm dropping. It is triggered by events evoking an emotional response: laughter, anger, upset, sadness, and so forth (35). Initially the patients, very often teenagers, present with long nocturnal sleep and great difficulty to arise in the morning. These symptoms typically progress over several years of evaluation along with a very clear nocturnal sleep disruption that adds to the daytime sleepiness. The patient typically shows very consistent timing, in which he or she is wide awake 3–4 hr after sleep onset and cannot fall asleep again for up to 60–90 min. These periods of complete awakenings induce a clear reduction of total nocturnal sleep time and nocturnal sleep deprivation (36–38). Patients know their nocturnal wake periods so well that they may plan routine activities or household chores, such as cleaning or ironing. But sleepiness will be very apparent during the daytime. The MSLT is always abnormal, with a mean sleep latency below 8 min (39), and two or more sleep-onset REM sleep periods (SOREMPS) during the five monitored and scheduled daytime naps. An abnormal absence of hypocretin (40) in the cerebrospinal fluid is detected in over 96% of the cases. This absence is related to the destruction or inactivity of the hypocretin cells in the hypothalamus. The amount of nocturnal sleep disruption and sleep deprivation appears to increase slightly over time. Longitudinal data are lacking; all narcoleptics receive treatment for daytime sleepiness and for cataplexy, if frequent. The interaction between the prescribed stimulant medication and the amount of nocturnal sleep disruption is unknown. But when patients are withdrawn from medications during drug holidays, nocturnal sleep disruption persists. Also, narcoleptics may present with periodic limb movements (41) that further disturb their nocturnal sleep and add to their nocturnal sleep deprivation. The nocturnal awakenings are an integral part of the narcolepsy syndrome, and this symptom has not responded to hypnotic medication (i.e., benzodiazepine or equivalents). It is too early to know whether the newly approved treatment for narcolepsy, sodium oxybate, will have an important impact on the nocturnal sleep deprivation. It is, however, the best therapeutic hope at this time.

### E. Insomnias

Insomnias are a cause of sleep deprivation. As indicated, there is no uniform underlying problem related to the report of poor nocturnal sleep. Insomnias have been subdivided based on the timing of lack of sleep: at sleep onset, during the night, or due to early-morning awakening (1). They have also been dissociated as part of a psychiatric syndrome, or independent from a psychiatric symptomatology such as major depressive disorder. The difficulty is that a patient with a psychiatric disorder may also present with a sleep disorder that contributes to the sleep disruption or that may have been the trigger of the psychiatric disorder. Finally, a nocturnal sleep disruption may lead, by its repetitiveness and its daytime impact, to fear of the next night and adverse conditioning toward sleep, with resultant increased anxiety close to sleep onset.

A syndrome resulting in repetitive nocturnal disruption will lead to more or less difficulty with falling asleep again. The preceding amount of sleep influences the ease of returning to sleep. Individuals also more easily return to sleep during the first third of the night owing to sleep pressure related to the homeostatic function of sleep. Factors such as the circadian influence, i.e., the position of the temperature cycle during the 24-hr period, also determine whether patients will have greater or lesser difficulty falling asleep again, and adverse conditioning may occur in the former case. Patients may react to the disruption and fragmentation by advancing their bedtime and delaying their out-of-bed time. They will begin to lose the relationship between their sleep-scheduling behavior, their own sleep/wake rhythm, and their sleep needs. They will develop fear and anxiety traits and will combine poor sleep hygiene, timing, and conditioning. Physicians often forget that what's waking someone up is frequently not what is maintaining wakefulness. The combination of these different factors will lead to sleep deprivation and daytime consequences. The fear of the consequences of the sleep deprivation will lead to requests for pharmacological treatment without appropriate investigation of the primary problem (i.e., what causes the awakenings). A drug dependency may be added to the problem.

The nonpsychiatric chronic insomnias often follow the above schema. In women, two events may be at the beginning of the abnormal conditioning: delivery and breast feeding, and menopause. An infant will build a day-night cycle during the first 6–10 weeks of life. The parent-child interaction, the location of the sleeping infant (cosleeping, bringing the infant inside the parent's bedroom, keeping the infant outside of the parent's bedroom), and the type and frequency of feedings during the night will determine the amount of sleep disruption inflicted by the infant on the mother. There will be sleep deprivation; it is seen in nearly all mothers during the first 3 months of infancy. The severity and duration of the sleep deprivation will vary depending on the mother's anxiety, her ability to set limits early on, her degree of personal gratification with breast feeding and body contact with the infant, her daytime response to her sleep deprivation (napping), the degree of induced circadian disruption, and spousal support during the night. These are some of the factors that will contribute to the conditioning of the mother's (and infant's) nocturnal sleep and sleep deprivation. These factors constitute the background upon which the chronic insomnia will occur.

Menopause is also associated with sleep disruption. Hot flashes and low-grade discomfort that may follow the temperature rhythm may lead to earlier morning awakenings and a reduction in total nocturnal sleep time, with daytime consequences and adverse conditioning resulting in a fear of sleep. The hormonal changes will also uncover mild sleep-disordered breathing with greater nasal congestion and slight enlargement of upper-airway mucosa. This will lead to more significant sleep fragmentation with a greater risk of difficulty falling asleep again in the early morning. A recent study showed that a very large percentage of postmenopausal women presented with mild SDB (42). A second study indicated that conditioning and SDB were involved in the daytime complaints related to the sleep deprivation. Treatment of each component in a random protocol demonstrated that different elements of the complaint were addressed by different treatments and demonstrated well the interaction of different components during the sleep deprivation and daytime consequences due to it (26).

## IV.  Conclusions

Major sleep disorders, independent of whether the dominant complaint is excessive daytime sleepiness or initiating or maintaining sleep, include a sleep deprivation component. Often the reaction to this component will lead to a worsening of abnormal sleep, impacting on sleep hygiene, circadian timing of sleep-wake, and/or conditioning against sleep. This will further worsen the sleep deprivation and daytime complaint. There are still many unknowns in our understanding of the different components leading to sleep deprivation and its daytime consequences. There are clear individual differences in sleep deprivation and further research is needed on all of these aspects.

### References

1.  American Sleep Disorders Association. The International Classification of Sleep Disorders. Rochester, MN: ASDA, 1990.
2.  American Psychiatric Association. Diagnostic and Statistical Manual of Mental Disorders (DSM-IV) 4th. ed Washington DC: American Psychiatric Press, 1994.
3.  American Sleep Disorders Association. EEG arousal: scoring rules and examples: a preliminary report from the Atlas Task Force of the American Sleep Disorders Association. Sleep 1992: 15;173–184.
4.  Pivik RT The several qualities of sleepiness: psychophysiological consideration. In: Monk TH, ed. New York: Wiley, 1991: 3–38.
5.  American Academy of Sleep Medicine Task Force. Sleep related breathing disorders in adults: recommendations for syndrome definition and measurements techniques in clinical research. Sleep 1999; 22:667–689.
6.  Poyares D, Guilleminault C, Rosa A, Ohayon M, Koester U. Arousal, EEG spectral power and pulse transit time in UARS and mild OSAS subjects. Clin Neurophysiol 2002; 113:1598–1606.
7.  Martin SE, Deary IJ, Douglas NJ. The effect of autonomic arousal on daytime function. Am J Respir Crit Care Med 1996; 153A:354.
8.  Guilleminault C, Stoohs R. Arousal, increased respiratory efforts, blood pressure and obstructive sleep apnea. J Sleep Res 1995; 4:s117–s124.

9. Moruzzi G. The physiologic properties of the brain-stem reticular system. In: Adrian ED, Bremmer F, Jasper HH, eds. Brain Mechanisms and Consciousness. Oxford: Blackwell, 1954:21–48.

10. Steriades M, McCarley RW Brainstem Control of Wakefulness and Sleep. New York: Plenum Press, 1990:203–229.

11. Symonds CP. Nocturnal myoclonus. J Neurol Neurosurg Psychiatry 1953; 16:166–171.

12. Lugaresi E, Coccagna G, Berti-Ceroni G. Restless leg syndrome and nocturnal myoclonus. In: Gastaut H, Lugaresi E, Berti-Ceroni, G Coccagna G, eds. The Abnormalities of Sleep in Man. Bologna: Aulo Gaggi,1968:285–294.

13. Guilleminault C, Raynal, D, Weitzman ED, Dement WC. Sleep related periodic myoclonus in patients complaining of insomnia. Trans Am Neurol Assoc 1975; 100:19–22.

14. Smith RC. Relationship of periodic movement in sleep (nocturnal myoclonus) and the Babinski sign. Sleep 1985; 8:239–243.

15. Borbely AA. A two process model of sleep modulation. Hum Neurobiol 1982; 1:195–204.

16. Ekbom KA. Restless legs. Acta Med Scand 1945: supl 158:1–123.

17. Montplaisir J, Boucher S, Poirier G, Lavigne G, Lapierre O, Lesperance P. Clinical polysomnographic and genetic characteristics of restless leg syndrome: a study of 133 patients diagnosed with new standard criteria. Movement Disord 1997; 12:61–65.

18. Trenkwalder C, Hening WA, Walters AS, Campbell SS, Rahman K, Chokroverty S. Circadian rhythm of periodic limb movements and sensory symptoms of restless legs syndrome. Movement Disord 1999; 14:102–110.

19. Sun ER, Chen CA, Ho G, Early CJ, Allen RP. Iron and the restless leg syndrome. Sleep 1998; 21:371–377.

20. Allen RP, Barker PB, Wehrl F, Song HK, Early CJ. MRI measurement of brain iron in patients with restless leg syndrome. Neurology 2001; 56:263–265.

21. American Academy of Sleep Medicine (AASM) Report: Standard of Practice Committee of the AASM: Practice parameters for the treatment of restless leg syndrome and periodic limb movement disorder. Sleep 1999; 22:961–968.

22. Guilleminault C, Black J, Palombini L, Ohayon M. Clinical investigation of obstructive sleep apnea syndrome and upper airway resistance syndrome patients. Sleep Med 2000; 1:51–56.

23. Carskadon MC, Dement WC. The Multiple Sleep Latency Test (MSLT): what does it measure? Sleep1982; 5:s67–s72.

24. Mitler MM, Gujavarty KS, Browman CP. Maintenance of Wakefulness Test: a polysomnographic technique for evaluating treatment efficacy in patients with excessive somnolence. Electroencephalogy Clin Neurophysiol 1982; 53:658–661.

25. Roth T, Hartse KM, Zorick F, Conway W. Multiple naps and evaluation of daytime sleepiness in patients with upper airway sleep apnea. Sleep 1980, 3:425–440.

26. Guilleminault C, Partinen M, Quera-Salva MA, Hayes B, Dement W.C, Nino-Murcia, G. Determinants of daytime sleepiness in obstructive sleep apnea. Chest 1988; 94:32–37.

27. Chervin RD, Kraemer HC, Guilleminault C. Correlates of sleep latency on the multiple sleep latency test in a clinical population. Electroencephalogr Clin Neurophysiol 1995: 95; 147–53.

28. Guilleminault C, Stoohs R, Clerk A, Cetel M, Maistros P. A cause of excessive daytime sleepiness: the upper airway resistance syndrome. Chest 1993; 104:781–787.

29. Black JE, Guilleminault C, Colrain IM, Carillo O. Upper airway resistance syndrome: central EEG power and changes in breathing effort. Am J Respir Crit Care Med 2000; 162:406–411.

30. Guilleminault C, Kim YD, Chowdhuri S, Horita M, Ohayon M Kushida C. Sleep and daytime sleepiness in upper airway resistance syndrome compared to obstructive sleep apnea syndrome. Eur Respir J 2001; 17:1–10.

31. Perlis ME, Giles DE, Bootzin RR, DikmanZV, Fleming GM, Drummond SP, Rose MW. Alpha sleep and information processing, perception of sleep, pain, and arousability in fibromyalgia. Int J Neurosci 1997; 89:265–280.

32. Guilleminault C, Palombini L, Poyares D, Chowdhury S. Chronic insomnia, post menopausal women, and SDB. Part 2. Comparison of non drug treatment trials in normal breathing and UARS post menopausal women complaining of insomnia. J Psychosomat Res 2002; 53:617–623.

33. Gold AR, Dipalo F, Gold MS, O'Hearn D. Symptoms and signs of upper airway resistance syndrome: a link to the functional somatic syndromes. Chest 2003. In press.

34. Guilleminault C, Dement WC, Passouant P, eds. Narcolepsy. New York: Spectrum Publication, 1976:1–689.

35. Guilleminault C, Heinzer R, Mignot E, Black J. Investigations into the neurologic basis of narcolepsy. Neurology 1998; 50(suppl 1):s8–15.

36. Rechtschaffen A, Wolpert E, Dement WC, Mitchell S, Fisher C. Nocturnal sleep of narcoleptics. Electroencephalogr Clin Neurophysiol 1963; 15:599– 609.

37. Montplaisir J, Billiard M, Takahashi S, Bell I, Guilleminault C, Dement WC. Twenty-four hour recordings in REM narcoleptics with special reference to nocturnal sleep disruption. Biol Psychiatr 1978; 13:73–89

38. Broughton R, Mullington J. Chronobiological aspects of narcolepsy. 1994; 17:s-35–s-44.

39. Van den Hoed J, Kraemer H, Guilleminault C, Zarcone V.P, Miles LE, Dement WC, Mitler MM. Disorders of excessive daytime somnolence: polygraphic and clinical data for 100 patients. Sleep 1981; 4:23–37.

40. Nishino S, Ripley B, Overeem S, Lammers GJ, Mignot E. Hypocretin (orexin) deficiency in human narcolepsy. Lancet 2000; 355:39–40.

41. Baker TL, Guilleminault C, Nino-Murcia G, Dement WC. Comparative polysomnographic study of narcolepsy and idiopathic central nervous system hypersomnia. Sleep 1986; 9:232–242.

42. Guilleminault C, Palombini L, Poyares D, Chowdhury S. Chronic insomnia, post menopausal women and sleep disordered breathing (SDB). Part 1. Frequency of SDB in a cohort. J Psychosom Res 2002; 53:611–615.

# 6

## Medical Conditions and Diseases

**NAOMI L. ROGERS**

**University of Pennsylvania School of Medicine, Philadelphia, Pennsylvania, U.S.A.**

**JACQUELINE D. KLOSS**

**Drexel University, Philadelphia, Pennsylvania, U.S.A.**

### I. Overview

Sleep disturbance occurs as a result of a number of medical disorders that at first glance have no direct association with the sleep-wake system. In many of these disorders sleep disturbance presents as a secondary or tertiary symptom, or indirectly as a result of other symptoms of the disorder, e.g., pain, fever. While hypnotic drugs may provide temporary relief from this sleep disturbance, they do not treat the underlying cause of the sleep loss. Treatment of the disorder and its symptoms will likely also produce an improvement in sleep consolidation and sleep quality. One caveat, however, is that many medications produce sleep disruption as an unwanted side effect. Therefore, it is important to consider not only pharmacological treatment of sleep disturbance associated with comorbid and causal medical disorders, but also cognitive and behavioral coping strategies. To better assess the most appropriate treatment regime, it may be useful to utilize a conceptual model for the treatment of non-disorder-specific secondary sleep disturbance.

Medical conditions based in nearly all physiological systems can produce coincident sleep disturbances and sleep deprivation. This includes disorders of the cardiovascular (chronic heart failure), pulmonary (asthma), gastrointestinal (hepatic failure), renal (urinary tract infections, polyuria), endocrine (diabetes, hypothyroidism, hyperthyroidism), and neurological (Parkinson's disease, fibromyalgia, migraine) systems, in addition to allergies, low-grade infections (influenza, common cold, fever), pain (cancer, arthritis), anxiety, and depression. In addition, pharmacological treatment of these disorders may augment sleep disturbance further. Some examples include anticonvulsants, beta-blockers, decongestants, opioids, interleukin-2, stimulants, and paradoxically sedative-hypnotics, if used for chronic periods, or after termination of treatment. In addition, substances such as alcohol, caffeine, and over-the-counter medications (e.g., melatonin) can also negatively affect sleep. Irrespective of the primary medical disorder, treatment of the associated sleep disruption can be addressed on a general level, rather than within the confines of the treatment for the individual disorder.

## II.  Impact of Sleep Deprivation Associated with Medical Conditions and/or Diseases

The effect of sleep loss associated with medical disorders can manifest in several ways. Several studies have reported on the detrimental effects of sleep restriction on neurobehavioral functioning. Following only one night of restricted sleep decreased neurobehavioral performance and increased subjective sleepiness and sleep propensity have been reported (1). When the number of nights of sleep restriction is extended beyond one, cumulative decrements in neurobehavioral functioning (2,3) and increased daytime sleepiness levels are evident (4).

Associated with sleep-loss-induced decreases in neurobehavioral functioning is an increased risk of and increased incidence of accidents. On-the-job and motor vehicle accidents have both been found to increase when individuals are sleep deprived. Although data are not consistently collected, it has been estimated that between 20% and 60% of single-vehicle motor accidents may be attributed to fatigue from sleep loss. While this includes sleep loss associated with working shiftwork and voluntary sleep loss, many of the individuals may experience sleep loss due to sleep and other medical disorders. Although the symptom of sleep disturbance with medical disorders is often recognized, the potential safety and public health impact may be overlooked.

Sleep deprivation has a significant impact on the optimal functioning of the immune system. Following one night of partial sleep deprivation, a decrease in natural killer (NK) cell activity, NK activity per number of NK cells, lymphokine-activated killer (LAK) cell activity, LAK activity per number of LAK cells, responsiveness to mitogen stimulation (5,6), and decreased IL-6 levels (7) have been reported. These findings suggest an attenuation of natural immune responses to challenge. An inability to adequately respond to immune challenges, especially in individuals already immunocompromised, can put individuals at greater risk for opportunistic infections, and have a detrimental effect on coping with primary medical disorders.

### III. Sleep Disturbance in a Selection of Medical Disorders

#### A. Neuromuscular-based Disorders

*Fibromyalgia*

Fibromyalgia (FM) is a rheumatoid syndrome of unknown etiology that is characterized by chronic musculoskeletal pain and generalized muscular tenderness (8). Approximately 2% of Americans, mostly women, are diagnosed with FM (9) and suffer chronically not only from pain, but also from fatigue, sleep disruption, and depressed mood (8,10,11). Given the extent to which these symptoms can negatively affect quality of life, it is disconcerting that the pathophysiology of FM is not clearly understood. Thus, understanding the interplay between sleep and the other symptoms of this disorder is of increasing theoretical import and clinical relevance.

Approximately 70–80% of individuals with FM complain of unrefreshing or non-restorative sleep (12,13), or describe themselves as "light sleepers." Their "light" sleep is often characterized by symptoms of insomnia, such as difficulty initiating and maintaining sleep, characterized by intermittent awakenings, and early-morning awakening (14). Not surprisingly, the daytime sequelae of sleep disruption in patients with FM are marked by morning stiffness, fatigue, cognitive impairment, and decreased mood (reviewed in Ref. 11,15). Clarifying the relationship between pain and sleep, albeit complex and somewhat controversial, becomes one pivotal means to direct treatment efforts. Ultimately this could help patients manage this debilitating syndrome and potentially further our understanding of the underlying etiology of FM.

Sleep in Fibromyalgia

A number of alterations in sleep architecture have been reported in individuals suffering from FM. Polysomonographic studies have revealed increased latencies to sleep onset (16,17), increased stage 1 sleep (17,18), an increased number of arousals (16,17,19), decreased sleep efficiency (20), and decreased amount of slow-wave sleep (SWS) (16,17). There is also evidence of a decrease in the percentage of REM sleep (17) and increased restless leg movements (20). The most striking pattern that has been identified among FM patients is an alpha-delta EEG activity pattern (17,18,21–23). The alpha-delta pattern, first identified in FM patients by Moldfosky et al., is characterized by alpha EEG waves present during NREM sleep. In addition, Drewes et al. (22) noted that low-frequency bands, which are typically associated with refreshing, good sleep quality, were diminished among FM patients. Taken together, these findings may account for the subjective experience of unrefreshing sleep among FM patients.

Not only may this EEG pattern be indicative of nonrestorative sleep, it may also be related to pain sensations. Three of six healthy, non-FM subjects underwent a sleep deprivation induction trial marked by the presentation of auditory stimuli during delta sleep (24). As a result, they experienced greater muscular tenderness at night and musculoskeletal pain (24). While this effect reversed following a refreshing night of sleep, this phenomenon supports a relationship between delta sleep and/or arousals with pain. Alpha-delta pattern has also been shown to correlate not only with pain at night, but also with daytime pain, energy, and mood levels (25) as well as the subjective experience of unrefreshing and disrupted sleep (26). In addition, Roizenblatt et al. (27) characterized specific alpha patterns of FM patients and demonstrated that the phasic alpha pattern, compared to the tonic and low alpha patterns, occurred most frequently among patients with FM and was most strongly correlated with pain symptoms, reports of morning pain/stiffness, and reports of nonrefreshing sleep. Despite this consistent pattern of alpha-EEG in FM patients, it is important to note that this phenomenon is not exclusively found in patients with FM; other patients with diagnoses such as rheumatoid arthritis, osteoarthritis, as well as other psychiatric conditions and chronic fatigue syndrome share this pattern (28). Consequently, the alpha-delta pattern may be a marker of pain-related disorders.

In a study examining pulmonary function, Sergi et al. (29) reported an increased incidence of periodic breathing in FM patients relative to normal controls, due to decreased transfer factors for carbon monoxide. The authors conclude that this may account for the daytime sequelae of FM patients, as opposed to the changes in sleep architecture reported above.

Further sleep disturbance in FM may be related to increased incidence of periodic limb movements in sleep, restless legs syndrome, or the presence of comorbid depression. Consequently, given that a number of factors contribute to the sleep disturbance in FM, it would appear prudent to undertake a multifactorial approach to best understand sleep complaints and daytime symptoms of FM patients. Consistent with this notion, the interaction between psychological variables, such as cognitive appraisals of pain and sleep, as well as emotional reactions ought to be more carefully examined to best understand this complex syndrome.

## Pathophysiology

*The Interplay of Pain and Sleep.*    As indicated earlier, disrupted or abnormal sleep patterns may represent a causal mechanism that contributes to the constellation of symptoms of the FM syndrome. That is, disrupted sleep leads to feelings of fatigue, increased pain or tenderness, or mood difficulties. While the notion that sleep affects pain is one viable pathway and potentially represents an underlying pathology, the alternative hypothesis is also convincing—i.e., pain symptoms can lead to disrupted sleep. Based on reports of sleep quality and pain intensity among female patients with FM, it appears that women complain of more pain following a poor night of sleep. Furthermore, women also report worsened sleep quality on nights following a day with high pain ratings (30). Thus, pain may get worse after a night of poor sleep and similarly worsen one's nighttime sleep quality. Given the degree to which FM individuals suffer from aches and pain, merely getting comfortable to fall asleep can be a challenge (11). Not only do patients suffer from the discomfort of their pain that makes it difficult for them to fall asleep or achieve refreshing sleep at night, they also are challenged by their already impaired daytime functioning due to the pain, which is worsened by the sequelae of disrupted sleep. Thus, the relationship between sleep and pain appears to be both bidirectional (31) and potentially synergistic: pain exacerbates sleep, and sleep can then exacerbate pain, representing a "vicious cycle" phenomena.

*Neurochemical and Neurobiological Processes.* The neurochemical processes that lead to altered sleep patterns have not been clearly delineated. As reviewed by Harding (15), low levels of cerebrospinal fluid (CSF), increased levels of Substance P, decreased growth hormone (GH), and reduced levels of serotonin are hypothesized to be responsible for some sleep abnormalities. Decreased serotonin may be related to decreases in delta sleep and may possibly account for the alpha-delta architecture. An intimate link between pain, mood, and sleep is apparent (32,33). Serotonin is one common denominator in each of these processes, and is one candidate that may explain the underlying pathophysiology. Research on the beneficial effects of antidepressants (reviewed below) also provides support for this notion. In addition, decreases in GH secretions have been implicated in the FM-associated sleep disturbances. To illustrate, Landis et al. (34) compared FM women to normal healthy controls on growth hormone and prolactin (PRL). Both these hormones were decreased in the FM patients compared to the controls. Their findings suggest neurohormonal dysregulation may also be one underlying pathophysiology of disturbed sleep among FM patients. Because of the degree of symptom overlap between individuals with FM and individuals with desynchronized circadian rhythms, disruption of the circadian system has also been hypothesized as one potential pathophysiological mechanism (35). However, no differences in circadian timing emerged between the women with FM and healthy female controls (35).

## Treatment

In general, the etiology of the syndrome of FM itself is not well established (36) and, at times, is controversial. Given the ambiguity around the pathophysiology of FM, clinical decision making is often a challenge. Rheumatoid specialists, primary-care providers, sleep specialists, and mental health providers are all likely to be confronted with patients with FM who present with a primary sleep complaint. Pharmacotherapies, physical therapies, and to some extent behavioral therapies offer promising means to manage the persistent symptoms associated with FM.

*Pharmacotherapy.* Despite the ambiguity around FM, antidepressants are a reasonable pharmacological candidate for treating FM for the following reasons: (a) depression is thought to mediate depressive symptoms; (b) as noted above, serotonin may underlie the pathophysiology of FM; and (c) tricyclic antidepressants tend to be efficacious in treating pain (39). Data from meta-analytic and review studies (37–40) suggest that tricyclics are likely to be most efficacious, whereas selective serotonin reuptake inhibitors (SSRIs) are not as robust. Tricyclics are likely to primarily improve sleep, and also reduce tenderness and stiffness. The degree to which antidepressants benefit FM has not been thoroughly studied and needs to be more carefully examined. One of the difficulties in determining the role of SSRIs in reducing FM complaints via mediating depression is that subtherapeutic doses, which may help pain, but may be ineffective for treating depression, have been used. Authors emphasize the need for double-blind, placebo-controlled, randomized trials, using therapeutic doses of antidepressants, and also examine the relationship between depression and FM. Using SSRIs to augment the effects of tricyclics should also be considered and researched more thoroughly (40).

Citera et al. (41) conducted a pilot investigation of melatonin administration to FM patients over a 4-week trial. Median values of tender point count pain severity, subjective sleep measures, using visual analog scales, and global assessment ratings by both patients and physicians were significantly improved, whereas there was a trend for other pain ratings and fatigue to be decreased. While the authors stress that randomized double-blind, placebo-controlled trials are warranted, this preliminary study provides encouraging data on the use of melatonin in FM patients.

In general, other pain-relieving medications and sleep agents are not encouraging. For example, the use of corticosteroids and nonsteroidal anti-inflammatory drugs (NSAIDS) has not been supported (reviewed in Ref. 38). Sedatives are contraindicated because of their high addictive potential and are unlikely to substantially reduce pain. Short-term administration of newer, shorter-acting sedative compounds may provide better outcomes. However, the long-term use and efficacy of hypnotic/sedative medications is questionable.

*Physical Therapies.*   In a review by Offenbacher and Stucki (42), a number of physical therapies reviewed were demonstrated to significantly reduce symptoms of fibromyalgia, such as pain, fatigue, and sleep. Such therapies, including cardiovascular fitness training, acupuncture, biofeedback, cryotherapy, and trigger point injection, may each have differential efficacies on various pain variables. While no single therapy is likely to be completely efficacious in relieving all symptoms significantly, the authors encourage a multidisciplinary approach where a combination of treatments are employed to tailor symptom relief to the specific needs of the patient.

Perhaps the role of cognitive-behavioral treatments ought to be tested, as both depression and chronic pain tend to be responsive to cognitive and behavioral interventions. To our knowledge, very few, if any, treatments have studied the combined effects of pharmacotherapy and behavioral or physical therapies. Given the complex nature of FM, a multifactorial approach may be the most effective (40) and an important area to explore with more scientific rigor.

## B. Neurological-based Disorders

*Chronic Fatigue Syndrome*

Chronic Fatigue Syndrome (CFS) is a condition of unknown etiology character-ized by fatigue that persists for more than 6 months (43) and presents with sev-eral of the following symptoms: impaired memory or concentration, pharyngitis, tender lymph nodes, muscle pain or joint pain, new headache patterns, non-restorative sleep, and malaise after physical exertion that extends beyond 24 hr. One distinguishing feature of clinical significance is that fatigue severity and malaise following physical exertion predict long-term fatigue (44). The diagnosis of CFS can be made when psychiatric conditions, substance abuse, or sleep dis-orders associated with excessive daytime sleepiness or fatigue, e.g., apnea or nar-colepsy, have been excluded.

### Chronic Fatigue Syndrome and Sleep Disturbance

Given that fatigue is the hallmark symptom of CFS, it is imperative that we exam-ine sleep to clarify its role in the pathophysiology and course of the syndrome. Patients complain of being exhausted, with an estimated 60% of patients report-ing disrupted sleep (45). Specifically, patients experience nonrestorative or unre-freshing sleep. In a study by Morriss et al. (46), sleep continuity was studied in the context of depressed mood, fatigue, and disability among CFS patients. The presence of a psychiatric condition did not appear to underlie the sleep com-plaints among patients with CFS. Difficulty with sleep continuity was a primary complaint, in contrast to sleep onset or early-morning awakening. Moreover, complaints of periodic limb movements (PLMS) were more common among CFS patients compared to healthy controls; however, these two groups did not com-plain differentially of obstructive sleep apnea syndrome symptoms. In addition, sleep continuity was correlated with daytime functional impairment. Thus, sleep disruption may represent an underlying pathophysiology or it may help us under-stand the pathophysiology or course of CFS. Comorbid psychiatric conditions also need to be carefully examined to determine the relative contributions of these factors and sleep in understanding the pathophysiology, onset, or course of CFS.

Polysomnographic data are limited to a few studies, but these data reveal anomalies in both sleep architecture and sleep continuity. Approximately 60% of patients' polysomnograms reveal the presence of a sleep disorder or clinically sig-nificant sleep abnormality (47). Similar to that experienced among patients with FM, patients with CFS also demonstrate increased alpha-EEG patterns during NREM sleep (48). In addition to alpha-EEG patterns, individuals with CFS also commonly demonstrate diminished sleep efficiency and reduced time in REM sleep (14,47–50). In another polysomnographic study, sleep maintenance diffi-culties were evident and correlated with CFS disability (51). The latter finding was further supported by a subsequent study, of subjective reports, that also sug-gested that sleep continuity was related to functional disability among CFS patients (46).

Pathophysiology

An identifiable cause for CFS has not yet been clearly identified. A variety of factors have been implicated, including viral infections, immune dysfunction, psychiatric conditions, allergic reactions, as well as dysfunction of the neuroendocrine, central nervous, and muscular systems. Although genetic vulnerabilities for fatigue were identified in one study (52), another study comparing monozygotic twins discordant for CFS did not find immune irregularities. Because sleep disruption is associated with each of the aforementioned conditions and with the hallmark symptom of fatigue, sleep disruption itself has been posed as the causative factor of chronic fatigue syndrome. As discussed in the fibromyalgia section, disrupted sleep lowers pain threshold the following day, even in healthy subjects. Sleep disruption has been associated with decreased pain threshold and increased levels of substance P—supporting the hypothesis that sleep disruption may play a role in the manifestation of CFS. However, it would be erroneous to conclude that sleep disruption is the sole etiological component responsible for fatigue and other symptomatology associated with the course of CFS.

Despite the high incidence of sleep disruption associated with CFS, not all patients report this symptom. A direct relationship between nocturnal sleep disruption and daytime fatigue is not well defined. Morris et al. (46) reported that only 20% of patients reporting fatigue associated this with disruption or discontinuity of their sleep. This is further strengthened by the observation that a sleep "fingerprint" or profile of sleep disruption unique to CFS has not been clearly demarcated (31). Despite these observations, subjective complaints of sleep disturbance serve as a marker of symptom relapse. For these reasons it is difficult to classify sleep disruption as the primary underlying pathophysiology of CFS. Nonetheless, changes in sleep patterns may still provide some insight into underlying pathophysiologies or potential etiologies of CFS. It appears evident that sleep is likely to play an integral role in the course of CFS, and the examination of sleep among CFS patients will likely lead to a better understanding of both its manifestation and treatment.

One way of understanding the relationship between sleep and CFS is through the immune system. While the evidence for a link between these variables is growing, the complexity of this relationship needs further investigation. Indeed it is well established that sleep deprivation leads to altered immune markers (reviewed in Refs. 53,54). These alterations may be mediated by neuroendocrine changes or be a direct result of sleep loss. Alternatively, sleep disruption may be a consequence of an underlying pathophysiological mechanism, for example an immune or infectious anomaly. To illustrate, allergic rhinitis is common in individuals with CFS and is known to disrupt sleep (reviewed in Ref. 55). Fatigue therefore may be secondary to such an immune reaction. More specific examinations may include the study of cytokine activity during immune dysregulation. It has been theorized that cytokines may play a role in the increased fatigue and sleepiness experienced by CFS patients (53,56).

One further factor that is known to interact with both immune and sleep-wake behavior is the neuroendocrine system. It has been suggested that down-regulation of the HPA axis may produce some of the pathophysiology of CFS. For example, an increase in nonspecific immune response has been reported in CFS patients (56). Cortisol is recognized to inhibit immune responses (e.g., Refs. 57–59); therefore a reduction in circulating cortisol would likely augment any immune responses occurring in these patients. In addition, a reduction in cortisol levels, for example in Addison's disease, is associated with increased fatigue levels (60), and both diseases are associated with an increased incidence of sleep disruption and mood disturbance (61). An increase in symptoms has been reported in CFS patients following experimental challenge tests, and also following non-experimental periods of emotional and physical stress, all of which are known to involve the HPA axis (reviewed in Refs. 62,63). It would appear reasonable, therefore, that inclusion of the neuroendocrine system with the immune system, in particular the HPA axis, in the assessment of CFS pathophysiology is essential.

Psychological factors (mood, behavior, and cognition) may also play a pivotal role in the course of CFS and the degree to which individuals experience impairment. For example, information-processing speed can be influenced by the somatic expression and attention to bodily sensations (64). Likewise, stress and immune function are likely to interact. For example, Cohen et al. (65) found an increase in colds among individuals who are stressed, and Wessely et al. (63) reported an exacerbation of CFS symptoms subsequent to stress. Again, this highlights the interplay between neuroendocrine and immune systems. Given the overlap between psychiatric symptoms and sleep disturbance, it is important to identify whether sleep continuity might be accounted for by depression. At least in one study (46), psychiatric difficulties, such as anxiety and depression, did not appear to be associated with worsened sleep continuity and quality in CFS patients. What Morriss et al. (46) did find, however, is that lifestyle factors may contribute to sleep continuity, and they hypothesize that sleep quality is likely to be accounted for by these factors, or fundamental to the manifestation of CFS itself. The role of depression, lifestyle factors, and cognitive factors requires further examination and should be accounted for and controlled for in future studies. Nonetheless, these findings highlight the significance of attending to psychological factors to better understand the mechanisms, potential interventions, and course of illness among CFS patients.

## CFS and FM

It is noteworthy to acknowledge the significant overlap between CFS and FM. Although these conditions have distinguishing features, patients with FM or CFS are both likely to suffer from and share many common manifestations of their conditions. Indeed many patients would meet criteria for both conditions. The study of the comorbidity from those who meet criteria for both CFS and FM may provide insight into the nature of each or both of these conditions. Given the degree of functional impairment it is imperative to evaluate the underlying pathophysiology, comorbid psychiatric conditions, and physical and neurocognitive impairment associated with these related conditions (66).

## Treatment

The objective of most therapies for CFS is aimed at helping patients cope with and manage symptoms, rather than providing a cure. Both cognitive-behavioral and pharmacological treatments, possibly in combination, are recommended (55). Behavioral strategies aimed at proper sleep hygiene, exercise, and nutrition, coupled with increasing adaptive thinking and enhancing one's cognitive coping styles, are emphasized. In addition, low-dose antidepressants and/or SSRIs may be tried. In Craig and Kakumanu's (55) review of treatments for CFS, tricyclic antidepressants were recommended to increase NREM sleep and reduce pain symptoms. Similar to the findings with FM patients, data supporting the usefulness of SSRIs for patients with CFS are limited at best (67). Preliminary evidence for nicotinamide-adenine dinucleotide (NADH) (68) and low-dose hydrocortisone (69) is also encouraging.

### Neurodegenerative Disorders: Parkinson's Disease and Related Disorders

Parkinsonism is the collective name for a group of disorders that share similar clinical characteristics, including tremor, rigidity of the limbs or trunk, bradykinesia, and postural instability. The most well known of these disorders is Parkinson's disease, which was first described in 1817 by James Parkinson in Essay on the Shaking Palsy (70). Parkinson's disease is also known as primary or idiopathic Parkinson's disease.

Other Parkinson's like disorders include: essential tremor, progressive supranuclear palsy, multisystem atrophy (including Shy-Drager, striatonigral degeneration, and olivopontocerebellar atrophy), Parkinson disease-amyotrophic lateral sclerosis of Guam, postencephalitic parkinsonism, drug- (in some cases reversible) or toxin-induced parkinsonism, arteriosclerotic parkinsonism, and Parkinson's co-occurring with other conditions, such as Alzheimer's disease, Creutzfeldt-Jakob disease, Huntington's disease, Wilson's disease, and Hallervorden-Spatz syndrome. Many of the other parkinsonism disorders strongly resemble Parkinson's disease, and initially may be mistakenly diagnosed as Parkinson's. Examination of the brains of individuals postmortem reveal the presence of Lewy bodies in patients suffering from Parkinson's, and the absence of Lewy bodies in all other disorders. In life, a lack of response to L-dopa treatment is the best means of distinguishing between Parkinson's and the other disorders.

Idiopathic Parkinson's, or Parkinson's, is a chronic and progressive disorder of the central nervous system, especially the motor control regions of the central nervous system. It is characterized by difficulty in initiating voluntary movements, decreased spontaneous movements, slowness of movements, muscular rigidity of the limbs and trunk, postural instability (especially an inability to maintain an upright position while standing or walking), bradykinesia, and tremor. It results from a loss of neurons in the substantia nigra, producing a decrease in the neurotransmitter dopamine. Treatment of Parkinson's disease typically involves pharmacological "replacement" of dopamine via administration of dopamine agonists, which are able to cross the blood-brain barrier and act directly on central dopamine receptors.

Parkinson's disease is primarily a disease of older age, with a reported incidence of between 0.6% and 0.9% in individuals aged 65–69 years and 2.6%-5% in individuals aged over 80 years (71,72). The peak age of onset for Parkinson's disease appears to be 60 years. There appears to be, however, an increasing incidence of early-onset Parkinson's disease, with approximately 10% of Parkinson's patients less than 40 years of age. Parkinson's disease is reported to affect a greater proportion of men than women (73,74).

It is thought that Parkinson's is primarily due to exposure to environmental toxins that results in accelerated cell death of the dopaminergic neurons in the substantia nigra. This theory was supported by the discovery that the chemical 1-methyl-4-phenyl-1,2,3,4-tetrahydropyridine (MPTP) produces Parkinsonian-like symptoms (75,76). MPTP enters the brain and causes the cell death of midbrain dopaminergic neurons that project to the basal ganglia. This results in symptoms akin to Parkinson's disease, including partial or complete paralysis, tremors, and abnormal postures, which degenerate across time. This compound is now used experimentally in animals to study progression of and treatments for Parkinson's disease.

Several studies have identified a genetic link in cases of familial Parkinson's disease, in a number of different families (77–85). A genetic mutation in the Parkin gene is responsible for the onset of disease in these families, with the typical degeneration of the substantia nigra and occurrence of Lewy bodies. In individuals with Parkinson's disease due to this genetic mutation, the average age of onset is between 35 and 40 years old (reviewed in Ref. 86).

Early symptoms of Parkinson's disease are subtle, occur gradually, and are not directly attributable to Parkinson's specifically. These early symptoms include increased tiredness and fatigue, difficulty in rising from chairs, feeling irritable or depressed for no apparent reason, losing track of thoughts and words, and shakiness. The primary symptoms of Parkinson's, which include rigidity, tremor, bradykinesia, and postural instability, are the result of specific impairment of the nervous system, in the motor control regions. The primary symptoms of Parkinson's disease occur as a result of the loss of dopamine from neurons in the substantia nigra and striatum. Neurons in the nigrostriatal tract are responsible for initiation and control of voluntary movements. These symptoms typically do not appear until a reduction of approximately 80% of the dopamine occurs in these regions (87). As dopamine continues to decrease over time, the rate of decline in and intensity of these symptoms will increase, and vary significantly from person to person.

Although many associate Parkinson's disease with tremor, this is the least common symptom. It typically occurs in only one hand or on only one side of the body, and is apparent when the patient is resting or under stressful conditions. Rigidity of the limbs or trunk is the most common symptom of Parkinson's disease, particularly in the early stages. This rigidity appears similar to arthritis with a stiffness of the joints, and patients have trouble with simple activities such as turning around, rising from chairs, fastening buttons. Bradykinesia, i.e., slowness or incompleteness of movement, is another common symptom of Parkinson's. Patients find walking an effort, having trouble initiating and maintaining movement. This symptom is probably the most disabling for Parkinson's patients. Postural instability describes an inability of Parkinson's patients to adjust the position of their body or limbs without conscious thought; for example, if they trip they are unable to reflexively prevent themselves from falling. A consequence of this instability is unsteadiness, and impaired balance and coordination, with patients often displaying a forward or backward lean with a stooped posture. In addition, walking style is often affected, with either a tendency to take quick, small steps, or a halting walk, with patients "freezing" while walking.

In addition to these primary symptoms, Parkinson's is associated with a large number of secondary symptoms that result from interactions between two or more primary symptoms. Secondary symptoms may include: lack of facial expression, altered posture, difficulty in maintaining balance and walking, light-headedness on standing, depression, anxiety, emotional changes, including increased fear, decreased motivation, memory loss, slowed thinking, and increased pessimism, dementia, cognitive impairment separate from dementia, symptoms relating to impairment of the autonomic nervous system, such as blood pressure, gut motility, and bladder function, constipation, difficulty swallowing and chewing, drooling, oily skin, increased sweating, difficulty with speech and handwriting, sexual dysfunction, and sleep disturbance with excessive daytime sleepiness.

## Comorbid Disorders

It is relatively common for individuals with Parkinson's disease to also have a number of comorbid disorders, including a number of sleep disorders, such as restless legs syndrome (RLS), PLMS, REM sleep behavior disorder, parasomnias (e.g., sleepwalking and sleep talking, circadian disruption). Approximately 30% of Parkinson's patients also have PLMS, which in some cases may be related to L-dopa therapy. This proportion tends to increase in patients aged 65 and older. Sleep-disordered breathing is more common in Parkinson's patients compared to age-matched controls. This increased incidence may be due to impaired respiratory muscle function due to muscle rigidity or impairment of the central control of breathing. Patients with autonomic dysfunction typically show increased occurrence of sleep-disordered breathing.

Sleep disturbance secondary to other disorders is common in Parkinson's. One common symptom associated with Parkinson's disease is dementia (88,89).

As a result, there is increased sleep disruption, excessive daytime sleepiness, inversion of sleep-wake rhythm, and sleep-wake schedule disturbance in many Parkinson's patients due to dementia. A large proportion (between 30 and 70%) of Parkinson's patients also experience depression (90,91). This depression may be independent of the Parkinson's part of the Parkinson's disease. In approximately 20% of Parkinson's patients, the Parkinson's-associated or endogenous depression is evident prior to the recognition of the motor-related primary symptoms of the disease. This endogenous depression is typically associated with feelings of hopelessness, pessimism, guilt, and remorse, and is not related to age of the patient, duration, or severity of disease. Depression is associated with sleep disturbance, including altered timing of REM sleep and early-morning awakening.

### Treatment of Parkinson's Disease

Neuronal input to the nigrostriatal tract is normally balanced between dopaminergic (inhibitory) and cholinergic (excitatory). Since dopaminergic neurons are lost in Parkinson's disease, many of the pharmacological therapies are aimed at augmenting dopamine levels in these areas. In addition, administration of anticholinergic compounds to inhibit cholinergic input and restore balance between the two systems may also be utilized (92).

The primary pharmacological treatment for Parkinson's disease is levodopa or L-dopa—short for levodihydroxyphenylalanine. This drug is the immediate precursor to dopamine, and, once it has crossed the blood-brain barrier, it enters cells of the substantia nigra where it is converted into dopamine and stored until released. Dopamine in the periphery cannot cross the blood-brain barrier.

L-dopa is effective in reducing essentially all Parkinsonian symptoms in approximately 80% of patients (92). In particular, the symptoms that are mitigated by L-dopa include bradykinesia, rigidity, resting tremor, difficulty walking, and microphagia. In addition, L-dopa therapy may reverse the Parkinson's-induced mood changes associated with the disease, resulting in an increased sense of well-being. L-dopa does not provide relief from the postural instability, action tremor, or difficulty swallowing. Treatment with L-dopa may also increase the severity of dementia when present, and is associated with nausea, vomiting, decreased blood pressure, increased involuntary movements, and restlessness.

Carbidopa is often coadministered with L-dopa to reduce the amount of L-dopa converted to dopamine in the periphery. Carbidopa thereby increases L-dopa's effectiveness and reduces its associated side effects, including nausea, vomiting, and loss of appetite. This compound blocks the action of the enzyme dopa-decarboxylase, which converts L-dopa into dopamine. Controlled-release Sinemet is a combination of L-dopa and carbidopa, with an extended half-life of immediate-acting combination products, producing an increased duration of effect. A combination of immediate-acting and controlled-release L-dopa and carbidopa is often used. In a number of patients, administration of the controlled-release pill only results in an insufficient conversion of central dopamine (93). The most common side effects associated with the administration of L-dopa/carbidopa medications include nausea, insomnia, abdominal pain, dyskinesia, headache, and depression (93).

Although L-dopa can increase dopamine levels in the brain, its effectiveness decreases across time, such that larger and more frequent doses are required for it to be effective. In addition, after only 2–5 years of L-dopa treatment, its duration of effect is reduced. Chronic administration of L-dopa has been reported to produce psychiatric symptoms, such as paranoia, mania, anxiety, depression, hallucinations as well as increased incidence of insomnia and nightmares (92). It is not clear whether these symptoms are associated with chronic L-dopa therapy or disease course, since the two are temporally related (94). Chronic L-dopa therapy may also produce a state where patients' response to administration fluctuates, such that they experience an on/off phenomena of L-dopa's effects. Additional symptoms of dyskinesias, e.g., involuntary twisting and writhing, are associated with this on/off phenomenon. Consequently, treatment with L-dopa is typically delayed until other treatments are no longer effective.

To reduce the impact of this on/off effect associated with prolonged L-dopa treatment, dopamine agonists, e.g., ropinirole, peroglide, may be prescribed. Dopamine agonists have a longer half-life than L-dopa; however, they may cause hallucinations and confusion with increasing age. Alternate drugs used in the treatment of Parkinsonian symptoms include anticholinergic compounds, monoamine oxidase-B (MAO-B) inhibitors, catechol-*O*-methyl transferase (COMT) inhibitors, and amantadine (originally developed as an antiviral medication), and are often administered as the disease and symptoms progress.

Prior to the discovery of the relationship between dopamine degradation and development of L-dopa, anticholinergic drugs were the most effective drugs to treat Parkinson's disease. These drugs are currently administered in patients who do not respond to dopaminergic-augmenting drugs, and may be administered in synergy with dopaminergic drugs; however, they can reduce the absorption of L-dopa, thereby reducing the efficacy of this drug. Although administration of anticholinergic drugs, or in some cases antihistaminergic drugs with anticholinergic properties, decreases tremor and drooling, they are also associated with increased sleepiness, dry mouth, blurred vision, constipation, mental confusion, and delirium, in particular with increasing age.

In the central nervous system, monoamine oxidase-B (MAO-B) is responsible for metabolizing dopamine in the synaptic cleft. Inhibition of the action of MAO-B reduces the rate of dopamine metabolism, thereby increasing the concentration in the cleft and prolonging the duration of effect (95). In addition to reducing the symptoms of Parkinson's disease, MAO-B inhibitors, such as selegiline, may also decrease the speed of disease progression (96). Administration of selegiline has been reported to decrease the need for L-dopa therapy (97), with research demonstrating that combination treatment with L-dopa and selegiline produces a reduction in the development of Parkinson's (98,99). A failure to reduce the dose of L-dopa during selegiline treatment can result in dyskinesia, insomnia, hallucinations, and orthostatic hypotension (96,100). Side effects directly attributable to selegiline include insomnia, fatigue, nausea, dizziness, constipation, and headache. COMT inhibitors are administered in combination with L-dopa to reduce the amount of L-dopa converted to the inactive metabolite 3-$O$-methyl-dopa in the periphery by catechol-$O$-methyl-transferase (COMT) (101). Possible side effects associated with COMT inhibitors include increased sleep disorders, gastrointestinal effects—including nausea, vomiting and diarrhea—and increased symptoms associated with elevated dopamine levels—dyskinesia, orthostatic hypotension, and hallucinations. Amantadine reduces dyskinesias, and is thought to stimulate the release of dopamine from intact dopaminergic neurons.

Treatment of Parkinson's does not necessarily improve sleep. In addition to the dopaminergic cells in the substantia nigra being lost in Parkinson's, other nondopaminergic nerve cells are destroyed. The loss of these nondopaminergic nerve cells may underlie some of the symptoms associated with Parkinson's, which may explain why treatment with dopaminergic drugs does not alleviate all the symptoms of Parkinson's disease.

### Sleep Disturbance Associated with Parkinson's Disease

Comorbid sleep problems are common in patients with Parkinson's disease (102–105), including difficulties in both initiating and maintaining sleep (105–107), excessive daytime sleepiness (104,105,108,109), and daytime naps (104,107). These sleep disturbances are primarily due to nocturnal vocalizations, nocturnal rigidity (resulting in difficulty in getting out of and returning to bed for bathroom visits, which occur with increased frequency, and difficulty in turning over in bed), hypokinesia, disruption of brain areas related to sleep regulation, depression, and pain (reviewed in Ref. 110). Further sleep disturbances include alterations in sleep architecture, respiratory disturbance, increased motor activity during sleep, and comorbid depression. One of the diagnostic and treatment challenges is differentiating whether the sleep disturbances are a direct result of Parkinson's disease per se or an adverse effect of pharmacotherapy.

It has been reported that the severity of waking motor symptoms is correlated with sleep-related events, including nightmares, sleepwalking, and excessive sweating during sleep, while the severity of Parkinson's-associated depression is correlated with difficulty in initiating and maintaining sleep (111). Consequently, in addition to the increased level of sleep disturbance associated with disease severity, an increase in excessive daytime sleepiness associated with disease severity has been reported (105,112).

Excessive daytime sleepiness is found in approximately 15% of Parkinson's patients (104). This is compared with an incidence of approximately 1% in the general population. Excessive daytime sleepiness is typically associated with the anti-Parkinson's medication being taken, such as L-dopa (113). The occurrence of daytime sleep attacks is not commonly associated with Parkinson's disease, but their incidence increases in association with administration of dopaminergic medications (104,113).

*Sleep Architecture.* Early studies in untreated and treated Parkinson's patients demonstrated significant alterations in sleep architecture that were typically of greater magnitude than those associated with healthy aging. These alterations include increased sleep latency and increased wake after sleep onset (WASO)—in both frequency and duration—and alterations in stage 1, slow-wave, and REM sleep (114–118). A relationship between the severity of daytime symptoms and difficulties in initiating and maintaining sleep has been reported (111,119). In addition, a relationship between the degree of daytime sleepiness and duration and severity of disease has been reported (120).

Several alterations in sleep architecture are associated with Parkinson's disease. A reduction in the amount of slow-wave and REM sleep has been reported by a number of authors (114,118), in addition to increased amounts of stage 1 sleep (114). Increased duration of stage 1 sleep and an increased number of awakenings have also been reported after commencement of dopaminergic medication (121). Alpha intrusion during REM sleep periods is common (122,123), and changes in phasic EMG activity prior to anti-Parkinson's treatment and changes in both phasic and tonic EMG activity following treatment with L-dopa are evident during REM periods (124).

Further disruption of REM sleep is related to the presence of hallucinations and REM sleep behavior disorder in Parkinson's patients. A decrease in REM sleep has been associated with nocturnal hallucinations (125), and REM intrusion during daytime hallucinations has been reported (126). More than one third of Parkinson's patients also suffer from REM sleep behavior disorder (RBD) (127,128) or REM sleep without atonia (128). In these patients, there is also a significant reduction in total sleep time. In many cases RBD is diagnosed several years prior to the onset of Parkinson's disease (129), although a link between disease severity and duration and the presence of RBD has also been reported (128). RBD is most often treated with the administration of clonazepam (104,129). Patients with comorbid dementia and depression also experience a high level of sleep disturbance, associated with nocturnal vocalizations and hallucinations (130). One side effect of many antidepressant medications, however, is insomnia and sleep disturbance (131).

*Respiratory Disorders.* Sleep disruption due to respiratory disturbance is common in Parkinson's patients who concurrently experience decreased respiratory and pulmonary function during waking periods. The increased levels of muscular rigidity and decreased level of effective muscular strength, in addition to changes in upper airway muscle tone, most likely underlie these respiratory disturbances (132). Treatment with L-dopa, however, is ineffective in relieving the nighttime symptoms of respiratory disturbance. Upper-airway dysfunction, producing reduced airflow in patients with extrapyramidal disorders, may also be due to changes in the musculature producing upper-airway obstruction (133). In Parkinson's patients the changes in upper-airway musculature may be due to the administration of dopaminergic compounds, in addition to the disease per se. Further respiratory disturbances during sleep in Parkinson's patients may be due to the presence of central or obstructive apneas and hypoventilation (116).

Another possible cause of respiratory-related disturbances in Parkinson's patients may be related to changes in cardiac autonomic control during sleep (134). Functional imaging studies reported the occurrence of selective cardiac sympathetic denervation in Parkinson's patients (135), though the clinical significance of this finding is still undetermined.

*Movement Disorders.* Although many of the debilitating symptoms of Parkinson's disease are present during the daytime waking hours, many, but not all, of the symptoms disappear with the onset of sleep. As mentioned earlier, some degree of respiratory sleep disturbance is associated with changes in muscle activity. In addition, the presence of tremor during the sleep period may contribute to difficulties with sleep maintenance. Despite the disappearance of tremor with sleep onset (136) and during slow-wave sleep, tremor may reappear during stages 1 and 2 sleep (137). In addition, tremor may also reappear during awakenings from sleep, with changes in body posture, sleep stage changes, and during or around the time of REM sleep periods (137).

Significant periods of movement are also evident during REM sleep periods, when REM sleep behavior disorder is present (117,138). These include vocalizations, increased muscle tone, and complex muscle movements. During NREM sleep, increased incidence of periodic limb movements is also evident in up to one third of Parkinson's patients (139). Muscle activity is often present in limbs that also express tremor during waking periods.

*Treatment of Sleep Disturbance Associated with Parkinson's Disease.* In a study of 220 Parkinson's patients, 215 reported sleep difficulties, with 29% of these patients using hypnotic or sedative drugs to assist their sleep (102). While administration of benzodiazepines or other nonbenzodiazepine drugs may assist with sleep initiation and maintenance, these drugs are typically recommended as only a short-term solution for insomnia, as with non-Parkinsonian patients. REM sleep behavior disorder is successfully treated with clonazepam (104,129), and in some cases nocturnal administration of L-dopa (138). An alternative therapy for sleep initiation difficulties is the use of tricyclic antidepressants with sedative properties. In addition to their sedating properties, these drugs exert anticholinergic effects, which may improve waking symptoms also. In Parkinson's patients with comorbid neurobehavioral impairment, however, these drugs are contraindicated, as they may produce nocturnal delirium.

As outlined earlier, many of the anti-Parkinson's medications concurrently produce insomnia or sleep disturbance while relieving other symptoms of the disease—e.g., L-dopa, combination L-dopa/carbidopa, MAO-B inhibitors, anticholinergic agents, and COMT inhibitors. Since much of the sleep disturbance may be attributed to the anti-Parkinsonian medications, adjustment of dosing regimens may provide some improvements in sleep. A balance between the alleviation of daytime symptoms and increased sleep quality is ultimately desirable, but not always achievable.

Nocturnal administration of L-dopa has been reported to improve subjective assessments of sleep and reduce the number of movements during sleep (140).

Similarly, administration of low doses of L-dopa and carbidopa (Sinemet) or dopaminergic drugs near bedtime is also useful in increasing sleep maintenance (141). These drugs may be readministered during the early hours of the morning (02:00–03:00 hr) if the patients awaken and have difficulty in returning to sleep. Dopamine agonists likely improve sleep by reducing the degree of muscular rigidity and bradykinesia, thereby reducing the difficulty in getting into and out of bed and turning in the bed, and also by reducing the number of limb movements during sleep (141,142).

Dopaminergic medications may be both sleep-inducing and sleep-disruptive, however. Although low doses of these drugs may assist in sleep initiation, large doses inhibit sleep initiation (113,140) and induce other sleep disturbances. In some Parkinson's patients, daytime administration of L-dopa or Sinemet has been associated with the onset of nightmares, vivid dreams, or night terrors (143). The occurrence of these sleep disruptions was associated with the duration of dopaminergic therapy. These drug-induced dreams and nightmares are more likely to occur in patients with comorbid dementia. In addition, chronic L-dopa therapy has been associated with increased daytime sleepiness (105), and increased incidence of limb movements during sleep and nocturnal myoclonus, due to disruption of the serotonin system (144–146), while dopaminergic and anticholinergic drugs have been reported to suppress REM sleep (113). In patients with chronic Parkinson's who experience on-off phenomenon associated with tolerance to L-dopa therapy, the incidence of sleep disturbance is further increased (125,147).

Some of the respiratory disturbances experienced by Parkinson's patients are similar in nature to that experienced by non-Parkinson's patients with sleep-related respiratory disturbances. Hence the same treatments may be used in both patient groups, depending on the stage of the Parkinson's. Continuous positive airway pressure (CPAP) can improve sleep in Parkinson's patients, but is not suitable during the advanced stages of Parkinson's. Alternatively, upper-airway surgery may provide some relief. Neither of these measures, however, alleviates the respiratory disturbance that may be due to the muscle rigidity associated directly with Parkinson's disease.

## C. Metabolically-based Conditions

### Diabetes

Diabetes is a chronic disease involving an inability by the body to produce or use insulin, resulting in hyperglcemia. There are three different forms of diabetes: type I, type II, and gestational. In type I (juvenile) diabetes, the pancreas is unable to produce sufficient levels of insulin. In type II (late-onset) diabetes, insulin production is normal; however, the cells are unable to convert the glucose to energy. Type II diabetes is typically associated with obesity, and the incidence of this disorder is increasing as the proportion of people with obesity also increases. Gestational diabetes occurs during pregnancy, and usually reverses following birthing; however, individuals are consequently at a greater risk for type II diabetes. Common symptoms of all three forms of diabetes include increased fatigue levels; increased hunger and thirst; increased frequency of urination; rapid weight loss; blurred vision; numbness in hands or feet; extended healing times for cuts and bruises; and dry, itchy skin.

## Sleep in Diabetes

Individuals with diabetes experience a myriad of symptoms that place them at risk for developing secondary sleep disorders, including obesity, hypertension, older age, nocturia, pain, decreased physical exercise, and hypoglycemia. Indeed, the prevalence of individuals with diabetes who have sleep disturbance is estimated at between 30% (148–150) and almost 60% (151). In one study, sleep logs of type II diabetes patients indicated that nearly 60% complained of sleep disruption, with 8% reporting sleep onsets > 30 min, 23% reporting intermittent awakenings lasting up to 25 min nightly, and 36% reporting both sleep-onset and maintenance difficulties (151). Despite the high incidence of sleep disturbance reported by diabetes patients, relatively few studies have examined the exact nature of sleep disruption associated with this disorder.

Although no alterations in sleep architecture pattern have been reported, symptoms of insomnia, periodic movements (152), and sleep-disordered breathing are of particular concern. The link between the obstructive sleep apnea syndrome (OSAS) and diabetes appears to be mediated by obesity. Given that central obesity is characteristic of individuals with diabetes and is furthermore predictive of OSAS, it is not surprising that individuals with diabetes concomitantly have OSAS. As Grunstein (153) speculates, not only may central obesity lead to OSAS, but OSAS may contribute to central obesity. Increased serotonergic deficiencies, decreased hormonal responses, and deficient insulin sensitivity are common pathways by which OSAS may lead to central obesity and potentially create a vicious cycle of obesity contributing to OSAS. Individuals who have obesity and sleep-disordered breathing may also be prone to hypoventilation. Phipps et al. (154) hypothesised that leptin, in particular hyperleptinemia, may be an underlying factor in predisposing obese individuals to hypoventialtion, more so even than body fat.

Hypertension and obesity are common symptoms of both diabetes and sleep-disordered breathing; the presence of these symptoms also represents an increased risk for cardiovascular disease. While a relationship between sleep-disordered breathing and cardiovascular disease has been well established, a link between diabetes and cardiovascular disease is less clear. It has been proposed that the cardiovascular autonomic neuropathy (CAN) common in diabetes may contribute to an increased risk for cardiovascular disease (155).

Not all patients with diabetes also have CAN; however, one quarter of diabetes patients with CAN also have OSAS, which has a significantly higher incidence than in diabetic patients without CAN (156). It is this correlation between sleep-disordered breathing and diabetic-associated CAN that suggests a link between diabetes and cardiovascular disease. The relationship between diabetes and cardiovascular disease may in fact be mediated via an increased incidence of sleep-disordered breathing in diabetic-CAN patients (157–159).

Of the aforementioned comorbid symptoms, hypoglycemia does not appear to significantly increase the number of awakenings or account for the increased sleep disruption (160,161). In a study of children with insulin-dependent diabetes mellitus, Matyka et al. (160) found that sleep was disrupted among children with diabetes, with an increased number of awakenings in the diabetic children, compared to controls. However, hypoglycemia did not appear to affect sleep in these children. In another study that assessed adult diabetes patients, path analyses revealed that nocturia and pain, such as the discomfort associated with neuropathy, accounted for much of the sleep disruption (151).

## Treatment

Intermittent awakenings and their potential effects on daytime cognitive and behavioral functioning are important to address. Clearly, the type of sleep disorder needs to be identified to tailor treatment to sleep-disordered breathing, pain, or nocturia, for example. Pain-reduction strategies and medications to improve nocturia may be the most efficacious for decreasing sleep complaints among individuals with diabetes and those prominent complaints (151). Continuous positive airway pressure (CPAP) therapy may be indicated in the course of sleep disturbances caused by OSAS. Alternatively, severely obese diabetic (type II) individuals who had undergone laporoscopic-adjustable gastric band surgery had their OSAS resolved at 1-year postsurgery, and both their sleep quality and daytime sleepiness improved.

### D.  Circadian-based Disorders

The circadian system plays an integral role in regulating nearly all of the physiological and behavioral systems in the body, including the timing of sleep and waking periods. When the timing of the endogenous circadian clock, located in the suprachiasmatic nuclei (SCN), is out of synchrony with the external environment, then disruption to the endogenously generated circadian rhythms may occur, as the body seeks to realign itself with the outside environment, e.g., jet lag. In some situations, however, the timing of the endogenous clock and external environment remain desynchronous. One example of this is seen in patients with delayed sleep-phase syndrome (DSPS).

### *Delayed Sleep-Phase Syndrome (DSPS)*

In patients with DSPS, a delay in the timing of physiological and behavioral systems that demonstrate circadian rhythmicity is reported, compared to normally entrained individuals. This delay is evident in a variety of functions, including secretion of the pineal hormone melatonin (e.g., Ref. 162), thermoregulation, and sleep-wake activity. Individuals with DSPS typically experience difficulty initiating and terminating sleep at the "correct" or "normal" time (163). When allowed, DSPS patients select later sleep (between 02:00 and 06:00 hr) and wake times (between 10:00 and 13:00 hr) compared to normally entrained individuals. The sleep architecture of these patients is otherwise normal.

Owing to waking commitments, such as schooling, employment, child care, and social activities, individuals are often required to curtail their sleep periods in order to participate. Despite the forced advance of their sleep termination times, and earlier exposure to phase-advancing zeitgebers under these circumstances, patients with DSPS typically are unable to advance their rhythms, and still experience difficulty in initiating sleep at a normal time. Consequently, these patients are exposed to chronic periods of sleep deprivation, or sleep restriction. As a result, this population reports increased daytime sleepiness, reduced alertness and attention, and reduced neurobehavioral and cognitive functioning.

There are no clear reports of the incidence of DSPS in the general population. In adolescents, there is a reported incidence of 7% (164,165), while in middle-aged adults it appears that the incidence is only 0.7% (166). In adolescents, the incidence of DSPS or a DSPS-like profile is higher compared to other age groups. A phase delay in the occurrence of daytime sleepiness, measured using the Multiple Sleep Latency Test (MSLT), has been reported in midpubertal children (167). In addition, observational studies have reported later bedtimes in adolescents compared to younger children and older adults, with forced early awakenings due to early school start times (168). When these adolescents are allowed to self-select their sleep and wake times, such as on weekends, both their bedtime and rising time are delayed compared to weekdays and compared to normally entrained individuals (168,169). In addition, these sleep periods on weekends are longer than those of weekdays, likely reflecting an increased sleep need due to cumulative sleep deprivation throughout the week. Although the basis for this transient period of DSPS-like behavior during adolescence is unknown, it is possibly due to a combination of developmental (pubertal) and environmental (late bedtimes) influences on the circadian system.

DSPS is typically diagnosed clinically via nocturnal polysomnography, with evidence of delayed sleep and REM onsets. DSPS can be further characterized, usually only experimentally, by using phase assessment, subjective sleep diaries or actigraphy, and morningness-eveningness questionnaires. It has been reported that individuals from one family with DSPS scored high on the eveningness scale (170). Hence, it has been suggested that there may be an underlying genetic basis for this disorder.

### Treatment

Treatment of DSPS is typically aimed at resynchronization of the circadian system, to restore balance between the endogenous and exogenous environments. A balance between these two environments may be achieved by delaying sleep by a few hours each night, until the desired sleep time relative to clock time is reached

(171). This treatment requires subjects to then maintain a rigid sleep-wake schedule to maintain correct light-dark exposure to avoid further phase shifts or relapse. Using light exposure as an entraining agent to resynchronize the circadian system in DSPS patients has produced mixed results. While one study reported on the success of light administration in advancing the circadian system (172), a further study reported little success with light therapy (173).

One further treatment that has been studied extensively to achieve resynchronization of the circadian system is the administration of melatonin. Endogenous melatonin is secreted from the pineal gland, primarily across the nocturnal or dark period. It has been proposed to play a role in the control of the circadian system (reviewed in Ref. 174) and potentially in the initiation of sleep (175,176). Studies that have administered exogenous melatonin, primarily during the daytime, have reported both chronobiotic (177) and soporific effects (178). Melatonin administration has been successful in studies examining the reentrainment of the circadian system after transmeridian flight or shiftwork (179). Similarly, the effectiveness of melatonin in reentraining the circadian system of those with DSPS to a normal day has been studied.

Phase advances of the circadian system and sleep-wake activity have been reported in a number of studies, with daily administration of melatonin (180–183). Termination of melatonin administration resulted in a reversal of the phase advances, with subjects reverting to their preadministration phase. Therefore, continued administration of melatonin may provide a means for those with DSPS to maintain a normal phase, and avoid the associated sleep deprivation due to having to live on a normal schedule. It is important to note, however, that at present the effective dose of melatonin to be administered and the safety of long-term melatonin administration have yet to be established (184). Therefore, melatonin should be thought of as a research compound and not a clinical solution to DSPS.

### E.  Infectious Diseases

Many infectious diseases are known to produce alterations in sleep-wake behavior, in particular in fatigue and alertness levels during waking periods and sleep physiology or architecture (185,186). Immunological compounds, such as cytokines, that are stimulated during an immune response also play a role in sleep regulation (187–189). During a bacterial or viral infection, secretion of these cytokines are elevated and may contribute to the changes in sleep that are observed throughout the infection.

Despite the co-occurrence of sleep disturbances with virtually all infectious diseases, relatively few studies have looked at the exact nature of sleep changes associated with infection. Reports of sleep during rhinovirus 23 infection (the cold virus) have included a decrease in sleep duration and sleep efficiency, with an associated reduction in neurobehavioral performance (vigilance) and a trend for reduced subjective vigor (Profile of Mood States, POMS) (190).

### HIV/ AIDS

A small number of studies have investigated alterations in sleep physiology following infection with the human immunodeficiency virus (HIV) and subsequent progression into acquired immune deficiency disease (AIDS). Infection with HIV may occur via the transfer of bodily fluids—blood, semen, or vaginal secretions. HIV infection then progresses through three distinct phases: acute infection, chronic infection, and AIDS. The first, and shortest, phase of HIV infection is the acute or clinical latency phase, where CD4 counts are greater than 400 cells/µL. The symptoms during this stage resemble the flu, typically with a fever and fatigue that lasts for 1–2 weeks. The chronic phase of HIV infection typically starts from 3 to 6 months postinfection, and may last for up to 10 years. During this phase there are few clinical symptoms; however, the immune system begins to deteriorate, with the number of CD4 T cells reducing over time, to between 400 and 200 cells/µL. The final stage of HIV infection, or AIDS, commences when CD4 T-cell counts reach a critical level (less than 200 cells/µL) or when patients experience an increase in opportunistic infections that the body is no longer able to combat. Similar to the chronic phase, AIDS has no symptoms itself; however, the symptomatology is representative of the opportunistic infections that patients contract.

It is estimated that approximately 42 million individuals worldwide are infected with HIV, with an estimated 5 million people becoming infected in 2002 (191). The proportion of men and women infected with HIV is about 50–50. During 2002, approximately 3.1 million people died from AIDS-related disorders.

### HIV Infection and Sleep Disturbance

Large numbers of patients infected with HIV also experience sleep difficulties and sleep disturbance (192–198). The degree of sleep disturbance increases with disease progression (192). Approximately 25% of patients with HIV infection have experienced significant sleep loss and resulting increased levels of daytime sleepiness and dysfunction (192,199). Between 10 and 20% of HIV patients report that their sleep loss is chronic and severe. The sleep loss associated with HIV infection is due to a number of different mechanisms, including the stage of the disease/level of immune function, symptoms from comorbid infections (especially during AIDS), and medications. Comparison of HIV+ and HIV- patients with depression demonstrated a greater degree of sleep disturbance in patients who were HIV+ (200,201). However, several studies have reported that the sleep disturbance experienced by HIV+ patients cannot be explained by the presence of depression or increased anxiety (199,201–204). Rubinstein and Selwyn (195) reported a higher incidence of insomnia in HIV+ patients with neurobehavioral impairment compared to those HIV+ patients without neurobehavioral impairment. In addition, many patients may experience sleep problems due to lifestyle factors, such as substance abuse (196), coping mechanisms, individual sleep-wake cycles, and sleep hygiene. During AIDS, much of the sleep loss and sleep problems are typically associated with the opportunistic infections, and may reflect the sleep problems in HIV- patients with these diseases.

Polysomnographic studies have characterized several changes in the sleep architecture of HIV+ patients. These changes represent a progressive deterioration of sleep. These changes begin to occur when HIV+ patients are asymptomatic, prior to the onset of AIDS (205). There is a decrease in total sleep time (TST) and sleep efficiency (SE), with an increased sleep onset latency (SOL) and increased number and duration of awakenings across the night (reviewed in Ref. 110). This increase in wake after sleep onset (WASO) results in significant amounts of cumulative sleep deprivation. Further changes in sleep architecture are also evident, with increased stage 1, decreased stage 2, and a decrease in the onset to REM sleep (reviewed in Refs. 110,186). Alterations in SWS are evident throughout the entire infectious period, even when patients are asymptomatic (195,199). Compared to HIV- subjects, HIV+ subjects have an increased amount of slow-wave sleep (SWS), with more even dispersion of SWS throughout the sleep period. Both SWS and REM sleep were found to occur in both the first and second halves of the sleep period (206).

In a study examining polysomnographic recordings in HIV+ male subjects collected at different stages of infection and disease progression, significant differences in sleep architecture were found. In one study in HIV+ patients, it was noted that TST and SE were increased, and the amount of SWS was elevated in the first stage of infection (207,208). Subsequent studies, however, have reported no difference in the amount of SWS relative to control subjects (205,209). During the first stage of infection, NREM-REM cycles across the sleep period become destabilized, and HIV+ patients have a more even distribution of SWS throughout the sleep period, particularly in the second half (210), with an increased incidence of alpha intrusion during NREM sleep relative to HIV- controls. No consistent changes in REM sleep have been reported, apart from the disruption of normal NREM-REM cycles and one report of reduced latency to REM in HIV+ patients (205). During the chronic phase of HIV infection, there is a decrease in SWS and a decrease in TST and sleep efficiency, due to increased sleep latency and increased number of awakenings, with an increased amount of stage 1 sleep (205). The NREM-REM cycles become even more disrupted. By the final stage of HIV infection, during AIDS, SWS is virtually absent, with sleep efficiency very low, owing to the high incidence of awakenings during sleep periods. NREM-REM cycles across the sleep period are absent (110,209,211).

It has been proposed that the changes in sleep-wake behavior during HIV infection may be due to an effect of the virus directly on the central nervous system (199,212). There is evidence that penetration of the blood-brain barrier by the virus occurs as early as the acute or clinical latency phase, prior to the development of symptoms (155). During the early stages of HIV infection, the sleep-promoting cytokines TNF-$\alpha$ and IL-1$\beta$ are elevated relative to normal (199,212). It has also been suggested that the changes in sleep physiology present in all stages of HIV infection may in some part be mediated via changes in the profile of growth hormone secretion (195).

Subjectively, compared to HIV- control subjects, HIV+ patients in the first stage of infection report mild sleep disturbances, with difficulty in initiating and maintaining sleep, and associated increased levels of fatigue and sleepiness. During the chronic phase of infection the incidence of sleep disturbance and daytime fatigue is increased, with patients also reporting difficulties in neurobehavioral functioning, including difficulty with concentration and memory. By the final stage of infection, sleep quality is markedly reduced, with high levels of fatigue throughout waking periods.

A similar pattern of sleep disturbance is observed in children and adolescents as in adults. In a study of children and adolescents an increase in WASO, with both an increased number of awakenings and increased duration of awakenings, more frequent daytime napping, and elevated evening sleepiness, was reported in HIV+ patients relative to control subjects (213).

In one study of 44 HIV+ women, 98% reported that their worst symptom was fatigue (197). The reduction in both sleep quality and duration intensified the daytime fatigue (196,198,214) and decreased the women's quality of life that typically is associated with HIV infection (196,198). In addition, the increased daytime fatigue may be reflective of a compromised immune system. It has been reported that lower CD4 counts are associated with increased daytime fatigue levels (193) and increased incidence of daytime napping (214). In addition, lower CD4 counts were associated with higher levels of both evening and morning fatigue (214). Further predictors of daytime fatigue levels include decreased mental health, weight loss, and longer duration of infection (193). In addition, it has been reported that the elevated levels of sleep disturbance and daytime fatigue increase disability and morbidity, particularly during the latter stages of infection (214).

## Treatment

At present, HIV infection or AIDS cannot be cured. One mechanism whereby the chronic phase of HIV infection may be extended and transition to AIDS delayed is via pharmacological treatment. Patients are typically prescribed a combination, or cocktail, of drugs that slow down the progression of the disease. Many of these drugs produce a myriad of side effects, including sleep disturbances.

Approximately one third of HIV+ patients in the United States who experience sleep loss seek medical assistance for it. Of these, 25% of patients use an over-the-counter treatment for insomnia, 27% use alcohol to help them sleep, and 15% use a hypnotic medication, with 61% of these patients using them on a chronic basis, for a period greater than 1 year. At present the most popularly prescribed hypnotic is temazepam. This drug is recommended only for short-term (1 week) use, with tolerance and decreased effectiveness associated with chronic use, and rebound insomnia following termination of administration.

## IV.  Summary and Conclusions

Although only a limited number of disorders are discussed in this chapter relative to the large number of disorders that produce or are related to sleep disturbance, it is evident that sleep deprivation secondary to medical disorders is prevalent. Other disorders that are associated with significant sleep disruption and sleep disturbance include cancer, chronic pain, dementia, depression, cystic fibrosis, reflux, cardiovascular disorders, asthma/respiratory disorders, and gastrointestinal disorders.

When thinking of sleep disturbance associated with medical disorders, it may be valuable to utilize a conceptual framework for the treatment of sleep disruption that is general in nature, and not specific to a particular disorder. Optimal treatment of secondary sleep disturbances may result in increased daytime functioning, increased quality of life, and improvement of disorder-associated symptoms. It is important for clinicians to be educated in the appropriate assessment and treatment of sleep disturbance that is associated with other medical disorders. This entails knowledge of the appropriate questions to be directed to patients, their partners, and/or caregivers, the interactions of the disorder with potential treatments, and the range of treatment options available.

Although significant differences exist between different disorders, including the cause, primary symptomatology, treatment, duration, and physiological systems involved, treatment of comorbid sleep disturbance may be approached using a common model. At the first level, the successful treatment of some disorders, e.g., influenza, arthritis, fibromyalgia, will result in improvement of sleep quality. With an acute illness such as influenza infection, much of the sleep disturbance is related to the complex bidirectional relationship that exists between the immune and sleep systems. Activation of various immunological pathways results in alterations in sleep-wake activity, which may in fact assist in the response of the body to the infection, and facilitate recovery. In addition, many of the medications used to fight viral infections contain soporific substances that promote sleep to promote healing.

For chronic disorders, the use of soporific or hypnotic compounds is not recommended for the treatment of comorbid sleep disturbance, just as these compounds are not recommended for the treatment of chronic insomnia. Alleviation of the pain associated with many disorders, including fibromyalgia and arthritis, results in a lessening of symptoms and improvement of sleep. Similar to how reduced sleep quality can amplify the symptoms of these disorders, and augment pain, which in turn produces reduced sleep quality and consolidation, improvement in sleep can improve the symptoms, which in turn helps maintain the increased sleep quality.

For some disorders, treatment is aimed at reducing the symptoms of the disorder to improve or maintain daytime functioning and slow down the progression of the disorder. This is especially the case with chronic (e.g., cancer, epilepsy, diabetes) or terminal disorders (e.g., HIV, Parkinson's disease). Although the treatment regimen may help manage the primary symptoms of these conditions, secondary symptoms (e.g., sleep disturbance) may persist. In this situation, direct treatment of the sleep disturbance may be necessary.

When treating sleep disturbance that is secondary to another medical condition, current pharmacological therapies may not be appropriate. Administration of hypnotic drugs, such as benzodiazepines, may inadvertently result in exacerbation of the primary medical disorder. This is especially likely in those disorders that have a central component to their manifestation, e.g., Parkinson's disease, HIV infection, depression. Consequently, multidisciplinary approaches may provide the most benefit in the management of sleep in patients with medical conditions. As an example, it may be more effective to treat sleep disturbance with treatments that are free from side effects typically associated with pharmacological interventions. These include sleep hygiene or cognitive behavior therapies, such as progressive relaxation, or stimulus control.

It is also important to recognize that with disorders that are degenerative, different treatments may be required at different stages of illness. This may be due to changes in the intensity of symptoms, or changes in the nature of symptoms associated with disease progression. In addition, it is common for the incidence of comorbid disorders, such as depression or OSAS, to increase in the later

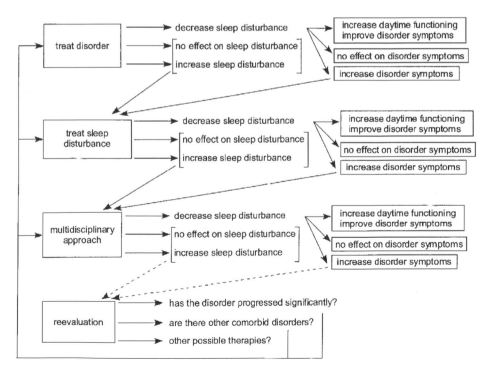

**Figure 1** Conceptual model for the treatment of sleep disturbance associated with medical disorders.

stages of many disorders. Consequently, the underlying mechanisms of the sleep disturbance may have multiple etiologies. A clear assessment of the nature of the sleep disturbance can best direct decision making with regard to the most appropriate treatment of the sleep disturbance.

Using a conceptual model such as that presented here (Fig. 1) could facilitate the diagnosis and appropriate treatment of sleep disturbances in a number of different medical disorders. This may ultimately result in improvements in daytime functioning, quality of life, and better management of the primary medical condition.

## Acknowledgments

The authors wish to thank Dr. Michael Dreher for his assistance with portions of this manuscript. This was supported by NIH R01-NR04281, NASA cooperative agreement NCC9-58 with the NSBRI, AFOSR F49620-00-1-0266, and the Institute for Experimental Psychiatry Research Foundation.

## References

1.  Devoto A, Lucidi F, Violani C, Bertini M. Effects of different sleep reductions on daytime sleepiness. Sleep 1999; 22:336–343.
2.  Dinges DF, Pack F, Williams K, Gillen KA, Powell JW, Ott GE, Aptowicz C, Pack AI. Cumulative sleepiness, mood disturbance, and psychomotor vigilance performance decrements during a week of sleep restricted to 4–5 hours per night. Sleep 1997; 20:267–277.
3.  Van Dongen HPA, Maislin G, Mullington JM, Dinges DF. The cumulative cost of additional wakefulness: dose-response effects on neurobehavioral functions and sleep physiology from chronic sleep restriction and total sleep deprivation. Sleep 2003; 26:117–126.
4.  Carskadon MA, Dement WC. Cumulative effects of sleep restriction on daytime sleepiness. Psychophysiology 1981; 18:107–113.
5.  Irwin M, Mascovich A, Gillin JC, Willoughby R, Pike J, Smith TL. Partial sleep deprivation reduces natural killer cell activity in humans. Psychosom Med 1994; 56:493–498.
6.  Irwin M, McClintick J, Costlow C, Fortner M, White J, Gillin JC. Partial night sleep deprivation reduces natural killer and cellular immune responses in humans. Fed of Am Soc Exp Biol J 1996; 10:643–653.
7.  Redwine L, Hauger RL, Gillin JC, Irwin M. Effects of sleep and sleep deprivation on interleukin-6, growth hormone, cortisol, and melatonin levels in humans. J Clin Endocrinol Metab 2000; 85:3597–3603.
8.  Wolfe F, Smythe HA, Yunus MB, Bennett RM, Bombardier C, Goldenberg DL, Tugwell P, Campbell SM, Abeles M, Clark P, et al. The American College of Rheumatology criteria for the classification of fibromylagia. Report of the multicenter criteria committee. Arthritis Rheumatol 1990; 33:160–172.

9. Wolfe F, Ross K, Anderson J, Russell IJ. Aspects of fibromyalgia in the general population: sex, pain threshold, and fibromyalgia symptoms. J Rheumatol 1995; 22:151–156.

10. Hudson JL, Pope HG Jr. The relationship between fibromylagia and major depressive disorder. Rheum Dis Clin N Amer 1996; 22:285–303.

11. Cudney SA, Butler MR, Weinert C, Sullivan T. Ten rural women living with fibromyalgia tell it like it is. Holistic Nurs Pract 2002; 16:35–45.

12. Drewes AM, Jennum P, Andersen A, Siol A, Nielsen KD. Self-reported sleep disturbances and daytime complaints in women with fibromylagia and rheumatoid arthritis. J Musculoskel Pain 1994; 2:15–31.

13. Yunus MB, Masi AT, Aldag JC. A controlled study of primary fibromyalgia syndrome: clinical features and association with other functional syndromes. J Rheumatol 1989 suppl; 19:62–71.

14. Schaefer KM. Sleep disturbances and fatigue in women with fibromyalgia and chronic fatigue syndrome. J Obstetric, Gynecologic, Neonat Nursi 1995; 24:229–233.

15. Harding SM. Sleep in fibromyalgia patients: subjective and objective findings. Am J Medi Sci 1998; 315:367–376.

16. Horne JA, Shackell BS. Alpha-like EEG activity in non-REM sleep and the fibromyalgia (fibrositis) syndrome. Electroencephalogr Clin Neurophysiol 1991; 79:271–276.

17. Branco J, Atalaia A, Paiva T. Sleep cycles and alpha-delta sleep in fibromyalgia syndrome. J Rheumatol 1994; 21:1113–1117.

18. Moldofsky H, Scarisbrick P, England R, Smythe H. Musculosketal symptoms and non-REM sleep disturbance in patients with "fibrositis syndrome" and healthy subjects. Psychosom Med 1975; 37:341–351.

19. Molony RR, MacPeek DM, Schiffman PL, Frank M, Neubauer JA, Schwartzberg M, Seibold JR. Sleep, sleep apnea and the fibromyalgia syndrome. J Rheumatol 1986; 13:797–800.

20. Wittig RM, Zorick FJ, Blumer D, Heilbronn M, Roth T. Disturbed sleep in patients complaining of chronic pain. J Nerv Ment Disord 1982; 170:429–431.

21. Drewes AM, Nielsen KD, Taagholt SJ, Bjerregard K, Svendsen L, Gade J. Sleep intensity in fibromyalgia: focus on the microstructure of the sleep process. Br J Rheumatol 1995; 34:629–635.

22. Drewes AM, Gade K, Nielsen KD, Bjerregard K, Taagholt SJ, Svendsen L. Clustering of sleep electroencephalographic patterns in patients with the fibromyalgia syndrome. Br J Rheumatol 1995; 34:1151–1156.

23. Shapiro CM, Devins GM, Hussain MRG. Sleep problems in patients with medical illness. Br Med J 1993; 306:1532–1535.

24. Moldofsky H, Scarisbrick P. Induction of neurasthenic musculoskeletal pain syndrome by selective sleep stage deprivation. Psychosom Med 1976; 38:35–44.

25. Moldofsky H, Lue FA. The relationship of alpha and delta EEG frequencies to pain and mood in "fibrositis" patients treated with chlorpromazine and L-tryptophan. Electroencephalogr Clin Neurophysiol 1980; 50:71–80.

26. Perlis ML, Giles DE, Bootzin RR, Dikman ZV, Fleming GM, Drummond SP, Rose MW. Alpha sleep and information processing, perception of sleep, pain, and arousability in fibromyalgia. Int J Neurosci 1997; 89:265–280.

27.  Roizenblatt S, Moldofsky H, Benedito-Silva AA, Tufik S. Alpha sleep characteristics in fibromyalgia. Arthritis Rheum 2001; 44:222–230.
28.  Drewes AM. Pain and sleep disturbances with special reference to fibromyalgia and rheumatoid arthritis. Rheumatology 1999; 38:1035–1038.
29.  Sergi M, Rizzi M, Braghiroli A, Puttini PS, Greco M, Cazzola M, Andreoli A. Periodic breathing during sleep in patients affected by fibromyalgia syndrome. Eur Respir J 1999; 14:203–208.
30.  Affleck G, Urrows S, Tennen H, Higgins P, Abeles M. Sequential daily relations of sleep, pain intensity, and attention to pain among women with fibromyalgia. Pain 1996; 68:363–368.
31.  Pascualy R, Buchwald D. Chronic fatigue syndrome and fibromyalgia. In: Kryger MH, Roth T, Dement WC, eds. Principles and Practice of Sleep Medicine. Philadelphia: WB Saunders, 2000:1040–1049.
32.  Agargun MY, Tekeoglu I, Gunes A, Adak. B, Kara H, Ercan M. Sleep quality and pain threshold in patients with fibromyalgia. Comprehensi Psychiatry 1999; 40:226–228.
33.  Moldofsky H. Sleep and fibrositis syndrome. Rheum Dis Clin N Amer 1989; 15:91–103.
34.  Landis CA, Lentz MJ, Rothermel J, Riffle SC, Chapman D, Buchwald D, Shaver JL. Decreased nocturnal levels of prolactin and growth hormone in women with fibromyalgia. J Clin Endocrinol Metab 2001; 86:1672–1678.
35.  Klerman EB, Goldenberg DL, Brown EN, Maliszewski AM, Adler GK. Circadian rhythms of women with fibromyalgia. J Clin Endocrinol Metab 2001; 86:1034–1039.
36.  Goldenberg DL. Fibromyalgia syndrome a decade later: what have we learned? Arch Intern Medi 1999; 159:777–785.
37.  O'Malley PG, Jackson JL, Tomkins GE, Santoro JA, Balden E, Kroenke K. Efficacy of antidepressants for physical symptoms: a critical review. J Family Practi 1999; 48:980–990.
38.  O'Malley PG, Balden E, Tomkins G, Santoro J, Kroenke K, Jackson JL. Treatment of fibromyalgia with antidepressants: a meta-analysis. J Gen Intern Med 2000; 15:659–666.
39.  Arnold LM, Keck PE, Jr., Welge JA. Antidepressant treatment of fibromyalgia: a meta-analysis and review. Psychosomatics 2000; 41:104–113.
40.  Lautenschlager J. Present state of medication therapy in fibromyalgia syndrome. Scand J Rheumatol 2000; Supplement 113:32–36.
41.  Citera G, Arias MA, Maldonado-Cocco JA, Lazaro MA, Rosemffet MG, Brusco LI, Scheines EJ, Cardinalli DP. The effect of melatonin in patients with fibromyalgia: a pilot study. Clin Rheumatol 2000; 19:9–13.
42.  Offenbacher M, Stucki G. Physical therapy in the treatment of fibromyalgia. Scand J Rheumatol 2000 Supplement; 113:78–85.
43.  Fukuda K, Straus SE, Hickie I, Sharpe MC, Dobbins JG, Komaroff A. The chronic fatigue syndrome: a comprehensive approach to its definition and study. International Chronic Fatigue Syndrome Study Group. Ann Intern Med 1994; 121:953–959.
44.  Taylor R, Jason LA, Curie CA. Prognosis of chronic fatigue in a community-based sample. Psychosom Med 2002; 64:319–327.
45.  Vercoulen JH, Swanink CM, Fennis JF, Galama JM, van der Meer JW, Bleijenberg G. Dimensional assessment of chronic fatigue syndrome. J Psychosom Res 1994; 38:383–392.

46. Morriss RK, Wearden AJ, Battersby L. The relation of sleep difficulties to fatigue, mood and disability in chronic fatigue syndrome. J Psychosom Res 1997; 42:597–605.

47. Krupp LB, Jandorf L, Coyle PK, Mendelson WB. Sleep disturbance in chronic fatigue syndrome. J Psychos Res 1993; 37:325–331.

48. Whelton C, Saskin P, Salit I, Moldofsky H. Post-viral fatigue syndrome and sleep. Sleep Res 1988; 17:307.

49. Whelton CL, Salit I, Moldofsky H. Sleep, Epstein-Barr virus infection, musculoskeletal pain, and depressive symptoms in chronic fatigue syndrome. J Rheumatol 1992; 19:939–943.

50. Buchwald D, Pascualy R, Bombardier C, Kith P. Sleep disorders in patients with chronic fatigue. Clin Infect Dis 1994; 18:S68–S72.

51. Morriss R, Sharpe M, Sharpley AL, Cowen PJ, Hawton K, Morris J. Abnormalities of sleep in patients with the chronic fatigue syndrome. Br Med J 1993; 306:1161–1164.

52. Buchwald D, Herrell R, Ashton S, Belcourt M, Schmaling K, Sullivan P, Neale M, Goldberg J. A twin study of chronic fatigue. Psychosom Med 2001; 63:936–943.

53. Mullington JM, Hinze-Selch D, Pollmacher T. Mediators of inflammation and their interaction with sleep: relevance for chronic fatigue syndrome and related conditions. Ann NY Acad Sci 2001; 933:201–210.

54. Rogers NL, Szuba MP, Staab JP, Evans DL, Dinges DF. Neuroimmunologic aspects of sleep and sleep loss. Semin in Clin Neuropsychiatry 2001; 6:295–307.

55. Craig T, Kakumanu S. Chronic fatigue syndrome: evaluation and treatment. Am Fam Physician 2002; 65:1083–1090.

56. Patarca R. Cytokines and chronic fatigue syndrome. Ann NY Acad Sci 2001; 933:185–200.

57. Katz P, Fauci AS. Autologous and allogeneic intercellular interactions: modulation by adherent cells, irradiation, and in vitro and in vivo corticosteroids. J Immunol 1979; 123:2270–2277.

58. MacDermott RP, Stacey MC. Further characterization of the human autologous mixed leukocyte reaction (MLR). J Immunol 1981; 126:729–734.

59. Rogers N, van den Heuvel C, Dawson D. Effect of melatonin and corticosteroid on in vitro cellular immune function in humans. J Pineal Res 1997; 22:75–80.

60. Riordan D, Farley D, Young W, Grant C, van Heerden J. Long term outcome of bilateral adrenalectomy in patients with Cushing's syndrome. Surgery 1994; 116:1088–1093.

61. Baxter JD, Tyrel JB. The adrenal cortex. In: Felig P. Baxter JD, Broadus AE, and Frohman LA. eds. Endocrinology and Metabolism. New York: McGraw-Hill, 1981:385–510.

62. Parker AJ, Wessely S, Cleare AJ. The neuroendocrinology of chronic fatigue syndrome and fibromyalgia. Psychol Med 2001; 31:1331–1345.

63. Wessely S, Hotopf M, Sharpe M. Chronic Fatigue and Chronic Fatigue Syndromes. Oxford: Oxford Unviersity Press, 1998.

64. van der Werf SP, de Vree B, van Der Meer JW, Bleijenberg G. The relations among body consciousness, somatic symptom report, and information processing speed in chronic fatigue syndrome. Neuropsychiatry Neuropsychol Behav Neurol 2002; 15:2–9.

65. Cohen S, Tyrrell DA, Smith AP. Psychological stress and susceptibility to the common cold. N Engl J Med 1991; 325:606–612.

66.   Aaron LA, Burke MM, Buchwald D. Overlapping conditions among patients with chronic fatigue syndrome, fibromyalgia, and temporomandibular disorder. Arch Intern Med 2000; 160:221–227.

67.   Vercoulen JH, Swanink CM, Zitman FG, Vreden SG, Hoofs MP, Fennis JF, Galama JM, van der Meer JW, Bleijenberg G. Randomised, double-blind, placebo-controlled study of fluoxetine in chronic fatigue syndrome. Lancet 1996; 347:858–861.

68.   Forsyth LM, Preuss HG, MacDowell AL, Chiazze L, Jr., Birkmayer GD, Bellanti JA. Therapeutic effects of oral NADH on the symptoms of patients with chronic fatigue syndrome. Ann Allergy Asthma Immunol 1999; 82:185–191.

69.   Cleare AJ, Heap E, Malhi GS, Wessely S, O'Keane V, Miell J. Low-dose hydrocortisone in chronic fatigue syndrome: a randomised crossover trial. Lancet 1999; 353:455–458.

70.   Parkinson J. Essay on the Shaking Palsy. London: Sherwood, Neely & Jones, 1817.

71.   de Rijk MC, Tzourio C, Breteler MM, Dartigues JF, Amaducci L, Lopez-Pousa S, Manubens-Bertran JM, Alperovitch A, Rocca WA. Prevalence of parkinsonism and Parkinson's disease in Europe: the EUROPARKINSON Collaborative Study. European Community Concerted Action on the Epidemiology of Parkinson's disease. J Neurol Neurosurg Psychiatry 1997; 62:10–15.

72.   de Rijk MC, Launer LJ, Berger K, Breteler MM, Dartigues JF, Baldereschi M, Fratiglioni L, Lobo A, Martinez-Lage J, Trenkwalder C, Hofman A. Prevalence of Parkinson's disease in Europe: a collaborative study of population-based cohorts. Neurologic Diseases in the Elderly Research Group. Neurology 2000; 54:S21–S23.

73.   Mutch WJ, Dingwall-Fordyce I, Downie AW, Paterson JG, Roy SK. Parkinson's disease in a Scottish city. Br Med J Clin Res Educ 1986; 292:534–536.

74.   Bower JH, Maraganore DM, McDonnell SK, Rocca WA. Incidence and distribution of parkinsonism in Olmsted County, Minnesota, 1976–1990. Neurology 1999; 52:1214–1220.

75.   Langston JW, Ballard P, Tetrud JW, Irwin I. Chronic Parkinsonism in humans due to a product of meperidine-analog synthesis. Science 1983; 219:979–980.

76.   Langston JW, Langston EB, Irwin I. MPTP-induced parkinsonism in human and non-human primates—clinical and experimental aspects. Acta Neurol Scandi 1984 suppl; 100:49–54.

77.   Polymeropoulos MH, Lavedan C, Leroy E, Ide SE, Dehejia A, Dutra A, Pike B, Root H, Rubenstein J, Boyer R, Stenroos ES, Chandrasekharappa S, Athanassiadou A, Papapetropoulos T, Johnson WG, Lazzarini AM, Duvoisin RC, Di Iorio G, Golbe LI, Nussbaum RL. Mutation in the alpha-synuclein gene identified in families with Parkinson's disease. Science 1997; 276:2045–2047.

78.   Kitada T, Asakawa S, Hattori N, Matsumine H, Yamamura Y, Minoshima S, Yokochi M, Mizuno Y, Shimizu N. Mutations in the parkin gene cause autosomal recessive juvenile parkinsonism. Nature 1998; 392:605–608.

79.   Kruger R, Kuhn W, Muller T, Woitalla D, Graeber M, Kosel S, Przuntek H, Epplen JT, Schols L, Riess O. Ala30Pro mutation in the gene encoding alpha-synuclein in Parkinson's disease. Nature Genet 1998; 18:106–108.

80.   Leroy E, Anastasopoulos D, Konitsiotis S, Lavedan C, Polymeropoulos M. Deletions in the Parkin gene and genetic heterogeneity in a Greek family with early onset Parkinson's disease. Hum Genet 1998; 103:424–427.

81.   Abbas N, Lucking CB, Ricard S, Durr A, Bonifati V, De Michele G, Bouley S, Vaughan JR, Gasser T, Marconi R, Broussolle E, Brefel-Courbon C, Harhangi BS,

Oostra BA, Fabrizio E, Bohme GA, Pradier L, Wood NW, Filla A, Meco G, Denefle P, Agid Y, Brice A. A wide variety of mutations in the Parkin gene are responsible for autosomal recessive parkinsonism in Europe. French Parkinson's Disease Genetics Study Group and the European Consortium on Genetic Susceptibility in Parkinson's Disease. Hum Mol Genet 1999; 8:567–574.

82. Satoh J, Kuroda Y. Association of codon 167 Ser/Asn heterozygosity in the Parkin gene with sporadic Parkinson's disease. Neuroreport 1999; 10:2735–2739.

83. Lucking CB, Durr A, Bonifati V, Vaughan J, De Michele G, Gasser T, Harhangi BS, Meco G, Denefle P, Wood NW, Agid Y, Brice A. Association between early-onset Parkinson's disease and mutations in the parkin gene. French Parkinson's Disease Genetics Study Group. N Engl J Med 2000; 342:1560–1567.

84. Teive HA, Raskin S, Iwamoto FM, Germiniani FM, Baran MH, Werneck LC, Allan N, Quagliato E, Leroy E, Ide SE, Polymeropoulos MH. The G209A mutation in the alpha-synuclein gene in Brazilian families with Parkinson's disease. Arq Neuro-Psiquiatria 2001; 59:722–724.

85. Lim KL, Dawson VL, Dawson TM. The genetics of Parkinson's disease. Curr Neurol Neurosci Rep 2002; 2:439–446.

86. Mayeux R. Epidemiology of neurodegeneration. Annl Rev Neurosci 2003; 26:81–104.

87. Dakof GA, Mendelson GA. Parkinson's disease: The psychological aspects of a chronic illness. Psychol Bull 1986; 99:375–387.

88. Levy G, Tang MX, Cote LJ, Louis ED, Alfaro B, Mejia H, Stern Y, Marder K. Motor impairment in PD: relationship to incident dementia and age. Neurology 2000; 55:539–544.

89. Levy G, Schupf N, Tang MX, Cote LJ, Louis ED, Mejia H, Stern Y, Marder K. Combined effect of age and severity on the risk of dementia in Parkinson's disease. Ann Neurol 2002; 51:722–729.

90. Brown RG, MacCarthy B, Gotham AM, Der GJ, Marsden CD. Depression and disability in Parkinson's disease: a follow-up of 132 cases. Psychol Medi 1988; 18:49–55.

91. Gotham AM, Brown RG, Marsden CD. Depression in Parkinson's disease: a quantitative and qualitative analysis. J Neurol Neurosurg Psychiatry 1986; 49:381–389.

92. Quinn N. Drug treatment of Parkinson's disease. Br Med J 1995; 310:575–579.

93. Block G, Liss C, Reines S, Irr J, Nibbelink D. Comparison of immediate-release and controlled release carbidopa/levodopa in Parkinson's disease: a multicenter 5–year study. The CR First Study Group. Eur Neurol 1997; 37:23–27.

94. Lewin R. More clues to the cause of Parkinson's disease. Science 1987; 237:978.

95. Knoll J. Rationale for (-)deprenyl (selegiline) medication in Parkinson's disease and in prevention of age-related nigral changes. Biomed Pharmacother 1995; 49:187–195.

96. Chrisp P, Mammen GJ, Sorkin EM. Selegiline. A review of its pharmacology, symptomatic benefits and protective potential in Parkinson's disease. Drugs Aging 1991; 1:228–248.

97. Myllyla VV, Heinonen EH, Vuorinen JA, Kilkku OI, Sotaniemi KA. Early selegiline therapy reduces levodopa dose requirement in Parkinson's disease. Acta Neurol Scand 1995; 91:177–182.

98. Larsen JP, Boas J, Erdal JE. Does selegiline modify the progression of early Parkinson's disease? Results from a five-year study. The Norwegian-Danish Study Group. Euro J Neurol 1999; 6:539–547.

99. Przuntek H, Conrad B, Dichgans J, Kraus PH, Krauseneck P, Pergande G, Rinne U, Schimrigk K, Schnitker J, Vogel HP. SHELDO: A 5–year long -term trial on the

effect of selegiline in early Parkinsonian patients treated with levodopa. Eur J Neurol 1999; 6:141–150.

100.  Heinonen EH, Myllyla V. Safety of selegiline (deprenyl) in the treatment of Parkinson's disease. Drug Safety 1998; 19:11–22.

101.  Kaakkola S. Clinical pharmacology, therapeutic use and potential of COMT inhibitors in Parkinson's disease. Drugs 2000; 59:1233–1250.

102.  Lees AJ, Blackburn NA, Campbell VL. The nighttime problems of Parkinson's disease. Clin Neuropharmacol 1998; 11:512–519.

103.  Karlsen KH, Larsen JP, Tandberg E, Maeland JG. Influence of clinical and demographic variables on quality of life in patients with Parkinson's disease. J Neurol Neurosurg Psychiatry 1999; 66:431–435.

104.  Larsen JP, Tandberg E. Sleep disorders in patients with Parkinson's disease: epidemiology and management. CNS Drugs 2001; 15:267–275.

105.  Kumar S, Bhatia M, Behari M. Sleep disorders in Parkinson's disease. Movement Disord 2002; 17:775–781.

106.  Factor SA, McAlarney T, Sanchez-Ramos JR, Weiner WJ. Sleep disorders and sleep effect in Parkinson's disease. Movement Disord 1990; 5:280–285.

107.  Stocchi F, Barbato L, Nordera G, Berardelli A, Ruggieri S. Sleep disorders in Parkinson's disease. J Neurol 1998; 245:S15–S18.

108.  Rye DB, Bliwise DL, Dihenia B, Gurecki P. Daytime sleepiness in Parkinson's disease. J Sleep Res 2000; 9:63–69.

109.  Happe S, Berger K, FAQT Study Investigators. The association of dopamine agonists with daytime sleepiness, sleep problems and quality of life in patients with Parkinson's disease—a prospective study. J Neurol 2001; 248:1062–1067.

110.  Jaffe SE. Sleep and infectious disease. In: Kryger MH, Roth T, and Dement WC, eds. Principles and Practice of Sleep Medicine. Philadelphia: WB Saunders, 2000:1093–1102.

111.  Happe S, Ludemann P, Berger K, investigators Fs. The association between disease severity and sleep-related problems in patients with Parkinson's disease. Neuropsychobiology 2002; 46:90–96.

112.  Tan EK, Lum SY, Fook-Chong SM, Teoh ML, Yih Y, Tan L, Tan A, Wong MC. Evaluation of somnolence in Parkinson's disease: comparison with age- and sex-matched controls. Neurology 2002; 58:465–468.

113.  Schafer D, Greulich W. Effects of parkinsonian medication on sleep. J Neurol 2000; 247:24–27.

114.  Kales A, Ansel RD, Markham CH, Scharf MB, Tan TL. Sleep in patients with Parkinson's disease and normal subjects prior to and following levodopa administration. Clin Pharmacol Ther 1971; 12:397–406.

115.  Bergonzi P, Chiurulla C, Gambi D, Mennuni G, Pinto F. L-Dopa plus dopa-decarboxylase inhibitor: sleep organization in Parkinson's syndrome before and after treatment. Acta Neurol Belg 1975; 75:5–10.

116.  Apps MC, Sheaff PC, Ingram DA, Kennard C, Empey DW. Respiration and sleep in Parkinson's disease. J Neurol Neurosurg Psychiatry 1985; 48:1240–1245.

117.  Schenck CH, Bundlie SR, Mahowald MW. Delayed emergence of a parkinsonian disorder in 38% of 29 older men initially diagnosed with idiopathic rapid eye movement sleep behavior disorder. Neurology 1996; 46:388–393.

118.  Moller JC, Stiasny K, Hargutt V, Cassel W, Tietze H, Peter JH, Kruger HP, Oertel WH. Evaluation of sleep and driving performance in six patients with Parkinson's

disease reporting sudden onset of sleep under dopaminergic medication: a pilot study. Movement Disord 2002; 17:474–481.

119. Friedman A. Sleep pattern in Parkinson's disease. Acta Med Polona 1980; 21:193–199.

120. Ondo WG, Dat Vuong K, Khan H, Atassi F, Kwak C, Jankovic J. Daytime sleepiness and other sleep disorders in Parkinson's disease. Neurology 2001; 57:1392–1396.

121. Brunner H, Wetter TC, Hogl B, Yassouridis A, Trenkwalder C, Friess E. Microstructure of the non-rapid eye movement sleep electroencephalogram in patients with newly diagnosed Parkinson's disease: effects of dopaminergic treatment. Movement Disord 2002; 17:928–933.

122. Mouret J. Differences in sleep in patients with Parkinson's disease. Electroencephalogr Clin Neurophysiol 1975; 38:653–657.

123. Wetter TC, Brunner H, Hogl B, Yassouridis A, Trenkwalder C, Friess E. Increased alpha activity in REM sleep in de novo patients with Parkinson's disease. Movement Disord 2001; 16:928–933.

124. Garcia-Borreguero D, Caminero AB, De La Llave Y, Larrosa O, Barrio S, Granizo JJ, Pareja JA. Decreased phasic EMG activity during rapid eye movement sleep in treatment-naive Parkinson's disease: effects of treatment with levodopa and progression of illness. Movement Disord 2002; 17:934–941.

125. Comella CL, Tanner CM, Ristanovic RK. Polysomnographic sleep measures in Parkinson's disease patients with treatment-induced hallucinations. Ann Neurol 1993; 34:710–714.

126. Arnulf I, Konofal E, Merino-Andreu M, Houeto JL, Mesnage V, Welter ML, Lacomblez L, Golmard JL, Derenne JP, Agid Y. Parkinson's disease and sleepiness: an integral part of PD. Neurology 2002; 58:1019–1024.

127. Gagnon JF, Bedard MA, Fantini ML, Petit D, Panisset M, Rompre S, Carrier J, Montplaisir J. REM sleep behavior disorder and REM sleep without atonia in Parkinson's disease. Neurology 2002; 59:585–589.

128. Wetter TC, Trenkwalder C, Gershanik O, Hogl B. Polysomnographic measures in Parkinson's disease: a comparison between patients with and without REM sleep disturbances. Wien Klini Wochenschr 2001; 113:249–253.

129. Ferini-Strambi L, Zucconi M. REM sleep behavior disorder. Clini Neurophysiol 2000; 111:S136–S140.

130. Smith MC, Ellgring H, Oertel WH. Sleep disturbances in Parkinson's disease patients and spouses. J Am Geriatr Soci 1997; 45:194–199.

131. Lemke MR. Effect of reboxetine on depression in Parkinson's disease patients. J Clin Psychiatry 2002; 63:300–304.

132. Hovestadt A, Bogaard JM, Meerwaldt JD, van der Meche FG, Stigt J. Pulmonary function in Parkinson's disease. J Neurol Neurosurg Psychiatry 1989; 52:329–333.

133. Vincken WG, Gauthier SG, Dollfuss RE, Hanson RE, Darauay CM, Cosio MG. Involvement of upper-airway muscles in extrapyramidal disorders: a cause of airflow limitation. N Engl J Med 1984; 311:438–442.

134. Ferini-Strambi L, Franceschi M, Pinto P, Zucconi M, Smirne S. Respiration and heart rate variability during sleep in untreated Parkinson patients. Gerontology 1992; 38:92–98.

135. Chaudhuri KR. Autonomic dysfunction in movement disorders. Curr Opin Neurol 2001; 14:505–511.

136.  Stern M, Roffwarg H, Duvoisin R. The parkinsonian tremor in sleep. J Nerv Ment Disord 1968; 147:202–210.
137.  Fish DR, Sawyers D, Allen PJ, Blackie JD, Lees AJ, Marsden CD. The effect of sleep on the dyskinetic movements of Parkinson's disease, Gilles de la Tourette syndrome, Huntington's disease, and torsion dystonia. Arch Neurol 1991; 48:210–214.
138.  Tan A, Salgado M, Fahn S. Rapid eye movement sleep behavior disorder preceding Parkinson's disease with therapeutic response to levodopa. Movement Disord 1996; 11:214–216.
139.  Aldrich MS. Parkinsonism. In: Kryger MH, Roth T, and Dement WC, eds. Principles and Practice of Sleep Medicine. Philadelphia: WB Saunders, 2000:1051–1057.
140.  Leeman AL, O'Neill CJ, Nicholson PW, Deshmukh AA, Denham MJ, Royston JP, Dobbs RJ, Dobbs SM. Parkinson's disease in the elderly: response to and optimal spacing of night time dosing with levodopa. Br J Clin Pharmacol 1987; 24:637–643.
141.  Askenasy JJ, Yahr MD. Reversal of sleep disturbance in Parkinson's disease by antiparkinsonian therapy: a preliminary study. Neurology 1985; 35:527–532.
142.  Lang AE, Quinn N, Brincat S, Marsden CD, Parkes JD. Pergolide in late-stage Parkinson disease. Ann Neurol 1982; 12:243–247.
143.  Sharf B, Moskovitz C, Lupton MD, Klawans HL. Dream phenomena induced by chronic levodopa therapy. J Neural Transmiss 1978; 43:143–151.
144.  Klawans HL, Goetz C, Bergen D. Levodopa-induced myoclonus. Arch Neurol 1975; 32:330–334.
145.  Vardi J, Glaubman H, Rabey JM, Streifler M. Myoclonic attacks induced by L-dopa and bromocryptin in Parkinson patients: a sleep EEG study. J Neurol 1978; 218:35–42.
146.  Vardi J, Glaubman H, Rabey J, Streifler M. EEG sleep patterns in Parkinsonian patients treated with bromocryptine and L-dopa: a comparative study. J Neural Transmiss 1979; 45:307–316.
147.  Menza MA, Rosen RC. Sleep in Parkinson's disease: the role of depression and anxiety. Psychosomatics 1995; 36:262–266.
148.  Gislason T, Almqvist M. Somatic diseases and sleep complaints: an epidemiological study of 3,201 Swedish men. Acta Med Scand 1987; 221:475–481.
149.  Schiavi RC, Stimmel BB, Mandeli J, Rayfield EJ. Diabetes, sleep disorders, and male sexual function. Biol Psychiatry 1993; 34:171–177.
150.  Sridhar GR, Madhu K. Prevalence of sleep disturbances in diabetes mellitus. Diabetes Res Clin Pract 1994; 23:183–186.
151.  Lamond N, Tiggemann M, Dawson D. Factors predicting sleep disruption in Type II diabetes. Sleep 2000; 23:415–416.
152.  Montplaisir J, Nicolas A, Godbout R, Walters A. Restless legs syndrome and periodic limb movement disorders. In: Kryger NH, Roth T, and Dement WC, eds. Principles and Practice of Sleep Medicine. Philadelphia: WB Saunders, 2000:742–752.
153.  Grunstein RR. Endocrine disorders. In: Kryger NH, Roth T, and Dement WC, eds. Principles and Practice of Sleep Medicine. Philadelphia: WB Saunders, 2000:1103–1112.
154.  Phipps PR, Starritt E, Caterson I, Grunstein RR. Association of serum leptin with hypoventilation in human obesity. Thorax 2002; 57:75–76.

155. Resnick L, Berger JR, Shapshak P, Tourtellotte WW. Early penetration of the blood-brain-barrier by HIV. Neurology 1988; 38:9–14.

156. Ficker JH, Dertinger SH, Siegfried W, Konig HJ, Pentz M, Sailer D, Katalinic A, Hahn EG. Obstructive sleep apnoea and diabetes mellitus: the role of cardiovascular autonomic neuropathy. Eur Respir J 1998; 11:14–19.

157. Rees PJ, Prior JG, Cochrane GM, Clark TJ. Sleep apnoea in diabetic patients with autonomic neuropathy. J Roy Soc Med 1981; 74:192–195.

158. Sobotka PA, Liss HP, Vinik AI. Impaired hypoxic ventilatory drive in diabetic patients with autonomic neuropathy. J Clin Endocrinol Metab 1986; 62:658–663.

159. Neumann C, Martinez D, Schmid H. Nocturnal oxygen desaturation in diabetic patients with severe autonomic neuropathy. Diabetes Res Clin Pract 1995; 28:97–102.

160. Matyka KA, Crawford C, Wiggs L, Dunger DB, Stores G. Alterations in sleep physiology in young children with insulin-dependent diabetes mellitus: relationship to nocturnal hypoglycemia. J Pediatr 2000; 137:233–238.

161. Porter PA, Byrne G, Stick S, Jones TW. Nocturnal hypoglycaemia and sleep disturbances in young teenagers with insulin dependent diabetes mellitus. Arch Dis Child 1996; 75:120–123.

162. Shibui K, Uchiyama M, Okawa M. Melatonin rhythms in delayed sleep phase syndrome. J Biol Rhythms 1999; 14:72–76.

163. Weitzman ED, Czeisler CA, Coleman RM, Spielman AJ, Zimmerman JC, Dement W, Richardson G, Pollak CP. Delayed sleep phase syndrome: a chronobiological disorder with sleep-onset insomnia. Arch Gen Psychiatry 1981; 38:737–746.

164. Pelayo RP, Thorpy MJ, Glovinsky P. Prevalence of delayed sleep phase syndrome among adolescents. J Sleep Res 1988; 17:392.

165. Regestein QR, Pavlova M. Treatment of delayed sleep phase syndrome. Gen Hosp Psychiatry 1995; 17:335–345.

166. Ando K, Kripke DF, Ancoli-Israel S. Estimated prevalence of delayed and advance sleep phase syndromes. J Sleep Res 1995; 24:509.

167. Carskadon MA. Patterns of sleep and sleepiness in adolescents. Pediatrician 1990; 17:5–12.

168. Link SC, Ancoli-Israel S. Sleep and the teenager. Sleep Res 1995; 24A:

169. Reid KJ, Zeldow M, Teplin LA, McClelland GM, Abram KA, Zee PC. Sleep habits of juvenile detainees in the Chicago area. Sleep 2002; 25:A433–A434.

170. Ancoli-Israel S, Schnierow B, Kelsoe J, Fink R. A pedigree of one family with delayed sleep phase syndrome. Chronobiol Int 2001; 18:831–840.

171. Czeisler CA, Richardson GS, Coleman RM, Zimmerman JC, Moore-Ede MC, Dement WC, Weitzman ED. Chronotherapy: resetting the circadian clocks of patients with delayed sleep phase insomnia. Sleep 1981; 4:1–21.

172. Rosenthal NE, Joseph-Vanderpool JR, Levendosky AA, Johnston SH, Allen R, Kelly KA, Souetre E, Schultz PM, Starz KE. Phase-shifting effects of bright morning light as treatment for delayed sleep phase syndrome. Sleep 1990; 13:354–361.

173. Regestein QR, Monk TH. Delayed sleep phase syndrome: a review of its clinical aspects. Am J Psychiatry 1995; 152:602–608.

174. Arendt J. Complex effects of melatonin. Therapie 1998; 53:479–488.

175. Dawson D, Encel N. Melatonin and sleep in humans. J Pineal Res 1993; 15:1–12.

176. Myers BL, Badia P. Changes in circadian rhythms and sleep quality with aging: mechanisms and interventions. Neurosci Biobehav Rev 1995; 19:553–571.

177. Dawson D, Armstrong SM. Chronobiotics—drugs that shift rhythms. Pharmacol Ther 1996; 69:15–36.

178. Wirz-Justice A, Armstrong SM. Melatonin: nature's soporific? J Sleep Res 1996; 5:137–141.

179. Arendt J. In what circumstances is melatonin a useful sleep therapy? Consensus statement, WFSRS focus group, Dresden, November 1999. J Sleep Res 2000; 9:397–398.

180. Dahlitz M, Alvarez B, Vignau J, English J, Arendt J, Parkes JD. Delayed sleep phase syndrome response to melatonin. Lancet 1991; 337:1121–1124.

181. Oldani A, Ferini-Strambi L, Zucconi M, Stankov B, Fraschini F, Smirne S. Melatonin and delayed sleep phase syndrome: ambulatory polygraphic evaluation. Neuroreport 1994; 6:132–134.

182. Dagan Y, Yovel I, Hallis D, Eisenstein M, Raichik I. Evaluating the role of melatonin in the long-term treatment of delayed sleep phase syndrome (DSPS). Chronobiol Int 1998; 15:181–190.

183. Nagtegaal JE, Kerkhof GA, Smits MG, Swart AC, Van Der Meer YG. Delayed sleep phase syndrome: a placebo-controlled cross-over study on the effects of melatonin administered five hours before the individual dim light melatonin onset. J Sleep Res 1998; 7:135–143.

184. Lewy AJ, Bauer VK, Ahmed S, Thomas KH, Cutler NL, Singer CM, Moffit MT, Sack RL. The human phase response curve (PRC) to melatonin is about 12 hours out of phase with the PRC to light. Chronobiol Int 1998; 15:71–83.

185. Moldofsky H. Sleep and the immune system. Int J Immunopharmacol 1995; 17:649–654.

186. Pollmacher T, Holsboer, F. Sleep-wake disturbances in HIV-infected patients: a potential model of the interactions between sleep and the immune system. Sleep Res Soc Bull 1996; 2:37–42.

187. Moldofsky H, Lue FA, Eisen J, Keystone E, Gorczynski RM. The relationship of interleukin-1 and immune functions to sleep in humans. Psychosom Med 1986; 48:309–318.

188. Krueger JM, Johannsen L. Bacterial products, cytokines and sleep. J Rheumatol 1989 suppl; 19:52–57.

189. Mullington J, Korth C, Hermann DM, Orth A, Galanos C, Holsboer F, Pollmacher T. Dose-dependent effects of endotoxin on human sleep. Am J Physiol 2000; 278:R947–R955.

190. Benham H, Roehrs T, Koskorek G, Fortier J, Rosenthal L, Roth T. Effects of rhinovirus type 23 on sleep and daytime function. Sleep 1998; 21:176.

191. Moeller AA, Oechsner M, Backmund HC, Popescu M, Emminger C, Holsboer F. Self-reported sleep quality in HIV infection: correlation to the stage of infection and zidovudine therapy. J AIDS 1991; 4:1000–1003.

192. Wilson IB, Cleary PD. Clinical predictors of declines in physical functioning in persons with AIDS: results of a longitudinal study. J AIDS 1997; 16:343–349.

193. Walker K. Depression. Profess Nurse 1997; 12:872–874.

194. Darko DF, Mitler MM, Miller JC. Growth hormone, fatigue, poor sleep, and disability in HIV infection. Neuroendocrinology 1998; 67:317–324.

195. Rubinstein ML, Selwyn PA. High prevalence of insomnia in an outpatient population with HIV infection. J AIDS 1998; 19:260–265.

196. van Servellen G, Sarna L, Jablonski KJ. Women with HIV: living with symptoms. West J Nurs Res 1998; 20:448–464.

197. Groopman JE. Fatigue in cancer and HIV/AIDS. Oncology 1998; 12:335–344.
198. Darko DF, Mitler MM, Henriksen SJ. Lentiviral infection, immune response peptides and sleep. Adv Neuroimmunol 1995; 5:57–77.
199. Penzak SR, Reddy YS, Grimsley SR. Depression in patients with HIV infection. Amer J Health Syst Pharm 2000; 57:376–386.
200. Fukunishi I, Matsumoto T, Negishi M, Hayashi M, Hosaka T, Moriya H. Somatic complaints associated with depressive symptoms in HIV-positive patients. Psychother Psychosom 1997; 66:248–251.
201. Perkins DO, Leserman J, Stern RA, Baum SF, Liao D, Golden RN, Evans DL. Somatic symptoms and HIV infection: relationship to depressive symptoms and indicators of HIV disease. Am J Psychiatry 1995; 152:1776–1781.
202. Cohen FL, Ferrans CE, Vizgirda V, Kunkle V, Cloninger L. Sleep in men and women infected with human immunodeficiency virus. Holistic Nurs Pract 1996; 10:33–43.
203. O'Dell MW, Meighen M, Riggs RV. Correlates of fatigue in HIV infection prior to AIDS: a pilot study. Disabil Rehabil 1996; 18:249–254.
204. Wiegand M, Moller AA, Schreiber W, Krieg JC, Fuchs D, Wachter H, Holsboer F. Nocturnal sleep EEG in patients with HIV infection. Eur Arch Psychiatry Clin Neurosci 1991; 240:153–158.
205. Norman SE, Resnick L, Cohn MA, Duara R, Herbst J, Berger JR. Sleep disturbances in HIV-seropositive patients. JAMA 1988; 260:922.
206. Norman SE, Demirozu MC, Chediak AD. Distorted sleep architecture (NREM-REM sleep cycles) in HIV healthy infected men. Sleep Res 1990; 19:340.
207. Norman SE, Demirozu MC, Chediak AD. Disturbed sleep architecture (NREM/REM sleep cycles) in HIV-infected healthy men. Sleep Research 1990; 19:339.
208. Norman SE, Chediak AD, Freeman C, Kiel M, Mendez A, Duncan R, Simoneau J, Nolan B. Sleep disturbances in men with asymptomatic human immunodeficiency (HIV) infection. Sleep 1992; 15:150–155.
209. White JL, Darko DF, Brown SJ, Miller JC, Hayduk R, Kelly T, Mitler MM. Early central nervous system response to HIV infection: sleep distortion and cognitive-motor decrements. AIDS 1995; 9:1043–1050.
210. Norman SE, Chediak AD, Kiel M, Cohn MA. Sleep disturbances in HIV-infected homosexual men. AIDS 1990; 4:775–781.
211. Darko DF, Mitler MM, Prospero-Garcia O, Henriksen SJ. Sleep and lentivirus infection: parallel observations obtained from human and animal studies. Sleep Res Soc Bull 1996; 2:43–51.
212. Franck LS, Johnson LM, Lee K, Hepner C, Lambert L, Passeri M, Manio E, Dorenbaum A, Wara D. Sleep disturbances in children with human immunodeficiency virus infection. Pediatrics 1999; 104:e62.
213. Lee KA, Portillo CJ, Miramontes H. The fatigue experience for women with human immunodeficiency virus. J Obstet Gynecol Neonat Nur 1999; 28:193–200.
214. Darko DF, McCutchan JA, Kripke DF, Gillin JC, Golshan S. Fatigue, sleep disturbance, disability, and indices of progression of HIV infection. Am J Psychiatry 1992; 149:514–520.

# 7

# Neonates

**PINGFU FENG**

Case Western Reserve University and Wade Park VA Medical Center, Cleveland, Ohio, U.S.A.

## I.  Behavior and Biology of Sleep-Wake States in the Postnatal Period

The newborns of birds including chickens and of some mammals such as guinea pigs and sheep can open their eyes, eat, and exhibit sleep-wake cycles similar to those found in adulthood (1–4); these animals are "precocial" species. The newborns of other mammals such as those of rats, cats, and rabbits are not able to open their eyes at birth and have very different sleep-wake states from their adulthood (4,5). These species are "altricial" mammals. There are also a variety of developmental and anatomical brain differences in altricial and precocial species that appear to relate to learning and experiential development (1).

Both the words "neonatal" and "postnatal" (PN) have been used in the study of early-life phenomena in rats. "Neonatal" refers to a period from birth to 2 weeks in the clinic. The developmental level of the newborn rat is equal to the third trimester of the human fetus and the 2-week old rat is equal to the human newborn (6). Landmarks in the rat are the eye opening and the end of so-called "stress hyporesponsive period" (SHRP) at this age (7). Thus, it is reasonable to call a rat "neonatal" at the age of 2 weeks or younger. There are more landmarks during the developmental period. One is that sleep-wake distribution nears adult level and the other is the appearance of sexual activity. Ages at these landmarks in the rat are approximately 1 month for the former and 2 months for the latter (4). Thus, it is important to consider the timing of neonatal rapid-eye-movement

(REM) sleep deprivation (RSD) and the potential that there are different effects depending on when an intervention is applied. Most studies of neonatal RSD are conducted between PN 8 and PN 21 and thus span a time when there are changes in the normal ontogeny of sleep.

### A.  Neonatal Sleep and Wakefulness

Sleep and the high frequency of phasic activities, particularly muscle twitches, dominate the daily life of altricial mammals and human neonates. "Active sleep" is the term that has been used to describe these behavioral phenomena in the rat, cat, and rabbit in comparison with a sleep state without phasic activities, which is called "quiet sleep" (4). Rapid eye movements (REMs) are recorded during active sleep but rarely during quiet sleep. Thus, visually scored active sleep is roughly the state of REM sleep. However, a small portion of visually scored active sleep (i.e., behaviorally "active" sleep) may show high-amplitude EEG at PN 10 or older in the rat if recorded by a polygraph. This type of sleep is first called "half-activated sleep" but is mostly scored as slow-wave sleep or non-REM (NREM) sleep (4,8). This implies that REM sleep could better distinguish the difference between sleep states when it applies, and the usage of active sleep should be limited to describe the sleep state in the neonatal period. Developmental features of sleep-wake states include: (1) REM sleep (active sleep) dramatically decreases, starting from a very high percent (>70%) and then replaced by wakefulness and NREM sleep; and (2) a high frequency of phasic activities occurs that dramatically decreases. The active (voluntary) behavioral activity during the wake state significantly increases as waking time is prolonged. Simultaneously, brain plasticity dramatically decreases (9).

The typical feature of neonatal REM sleep is that it starts from the highest percentage shortly after birth and then decreases as maturation proceeds (Fig. 1). According to Jouvet-Monier et al., the neonatal rat spends 72% of time in REM sleep in the first 10 days of life and this percentage dramatically drops to 40% or less during the second week (4). About one third of time is distributed almost equally into each state of wake, REM sleep, and NREM sleep by the end of the second week, according to our study using a long-term, continuous polysomnographic recording method (10). Over the third and fourth week, REM sleep continues to decrease and reaches the level (14%) near adulthood by the end of the fourth week (4,10). Thus, REM sleep drops 80% over the first month of life. In addition to the change in REM sleep percentage, there is a decrease in the number of REM sleep episodes, mean REM period duration, and number of sleep-onset REM periods. REM latency also dramatically increases during this period. All of these changes are closely correlated with the change of age. It may be noteworthy that the number of REM episodes and the mean duration of each REM period decrease together. Thus, propensity to initiate REM sleep episodes and the propensity to sustain REM sleep episodes decrease monotonically from age 2 weeks to age 4 weeks (10,38).

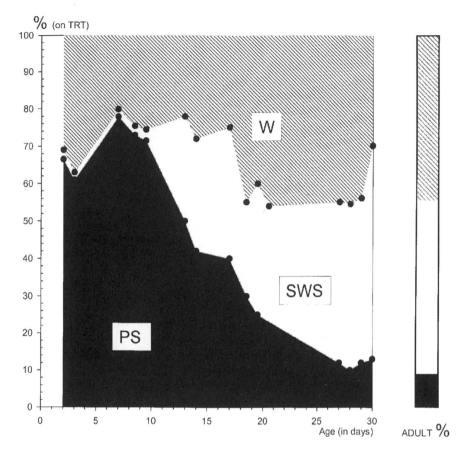

**Figure 1** Ontogeny of sleep-wake states in the first month of life in the rat. REM sleep dominates daily life in the first postnatal week. Waking without eyes open is about 30% or less. NREM sleep, however, is almost zero during this period of time. Thereafter, REM sleep is dramatically decreased while wake and NREM sleep increase. (From Ref. 4.)

Quiet sleep, used to describe a sleep state without phasic movements in the first 2 weeks of life, is behaviorally and polysomnographically identical to NREM sleep (4). The actually scored NREM sleep, however, includes the part of half-activated sleep, which comprises a small portion of total NREM sleep (4,8). This type of sleep is found to be almost nonexistent in the first week and increases to about 15% in the second week. By PN 12, NREM sleep is identified by high-amplitude EEG, and increases, rapidly paralleling the increase of wakefulness. Newborn rats do not open their eyes until PN 14. Their wake state is identified as behavioral waking, such as walking and eating without eyes open. This state is only 10–30% in the first 2 weeks of life. Similar to REM sleep development, all states develop to a near-adult level at the end of the fourth week (4).

Considering the fact that an increase in the percentage of wake parallels the decrease of REM sleep, the wake/REM (W/R) ratio might be an important index to describe the developmental levels in altricial mammals. This ratio is about 0.4 (28%/72%) in the first 10 days of life in the rat (4), dramatically increases to 1.77 at PN 21, 3.99 at PN 26 (9), and 8.1 in adulthood (calculated from Ref. 152). This ratio is 1.0 in the human newborn and is 2.6, 10.3, and 11 at PN 1, PN 14–18, and adult, respectively (calculated from Ref. 12). The developmental features of sleep-wake states suggest that the strong REM sleep propensity in neonates is progressively suppressed or that a REM sleep inhibitory process is immature in neonatal rats.

Phasic muscle twitches are one of the major REM phasic activities in neonates and also comprise prominent neonatal behavior. A similar feature is found not only in rats but also in other rodents and humans. The period that shows frequent muscle twitches is the first 4 weeks in the rat (4), the first 40 days in the kitten (8), and the first 8 months in the human newborn (13). In humans, this feature is more typical in the premature fetus (14). This activity appears primarily during REM sleep but also in a small portion of NREM sleep, i.e., "half-activated" sleep (4). The rate of muscle twitches is only 1.5/min and 0.3/min during quiet sleep compared to the rate of 7.5/min and 3/min, respectively, during REM sleep at the same age in PN 10 and PN 20 kittens (8). The number of phasic events dramatically decreases as animals mature (8,9,13,15). It is of interest to note that the dramatic reduction of phasic activities in REM sleep is associated with the increase of wakefulness.

### B.  Neural Substrates for Neonatal REM Sleep

One of the major concerns in neonatal regulation of sleep-wake states is the neuronal and molecular mechanism for generation of the high percentage of REM sleep because this is the major difference in sleep-wake states between neonates and adults. One viewpoint of the decline of REM sleep is that a REM-inhibitory system develops as the rat matures (10). It is very likely that this inhibitory system is the same one as the wake generation system because most wake-promoting neurotransmitters and peptides suppress REM sleep in adult observations (9,16–18). At any rate, the explanation of the high percentage and progressive decrease of REM sleep remains a puzzle.

Laterodorsal and pedunculopontine tegmental (LDT/PPT) cholinergic neurons have been identified as the REM sleep generation neurons in adults (11). Cholinergic neurons in the LDT/PPT project to and provide acetylcholine (Ach) to cholinoceptive medial pontine reticular formation (mPRF) neurons (17,19–21). Muscarinic (M) cholinergic receptors have been identified in at least five subtypes (M1–M5). M2 and M4 receptors are believed to contribute to cholinergic REM sleep generation. M2 autoreceptors regulate Ach release within the mPRF, and mPRF microinjections have shown that components of the signal transduction pathway modulated by M2/M4 receptors participate in cholinergic REM sleep generation. Cholinergic LDT/PPT neurons can be phenotypically defined based on the presence of the Ach synthetic enzyme choline acetyltransferase (ChAT) and the presence of a vesicular Ach transporter (VAchT) (22,23).

Rat PPT neurons are capable of responding to stimulation and treatment with cholinergic drugs when tested at the age of PN 12 and 21 (24). This indicates that the cholinergic system may play a role in REM sleep regulation in neonates similar to that of adulthood. Provided that REM sleep and phasic activities are driven by certain neuronal or humoral systems, the functional indication of this system, such as the level of the transmitters or the density of receptors or critical enzymes involved in this mechanism, should have a developmental pattern similar to that of REM sleep, i.e., showing the highest level in the neonate and then progressively decreasing as maturation proceeds. Actual findings from ontogeny studies are that brain levels of Ach and acetylcholinesterase (AchE) activity are low in neonates and gradually increase. The Ach level attains adult values at the seventieth day and AchE activity shows a rapid increase between the seventh and thirtieth days (25). The time course of the increase in ChAT activity correlates to that of the decrease in the amount of REM sleep or phasic activities after birth (26). None of the M1–M5 receptors in the brain regions of cortex, hippocampus, basal forebrain, and striatum exhibits the changing pattern similar to that of REM sleep (27–31). In fact, M1 receptors are expressed at 31% of adult levels, M2 receptors at 32% of adult levels, M3 receptors at 36% of adult levels, and M4 receptors at 20% of adult levels in 3–4-day-old neonates. The combined M2/M4 receptor density increases at a uniform rate during development from 173 to 757 fmol/mg (28). These observations suggest that cholinergic function may not be the major driving force to the high percentage of REM sleep, but rather plays a critical role in the executive generation of REM sleep during the neonatal period.

Looking into other neural systems involved in sleep-wake regulation, none of the 5-HT, dopaminergic, noradrenergic, and GABAergic systems or orexinergic neurons seems to promote REM sleep (18,32,33). Adenosine neurons were recently found to promote NREM but not REM sleep (34). Glutamate is one of the major excitatory neurotransmitters in the brain and exhibits cholinergic LDT/PPT exciting effect (35). However, it does not stimulate cholinergic PPT neurons in the rat between PN 12 and PN 21 (24). Therefore, there is still no evidence to address the question of neonatal regulation of sleep-wakefulness including the driving force for the high percentage of REM sleep.

## II.   Neonatal REM Sleep Deprivation: Methodological Considerations

Only RSD has been studied in neonates. Three reasons may apply: (a) REM sleep may have more attraction for its special feature as a driving force for neural development. (b) REM sleep occupies about 70% of time followed by wakefulness, and NREM sleep occupies only a very small proportion of daily behavior. (c)

Total sleep deprivation may not be performed easily because wake capacity is very low in neonates. The method of RSD by nondrug means has been developed and proven to be equally effective as RSD by drug. Since neonates are very sensitive to all kinds of stimulation and instrumental RSD (IRSD) has unavoidable mechanical stimulation, the application of IRSD in the neonate must be accompanied by a reasonable yoked control. Computer-controlled IRSD may not be applied before PN 12 because NREM sleep is undetectable before this age.

### A.   Environmental Confounders

Even though there is evidence of the existence of neuronal plasticity in adulthood, the developing brain is more sensitive to exogenous and endogenous stimulation. Maternal separation, social isolation, maternal handling, and enriched or improvised environments all affect brain and behavioral development (36,37). Factors that are not strong enough to produce effects on adult brain may be strong enough to produce significant effects on neonates (38). Three to six hours of daily maternal deprivation for 10 days produces persistent behavioral, humoral, and neuronal changes including an elevated hypothalamic-pituitary-adrenal (HPA) axis, underfunctional brain monoaminergic systems, and stress-like behaviors (36,37,39–47). In contrast, maternal handling produces behavioral and molecular effects against maternal deprivation (7,47). Maternally handled adult rats had significantly lower levels of corticotrophin-releasing factor (CRF) in the median eminence in basal and stress conditions compared to nonhandled control rats and maternally deprived adult rats, which had significantly increased basal and stress levels of CRF (47,48).

### B.   Drug RSD

Drug administration is a common method to study neonatal RSD. Both subcutaneous injection and oral administration are applicable. The consequence of neonatal RSD by drug depends on the dose and the way that the drug was administered, such as the treatment duration (38,49). In contrast to an adult response, RSD in the rat at age 2 weeks or younger does not produce a REM rebound to REM suppression (50). Therefore, a dose-response relationship between drug and REM suppression is not as easy to differentiate as in adult models. For uniformity, an injection of a full dose once a day may not produce the same result as an injection of this dose split into a twice-daily dose (51). One to two weeks of total treatment duration with appropriate doses has been proven to be effective in producing long-term developmental abnormalities (38).

The magnitude of behavioral abnormalities produced by neonatal treatment with RSD drug depends on the dose of the drug. Vogel et al. reported that abnormalities of six sexual variables are found to be dependent on the neonatal treatment dose of clomipramine (CLI). The 30 mg/kg/day dose caused deficiencies in some, but not all, sexual behavior measures; higher doses caused deficiencies in all measures of sexual behavior (49). There is also a dose-response characteristic corresponding to the age of treatment. One week or longer treatment of RSD conducted either in the PN first or third week produced persistent effect on the brain aminergic system (52,53). Similar treatment started after the third week, however, was not able to produce such an effect (38). This fact indicates that the rat is more susceptible to RSD during the period from birth to the third week. This "sensitive" period corresponds to the evolution of sleep-wake states since by PN 28–30, an adult type of sleep-wake pattern and percentage of sleep-wake distribution has emerged (4). However, a sensitive period may be different depending on the stimulation and the measured outcomes. For example, the reactive secretion of hypophyseal adrenocorticotropic hormone (ACTH) induced by the stimulation of saline injection is larger in older than in younger rats in the first 2 weeks of life (54). Hence, the long-term pathological effect produced by neonatal RSD may depend on the total REM sleep reduction as well as the timing of the intervention. Since REM sleep shows the highest percentage and the most occurrence of phasic activities in PN 0–8, the same dose of drug would result in more REM sleep loss in younger rats than in older ones (9). Alternatively, the susceptibility of the neonates could coincide with the development of wakefulness.

### C. Instrumental Method for RSD

To overcome the confounding effect of drug RSD, an instrumentally aroused animal would be an ideal alternative. Mirmiran and colleagues tried the pendulum method for RSD (55). However, when applied to neonatal rats, the method does not achieve the level of RSD produced by drugs. It also substantially decreased total sleep time, thus confounding the effects of RSD with the effects of total sleep deprivation. Marks and colleagues used a variant of the small-platform-above-water method to REM-sleep-deprive kittens (56). However, neonatal rats are too small (i.e., thumb-sized) for this method. In 1990, Shaffery et al. reported RSD of one kitten by a combination of vertical vibration of the kitten's cage at REM sleep onsets for 18 hr/day and total sleep deprivation by gentle experimental handling for 6 hr/day (57). The total sleep deprivation is done in four 1 1/2-hr sessions for feeding. This is also not applicable for long-term nonstop REM sleep deprivation in the neonatal rat because the head plug may not be able to last for a lengthy time period.

The ideal IRSD would require: (1) continuous sleep recording with online sleep-wake recognition, and (2) standardized intervention to produce REM sleep reduction. Obviously the former is crucial to the success of IRSD. For many years, animal sleep has been recorded through bipolar recording from electrodes that are screwed in and cemented to the skull with dental acrylic. The developmental characteristic in the neonatal period makes automatic IRSD extremely difficult. This method, thus, does not work for the neonate because the neonatal rat skull is thin, soft, fragile, and growing. In addition, the neonatal rat typically could not survive either surgical removal of the head plug or leaving the fixed head plug and screws in place as the skull grows. Thus, the new method needs to be developed that allow continuous, chronic, neonatal sleep recording and that permit neonatal rat survival into adulthood after RSD.

A new method was developed that does not use screws as electrodes and does not cement a connector to a hard head plug on the skull; thus, it is called the soft-head-plug (SH) method. In the SH recording system, the electrode is a thin, pliable microwire instead of the screw used in the conventional recording method. The uncoated end of the wire serves as the contact electrode with tissue for both EEG and EMG recordings. Two such microwire implants are needed to make a bipolar recording. All wires exit the skin through a soft guide tube (Silastic tubing), which connects to a small connector suspended about 3 inches above the skull. After implantation of electrodes (microwires), rat pups have to be housed singly to avoid the possible damage that may result from the dam's (i.e., mother's) care. A rat cage can be separated into two compartments by a vertical wall. An IRSD rat and a yoked control rat are housed in each compartment. The cage is mounted on a test tube shaker for IRSD. Milk access and extra manual feeding are necessary. An ambient temperature of 27–28°C is the best temperature range that maintains a rat pup's body temperature consistent with an age of 2 weeks. Higher ambient temperature will bring the body temperature higher, and lower ambient temperature will bring the body temperature lower. Since rats open their eyes at PN 14, full manual feeding may be needed in a rat younger than 2 weeks, and partial manual feeding may also be needed in the PN third week (58,59).

Electrode implantation is nontraumatic to the rat. The electrodes can be left in place for weeks and can be removed without trauma. Signals from the connector are sent to a polygraph, a data processor, and a computer for paper and/or paperless recording. When the computer detects REM sleep onset in the IRSD rat, it turns the shaker on for 5 sec. In most cases, REM sleep is terminated and the IRSD rat returns to NREM sleep. The yoked control rat may have REM sleep during the period when the IRSD rat is not in REM sleep. Any data collection circuit board and compatible software that is capable of recognizing sleep-wake states and has the output control function online may be used for neonatal IRSD. A data processor (e.g., Dap 3000a/212, Microstar Lab) with customized software has been successfully used to perform neonatal IRSD (58,60).

### D.  Polysomnographic Data Analysis

The appearance of high-amplitude EEG at PN 12 makes polysomnographic data collected from the rat at PN 12 or older capable of being scored by a computer. Frequent muscle twitches occurring during REM sleep increase the total power of EMG in REM sleep. As a consequence, REM sleep may be underscored as wakefulness. Data collected during RSD, however, may not be scored by a computer program because of the artifact generated by cable movements during the shaking used to keep the IRSD rat awake in the RSD apparatus. Efforts have been made to solve this problem in several ways but are currently unsuccessful. In our studies, sleep-wake states are scored in 30-sec epochs by the following criteria:

wake is low-amplitude EEG with high-amplitude EMG; REM sleep is low-amplitude EEG with low-amplitude EMG; NREM sleep is high-amplitude EEG with low-amplitude EMG.

## III. Short-Term Effects of Neonatal REM Sleep Deprivation

The decrease of REM sleep without a corresponding increase of wakefulness might be one of the most important features in the short-term effects of neonatal RSD. This fact indicates the immature wake generator or a low waking capacity in the neonatal period. A similar observation was first reported by Mirmiran et al. (61) and described as an increase of NREM (quiet) sleep during neonatal RSD by CLI, without emphasizing its importance.

### A. Neonatal RSD Results in a Large Decrease of REM Sleep and a Small Increase of Wakefulness

During 2 days of neonatal IRSD, the mean of waking percent (of total time) increased (as total sleep decreased) 4.95%, 5.16%, and 8.86%, compared to a REM sleep reduction of 23.39%, 18.41%, and 7.93% in the same group and same time period, at age 2, 3, and 4 weeks, respectively. The amount of lost REM sleep is about threefold higher as wake increases in the same time period of the second and third week. Most of the lost REM sleep is replaced by NREM sleep at age 2 and 3 weeks, but not at 4 weeks (50). A similar result is seen in 6-day RSD by CLI and by instrumental method from the age of 2 weeks, which produces a larger REM reduction and a larger NREM sleep increase simultaneously during the treatment (Fig. 2). Lost REM sleep during neonatal RSD is compensated almost fully by NREM sleep (9). RSD by CLI increases wakefulness in adults but not in neonates (9). This is one of the major differences between RSD in adults and neonates. This suggests that the activity lost in the reduction of REM sleep during RSD in neonates cannot be replaced by the increase of behavioral activity as a general consequence of wakefulness increase. The significance of this finding is that it implicates a net loss of phasic activities during neonatal RSD (Fig. 3).

Strong stimulation by shaking in IRSD or a larger dose of CLI that is effective to increase wakefulness in adults does not increase wakefulness correspondingly in neonates. This fact indicates that the wake capacity is either very low or wake generation systems are very immature in the first 2 weeks. This is consistent with the finding that orexinergic neurons that promote wakefulness through releasing peptides of orexin A and orexin B are very immature in the neonate (18,62). The neural system responsible for the generation of NREM sleep is not known. The compensative increase of NREM sleep during neonatal RSD indicates that the capacity of NREM sleep is not low during this period of time and the NREM sleep might be a "default setting" of the neural system (9). These find-

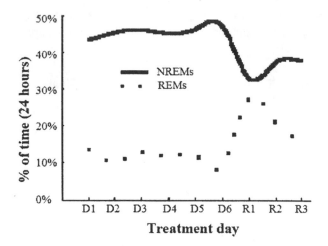

**Figure 2**  Relationship of REM sleep (REMs) and NREM sleep (NREMs) during and after RSD by clomipramine (CLI). D1–D6 means day 1–day 6 during RSD and R1–R3 means recovery day 1–3. The curved dual lines show that NREM sleep increases while REM sleep decreases, and NREM sleep decreases while REM sleep increases, indicating a well-balanced total of sleeping-waking. (From Ref. 9.)

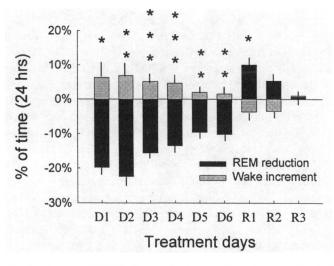

**Figure 3**  Daily changes of REM sleep and corresponding changes of wakefulness during 6 days of RSD by clomipramine (CLI) and 3 days of recovery. During CLI treatment, a larger REM sleep reduction corresponds to a smaller portion of waking changes across treatment and posttreatment days. (From Ref. 9).

ings indicate that the wake generation system develops later than the REM and NREM sleep generation systems and suggest that the increase of waking capacity is one of the most important processes during brain maturation.

### B. Neonatal RSD and REM Rebound

Another feature of RSD in the neonate is that REM rebound post-RSD does not exist at age 2 weeks, exists weakly at 3 weeks, and reaches a near-adult level at 4 weeks (50). This observation suggests that maturation of a group of neurons may play a crucial role in the generation of REM rebound. The finding that RSD produces a larger increase of NREM sleep at 2 and 3 weeks indicates that the neural mechanism responsible for NREM sleep generation exists at these ages and that the appearance of REM rebound does not positively correlate with the decrease of NREM sleep or the maturation of NREM generation. The largest REM sleep reduction during RSD at age 2 weeks does not produce a REM rebound and the smallest percentage of REM sleep reduction at age 4 weeks does produce the largest REM rebound. However, the trend of wake increase during 2 days of RSD from age 2 to 4 weeks seems to have the similar pattern as a REM rebound increase. This indicates that the increase of waking capacity and wake time during RSD may play a decisive role in the generation of REM rebound and that "wake homeostasis" seems more reasonable than sleep homeostasis in describing neonatal sleep-wake balance.

In summary, the effects of RSD in neonates are totally different from those in adults. The major features include the findings that neonatal RSD produces significant and large increases of NREM sleep rather than increases of compatible amounts of wakefulness, and that neonatal RSD results in REM rebound in older but not in younger rats. These findings indicate that REM sleep-driving neurons develop earlier than wake generation neurons and that the neural mechanism driving REM rebound is not the one that drives the high percentage of REM sleep. These findings suggest that REM rebound may depend on the maturation of the wake generation system or the increase of wake time.

## IV. Adult Consequences of Neonatal REM Sleep Deprivation

Mirmiran and colleagues (61) first studied the adult behavioral effects of neonatal RSD in rats by administering CLI, an antidepressant and a powerful REM sleep suppressant, from PN 8 through PN 21. They found an increased REM propensity and sexual behavior deficits in adult rats neonatally treated with CLI (CLI rats). Vogel and Vogel (63) hypothesized that the adult CLI rat is a model of human endogenous depression, now called melancholia, and they systemically studied the behavioral abnormalities of CLI rats thereafter (64). Similar behavioral changes are also found in adult rats neonatally treated with other REM sleep suppressants and RSD by instrumental methods (65). Application of molecular techniques brought the findings from behavioral level to neuronal level in CLI rats. The latest findings from CLI rats show that neonatal RSD may also result in defective development of wakefulness.

## A.  Adult Behavioral and Physiological Consequence of Neonatal RSD

Drug administration has been a major means of neonatal RSD in the previous studies. It has been well duplicated and documented that the neonatally REM-sleep-deprived adult rat has multiple behavioral, physiological, monoaminergic, and HPA abnormalities comparable to those of human depression (66–69). The major behavioral abnormalities found in these rats include: (a) diminished pleasure-driven behavior including diminished sexual activity (38,55,61,67–69) and decreased pleasure-seeking behavior (70); (b) dysfunctional motor activity including decreased fighting power indicated by loss in a shock-induced fighting test (71) and increased immobility (72,73); (c) increased anxiety-like behavior including increased locomotor activity (66,74,75); (d) delayed response to stimulation including increased mount latency and increased latency in a passive avoidance reaction (76); and (e) increased desire of psychostimulation indicated by increased alcohol intake (73,77,78). The sexual deficits found in the CLI rat are dose-dependent with respect to neonatal drug treatment (49).

These behavioral abnormalities also existed in the adult rat neonatally REM-sleep-deprived by an instrumental method (65). Five treatment groups were studied: an IRSD group; a yoked control (YC) group; a nonshaken, maternally separated (MS) control group; and CLI and saline-treated (SAL) home cage control groups. All treatments began at PN 14 and lasted for 7 days. Adult behavioral measurements, including those of sexual activity, locomotor activity, sleep, and shock-induced fighting, were subsequently performed. In addition to the expected findings from rats neonatally injected with CLI, the major findings were: (1) Compared with yoked control rats, IRSD rats demonstrated diminished sexual and aggressive behavior and an increased percentage of REM sleep. (2) Compared with saline-treated home cage controls, IRSD and YC rats both showed increased sexual activity and increased offensive behavior. First, these findings are compatible with the findings from neonatal RSD by CLI and support the hypothesis that RSD is the mediator of adult depressive behavior because the behavioral changes between IRSD and YC rats are similar to the differences between CLI and SAL rats. Second, the findings from comparison of YC, IRSD, and SAL rats, i.e., increased sexual activity and increased aggression, demonstrate that shaking, a nonspecific stimulant administered during the neonatal period, may contribute to the signs of this manic behavior. As discussed before, neonatal manipulation by handling resulted in adult behavioral changes that are against the maternal deprivation (7,47). Nevertheless, findings from IRSD rats demonstrate that neonatal RSD by a nondrug method produces behavioral pathological changes similar to those produced by a drug method.

Adult CLI rats also show decreased food intake (79) and hypothermia (80). Neonatal RSD by scopolamine, which acts on cholinergic neurons, and by clonidine, which acts on the adrenergic system, produce defective function in respiration (53). Both clonidine- and scopolamine-exposed animals have lower tidal volumes and respiratory quotients. In addition, clonidine-injected adult rats exhibit a higher breathing frequency (53). These findings are consistent with the findings that adult CLI rats have a decreased power of fighting and increased immobility in forced swimming tests, in terms of the function of respiration.

The first study of neonatal RSD by Mirmiran et al. reported that adult CLI rats have disinhibited REM sleep (61). Thereafter, more studies confirmed these findings. CLI rats have increased REM sleep percentages of total sleep (61,81), decreased REM latency, increased sleep-onset REM periods, increased muscle twitches during REM sleep (55,61), and more REM-rebound post-RSD (81). Unfortunately, there are no data about wake changes. According to the mean of total sleep time (333 min in adult control rats and 354 min in adult CLI rats for 8-hr recordings) and REM sleep time (28 min in control rats and 49 min in CLI rats for 8-hr recordings) presented in Mirmiran et al.'s study, the W/R ratio is 2.57 in CLI rats and 5.36 in control rats (55). Statistics, however, are not possible without original data. These findings nevertheless show that the defective development of neurons responsible for wakefulness is one of the major pathological consequences of neonatal RSD.

### B. Cellular and Molecular Correlates

Neonatal RSD has been shown to result in reduced size of brain cells and decreased protein content in the brain (56,61). Downregulated monoaminergic neuronal transmission is one of the major and consistent pathological changes in neonatally REM-sleep-deprived rats. These findings can be seen not only from neonatal RSD by CLI, but also by clonidine and scopolamine (55). The findings include: (a) reduced dorsal raphé nucleus (DRN) neuronal activity in the anesthetized CLI rat (82); (b) decreased levels of 5-HT in the frontal cortex, hypothalamus, hippocampus, and brainstem (79,83); and (c) hyporeaction of 5-HT neurons to 5-HT reuptake blocker (84). The level of noradrenaline in CLI rats is also decreased in the frontal cortex, hippocampus, brainstem, septum, and hypothalamus, but the level of dopamine is decreased only in the hippocampus (79). Neonatal RSD by scopolamine and clonidine produces similar effects on brain levels of 5-HT compared to those of CLI (53). Our preliminary findings indicate that junior CLI rats have decreased brain levels of orexin B in multiple brain regions including frontal cortex, hippocampus, and thalamus (85). These findings indicate that CLI rats have a decreased waking capacity possibly because B is a very powerful wake-promoting peptide (18). In addition, a have increased blood levels of ACTH and corticosterone, indicating hibited HPA axis (86) mechanism might also play a role.

CLI rats exhibit defective cell signal transduction in the frontal cortex and hippocampus. A common cellular response to monoamines is the activation of extracellular signal-regulated kinase (ERK), which belongs to the mitogen-activated protein kinase (MAPK) family and is involved in neuronal survival, differentiation, growth, and plasticity. The p44 ERK (ERK1) and p42 ERK (ERK2) are activated by phosphorylation in response to the neurotransmitters, including 5-HT, norepinephrine, dopamine, and neurotrophins (87–93). The phosphorylation of ERK1 and ERK2 is mediated by the MAPK/ERK kinase (MEK) (94,95). Protein phosphatases, including protein phosphatase 1 (PP1) and MAPK phosphatase-2 (MKP-2), are involved in the reversion of phosphorylated ERK (pERK) to ERK. The alterations found in adult CLI rats are decreased levels of pERK1, pERK2 in the frontal cortex, and ERK2 in the frontal cortex and hippocampus, and increased levels of PP1 in both the frontal cortex and hippocampus. However, there are no significant changes in levels of pERK1/2 in the temporal cortex, occipital cortex, parietal cortex, midbrain, or medulla (146). Findings from neonatal RSD studies indicate that a deficiency in the ERK signaling pathway is involved in the display of depressive behaviors. The defective cell signal transduction in the frontal cortex may result from decreased levels of 5-HT, because 5-HT levels are decreased in the CLI rat, and the frontal cortex has the highest density of 5-HT receptors (79,83). These findings indicate that the frontal cortex is severely impacted in CLI rats. Findings from CLI rats are similar to the findings from depressed, suicidal subjects, in which levels of pERK1/2, the levels of ERK1/2, and the expression of ERK1/2 mRNA are significantly decreased in the frontal cortex and hippocampus (96).

## C.  RSD and Depression

The up-to-date findings from neonatally REM-sleep-deprived adult rats support Vogel's hypothesis that these rats are models of human major depression with melancholic features. It has been well summarized that the CLI rat has persistent decreased pleasure-seeking behavior, prolonged responsive latency to stimulation (female rat), disinhibited REM sleep, and a decreased capacity of swimming and loss in shock-induced fighting (64,97). Reports indicate that 40–75% of human depression includes dysfunctional sexual activity (98–101). Disinhibited REM propensity, indicated by the shorter REM latency found in the adult CLI rat, is also a reliable indicator in human major depression. An elevated HPA axis, indicated by increased blood ACTH and corticosterone, is found in human depression and in the adult CLI rat (86). At the cellular level, a reliable change found in human depression is a dysfunctional 5-HT system (79,82,84,95), which is also the major pathological change in the CLI rat. At the molecular level, CLI rats share the similar pathology of defective cell signal transduction with that of suicidally depressed humans (96). Consequences of neonatal RSD may be far beyond the pathology and symptoms found in human depression. Neonatal RSD rats also display behavioral changes seen in other type of human disease, such as the limb jerks seen in attention deficit/hyperactivity disorder (ADHD) (102), restless legs syndrome (103), and sleep apnea (104); the increased phasic REM sleep seen in depression (97); and the wake-sleep disturbance seen in insomnia and circadian rhythm disorders. Neonatal RSD may also provide one of the explanations for the widespread depressive syndromes in patients who are not originally diagnosed as having depression.

Evidence also supports the hypothesis of Vogel et al. (64,97) that the consequence of neonatal RSD by CLI is mediated by RSD rather than the direct effect of CLI. CLI is a 5-HT reuptake inhibitor and may increase the effect of natural 5-HT. In adults, upregulation of 5-HT neural transmission by local and systemic application of 5-HT1a receptor agonists increase wakefulness and inhibit REM sleep (105). This effect in neonates, however, is turned into suppressing REM sleep without the increase of wakefulness, because of the immature cortex (9). One explanation for this effect is that neurons served for REM drive are much more mature than those served for wake generation. Therefore, upregulation of the 5-HT system by CLI exhibits the normal function on REM sleep suppression but not on the wake system. Adult consequences of neonatal treatment with CLI do not result from the direct effect of increasing natural 5-HT because 5-HT plays a neurotrophic role in neuronal growth (106–110). Additional support to our hypothesis is that neonatal RSD by scopolamine and clonidine results in the same effects on the brain levels of 5-HT as by CLI (53). The final support is that neonatal RSD by the instrumental method produces effects on neonatal sleep and adult behavioral abnormalities comparable to neonatal RSD by CLI (77). Hence, evidence supports our hypothesis that RSD is the common pathway through which neonatal RSD by drug produces adult pathological changes.

### D. The "RSD Paradox"

The prior section concluded that neonatal RSD produces adult depression-like behavior. Interestingly, most of the effective antidepressant agents suppress REM sleep. In Vogel's review (52), about 25 of 30 antidepressant drugs produce an arousal-type of RSD. Like RSD by arousals, these drugs produce a large, sustained RSD followed by a REM rebound. Patients with endogenous depression (major depression with melancholic features) not improved by RSD via arousals were not improved by imipramine. Thus, although a few antidepressant drugs may work by mechanisms other than RSD, the evidence suggests that most antidepressant drugs improve depression by arousal-type RSD. Sleep deprivation has been shown in more than three dozen studies published in the last three decades to produce marked and acute antidepressant effects in the majority of depressed individuals (111,112). These facts and the findings from neonatal RSD demonstrate that the effect of neonatal RSD is paradoxical to the effect of adult RSD, the so-called "RSD paradox" (97). The mechanism of RSD paradox is not known.

Crucial in the understanding of the RSD paradox is that the effect of RSD on sleep-wake states in neonates differs from that in adults (9). In adult humans,

CLI significantly reduces REM sleep and increases the number of waking episodes and waking time (105,113). In adult humans, CLI administration also shifts deep NREM sleep (stages 3 and 4; slow-wave sleep) to light NREM sleep (stages 1 and 2) and increases intrasleep restlessness (114–116). In the adult rat, ventromedial hypothalamic superinfusion of CLI produces a significant reduction of REM sleep (1.0% in the CLI group compared to 6.6% in the control group) and total sleep (16.4% in the CLI group compared to 67.0% in the control group) (105). In contrast, RSD in the neonatal rat reduces REM sleep without a comparable increase of wakefulness and results in a net loss of phasic activities; these phasic activities might be a critical drive to stimulate the development of brain and behavior.

In summary, neonatal RSD produces adult depression-like changes and behavioral changes beyond depression. In general, neonatal RSD slows the overall development of brain and behavior. At the cellular and molecular levels, neonatal RSD yields the immature features of a low-waking capacity and less voluntary movements.

## V.  New Understandings of Neonatal Sleep-Wake States

Extremely high percentages of REM sleep and frequent nonvoluntary movements (jerks) are near-mythic phenomena in neonates. Understanding the molecular mechanism of neonatal REM sleep may be crucial in understanding why the amount of REM sleep is so high in neonates.

### A.  The Driving Force of Neonatal REM Sleep

The prior sections indicate that cholinergic neurons may not be the driving force for the high percentage of REM sleep in the neonatal period. This is because the developmental patterns of the cholinergic neurotransmitters and receptors do not show a positive correlation with the change in neonatal REM sleep amounts. One interesting piece of evidence is that CRF mRNA expression does exhibit such a developmental pattern. CRF is a 41-amino-acid peptide 36, which plays an important neuroendocrine role in the regulation of the HPA axis (117), and is involved in the coordination of various responses to stress (118–120). It acts via the secretion of ACTH, which stimulates the release of adrenal glucocorticoids. In the brain, CRF induces different autonomic, electrophysiological, and behavioral effects, indicating that this peptide serves as a neuromodulator (121,122). CRF neurons are located in the hypothalamic paraventricular nucleus (PVN) and have the highest activity and secretion at the beginning of life. Birth in most animal species is triggered by the fetus through activation of the fetal HPA axis (123). CRF binding shows the highest level in the first week after birth and decreases significantly in the hippocampus and striatum from PN 7 to PN 21 (124). CRF receptor mRNA in hippocampal CA1, CA2, and CA3a increases to 300–600% of adult levels by PN 6 with a subsequent decline. In the amygdala,

CRF receptor mRNA abundance increases steadily between PN 2 and PN 9, to levels twice higher than those in the adult. In the cortex, CRF receptor mRNA levels are high on PN 2 and are decreased to adult levels by PN 12 (125).

The high levels of CRF and CRF receptor mRNA in the first 2 weeks of life in the rat co-occur with the extremely high percent of REM sleep (>70%) and phasic activities (4). Adult findings indicate a relationship between elevated HPA axis and disinhibited REM propensity. The prenatally stressed adult rat shows increased amounts of paradoxical sleep, positively correlated with plasma corticosterone levels (126). Sleep deprivation results in a stressful reaction, including elevated HPA axis and an increased REM rebound (127,128). Increased blood levels of ACTH and corticosterone are found in rats that exhibit high REM propensity (86,129). Increased cerebrospinal fluid levels of CRF, blood ACTH, and cortisol are also found in human depression (130), which has reliable signs of increased REM propensity (113). Furthermore, intracerebroventricular injection of CRF to rats after 72 hr of sleep deprivation markedly increases REM sleep (131), and a CRF antagonist blocks the sleep-deprivation-induced REM sleep rebound (132). Intracerebroventricular injection of CRF increases locomotion in the chick (133) and fish (134). The criticism may be that the increase of CRF has mostly demonstrated an increase of wakefulness in the adult (135). The arguments are: (1) The data that show CRF results in increasing wakefulness are acquired from adult animals. (2) The difference between adults and neonates is that the HPA loop is open in neonates because cells that secrete ACTH and corticosterone are immature (136). (3) Adult CLI rats and humans with depression who have elevated HPA axis and disinhibited REM propensity also have dysfunctional 5-HT systems and semiopen loops of the HPA axis as indicated by signs of a dysfunctional glucocorticoid receptor in the hypothalamus (7,86,137). Thus, evidence supports my hypothesis that CRF may play a crucial role in driving the high percentage of neonatal REM sleep and their phasic activities, especially under conditions of dysfunctional end products of the HPA axis such as glucocorticoid and corticosterone. However, empirical tests of this hypothesis are needed.

## B. Molecular Alterations During Neonatal REM Sleep

Neonatal REM sleep has been hypothesized to play a role in stimulating brain development (12). However, the alteration of molecules during neonatal REM sleep is still unknown. Recent study indicates that both 5-HT dorsal raphé nuclei (DRN) neurons and noradrenergic locus ceruleus (LC) neurons are locomotor-activity dependent (138,139). Atonia induced by electrical stimulation of the pontine inhibitory area and gigantocellular reticular nucleus causes a reduction in the activity of the LC (139). 5-HT DRN neurons cease firing by disfacilitation during REM sleep (140). These findings suggest that abundant phasic activities, which appear during neonatal REM sleep, may result in higher levels of brain 5-HT, noradrenaline, and other neurotrophic factors such as nerve growth factors

(NGF) and brain-derived neurotrophic factors (BDNF) compared with the levels in quiet sleep. The release of 5-HT, neurotrophic factors, and perhaps other unknown signal pathways stimulated by REM phasic activities facilitate the development of neural systems involved in the regulation of wake capacity and voluntary behavioral activity-related subservice systems, such as respiration and cardiovascular function. This hypothesis may not be easily accepted because 5-HT level is lowest during REM sleep, higher during NREM sleep, and is the highest during wakefulness in adulthood. The argument is that the evidence that 5-HT level is the lowest during REM sleep is acquired in adulthood, and that abundance of REM-phasic activities is a feature of the neonate rather than the adult. However, this hypothesis needs to be empirically tested.

Many studies demonstrate that neurotrophic factors play a critical role in cell's growth (141). The early appearance of monoamine systems in the developing mammalian central nervous system suggests that they may also play a role in neural development (142). 5-HT receptor activation enhances neurite outgrowth of thalamic neurons in rodents. Changes of 5-HT concentration, both in vivo and in vitro, influence neuronal development (106–110). 5-HT increases the length of the primary process, the total length of all processes, total neurites per cell, number of branch points per cell, and branch points on the primary neurite in the cultured ventrobasal thalamic neurons harvested from newborn rats (110). The depletion of cortical 5-HT during development results in a decrease in the size of the patches of thalamocortical afferents to the primary somatosensory cortex (143,144). 5-HT enhances neurite outgrowth of thalamic neurons by activating the 5-HT1b receptor. The sodium channel blocker tetrodotoxin (TTX) blocks these effects, whereas the selective 5-HT1B agonist CGS-12066A maleate reproduces 5-HT's effects (110). 5-HT plays a facilitatory role in activating the cortex through the activation of $5\text{-HT}_{2A}$ receptors on thalamocortical neurons, and thereby increases glutamate release, which in turn activates cortical neurons as indicated by an increase of c-Fos expression (145).

In summary, the above evidence supports my hypothesis that neonatal REM sleep may increase the release of 5-HT and neurotrophic factors and may facilitate the development of multiple brain systems through the increase of 5-HT and neurotrophic factors. However, this hypothesis needs to be empirically tested.

## C.   REM Sleep Suppression and Maturation of the Wake System

Findings from the ontogeny of neonatal REM sleep indicate that the change in six REM-related variables (including tonic REM sleep, phasic REM sleep, mean REM sleep period duration, number of REM sleep periods, REM sleep latency, and percentage of wake-onset REM sleep periods) parallels age. This indicates that the REM propensity is developed and becomes stronger from age 2 to 4 weeks. One of the potential candidates for the substrates of the REM-inhibitory processes is the set of wake-related neurons including orexinergic, monoaminergic systems and the maturation of cortex particularly the frontal cortex. In adults, upregulation of dopaminergic, serotonergic, and noradrenergic neuronal transmission inhibits REM sleep and CRF. These neural systems are immature in neonates and mature progressively as the rat ages. Brain levels of 5-HT, noradrenaline, and dopamine are very low in neonates and increase to near the adult level by the end of first the month, and reach the adult level in the second month. Orexin A- and B-like immunopositive cells and fibers are not detected from PN 0 to 10, but are observed after PN 15 (62). Thus, the suppression of REM sleep during this period of time is very limited. The limited suppression, however, increases progressively as the rat ages (Fig. 4). The increase of maturation level of monoaminergic, orexinergic, and cortical neurons results in a progressive decrease of REM sleep and brain level of CRF. Simultaneously, W/R ratio increases progressively. Decreased W/R ratio and/or disinhibited REM sleep may indicate a defective or underfunctioned wake system (Fig. 4). An interesting phenomenon is that the development of NREM sleep almost parallels that of wakefulness. Whether this is just a coincidence or some unknown intrinsic correlation remains to be discovered.

Figure 4 illustrates my hypothesis of neonatal regulation of sleep-wake states. Under an immature wake system, the high level of CRF in the neonate plays a critical role in driving the high percentage of neonatal REM sleep and the phasic activities. The phasic activities may stimulate the release of 5-HT and other neurotrophic factors such as BDNF and NGF. These biomolecules facilitate the development of neurons involved in the regulation of waking capacity and voluntary movement. In turn, maturation of waking and voluntary-movement-related neurons inhibits the release of CRF.

### D. A Function of Neonatal REM Sleep

The function of neonatal REM sleep lies in the neurotrophic role played by the neural and molecular signals generated during neonatal REM sleep. The discovery of electrophysiological signals and molecular alterations generated during REM sleep will be critical in understanding the function of neonatal REM sleep. Unfortunately, available data are still insufficient. Findings from neonatal RSD, however, fill the gaps to a certain degree. Summary of findings from neonatal RSD suggests that neonatal REM sleep plays an important role in supporting the development of monoaminergic, orexinergic systems and frontal cortex. The normal maturation of these neural systems and frontal cortex is crucial in: (a) the regulation of waking capacity and voluntary activity, (b) the suppression of REM sleep and CRF, and (c) the possible coordination of the subservice systems, such as respiratory and cardiovascular functions. These are indicated by the fact that neonatal RSD results in reduced pleasure-seeking behavior and dysfunctional sexual activity. It also results in lower fighting power indicated by loss in shock-induced fighting (decreased offensive behavior), lower body temperature, and abnormal respiration. Findings in cellular and molecular levels indicate that the rat model of neonatal RSD is similar to suicidal depression.

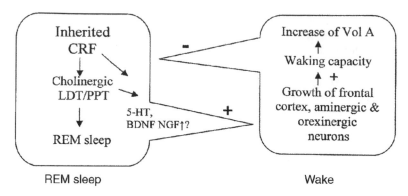

**Figure 4**  The hypothesized neonatal regulation of sleep-wake state. Vol A: voluntary activities. Strong REM sleep propensity is driven by the inherited high expression of CRF under conditions of immature neurons that secrete ACTH and corticosterone, and neurons of 5–HT, orexin, and cortex. REM phasic activities stimulate the release of 5–HT and other neurotrophic factors that play a crucial role in supporting the growth of waking-related neurons. In addition, CRF may play a direct role in supporting the growth of the waking-related neural system. During development, highly expressed CRF is suppressed by the maturation of the waking system. This may include the roles of those items produced by the waking product, including hormones (such as corticosterone), neurotransmitters (such as adenosine), and intracellular environmental changes (such as pH and glucose). The maturation of waking capacity-related neural systems precedes the voluntary behavioral activities. Both the maturation of waking systems and the increased voluntary behavioral activities suppress CRF and REM sleep progressively. This hypothesis suggests that neonatal RSD and neonatal blockage of CRF produce defective development of the waking system and voluntary behavior, as well as a decreased W/R ratio. This hypothesis is supported by findings from the consequence of neonatal RSD discussed in the text, and that neonatal treatment with dexamethasone might have a direct suppression on CRF, producing a later life of increased immobility (151).

The specific changes include a downregulated monoaminergic system and a defective orexinergic system as well as defective cell signal transduction in the frontal cortex and hippocampus. The loss of interest found in human depression and decreased pleasure-seeking behavior resulting from neonatal RSD indicate that a defective pleasure sensation exists in human depression and has the consequence of neonatal RSD. One possibility of the molecular changes may be that neonatal RSD results in a poor connection between the sensory system and the motor system at the level of the motor cortex, indicated by the decreased level of protein in the frontal cortex. Another possibility is that neonatal RSD results in an elevated threshold of pleasure sensation indicated by the larger decrease of pERK and 5-HT in the frontal cortex, and the decrease of orexin B in the frontal cortex and thalamus. The basic function of the frontal cortex is the control of voluntary movements (146). Voluntary movement is certainly a behavior that requires the conscious state. Thus, the threshold of cortical sensation seems closely related to the level of vigilance and is regulated by monoaminergic and orexinergic systems.

Another function of neonatal REM sleep may be the suppression of REM sleep and CRF as a subsequent function of facilitating the development of monoaminergic and orexinergic systems and the frontal cortex. Monoamines and orexin peptides suppress REM sleep and CRF (18,147). 5-HT suppresses REM sleep (16,17), and may promote corticosterone (148) to suppress CRF. Thus, the progressive increase of the W/R ratio is one of the indicators of normal development of brain and behavior. Dysfunctional monoaminergic and orexinergic systems result in the disinhibited REM propensity and disinhibited HPA system. The disinhibited REM propensity and HPA axis are typically seen in many psychiatric illnesses such as depression and schizophrenia (130,149,150). Disinhibited REM propensity and HPA axis may elevate the risk level of sleep apnea and cardiac disease patients, because sleep apnea and myocardial infarctions appear during REM sleep.

Although evidence strongly supports the aforementioned hypothesis, empirical tests are needed to clarify the cellular and molecular effect of neonatal REM sleep, i.e., the cellular and molecular alteration during neonatal REM sleep and the molecular mechanism, and to determine the driving force of the high percentage of neonatal REM sleep. Molecular alteration during neonatal RSD remains a crucial subject for further study in understanding the function of neonatal REM sleep. Successful completion of these studies may provide strong evidence in supporting or denying the proposed hypothesis and understanding human depression.

## VI. Summary and Conclusions

This chapter reviews the short-term and long-term adult effects of neonatal RSD in rats. Neonatal sleep-wake states in human and altricial mammals are characterized by a high percentage of and then a progressive decline in REM sleep. This decline has a negative correlation with brain levels of monoamines, acetylcholine, and orexin peptides, and has a positive correlation with brain mRNA expression of CRF. Waking capacity develops much later than REM and NREM sleep. Neonatal RSD is remarkable in that the neonate does not increase wakefulness percentage correspondingly, and the decline of REM sleep during RSD is mostly compensated by NREM sleep rather than by wakefulness. Such a behavioral response is accompanied by a loss of REM-related motor stimulation. Although RSD in adulthood shows antidepressant effects, neonatal RSD, either by drug or by instrumental means, produces adult behaviors described as depression-like consequences. Neonatal RSD by drug produces downregulated monoaminergic neurotransmission, decreased levels of orexin B, and defective cellular signal transduction in the frontal cortex, and also produces disinhibited REM propensity and disinhibition of the hypothalamic-pituitary-adrenal (HPA) axis. Thus it appears that the developmental trajectory of waking capacity might play a decisive role in explaining the paradoxical effect of RSD in neonates and adults. Studies on neonates show that neonatal REM sleep is needed for the development of normal waking capacity, the pleasure sensation-based voluntary movements, and the inhibition of REM propensity and the HPA axis.

## Acknowledgments

I thank Dr. Kingman P. Strohl (Case Western Reserve University) and Dr. Jidong Fang (Pennsylvania State University) for their review of the manuscript and their extremely helpful comments.

## References

1.  Speciale SG, Nowaczyk T, Jouvet M. A longitudinal study of bioelectric activity in the pre- and post-hatch chick. Dev Psychobiol 1976; 9:539–547.
2.  Ruckebusch Y, Development of sleep and wakefulness in the foetal lamb. EEG Clin Neurophysiol 1972; 32:119–28.
3.  Ioffe S, Jansen AH, Russell BJ, Chernick V. Sleep, wakefulness and the monosynaptic reflex in fetal and newborn lambs. Pflugers Arch Eur J Physiol 1980; 388:149–57.
4.  Jouvet-Mounier D, Astic L, Lacote D. Ontogenesis of states of sleep in rat, cat, and guinea pig during first postnatal month. Dev Psych 1970; 2:216–239.
5.  Shimizu A, Himwich HE. The ontogeny of sleep in kittens and young rabbits. EEG Clin Neurophysiol 1968; 24:307–318.
6.  Romijn HJ, Hofman MA, Gramsbergen A. At what age is the developing cerebral cortex of the rat comparable to that of the full-term newborn human baby? Early Hum Dev 1991; 26:61–67.
7.  Levine S. Primary social relationships influence the developmenment of the hypothalamicpituitary—adrenal axis in the rat. Physiol Behav 2001; 73:255–260.
8.  McGinty DJ, Stevenson M, Hoppenbrouwers T, Harper RM, Sterman MB, Hodgman J. Polygraphic studies of kitten development: sleep state patterns. Dev Psychobiol 1977;10:455–469.
9.  Feng P and Ma Y. Clomipramine suppresses postnatal REM sleep without increasing wakefulness: implications for the production of depressive behavior. Sleep 2002; 25:177–184.
10.  Vogel GW, Feng P, Kinney GG. Ontogeny of REM sleep in rats: possible implications for endogenous depression. Physiol Behav 2000; 68:453–461.
11.  Capece ML, Baghdoyan HA, Lydic R. New direction for the study of cholinergic REM sleep generation: specifying pre- and postsynaptic mechanisms. In: Mallick BN, Inoue S, eds. Rapid Eye Movement Sleep. London: Narasa Publishing House, 1999:123–141.
12.  Roffwarg HP, Muzio JN, Dement WC. Ontogenetic development of the human sleep-dream cycle. Science 1966; 152:604–619.
13.  Kohyama J. A quantitative assessment of the maturation of phasic motor inhibition during REM sleep. J Neurol Sci 1996; 143: 150–155.

14. Dreyfus-Brisac C. Sleep ontogenesis in early human prematurity from 24 to 27 weeks. Dev Psychol 1968; 1:162–169.
15. Denenberg VH, Thoman EB. Evidence for a functional role for active (REM) sleep in infancy. Sleep 1981; 4: 185–191.
16. Horner RL, Sanford LD, Annis D, Pack AI, Morrison AR. Serotonin at the laterodorsal tegmental nucleus suppresses rapid-eye-movement sleep in freely behaving rats. J Neurosci 1997; 17):7541–7552.
17. Jones BE. Influence of the brainstem reticular formation, including intrinsic monoaminergic and neurons, on forebrain mechanism of sleep and waking: In Mancia M, Marini G, eds. The Diencephalons and Sleep. New York: Raven Press, 1990:31–48.
18. Taheri S, Zeitzer JM, Mignot E. The role of hypocretins (orexins) in sleep regulation and narcolepsy. Annu Rev Neurosci 2002; 25:283–313.
19. Mitani A, Ito K, Hallanger AE, Wainer BH, Kataoka K, McCarley RW. Cholinergic projections from the lateral and pedunculopontine tegmental nuclei to the pontine gigantocellular tegmental field in the cat. Brain Res 1988; 451:397–402.
20. Semba K. Aminergic and cholinergic afferents to REM sleep induction regions of the pontine reticular formation in the rat. J Comp Neurol 1993; 330:543–556.
21. Shiromani PJ, Armstrong DM, Gillin JC. Cholinergic neurons from the dorsolateral pons project to the medial pons: a WGA-HRP and choline acetyltransferase immunohistochemical study. Neurosci Lett 1988; 95:19–23.
22. Parsons SM, Bahr BA, Rogers GA, Clarkson ED, Noremberg K, Hicks BW. Acetylcholine transporter-vesamicol receptor pharmacology and structure. Prog Brain Res 1993; 98:175–181.
23. Parsons SM, Prior C, Marshall IG. Acetylcholine transporter, storage, and release, Int Rev Neurobiol 1993; 35:279–390.
24. Homma Y, Skinner RD, Garcia-Rill E. Effects of pedunculopontine nucleus (PPN) stimulation on caudal pontine reticular formation (PnC) neurons in vitro. J Neurophysiol 2002; 87:3033–3047.
25. Hrdina PD, Ghosh PK, Rastogi RB, Singhal RL. Ontogenic pattern of dopamine, acetylcholine, and acetylcholinesterase in the brains of normal and hypothyroid rats. Can J Physiol Pharm 1975; 53:709–715.
26. Ninomiya Y, Koyama Y, Kayama Y. Postnatal development of choline acetyltransferase activity in the rat laterodorsal tegmental nucleus. Neurosci Lett 2001; 308:138–140.
27. Mechawar N, Watkins KC, Descarries L. Ultrastructural features of the acetylcholine innervation in the developing parietal cortex of rat. J Comp Neurol 2002; 443:250–258.
28. Wall SJ, Yasuda RP, Li M, Ciesla W, Wolfe BB. The ontogeny of m1–m5 muscarinic receptor subtypes in rat forebrain. Brain Res Dev Brain Res 1992; 66:181–185.
29. Buwalda B, de Groote L, Van der Zee EA, Matsuyama T, Luiten PG. Immunocytochemical demonstration of developmental distribution of muscarinic acetylcholine receptors in rat parietal cortex. Brain Res Dev Brain Res 1995; 84:185–191.
30. van Huizen F, March D, Cynader MS, Shaw C. Muscarinic receptor characteristics and regulation in rat cerebral cortex: changes during development, aging and the oestrous cycle. Eur J Neurosci 1994; 6:237–243.

31.  Balduini W, Cimino M, Reno F, Marini P, Princivalle A, Cattabeni F. Effects of postnatal or adult chronic acetylcholinesterase inhibition on muscarinic receptors, phosphoinositide turnover and m1 mRNA expression. Eur J Pharm 1993; 248:281–288.

32.  Gottesmann C. The neurochemistry of waking and sleeping mental activity: the disinhibition-dopamine hypothesis. Psychiatr Clin Neurosci 2002; 56:345–354.

33.  Lancel M, Langebartels A. gamma-aminobutyric Acid(A) (GABA(A)) agonist 4,5,6,7-tetrahydroisoxazolo[4,5-c]pyridin-3-ol persistently increases sleep maintenance and intensity during chronic administration to rats. J Pharm Exp Ther 2000; 293:1084–1090.

34.  Benington JH, Kodali SK, Heller HC. Stimulation of A1 adenosine receptors mimics the electroencephalographic effects of sleep deprivation. Brain Res 1995; 692:79–85.

35.  Datta S. Evidence that REM sleep is controlled by the activation of brain stem pedunculopontine tegmental kainate receptor. J Neurophysiol 2002; 87:1790–1798.

36.  Plotsky PM, Meaney MJ. Early, postnatal experience alters hypothalamic corticotropin-releasing factor (CRF) mRNA, median eminence CRF content and stress-induced release in adult rats. Brain Res Mol Brain Res 1993; 18:195–200.

37.  Cirulli F. Role of environmental factors on brain development and nerve growth factor expression. Physiol Behav 2001; 73:321–330.

38.  Feng P, Ma Y, Vogel GW. The critical window of brain development from susceptive to insusceptive: effects of clomipramine neonatal treatment on sexual behavior. Dev Brain Res 2001; 129:107–110.

39.  Francis DD, Meaney MJ. Maternal care and the development of stress responses. Cur Opin Neurobiol 1999; 9:128–134.

40.  Ladd CO, Owens MJ. Nemeroff CB. Persistent changes in corticotropin-releasing factor neuronal systems induced by maternal deprivation. End 1996;137:1212–1218.

41.  Matthews K, Dalley JW, Matthews C, Tsai TH, Robbins TW. Periodic maternal separation of neonatal rats produces region- and gender-specific effects on biogenic amine content in postmortem adult brain. Syn 2001; 40:1–10.

42.  Vazquez DM, Lopez JF, Van Hoers H, Watson SJ, Levine S. Maternal deprivation regulates serotonin 1A and 2A receptors in the infant rat. Brain Res 2000; 855:76–82.

43.  Sibug RM, Oitzl MS, Workel JO, de Kloet ER. Maternal deprivation increases 5-HT(1A) receptor expression in the CA1 and CA3 areas of senescent Brown Norway rats. Brain Res 2001; 912:95–98.

44.  Heidbreder CA, Weiss IC, Domeney AM, Pryce C, Homberg J, Hedou G, Feldon J, Moran MC, Nelson P. Behavioral, neurochemical and endocrinological characterization of the early social isolation syndrome. Neuroscience 2000; 100:749–768.

45.  Hall FS, Wilkinson LS, Humby T, Robbins TW. Maternal deprivation of neonatal rats produces enduring changes in dopamine function. Syn 1999; 32:37–43.

46.  Kehoe P, Shoemaker WJ, Arons C, Triano L, Suresh G. Repeated isolation stress in the neonatal rat: relation to brain dopamine systems in the 10-day-old rat. Behav Neurosci 1998;112:1466–1474.

47.  Costela C, Tejedor-Real P, Mico JA, Gibert-Rahola J. Effect of neonatal handling on learned helplessness model of depression. Physiol Behav 1995; 57:407–410.

48. Liu D, Diorio J, Tannenbaum B, Caldji C, Francis D, Freedman A, Sharma S, Pearson D, Plotsky PM, Meaney MJ. Maternal care, hippocampal glucocorticoid receptors, and hypothalamic-pituitary-adrenal responses to stress. Science 1997; 277:1659–1662.

49. Vogel G, Hagler M, Hennessey A, Richard C. Dose-dependent decrements in adult male rat sexual behavior after neonatal clorimipramine treatment. Pharm Biochem Behav 1996;54:605–609.

50. Feng P, Ma Y, Vogel GW. Ontogeny of REM rebound in neonatal rats. Sleep 2001; 24:645–653.

51. Yoo HS, Bunnell BN, Crabbe JB, Kalish LR, Dishman RK. Failure of neonatal clomipramine treatment to alter forced swim immobility: chronic treadmill or activity–wheel runing and imipramine. Physiol Behav 2000; 70:407–411.

52. Vogel GW, Buffenstein A, Minter K, Hennessey A. Drug effects on REM sleep and on endogenous depres sion. Neurosci Biobehav Rev 1990;14:49–63.

53. Thomas AJ, Erokwu BO, Yamamoto BK, Ernsberger P, Bishara O, Strohl KP. Alterations in respiratory behavior, brain neurochemistry and receptor density induced by pharmacologic suppression of sleep in the neonatal period. Brain Res Dev Brain Res 2000; 120:181–189.

54. Levine S, Huchton DM, Wiener SG, Rosenfeld P. Time course of the effect of maternal deprivation on the hypothalamic-pituitary-adrenal axis in the infant rat. Dev Psychobiol 1991; 24:547–558.

55. Mirmiran M, Scholtens J, van de Poll NE, Uyling HBM, van der Gugsten J, Boer GJ. Effects of experimental suppression of active (REM) sleep during early development upon adult brain and behavior in the rat. Dev Brain Res 1983;7:277–236.

56. Marks GA, Shaffery JP, Oksenberg A, Specimle SG, Roffwarg HP. A functional role for REM sleep in brain maturation. Behav Brain Res 1995; 69:1–11.

57. Shaffery JP, Marks GA, Specigle SC, Roffwarg HP. REM sleep deprivation on a vibrating platform: automating a standard technique. Sleep Res 1990; 19:110.

58. Feng P, Vogel GW. A new method for continuous, long term polysomnographic recordings of neonatal rats. Sleep 2000; 23:9–14.

59. Vogel GW, Feng P. A reply to Frank and Heller about neonatal active sleep. Sleep 2000; 23:1005–1011.

60. Feng P, Obermeyer W, Vogel GW. An instrumental method for long term continuous REM sleep deprivation of neonatal rats. Sleep 2000; 23:175–183.

61. Mirmiran M, van de Poll NE, Corner MA, van Oyen HG, Bour HL. Suppression of active sleep by chronic treatment with chlorimipramine during early postnatal development: effects upon adult sleep and behavior in the rat. Brain Res 1981; 204:129–146.

62. Yamamoto Y, Ueta Y, Hara Y, Serino R, Nomura M, Shibuya I, Shirahata A, Yamashita H. Postnatal development of orexin/hypocretin in rats. Brain Res Mol Brain Res 2000; 78:108–119.

63. Vogel GW, Vogel FA. A new animal model of human endogenous depression. Sleep Res 1982; 11:222.

64. Vogel G, Neill D, Hagler M, Kors D. A new animal model of endogenous depression: a summary of present findings. Neurosci Biobehav Rev 1990; 14:85–91.

65. Feng P, Ma Y, Vogel GW. Instrumental REM sleep deprivation in neonates: depression or mania? Sleep 2001; 24(suppl):A236.

66. Hartley P, Neill D, Hagler M, Kors D, Vogel G. Procedure- and age-dependent hyperactivity in a new animal model of endogenous depression. Neurosci Biobehav Res 1990; 14:69–72.

67.  Neill D, Vogel G, Hagler M, Kors D, Hennessey A. Diminished sexual activity in a new animal model of endogenous depression. Neurosci Biobehav Rev 1990; 14:73–76.

68.  Bonilla-Jaime H, Retana-Marquez S, Velazquez-Moctezuma J. Pharmacological features of masculine sexual behavior in an animal model of depression. Pharm Biochem Behav 1998; 60:39–45.

69.  Velazquez-Moctezuma J, Aguilar-Garcia A, Diaz-Ruiz O. Behavioral effects of neonatal treatment with clomipramine, scopolamine, and idazoxan in male rats. Pharm Biochem Behav 1993; 46:215–217.

70.  Vogel G, Neill D, Hagler M, Kors D, Hartley P. Decreased intracranial self-stimulation in a new animal model of endogenous depression. Neurosci Biobehav Rev 1990; 14:65–68.

71.  Vogel G, Hartley P, Neill D, Hagler M, Kors D. Animal depression model by neonatal clomipramine: reduction of shock induced aggression. Pharm Biochem Behav 1988; 31:103–106.

72.  Velazquez-Moctezuma J, Diaz Ruiz O. Neonatal treatment with clomipramine increased immobility in the forced swim test: an attribute of animal models of depression. Pharm Biochem Behav 1992; 42:737–739.

73.  Hilakivi LA, Taira T, Hilakivi I, Loikas P. Neonatal treatment with monoamine uptake inhibitors alters later response in behavioural "despair" test to beta and GABA-B receptor agonists. Pharm Toxicol 1988; 63:57–61.

74.  Hilakivi LA, Taira T, Hilakivi I, MacDonald E, Tuomisto L, Hellevuo K. Early postnatal treatment with propranolol affects development of brain amines and behavior. Psychopharmacology 1988; 96:353–359.

75.  Mirmiran M, Scholtens J, van de Poll NE, Uylings HB, van der Gugten J, Boer GJ. Effects of experimental suppression of active (REM) sleep during early development upon adult brain and behavior in the rat. Brain Res 1983; 283:277–786.

76.  Prathiba J, Kumar KB, Karanth KS. Effects of neonatal clomipramine on cholinergic receptor sensitivity and passive avoidance behavior in adult rats. J Neural Trans Gen Sec 1995; 100:93–99.

77.  Dwyer SM, Rosenwasser AM. Neonatal clomipramine treatment, alcohol intake and circadian rhythms in rats. Psychopharmacology 1998; 138:176–183.

78.  Hilakivi LA, Sinclair JD, Hilakivi IT. Effects of neonatal treatment with clomipramine on adult ethanol related behavior in the rat. Brain Res 1984; 317:129–132.

79.  Vijayakumar M, Meti BL. Alterations in the levels of monoamines in discrete brain regions of clomipramine-induced animal model of endogenous depression. Neurochem Res 1999; 24:345–349.

80.  Prathiba J, Kumar KB, Karanth KS. Effects of REM sleep deprivation on cholinergic receptor sensitivity and passive avoidance behavior in clomipramine model of depression. Brain Res 2000; 867:243–245.

81.  Vogel G, Neill D, Kors D, Hagler M. REM sleep abnormalities in a new animal model of endogenous depression. Neurosci Biobehav Rev 1990; 14:77–83.

82.  Kinney GG, Volgel GW, Feng P. Decreased dorsal raph'l nucleus neuronal activity in adult chloral hydrate anesthetized rats following neonatal clomipramine treatment: implications for endogenous depression, Brain Res 1997; 756:68–75.

83.  Feenstra MG, van Galen H, Te Riele PJ, Botterblom MH, Mirmiran M. Decreased hypothalamic serotonin levels in adult rats treated neonatally with clomipramine. Pharm Biochem Behav 1996; 55:647–652.

84. Maudhuit C, Hamon M, Adrien J. Effects of chronic treatment with zimelidine and REM sleep deprivation on the regulation of raph'l neuronal activity in a rat model of depression. Psychopharmacology 1996; 124:267–274.

85. Feng P. Brain levels of orexin B are decreased in junior rats neonatally treated with REM sleep suppressant of clomipramine. Sleep 2003; 26:A35–A36.

86. Prathiba J, Kumar KB, Karanth KS. Hyperactivity of hypothalamic pituitary axis in neonatal clomipramine model of depression. J Neural Trans (Bud) 1998;105:1335–1339.

87. Suzuki T, Mitake S, Murata S. Presence of up-stream and downstream components of a mitogen-activated protein kinase pathway in the PSD of the rat forebrain. Brain Res 1999; 840:36–44.

88. Suzuki T, Okumura-Noji K, Nishida E. ERK2–type mitogen-activated protein kinase (MAPK) and its substrates in postsynaptic density fractions from the rat brain. Neurosci Res 1995; 22:277–285.

89. Yuen EC, Mobley WC. Early BDNF, NT-3, and NT-4 signaling events. Exp Neurol 1999; 159:297–308.

90. Ambrosini A, Tininini S, Barassi A, Racagni G, Sturani E, Zippel R. cAMP cascade leads to Ras activation in cortical neurons. Brain Res Mol Brain Res 2000; 75:54–60.

91. Cai G, Zhen X, Uryu K, Friedman E. Activation of extracellular signal regulated protein kinases is associated with a sensitized locomotor response to D(2) dopamine receptor stimulation in unilateral 6–hydroxydopamine?lesioned rats. J Neurosci 2000; 20:1849–1857.

92. Mukhin YV, Garnovskaya MN, Collinsworth G, Grewal JS, Pendergrass D, Nagai T, Pinckney S, Greene EL, Raymond JR. 5–Hydroxytryptamine1A receptor/gibetagamma stimulates mitogen-activated protein kinase via NAD(P)H oxidase and reactive oxygen species upstream of src in chinese hamster ovary fibroblasts. Biochem J 2000; 347 (Pt 1):61–67.

93. Valjent E, Corvol JC, Pages C, Besson MJ, Maldonado R, Caboche J. Involvement of the extracellular signal regulated kinase cascade for cocaine rewarding properties. J Neurosci 2000; 20:8701–8709.

94. Grewal SS, York RD, Stork PJ. Extracellular-signal-regulated kinase signalling in neurons. Curr Opin Neurobiol 1999; 9:544–553.

95. Stariha RL, Kim SU. Protein kinase C and mitogen-activated protein kinase signaling in oligodendrocytes. Microscopy Res Tech 2001; 52:680–688.

96. Dwivedi Y, Rizavi HS, Roberts RC, Conley RC, Tamminga CA, Pandey GN. Reduced activation and expression of ERK1/2 MAP kinase in the post-mortem brain of depressed suicide subjects. J Neurochem 2001; 77:916–928.

97. Vogel GW. REM sleep deprivation and behavioral changes. In: Mallick BN, Inoue S, eds. Rapid Eye Movement Sleep. London: Narasa Publishing House, 1999:355–366.

98. Kennedy SH, Dickens SE, Eisfeld BS, Bagby RM. Sexual dysfunction before antidepressant therapy in major depression. J Affect Disord 1999; 56:201–208.

99. Bartlik B, Kocsis JH, Legere R, Villaluz J, Kossoy A, Gelenberg AJ. Sexual dysfunction secondary to depressive disorders. J Gender-Specif Med 1999; 2:52–60.

100. Clayton AH. Recognition and assessment of sexual dysfunction associated with depression. J Clin Psychiatry 2001; 62(Suppl 3):5–9.

101. Phillips RL Jr, Slaughter JR. Depression and sexual desire. Am Family Physician 2000; 62:782–786.

102. Kim EY, Miklowitz DJ. Childhood mania, attention deficit hyperactivity disorder and conduct disorder: a critical review of diagnostic dilemmas. Bipolar Disord 2002; 4:215–225.

103. Desautels A, Turecki G, Montplaisir J, Brisebois K, Sequeira A, Adam B, Rouleau GA. Evidence for a genetic association between monoamine oxidase A and restless legs syndrome. Neurology 2002;59:215–219.

104. Schechter MS. Section on Pediatric Pulmonology, Subcommittee on Obstructive Sleep Apnea Syndrome. Technical report: diagnosis and management of childhood obstructive sleep apnea syndrome. Pediatrics 2002; 109:e69.

105. Danguir J, Elghozi JL. Superfusion of clomipramine within the ventromedial hypothalamus selectively suppresses paradoxical sleep in freely moving rats. Brain Res Bull 1985; 15:1–4.

106. Young-Davies CL, Bennett-Clarke CA, Lane RD, Rhoades RW. Selective facilitation of the serotonin (1B) receptor causes disorganization of thalamic afferents and barrels in somatosensory cortex of rat. J Comp Neurol 2000; 425:130–138.

107. Bennett-Clarke CA, Leslie MJ, Lane RD, Rhoades RW. Effect of serotonin depletion on vibrissa-related patterns of thalamic afferents in the rat's somatosensory cortex. J Neurosci 1994; 14:7594–7607.

108. Bennett-Clarke CA, Hankin MH, Leslie MJ, Chiaia NL, Rhoades RW. Patterning of the neocortical projections from the raphe nuclei in perinatal rats: investigation of potential organizational mechanisms. J Comp Neurol 1994; 348:277–290.

109. Boylan CB, Bennett-Clarke CA, Chiaia NL, Rhoades RW. Time course of expression and function of the serotonin transporter in the neonatal rat's primary somatosensory cortex. Somatosensory Motor Res 2000; 17:52–60.

110. Lotto B, Upton L, Price DJ, Gaspar P. Serotonin receptor activation enhances neurite outgrowth of thalamic neurones in rodents. Neurosci Lett 1999; 269:87–90.

111. Szuba MP, O'Reardon JP, Evans DL. Physiological effects of electroconvulsive therapy and transcranial magnetic stimulation in major depression. Dep Anx 2000; 12:170–177.

112. Wirz-Justice A, Van den Hoofdakker RH. Sleep deprivation in depression: what do we know, where do we go? Biol Psychiatry 1999; 46:445–453.

113. Riemann D, Berger M. The effects of total sleep deprivation and subsequent treatment with clomipramine on depressive symptoms and sleep electroencephalography in patients with a major depressive disorder. Acta Psychiatr Scand 1990; 81(1):24–31.

114. Dunleavy DL, Brezinova V, Oswald I, Maclean AW, Tinker M. Changes during weeks in effects of tricyclic drugs on the human sleeping brain. Br J Psychiatry 1972; 120:663–672.

115. Passouant P, Cadhilac J, Billiard M. Withdrawal of the paradoxal sleep by the clomipramine, electrophysiological, histochemical and biochemical study. Int J Neurol 1975; 10:186–197.

116. Steiger A. Effects of clomipramine on sleep EEG and nocturnal penile tumescence: a long-term study in a healthy man. J Clin Psychopharm 1988; 8: 349–354.

117. Vale W, Spiess J, Rivier C, Rivier J. Characterization of a 41–residue ovine hypothalamic peptide that stimulates secretion of corticotropin and beta-endorphin. Science 1981; 213:1394–1397.

118. Laatikainen TJ. Corticotropin-releasing hormone and opioid peptides in reproduction and stress. Ann Med 1991; 23:489–496.

119. Rivier C, Rivest S. Effect of stress on the activity of the hypothalamic-pituitary-gonadal axis: peripheral and central mechanisms. Biol Reprod 1991; 45:523–532.

120. Webster EL, Grigoriadis DE, De Souza EB. Corticotropin-releasing factor receptors in the brain-pituitary-immune axis. In: McCubbin JA, Kaufmann PJ, Nemeroff

CB, eds. Stress, Neu-ropeptides, and Systemic Disease. San Diego: Academic Press, 1991:233–260.

121. Dunn AJ, Berridge CW. Physiological and behavioral responses to corticotrophin-releasing factor administration: is CRF a mediator of. anxiety or stress responses? Brain Res Rev 1990; 15: 71–100.

122. Owens MJ, Nemeroff CB. Physiology and pharmacology of corticotropin-releasing factor. Pharm Rev 1991; 43:425–473.

123. Challis J, Sloboda D, Matthews S, Holloway A, Alfaidy N, Howe D, Fraser M, Newnham J. Fetal hypothalamic-pituitary adrenal (HPA) development and activation as a determinant of the timing of birth, and of postnatal disease. Endocr Res 2000; 26:489–504.

124. Pihoker C, Cain ST, Nemeroff CB. Postnatal development of regional binding of corticotropin-releasing factor and adenylate cyclase activity in the rat brain. Prog Neuro-Psychopharm Biol Psychiatry 1992; 16:581–586.

125. Avishai-Eliner, Sarit; Su-Jin, Yi; Baram, Tallie Z. Developmental profile of messenger RNA for the corticotropin-releasing hormone receptor in the rat limbic system. Dev Brain Res 1996; 91:159–163.

126. Dugovic C, Maccari S, Weibel L, Turek FW, Van Reeth O. High corticosterone levels in prenatally stressed rats predict persistent paradoxical sleep alterations. J Neurosci 1999; 19:8656–8664.

127. Meerlo P, Koehl M, van der Borght K, Turek FW, Investigator: Turek FW. Sleep restriction alters the hypothalamic-pituitary-adrenal response to stress. J Neuroendocrinol 2002; 14:397–402.

128. Hairston IS, Ruby NF, Brooke S, Peyron C, Denning DP, Heller HC, Sapolsky RM. Sleep deprivation elevates plasma corticosterone levels in neonatal rats. Neurosci Lett 2001; 315:29–32.

129. Vogel G, Neill D, Kors D, Hagler M. REM sleep abnormalities in a new animal model of endogenous depression. Neurosci Biobehav Rev 1990; 14:77–83.

130. Arborelius L, Owens MJ, Plotsky PM, Nemeroff CB. The role of corticotropin-releasing factor in depression and anxiety disorders. J Endocr 1999; 160:1–12.

131. Marrosu F, Gessa GL, Giagheddu M, Fratta W. Corticotropin-releasing factor (CRF) increases paradoxical sleep (PS) rebound in PS-deprived rats. Brain Res 1990; 515:315–318.

132. Gonzalez MM, Valatx JL. Involvement of stress in the sleep rebound mechanism induced by sleep deprivation in the rat: use of alpha-helical CRH (9–41). Behav Pharm 1998; 9:655–662.

133. Ohgushi A, Bungo T, Shimojo M, Masuda Y, Denbow DM, Furuse M. Relationships between feeding and locomotion behaviors after central administration of CRF in chicks. Physiol Behav 2001; 72:287–289.

134. Clements S, Schreck CB, Larsen DA, Dickhoff WW. Central administration of corticotropin-releasing hormone stimulates locomotor activity in juvenile chinook salmon (*Oncorhynchus tshawytscha*). Gen Comp Endocr 2002; 125:319–337.

135. Opp MR. Corticotropin-releasing hormone involvement in stressor-induced alterations in sleep and in the regulation of waking. Adv Neuroimmunol 1995;5:127–113.

136. Ordyan NE, Pivina SG, Rakitskaya VV Shalyapina VG. The neonatal glucocorticoid treatment-produced long-term changes of the pituitary-adrenal function and brain corticosteroid receptors in rats. Steroids 2001; 66:883–888.

137. Pariante CM, Miller AH. Glucocorticoid receptors in major depression: relevance to pathophysiology and treatment. Biol Psychiatry 2001;49:391–404.

138. Jacobs BL. Single unit activity of locus coeruleus neurons in behaving animals. Prog Neurobiol 1986; 27:183–194.

139. Mileykovskiy BY, Kiyashchenko LI, Kodama T, Lai YY, Siegel JM. Activation of pontine and medullary motor inhibitory regions reduces discharge in neurons located in the locus coeruleus and the anatomical equivalent of the midbrain locomotor region. J Neurosci (Online) 2000; 20: 8551–8558.

140. Sakai K, Crochet S. Serotonergic dorsal raphe neurons cease firing by disfacilitation during paradoxical sleep. Neuroreport 2000; 11:3237–3241.

141. Lu B, Figurov A. Role of neurotrophins in synapse development and plasticity. Rev Neurosci 1997; 8:1–12.

142. Levitt P, Harvey JA, Friedman E, Simansky K, Murphy EH. New evidence for neurotransmitter influences on brain development. Trends Neurosci 1997; 20:269–274.

143. Fujimiya M, Kimura H, Maeda T. Postnatal development of serotonin nerve fibers in the somatosensory cortex of mice studied by immunohistochemistry. J Comp Neurol 1986; 246:191–201.

144. Rhoades RW, Chiaia NL, Lane RD, Bennett-Clarke CA. Effect of activity blockade on changes in vibrissae-related patterns in the rat's primary somatosensory cortex induced by serotonin depletion. J Comp Neurol 1998; 402:276–283.

145. Scruggs JL, Patel S, Bubser M, Deutch AY. DOI-Induced activation of the cortex: dependence on 5–HT2A heteroceptors on thalamocortical glutamatergic neurons. J Neurosci 2000; 20:8846–8852.

146. Feng P, Guan Z, Yang X, Fang J. Changes of sexual activity, ERK, pERK, PP1 and MPK-2 in rat model of depression. Sleep 2002; 25:A17–18.

147. Samson WK, Taylor MM. Hypocretin/orexin suppresses corticotroph responsiveness in vitro. Am J Physiol Reg Int Comp Physiol 2001; 281:R1140–1145.

148. Hemrick-Luecke SK, Evans DC. Comparison of the potency of MDL 100,907 and SB 242084 in blocking the serotonin (5–HT)(2) receptor agonist-induced increases in rat serum corticosterone concentrations: evidence for 5–HT(2A) receptor mediation of the HPA axis. Neuropharmacology 2002; 42:162–169.

149. Duman RS. Novel therapeutic approaches beyond the serotonin receptor. Biol Psychiatry 1998; 44:324–335.

150. Ressler KJ, Nemeroff CB. Role of serotonergic and noradrenergic systems in the pathophysiology of depression and anxiety disorders. Depress Anxiety 2000; 12(suppl 1):2–19.

151. Felszeghy K, Sasvari M, Nyakas C. Behavioral depression: opposite effects of neonatal dexamethasone and ACTH-(4–9) analogue (ORG 2766) treatments in the rat. Horm Behav 1993; 27:380–396.

152. Feng PF, Bergmann BM, Rechtschaffen A. Sleep deprivation in rats with preoptic/anterior hypothalamic lesions. Brain Res 1995; 703:93–99.

# 8

# Inadequate Sleep in Children and Adolescents

**CHRISTINE ACEBO**

E. P. Bradley Hospital/Brown Medical School, East Providence,
Rhode Island, U.S.A.

**AMY R. WOLFSON**

College of the Holy Cross, Worcester, Massachusetts, U.S.A.

## I. Introduction

We are using the term "inadequate sleep" instead of "sleep deprivation" in our title for a number of reasons. First, few studies have aimed specifically to deprive children or adolescents of sleep. We describe some research on experimental sleep restriction in children but most of these studies fall far short of common deprivation paradigms in animals or even adult humans. Instead, most research in younger humans has assessed outcome measures such as school grades, self-reported sleepiness, and so forth as a function of variations in self-selected or  usual sleep patterns with the expectation that children and adolescents who obtain lower than normal amounts of sleep will manifest deficits. Thus, inadequate sleep is defined by sleep characteristics of a sample. We also wanted to note some of the literature on sleep that is disturbed or disrupted due to disease processes such as apnea or periodic leg movements; the duration of sleep in sleep disorders may or may not be shortened or restricted although it is likely fragmented and otherwise abnormal. We decided on the term "inadequate sleep' with the hope that it would encompass these different areas of concern.

Of course, a notion that sleep can be inadequate implies that there is such a thing as adequate sleep. The question of how much or what quality of sleep is required for humans to function optimally or even adequately seems simple. Yet a convincing answer to this question has eluded philosophers, researchers, clinicians, and parents over the centuries, and considerable scientific debate has occurred about how much or what kind of sleep is required to prevent measurable deficits in performance (see, for example, Refs. 1–3; Chaps. 25 and 28). Few dispute that the range of domains affected by severe sleep loss is wide, from cognitive to metabolic functions, and few deny the importance of adequate sleep for optimal functioning. The constructs of adequate and inadequate sleep, however, remain difficult to operationalize and assess. A persistent finding noted in sleep restriction studies in adults is that individuals show marked differences in their responses to sleep amounts that are "on average" inadequate. Explanations for these differences include: (a) individual differences in sleep need (4,5) and (b) individual differences in the ability to compensate for sleep loss (6). Both of these potential variables, sleep need and differential response to sleep loss, may add unexplained variance in sleep restriction studies. When the participants of studies are children and adolescents, developmental differences are also important to take into account. Additional factors that add complexity include the domain and sensitivity of outcome measures, and the influence of the circadian system on both sleep and wakefulness. The number and interactive nature of these mitigating variables make difficult the assessment of deficits or dysfunction resulting from decreased sleep duration or disruption.

### A. Developmental Changes and Individual Differences in Sleep Duration

The average newborn sleeps about 16 out of every 24 hr in bouts of 1–4 hr (7). Sleep decreases to about 13 hr at 1 year and consists of nocturnal sleep plus two daytime naps. By 4–5 years old, most children have given up naps and spend at least 10 hr asleep at night (8). We believe that older children and adolescents need at least 9 hr of sleep, although most obtain far less than that amount. These familiar generalizations about changes in sleep duration across age are based on studies in both naturalistic settings and the laboratory. Rarely, however, is the construct of sleep need addressed directly and we must be careful not to confuse usual sleep duration with sleep need.

Individuals at all ages vary in the amount of sleep they consume. Parmelee and co-workers (7) described sleep over the first 3 days of life in 75 full-term neonates. The group average was 16.6 hr; however, average sleep for individual infants ranged from 10.5 to 23 hr. Kleitman and Engelmann (9) also reported wide inter- and intra-infant variability in sleep duration per 24 hr in 19 infants repeatedly studied over the first 6 months of life. Average 24-hr sleep for the group of infants decreased from 14.8 to 13.9 hr over the 6 months. Sleep times for individual infants, however, ranged from 7 to 21 hr on any given 24-hr period, and individual infants' overall averages ranged from just under 12 to over 16 hr out of 24. Studies of older infants, children, and adolescents have also reported wide individual differences in sleep durations; standard deviations of 30–90 min indicate ranges of 2–6 hr (see, for example, Refs. 10–14). We note that much of the available normative data have been obtained from children and adolescents screened for medical and sleep problems and studied on their "usual" schedules. Thus, parental schedules and expectations and other constraints may have affected sleep duration measures (and the range of values). Studies by Carskadon and colleagues (11), however, indicate that even when 10-hr sleep opportunities are provided to adolescents in the laboratory, standard deviations are generally around 30 min, indicating a range of about 2 hr. In a more recent study, adolescents were provided three consecutive nights of 18-hr sleep opportunities in the laboratory following a week at home on a schedule involving 10 hr of scheduled sleep. Total sleep on the third "long night" averaged 606 min with a standard deviation of 57 min and almost a 4-hr range (15). Thus, adolescents provided what may be considered optimal opportunities for sleep show marked individual differences in the amount of sleep they actually consume in these conditions. We do not know whether individual differences in sleep under optimal conditions reflect differences in sleep "need," however, or differences in some other variable such as an ability to extend usual sleep past what is needed.

Many of the studies described in this chapter have obtained usual sleep duration variables from self-report or home measurement with actigraphy with the expectation that lower sleep durations will be linked to deficits in functioning. Yet we have no information about how the amount of sleep consumed is related to the amount required for optimal functioning at the level of the individual child or adolescent. *Should we expect the same amount of dysfunction following a night of 5 hr of sleep from a child who needs 12 hr of sleep and a child who needs 8 hr of sleep? How do we determine how much sleep an individual child needs? Does the amount of sleep needed vary as a function of the task required? How do we incorporate individual differences in sleep need into analytical models?* Additionally, individual differences in vulnerability to sleep loss have been described in studies of adults subjected to restricted sleep and some researchers are actively pursuing attempts to identify individuals with high or low vulnerability (6,16). *Are sleep need and vulnerability to sleep loss linked? Are they stable characteristics of individuals? How best can we measure them?* These issues have not been studied actively in children and adolescents, and these and other questions provide a larger context for what we know from the research summarized in the rest of this chapter.

## B. Who Do We Measure and in What Contexts?

Infants, school-age children, and adolescents have been studied in the laboratory, hospital nurseries, schools, institutions, and their homes with polysomnography, time-lapse video monitors, activity monitors, diaries, and self- and parent-report instruments. Children both with and without sleep disorders have been evaluated with these various assessment procedures, and researchers have used a wide range of study designs to investigate the impact of inadequate sleep. For example, in laboratory studies children and adolescents have been assessed on their usual (often arguably inadequate) schedules as well as on study-defined optimized and restricted schedules. Other studies have relied on experiments of nature. Variations in school start times, work hours, cosleeping arrangements, disasters and wars, socioeconomic status, and so forth have been related to sleep quantity, sleep quality, and daytime functioning using measures obtained from interviews, self-report questionnaires, and increasingly actigraphy. Furthermore, both laboratory and survey studies have been conducted to evaluate the impact of sleep disorders, physical or mental illness, and parent and family characteristics on sleep schedules, sleep durations, and daytime behaviors. A few studies have incorporated measures of parents' sleep patterns or schedules as a context for understanding children's sleep.

## C.  How Do We Measure Sleep and Sleep Patterns?

Historically, a variety of strategies have been used to assess children and adolescents' sleep/wake patterns, ranging from self- or parent report instruments to polysomnography. Self-report questionnaires are relatively easy to use but are limited by their subjectivity. These measures often give a broad overview of a child's sleep/wake patterns at one time point (i.e., usually retrospective or current). Daily sleep diaries or logs also rely on self-report although they are generally viewed as more accurate than subjective impressions obtained from a one-time survey. In comparison to questionnaires, daily sleep diaries depend less on memory and allow quantitative measurements of sleep length and sleep/wake schedules across a series of daily reports (17). Sleep diary assessments tend to be correlated with objective measures of sleep such as polysomnographic recordings, although respondents tend to underestimate sleep duration and number of night wakings, and overestimate sleep latency in diary reports (18,19). Parents and younger children in particular are not always aware of the length or timing of night wakings or the precise times of sleep onset or offset.

Another approach for assessing sleep patterns is to use more objective methodologies and thus increase precision and reliability and reduce error variance resulting from human judgment and interpretation. Actigraphy (activity-based monitoring) has been established as a valid and reliable method of assessing current sleep-wake patterns in children and adolescents; comparisons of actigraph measures with concurrent polysomnography typically yield overall agreement rates in the range of 78–90% for children, adolescents, and adults (17,20–22). This method is useful for describing behavioral sleep patterns over extended periods of time in natural settings and is well accepted by even very young children (23). It is also a good technique for documenting compliance with study-guided at-home sleep schedules (24).

Polysomnography has been used in both laboratory and home-based studies of children and adolescents to obtain measures of sleep and sleep-related events (10,25–31), and also measures of daytime sleepiness from the Multiple Sleep Latency Test (MSLT) procedure (11). Because polysomnography is so expensive, most of these studies have obtained only one or a few nights of study for cross-sectional samples of children and adolescents at different ages or developmental stages. A few longitudinal studies have been conducted, however (11,13,32), and some laboratory studies have obtained extensive recordings over days and weeks of continuous study in the laboratory in older children and adolescents (15,33,34). Limitations of some laboratory polysomnography studies include scheduling sleep recording time in the laboratory based on subject's reports of "usual" schedule, which may or may not be representative, scheduling sleep recording time based on laboratory convenience, failing to document sleep history for prestudy nights, and relying on single-night recordings for measures. For example, the earliest studies reporting validity and reliability of polysomnographic measures documented the importance of obtaining multiple nights to obtain reliable measures (35–40), yet few studies have recorded children or adolescents in the laboratory for more than one or two nights.

Other objective measures that have been used for very young children include direct behavioral observation (41,42), video recordings (43), and mattress or crib recordings (44,45). The strengths and weaknesses vary for all of the techniques mentioned above (46).

### D. What Are Outcome Measures of Inadequate Sleep?

Most sleep scientists and clinicians believe that inadequate sleep in children and adolescents leads to decreased functioning in a broad range of domains, including daytime alertness, school performance, motor skills, attention/concentration, memory, problem solving, emotional regulation, and mood. Increased caffeine, nicotine, and other substance use; higher rates of accidents and injuries; and impairment in skills such as driving have also been investigated as outcome measures of inadequate sleep. These assorted variables have been measured with variable precision, most often with self-, parent-, or teacher-report instruments, but occasionally with more objective laboratory procedures. Some procedures that have been valuable in studies of adult sleep restriction or deprivation have been incorporated into studies of younger humans. These include motor skills, attention, and problem-solving measures (47–51). Other performance measures developed specifically for children and adolescents have been incorporated into sleep restriction studies (50). Experimental measures of performance are valued because they are presumed to tap neurobehavioral function. Some of these measures, however, are prone to confounding influences such as practice effects, and motivation, aptitude, and developmental differences. Finally, the MSLT, an objective measure of daytime sleepiness, was developed for adults and children simultaneously (11). This measure has been associated consistently with inadequate sleep in children and adolescents.

### E. When Do We Measure?

Enormous changes in the timing of sleep occur from infancy to adulthood. In early infancy sleep is organized in short (about 4 hr) bouts throughout the day and night. Sleep is gradually consolidated over the first years and by 5 years of age, sleep occurs only during nighttime hours for the majority of children most of the time. Sleep duration gradually decreases throughout childhood and adolescence primarily as a function of an increasingly later bedtime (e.g., Ref. 52). These changes in the timing of sleep throughout the life span provide an important context for assessment of sleep and daytime functioning. The duration and boundaries of both "daytime" and "nighttime" are different for infants, teenagers, and older adults. The biological processes underlying the expression of sleep and waking behavior may also differ as a function of developmental stage (53).

Timing of sleep in adults is conceptualized as an interaction of the circadian system and a sleep-dependent homeostatic process (54–58). The circadian process is modeled as an oscillatory function with a period of about 24 hr that reflects variations in a clock-dependent alerting process. The homeostatic process reflects sleep pressure or sleep need, which increases during waking and then decreases during sleep. These processes interact and oppose each other, resulting in the systematic ebb and flow of alertness and onset and offset of sleep. Along with sleep tendency, many of the variables that have been used as outcome measures in experimental studies of sleep deprivation—such as subjective sleepiness/alertness; recovery sleep measures; and motor, cognitive, memory, and physiological measures—have been shown to vary in adults both as a function of length of time awake and as a function of circadian phase (reviewed in Refs. 59,60). Less attention has been given to circadian variation of daytime functioning in children and adolescents although some studies using constant routine or forced desynchrony procedures have described circadian and homeostatic patterns in older children and adolescents (33,61).

A consistent finding over the last few decades is a marked delay in the timing of sleep over the adolescent years (62–67). The tendency for adolescents to go to bed later and wake up later than preadolescents is likely due, in part, to changes in the psychosocial environment. In addition, however, evidence is accumulating that changes in the circadian timing system could interact with the sleep-dependent homeostatic process to drive or permit the phase delay in sleep seen during pubertal development (33,53,61,63,68). The results of studies demonstrating the influence of the circadian system on variation in functioning over the day mandate careful consideration of time of day when designing studies and analyzing and reviewing data from sleep-restricted or sleep-deprived individuals. Developmental changes in timing of sleep and wakefulness add another level of complexity for cross-sectional studies. Finally, the circadian system has influences on sleep itself; individuals have less and lower-quality sleep when sleeping at the wrong circadian time (e.g., Ref. 69). Thus, *when* sleep occurs may influence its "restorative" properties.

In the following sections we briefly review some of the literature related to inadequate sleep in young humans with an emphasis on older children and adolescents. This is not intended to be a comprehensive review but we hope we have provided a sense of the directions of previous research and indications of unanswered questions.

## II. Social/Environmental Constraints: Sleep as a Dependent Variable

Available time to sleep for infants, children, and adults is influenced by a range of environmental and societal factors. In infancy, caretaking practices affect sleep; infants sleeping with their mothers have more arousals and less quiet sleep (70), and breast-fed infants wake up more often during the night to nurse (71). Additionally, a small number of researchers have reported that socioeconomic status and other family factors may have an impact on children's sleeping patterns. For example, Sadeh and colleagues (72) assessed the sleep patterns, disruptions, and sleepiness in 140 7–13-year-olds from two-parent, upper-middle-class Israeli families through the use of actigraphy and diaries. A child's age was the best predictor of sleep schedule and duration (e.g., older children displayed more delayed sleep, more daytime sleepiness, shorter sleep periods, morning drowsiness, and more unplanned naps). However, parental age, parental education, and family stress also predicted sleep quality. Similarly, Tynjala and colleagues (73) observed the sleep habits of nearly 3,000 Finnish adolescents and found that geographic location influenced sleep patterns. Specifically, teenagers living in rural areas slept longer than those in urban environments. Family size and schedules may also affect the amount and scheduling of sleep (74). The sleep of a child or adolescent, in particular, tends to be governed by societal or environmental constraints, such as school schedules, parent work schedules, television and computer use, and so forth. Some constraints are more or less negotiable.

Over the last 20 years, Carskadon and colleagues and other researchers have demonstrated the following with regard to changes in sleep patterns in older children and adolescents (61): (a) Sleep "need" does not seem to change from 10 to 17 years of age and, if anything, older adolescents sleep more than younger adolescents when given the unconstrained opportunity (e.g., Refs. 75–77). (b) Across age, sex, and Tanner stage, polysomnographic sleep length is about 9 hr (11,75,78). (c) Slow-wave sleep (SWS) decreases by 40% from ages 10 to 17 years, even though total sleep does not change. (d) On the MSLT, adolescents show an increased daytime sleep tendency at approximately midpuberty. However, numerous studies across a variety of geographic and cultural settings point out that middle-school- and high-school-age adolescents in the "real world" are not obtaining an adequate amount of sleep and get significantly less sleep than younger, elementary-school-age children (e.g., 62,65,79–81). Studies have shown that teenagers usually obtain much less sleep than elementary-school-age children, from 10 hr during middle childhood to less than 7 hr by the end of high school (65,75,82–84). Adolescents tend to stay up increasingly later over the middle- and high-school years, get up early for school, and, as a result, get progressively less sleep over the course of adolescence (65,75,84,85).

The social pressures of the teen years—staying up late to watch TV, chatting on the phone endlessly with friends, or doing homework—when combined with the need to arise early in the morning for school and possibly afterschool employment, can easily create a situation in which the adolescent chronically obtains inadequate sleep. Historically, schools have started early in the morning throughout the United States as well as elsewhere. Additionally, many U.S. school districts use a three- or four-bell schedule where high schools open first, followed by middle or junior-high schools, and then elementary schools with one or two starting times (86). In a preliminary survey of 40 high-school schedules posted on the Internet from throughout the United States for the 1996–1997 academic year, 48% started at 7:30 A.M. or earlier, whereas only 12% started between 8:15 and 8:55 A.M. (87). More recently, in 2001-2002, nearly 50% ($N = 50$ schools) started between 7:31 and 8:14 A.M., 35% prior to 7:30 A.M., and only 16% started the day between 8:15 and 8:55 A.M.

Earlier middle- and high-school start time is a major externally imposed constraint on teenagers' sleep-wake schedules. Early-morning school demands often significantly constrict the hours available for sleep. For example, Szymczak and colleagues (88) followed Polish students aged 10 and 14 years for over a year and found that all slept longer on weekends and during vacations as a result of waking up later. These investigators concluded that the school duty schedule was the predominant determinant of awakening times for these students.

Epstein and colleagues (89) surveyed over 800 Israeli preadolescents who attended schools with starting times that ranged from 7:10 to 8:30 A.M. The investigators compared those that started at least 2 days per week at 7:15 A.M. or earlier with those that started regularly at 8:00 A.M. Mean total sleep times of the students attending the schools with early start times were significantly shorter than those of students at the later starting schools. Similarly, several surveys of high-school students found that students who start school at 7:30 A.M. or earlier obtain less total sleep on school nights owing to earlier rise times (83,90,91).

Wahlstrom (92) also examined differences among districts with different high-school start times. This researcher compared sleep habits and daytime functioning of high-school students ($N = 7168$) from three school districts in the Minneapolis/St. Paul, Minnesota area. District A started classes each day at 8:30 A.M., whereas Districts B and C started at 7:25 A.M. and 7:15 A.M., respectively. High-school students in District A reported similar bedtimes to students in Districts B and C; however, they reported getting up about 1 hr later and obtaining about an hour more sleep on school nights. Weekend sleep habits did not differ among students in these districts.

Finally, Carskadon and her colleagues evaluated the impact of a 65-min advance in school start time on approximately 40 ninth graders across the transition to tenth grade (91). Specifically, junior high school started at 8:25 A.M. and high school started at 7:20 A.M. in this large urban school district. The following results were obtained: (a) Only 62% of the students in ninth grade and fewer than half the students in tenth grade got an average of even 7 hr of sleep on school nights. (b) Students woke earlier on school days in tenth grade than in ninth grade. (c) They had shorter sleep latencies on the MSLT in the tenth than in ninth grade, particularly on the 8:30 A.M. assessment. (d) Sixteen percent of participants experienced two REM episodes on MSLT in tenth grade (one REM episode occurred in 48%). Certainly, the imposition of an early school start time may require impractical and infeasible bedtimes to provide enough time for sleeping.

We have much to learn from the research on work hours, schedules, and sleep/wake patterns. Rosa (93) documents that the circadian timing of work (i.e., early work or school start times) and the total number of hours worked (e.g., school plus work hours) both reduce sleep length and increase morning sleepiness. In one study, Rosa and his colleagues (94) demonstrated that an early-morning job start time (e.g., 6:00 vs. 7:00 A.M.) decreased sleep time since it was difficult to advance bedtime enough on the night before work. Similarly, working a 12-hr shift in comparison to an 8-hr shift made it difficult for the employees to get adequate sleep because the extended hours either directly overlapped with the nighttime sleep period or forced them to take care of their daytime responsibilities during that time (95).

Similar to early work start times, early school start times increase the likelihood of shortening morning sleep and increasing daytime sleepiness during school hours. Likewise, extended workdays are analogous to high-school students attending school 35 hr/week and while working 20 hr/week in an after-school job (93). Carskadon (96) and Wolfson (87) documented a disconcerting relationship between hours spent at jobs, sleep patterns, and daytime sleepiness. Specifically, in both studies, the students who reported working more than 20 hr/week, in comparison to those working less than 20 hr/week or not at all, reported more symptoms of daytime sleepiness. These symptoms included struggling to stay awake while driving; difficulty staying awake in their classes, studying, or doing homework; and increased sleep/wake behavior problems (for example, arriving late to class owing to oversleeping; feeling tired, dragged out, or sleepy during the day). They also reported greater use of caffeine, alcohol/drugs, and tobacco.

### III. Mental Health Difficulties with Sleep Problems as Outcomes

Children with inadequate sleep are often diagnosed with behavioral and mental health difficulties. The development, regulation, and timing of sleep can be altered by behavioral/emotional disorders, while cognitive, behavioral, and emotional control during daytime hours can be influenced by the way children and adolescents sleep (97). Additionally, medications used to treat psychiatric disorders often affect sleep, and sleep loss can exacerbate mood and behavioral symptoms. In an earlier review, Wolfson and colleagues point out that it can be extremely difficult to tease apart the boundaries of these overlapping and interacting domains in clinical settings. For example, it can be impossible to retrospectively determine whether disturbed sleep symptoms antedated symptoms of depression or vice versa. Sleep interacts with both internalizing disorders (i.e., the primary symptoms are directed internally—such as depression, anxiety) and externalizing disorders [i.e., the primary symptoms are externally directed problems with behavior—such as attention deficit/hyperactivity disorder (ADHD) and conduct problems].

Many researchers believe that mood disorders in children and adolescents represent one of the most underdiagnosed emotional disorders in the mental health field. Population studies report prevalence rates of depression in children between 0.4 and 2.5% and in adolescents between 4 and 8.5% (reviewed in Ref. 98). Subjective sleep complaints are very common in children and adolescents diagnosed with major depressive disorder (MDD). Symptoms include insomnia (75% of cases) and hypersomnia (25%). Hypersomnia difficulties are reported more frequently after puberty. Insomnia symptoms usually include difficulty falling asleep and a subjective sense of not having slept deeply all night. Early-morning awakenings are less prevalent in children and adolescents than in adults with depression. Clinicians and researchers have seen increasingly more adolescents with overlapping phase delay disorders and/or other sleep/wake schedule disorders with depression. Studies suggest that depressed adolescents may have difficulty falling asleep and maintaining sleep, are unable to get up or refuse to go to school, sleep in late in the day, complain of daytime tiredness, and, over time, shift to increasingly more delayed sleep/wake schedules (e.g., Refs. 99,100).

Moreover, children and adolescents diagnosed with ADHD and related externalizing disorders also seem to experience inadequate and/or disrupted sleep. Numerous clinicians and researchers have commented on the complex relationships between sleep and ADHD symptoms. There are four primary observations regarding this relationship: (a) Children diagnosed with ADHD have high rates of subjective sleep complaints (and some evidence of sleep disturbances). (b) Children obtaining inadequate sleep or with sleep disruption often show signs of inattentiveness (sometimes including hyperactivity). (c) Stimulant medications used to treat attention deficit disorders can also interfere with sleep. (d) Behavioral problems associated with the ADHD (as well as conduct disorder and oppositional defiant disorder) can interfere with bedtime organization and scheduling and thus can contribute to insufficient sleep from late and erratic bedtimes (reviewed in Ref. 97).

In addition, there is some debate regarding the degree of sleep disruption associated with ADHD (101). Although questionnaire and survey data of ADHD children and controls show very high rates of sleep problems and complaints, in general, the more objective the study (including structured interviews, actigraphy, and EEG studies), the weaker is the evidence for sleep abnormalities associated with ADHD (97,102). One apparent misconception is the suggestion that ADHD children *need* less sleep than normal age-matched children. The data indicate that ADHD children are more difficult to wake up on school mornings, suggesting that, if anything, ADHD children are getting less sleep than they require. Increasingly more studies, however, have shown evidence for sleep disruption in some ADHD children (e.g., increased rates of snoring, sleep apnea, as well as periodic limb movements [103]). Clearly, additional well-controlled studies in these areas are necessary to explain the relationship between ADHD and inadequate and/or disrupted sleep (101).

Moreover, there is evidence for increased rates of ADHD symptoms in clinical populations of children with sleep disorders, including children with the obstructive sleep apnea syndrome (OSAS), periodic limb movements of sleep (PLMS), narcolepsy, and sleep-wake schedule disorders. Studies indicate that treating the primary sleep disorder can produce significant improvement in ADHD symptoms (103).

## IV.  Sleep Disorders with Sleep Disruption and Disrupted Sleep

Inadequate sleep may also be associated with sleep disorders in adolescents. It is estimated that almost half of adult Americans and 20–30% of children have difficulty sleeping (104). This occurs not because they do not want to sleep but because they cannot sleep owing to various sleep-related disorders. A number of sleep disorders may also contribute to inadequate sleep and difficulties during the day. In comparison to adult sleep disorders, far less is known about the incidence of diagnosable sleep disorders among adolescents. However, increasingly more clinicians are reporting apnea, narcolepsy, insomnia, and phase delay disorders among adolescents. Ohayon and colleagues estimate the prevalence of DSM-IV insomnia to be 4% and incidence of phase delay disorder at 1% for 15–18 year-olds; however, approximately 25% report insomnia symptoms (105). In an earlier study, Morrison and colleagues (106) used DSM-III to evaluate 15-year-old adolescents and estimated that approximately 15% experienced insomnia.

Sleep disorders such as sleep apnea, narcolepsy, delayed sleep-phase syndrome (DSPS), and insomnia can cause problem sleepiness and difficulty functioning during the day for adolescents (103). Over the course of several studies, Roberts and colleagues have shown that insomnia and related sleep problems have adverse consequences for the future functioning of adolescents (107,108). In particular, insomnia symptoms such as nonrestorative sleep, difficulty initiating sleep, and daytime sleepiness predicted self-esteem difficulties, interpersonal relationship problems, and symptoms of depression, along with somatic complaints (108).

DSPS is especially troublesome for adolescents (103,109). DSPS is manifested by sleep onset times that are delayed several hours relative to conventional bedtimes. Conversely, the normal time to wake up drifts to correspondingly later in the morning. Since school must be attended, these teens often come home from school and crash for a nap, then later stay up until all hours of the night in a repetitive cycle. There seems to be a strong relationship between depression and DSPS. One study of adolescents with DSPS found that 36% had features of depression (110). And, in a more recent study of older adolescents (first-year college students), the researchers concluded that the sleep/wake patterns associated with DSPS and chronic insufficient sleep tend to result in lowered academic performance, depressed mood, and other daytime difficulties. The relationship between DSPS and mood difficulties is poorly understood in that the inadequate sleep associated with DSPS may give rise to depression, or there may be a primary mood disorder that evokes the symptoms of DSPS (111).

Neurologically based disorders of hypersomnolence often have their onset in adolescence and can have a profound impact on the young person's academic and social functioning. Such disorders are often unrecognized and can cause the perception that adolescents are lazy, unmotivated, or learning-disabled. Narcolepsy involves a classic tetrad of symptoms: sleep attacks (i.e., irresistible urges to fall asleep), sleep-onset paralysis, sleep-onset hallucinations, and cataplexy. Many young people with this disorder receive an initial diagnosis of either ADHD or depression.

Adults with sleep apnea will be aware of snoring and insufficient refreshment from sleep. Adult sleep apnea has been well publicized in recent years. Less well discussed is that adolescents can and do develop a similar problem. The usual causes of sleep-related breathing disturbances in young people are chronic allergies, obesity, tonsils and/or adenoids large enough or positioned in such a way as to affect breathing during sleep, or, on occasion, a broken nose. This common sleep disorder can produce daytime problems that are often thought to be solely psychological in origin: difficulty waking up in the morning and reluctance to go to school, depression, having an "attitude," and even difficulties in school or with a peer group (103).

Undoubtedly, there is growing evidence for an association between disturbed sleep and impaired adolescent functioning; however, more attention needs to be directed toward identifying possible causal paths and possible strategies for intervention. Furthermore, clinicians need to become more aware of the potential role of sleep disorders when evaluating children with neurobehavioral deficits.

The research described above illustrates the large number of factors that can influence sleep quantity and quality. Next, we describe studies that relate variations in sleep variables to other measures of functioning.

## V. Sleep Duration and Schedules: Sleep as an Independent Variable

Problems related to inadequate sleep in children and adolescents are fairly common. Studies have shown that inadequate or irregular sleep usually results in some variation of daytime sleepiness, but may also result in behavior problems, difficulties with alertness, concentration, attentiveness, problem solving, memory, school problems, and other daytime behavior problems. Adolescents' health may also be compromised by poor sleep/wake habits, with increased irritability and depressed moods, substance abuse, and risk for falling-asleep-at-the-wheel and drowsy-driving accidents.

### A. Academic Performance

Cognitive function and psychomotor skills are closely related to sleep, and numerous studies have correlated sleep loss with significant decreases in performance in these areas (112). Most recently, studies have shown that when young adults learn a new skill, their performance does not improve until after they have had 6 and preferably 8 hr of sleep (113). According to Stickgold and colleagues, at least 6 hr of sleep, where an individual obtains both the NREM sleep from early in the night and the later hours of REM sleep, are needed to integrate and consolidate learning from the previous day. Their data show that college-age students who do not get an adequate total amount of sleep will have significant difficulty with tasks that require skilled movements and memories for procedures, such as mastering a sport, playing a musical instrument, driving a car, working at the computer, etc. It is not surprising that sleepy adolescents—that is those with inadequate sleep—seem to encounter increased academic difficulties. Wolfson and Carskadon (114) reviewed and critiqued studies that assessed the relation between sleep patterns, sleep quality, and school performance of adolescents attending middle school, high school, and/or college. The majority of studies relied on self-report, yet researchers approached the question with different designs and measures. The findings strongly indicated that self-reported shortened total sleep time, erratic sleep/wake schedules, late bed and rise times, and poor sleep quality are negatively associated with academic performance for adolescents from middle school through the college years. For example, several surveys of high-school students reported that more total sleep, earlier bedtimes, and later weekday rise times were associated with better grades in school (65,83,115).

Similarly, persistent sleep problems have also been associated with learning difficulties throughout the elementary-high-school years (116). Studies of excessive sleepiness in children and adolescents due to DSPS, narcolepsy, or sleep apnea have also reported negative effects on learning, school performance, and behavior (117–119). Students who get more sleep and maintain more consistent school/weekend sleep schedules may obtain better grades because of their ability to remain alert and to pay greater attention in class and on homework.

### B. Emotional and Behavioral Well-Being

Research is in the early stages of investigating the complex relationship between adolescents' sleep patterns and behavioral well-being. Studies have shown that sleep-disturbed older elementary-school-age children experienced a greater number of stresses (e.g., maternal absence due to work/school, family illness/accident, maternal depressed mood) than non-sleep-disturbed children (120). Likewise, sleepy school-age children may have poorer coping behaviors (e.g., more difficulty recognizing, appraising, and adapting to stressful situations) and display more behavior problems at home and in school (121,122). Aronen and colleagues (123) monitored 7–12 year-olds for 72 consecutive hours with activity monitors and assessed psychiatric symptoms through parent and teacher reports. Quantity of sleep was significantly associated with both externalizing and internalizing symptoms, particularly teacher-reported symptoms. Clearly, inadequate sleep contributes to behavioral problems for elementary- and middle-school-age children.

Furthermore, Wolfson and Carskadon (65) found that high-school students who adopted more adequate sleep habits (defined as longer total sleep times and more regular sleep schedules across the week) reported lower levels of depressed mood, fewer complaints of daytime sleepiness, and fewer problematic sleep behaviors in comparison to students with inadequate sleep habits. Likewise, students with more irregular sleep schedules had more behavior problems and increased substance abuse [e.g., cigarettes, drugs, such as marijuana (87)]. Researchers in New Zealand, France, and Quebec, Canada reported analogous findings. Morrison and colleagues (106) compared four groups of 13- and 15–year-olds in New Zealand: (1) those with no sleep problems, (2) those indicating they needed more sleep only, (3) those reporting difficulties falling asleep or maintaining sleep, and (4) those with multiple sleep problems. These authors concluded that adolescents in the three sleep-problem groups were more anxious, had higher levels of depression, and had lower social competence than those in the no-sleep-problem group did. These studies all strongly suggest that adolescents with inadequate total sleep, irregular school-night-to-weekend sleep/wake schedules, and/or sleep disturbances struggle with emotional/behavior problems and/or academic difficulties.

### C.  Safety, Health, and Well-Being

Research suggests that the consequences of chronic sleep deprivation may be much worse than simply diminished mental sharpness, moodiness, and/or excessive daytime sleepiness. Spiegel and colleagues (124) found that even in healthy young adults, as little as a weeklong sleep debt of 3 or 4 hr each night has adverse effects on the body's ability to process carbohydrates, manage stress, maintain a proper balance of hormones, and fight off infections. Although this study was not conducted with young adolescents, undoubtedly adequate sleep is important for adolescents' health as well. A small number of studies have found that adolescents with disrupted or inadequate sleep report more fatigue, less energy, symptoms of headache, stomachache, and backache, and worse perceived health (125–127).

Furthermore, accidents and injuries are leading health concerns for child and adolescent populations (e.g., Ref. 128). In fact, unintentional injuries are among the leading causes of death for adolescents (129,130). Adolescents who are not able to obtain adequate sleep may struggle with lapses in attention and delayed responses that can affect their ability to safely operate hazardous or technical equipment, such as stoves, automobiles, Bunsen burners, lawn mowers, snow blowers, etc. In two different surveys, nearly 10% of high-school students reported being sleepy while driving a car (87,96) and teenagers with low amounts and irregular timing of sleep are more likely to report increased accidents and injuries ranging from cuts to gunshots (131). While there is minimal research on the impact of chronic sleep deprivation on middle-school-age youngsters' functioning and health, it is reasonable to believe that a developing pattern of inadequate sleep will have adverse consequences.

Although few researchers have looked at the use of cigarettes, other nicotine products, caffeine, and other stimulants in relationship to adolescents' sleep patterns, it is clear that increasingly more middle- and high-school students are smoking cigarettes and drinking caffeinated beverages to keep themselves alert (132). Specifically, 80% of smokers begin before age 18, and approximately 36% of high-school students were current smokers in 1997, an increase of about one third from 1991 (133). The Centers for Disease Control (134) reported that the overall prevalence of any current tobacco use among students in grades 6–8 was nearly 13%. In the Rhode Island survey of over 3000 high-school students, many of the teenagers complained about feeling depressed, fatigued, and falling asleep in classes, and noted that they used a variety of mood-altering substances (87). Specifically, about half of the 9th–12th graders reported that they felt tired or dragged out nearly everyday, 30% rarely had a good night's sleep in the last 2 weeks, just over 25% admitted that they fell asleep and/or struggled to stay awake while in class, and 34% reported that they use two to four substances [e.g., caffeine, alcohol, cigarettes at least once a day (87)]. Similarly, Phillips and Danner (135) found that adolescent and adult smokers, in comparison to nonsmokers, reported more problems falling asleep and maintaining sleep during the night as well as increased daytime sleepiness, accidents, depressed mood, and caffeine intake. Likewise, Patten and colleagues (100) demonstrated that depressive symptoms and/or cigarette smoking predicted the development and persistence of sleep problems (e.g., difficulty falling asleep and/or maintaining sleep) among 12–18 year-old teenagers.

Other types of substance abuse among adolescents are unfortunately widespread and often initially undetected or even unsuspected. Marijuana, alcohol, and cocaine all cause disturbances of normal sleep rhythms and can produce daytime sleepiness. Similarly, prescription medications (e.g., antihistamines, antiseizure medications, antidepressants, etc.) and over-the-counter drugs can influence sleep patterns or lead to daytime sleepiness. Among adolescents, sleep problems and substance use have received little attention. Not surprisingly, however, a few studies have found that the use of cigarettes, alcohol, and other illicit drugs (e.g., marijuana, cocaine, inhalants) is associated with sleep problems such as needing more sleep, difficulty falling asleep, and/or maintaining sleep (125,136). However, the nature of the associations between inadequate sleep and use of drugs is complex and requires further study. As Johnson and Breslau (136) emphasized, whether the independent association of sleep problems with use of various drugs is due to lifestyle factors connected to substance use, such as more erratic sleep/wake schedules, or an effect of the substances themselves is ambiguous.

## VI.  Experimental Studies of Sleep Restriction/Disruption and Circadian Timing

As we have shown earlier, survey studies and studies of clinical samples have provided a large body of evidence relating inadequate or disturbed sleep to various measures of functioning. Very few studies, however, have employed experimental designs to study consequences of inadequate or restricted sleep. Parents are often reluctant for their children to lose sleep or to stay overnight in a laboratory. In addition, preparing laboratory and staff for the needs of children adds another layer of complexity to laboratory studies. The few experimental studies have provided mixed results and much more research is required. New evidence that school-age children can comply with imposed sleep schedules at home for days and weeks may facilitate additional studies (137).

To date, the variable most consistently associated with experimental sleep restriction in children and adolescents is sleepiness as measured by the MSLT. These studies restricted sleep in children aged 8–15 years for 1 night to up to 7 nights with nocturnal sleep opportunities ranging from 4 to 7 hr (47,49,50,137); one older study deprived children aged 11-14 years of sleep for 38 hr (48). As mentioned earlier, Carskadon and colleagues (91) studied adolescents during the transition from ninth to tenth grade to assess the effects of a shift to an earlier school start time. In this more naturalistic study, sleep at home was assessed with actigraphy and sleep diaries for 2 weeks at each assessment. Students woke earlier on school days in tenth than in ninth grade, but did not go to sleep earlier. The consequent decrease in sleep was associated with an increase in sleep latency scores from MSLTs after overnight sleep monitoring. Finally, longitudinal studies of children undergoing pubertal development demonstrated decreased MSLT scores (increased sleepiness) as children matured, despite the fact that they were allowed 10-hr sleep opportunities for 3 consecutive nights during every visit (11). The participants in this study did not sleep less over the yearly visits, yet they showed increased sleepiness during midday tests as they reached midpuberty. Carskadon and colleagues have argued that these results indicate that postpubertal adolescents actually need more sleep to maintain prepubertal levels of alertness.

The results from the studies described above indicate that the MSLT provides a robust measure of sleepiness that is sensitive to sleep restriction in children and adolescents (112). Patterns of sleep latency from repeated naps during constant routine protocols or forced desynchrony protocols in older children and adolescents also illustrate the influences of both homeostatic and circadian processes on sleepiness/alertness and provide evidence for the hypothesis that changes in these systems either drive or permit the adolescent phase delay in sleep timing (53,61,138).

Results from other variables assessed in sleep restriction studies are less consistent. For example, some studies have found no deficits in tasks assessing motor skills (48,49), auditory attention (47,48), sustained attention and response inhibition (50), memory tasks (47,49,139), and computational accuracy (47,48,139) after acute or extended sleep restriction. On the other hand, decrements in performance have been demonstrated for reaction time (51), impaired verbal fluency, creativity (49,139), computational speed (47,48,139), and abstract problem solving following acute or extended sleep restriction. Decrements in performance have also been shown in reaction time, other motor skills tasks such as balance and agility, and memory tasks after 38 or 50 hr of sleep deprivation (47,48,140). Clearly, more experimental research is needed to tease apart the developmental influences of sleep restriction and/or disruption on a range of daytime functioning behaviors and cognitive skills. Additionally, studies are needed that restrict sleep for extended periods of time to identify deficits that may be associated with the typical sleep patterns of children and adolescents.

## VII.  Summary, Conclusions, and Future Directions

In this chapter, we have described considerable empirical evidence that relates inadequate or disturbed sleep in children and adolescents to a variety of impairments and potential risks. Inadequate sleep is clearly a concern for parents, teachers, and children and the consequences have important social, educational, and medical ramifications. Less evidence is available regarding the effects on specific functional domains using experimental techniques. As we have argued, mixed and ambiguous results from studies relating outcome measures to sleep and sleep pattern measures may be a result of variability due to a number of factors, including: individual and developmental differences in sleep need or vulnerability to sleep loss, insensitivity of measures (e.g., subjective measures and reports), practice, motivation, or time-of-day effects, and unsuitability of procedures for children. An additional difficulty is that a given amount of sleep restriction may lead to decreased function in one domain, such as emotional regulation, but no change in functions such as reaction time or cognitive performance. Thus, sleep that is inadequate for some tasks may be adequate for others. Much work remains to sort out the reasons for negative and mixed results, including evaluation of measures and procedures for their use in sleepy children and, as noted above, incorporation of potentially important covariates such as sleep need and vulnerability to sleep loss. Experimental paradigms that might prove useful include sleep restriction and sleep extension studies, particularly those with multiple nights of restriction/extension and multiple measures of performance obtained throughout waking intervals, and longitudinal or multisession studies to assess the stability of measures of sleep need or vulnerability to sleep loss. In addition, studies using complex protocols such as constant routines and forced desynchrony, though expensive, time-consuming, and difficult, hold the promise of elucidating underlying biological processes. Finally, as with any complex system, understanding will be fostered by the use of multiple measures and multiple informants within studies in a variety of laboratory and field environments.

A number of other important research and clinical issues and questions have not been addressed for children and adolescents. *How much napping occurs in school and out of bed? What are the effects of sleep loss on metabolic processes, the immune system, and health outcomes in children and adolescents? How do light exposure patterns affect sleep patterns and processes in children and adolescents? How much and when do parents sleep and what role does a family's schedule of activities play in children's and adolescents' sleep patterns? What outcome measures have not been studied that are particularly important to parents and children? What does sleep look like in underprivileged children and adolescents?* The list is long.

Finally, though we cannot map precisely a landscape of destruction that follows the disruption or restriction of sleep, an abundance of smaller pieces of evidence indicates that many children and adolescents are not functioning as well as they might and inadequate sleep might be one of the significant reasons. Furthermore, the demands and pressures of an increasingly complex world are unlikely to lessen. We need to develop interventions that are effective for increasing sleep opportunities, clinical support for sleep disorders, countermeasures when adequate sleep cannot be obtained, and education programs to increase support of sleep by parents, health care practitioners, and society. The complexities and risks of today's and tomorrow's world require as much vigilance as we can muster.

## References

1. Webb W, Agnew H. Are we chronically sleep deprived? Bull Psychon Soc 1975; 6:47–48.
2. Horne JA. Why We Sleep: The Functions of Sleep in Humans and Other Mammals. New York: Oxford University Press, 1988.
3. Carskadon MA, Roth T. Sleep restriction. In: Monk TH, ed. Sleep, Sleepiness and Performance. New York: Wiley, 1991:155–67.
4. Aeschbach D, Cajochen C, Landolt H, Borbely AA. Homeostatic sleep regulation in habitual short sleepers and long sleepers. Am J Physiol 1996; 270:R41-R53.
5. Aeschbach D, Postolache TT, Sher I, Mathews JR, Jackson MA, Wehr TA. Evidence from the waking elecroencephalogram that short sleepers live under higher homeostatic sleep pressure than long sleepers. Neuroscience 2001; 102:493–502.
6. Dinges DF, Achermann P. Commentary: Future considerations for models of human neurobehavioral function. J Biol Rhythms 1999; 14:598–601.
7. Parmelee AH, Jr., Schulz HR, Disbrow MA. Sleep patterns of the newborn. J Pediatr 1961; 58:241-250.

8.  Kleitman N. Sleep and Wakefulness, rev. ed. Chicago: University of Chicago Press, 1967.
9.  Kleitman N, Engelmann TG. Sleep characteristics of infants. J Appl Physiol 1953:6:269–282.
10. Kahn A, Fisher C, Edwards A, Davis A. Twenty-four hour sleep patterns: comparison between 2– to 3–year old and 4– to 6–year-old children. Arch Gen Psychiatry 1973; 29:380–385.
11. Carskadon MA, Harvey K, Duke P, Anders TF, Litt I, Dement WC. Pubertal changes in daytime sleepiness. Sleep 1980; 2:453–460.
12. Coble PA, Kupfer DJ, Taska LS, Kane J. EEG sleep of normal healthy children. Part I. Findings using standard measurement methods. Sleep 1984; 7(4):289–303.
13. Louis J, Cannard C, Bastuji H, Challamel M-J. Sleep ontogenesis revisited: a longitudinal 24 hour home polygraphic study on 15 normal infants during the first two years of life. Sleep 1997; 20(5):323–333.
14. Acebo C, Sadeh A, Seifer R, Tzischinski O, Hafer A, Carskadon MA. Sleep/wake patterns in one to five year old children from activity monitoring and maternal reports. Sleep 2000; 23:A30.
15. Carskadon MA, Acebo C, Seifer R. Extended nights, sleep loss, and recovery sleep in adolescents. Arch Itali Biol 2001; 139:301-312.
16. Van Dongen HPA, Maislin MS, Mullington JM, Dinges DF. The cumulative cost of additional wakefulness: dose-response effects on neurobehavioral functions and sleep physiology from chronic sleep restriction and total sleep deprivation. Sleep 2003; 26:117–126.
17. Wolfson AR, Carskadon MA, Acebo C, Seifer R, Fallone G, Labyak SE, Martin JL. Evidence for the validity of a sleep habits survey for adolescents. Sleep 2003; 26(2):213–216.
18. Chambers MJ. Actigraphy and insomnia: a closer look. Part I. Sleep 1994; 17:405–408.
19. Sadeh A, Sharkey KM, Carskadon MA. Activity-based sleep-wake identification: an empirical test of methodological issues. Sleep 1994; 17:201-207.
20. Sadeh A, Lavie P, Scher A, Tirosh E, Epstein R. Actigraphic home-monitoring sleep-disturbed and control infants and young children: a new method for pediatric assessment of sleep-wake patterns. Pediatrics 1991; 87:494-9.
21. Sadeh A, Acebo C, Seifer R, Carskadon MA. Activity-based assessment of sleep-wake patterns during the first year of life. Infant Behav Dev 1995; 18(3):329–337.
22. Acebo C, Sadeh A, Seifer R, Tzischinsky O, Wolfson AR, Hafer A, Carskadon MA. Estimating sleep patterns with activity monitoring in children and adolescents: how many nights are necessary for reliable measures? Sleep 1999; 22(1):95–103.
23. Sadeh A, Acebo C. The role of actigraphy in sleep medicine. Sleep Med Rev 2002; 6:113–124.
24. Fallone G, Seifer R, Acebo C, Carskadon MA. How well do school-aged children comply with imposed sleep schedules at home? Sleep 2002; 25:739–745.
25. Roffwarg HP, Dement WC, Fisher, C. Preliminary observations of the sleep-dream pattern in neonates, infants, children, and adults. In: Harms, E, ed. Problems of Sleep and Dreams in Children. Monographs on Child Psychiatry, no. 2. New York: Pergamon Press, 1964:60–72.

26. Kohler WC, Coddington D, Agnew HW. Sleep patterns in 2–year-old children. J Pediatr 1968; 72:228–233.

27. Williams R, Karacan I, Hursch C. EEG of Human Sleep. New York: Wiley, 1974.

28. Hoppenbrouwers T, Hodgman JE, Harper RM, Sterman MB. Termporal distribution of sleep states, somatic activity and autonomic activity during the first half year of life. Sleep 1982; 5:131-144.

29. Fagioli I, Salzarulo P. Sleep states development in the first year of life assessed through 24–hr recordings. Early Hum Dev 1982; 68:215–228.

30. Coble P, Kupfer D, Reynolds C, Houck R. EEG sleep of healthy children 6 to 12 years of age. In: Guilleminault, C, ed. Sleep and Its Disorders in Children. New York: Raven Press, 1987:29–41.

31. Carskadon MA, Keenen S, Dement WC. Nighttime sleep and daytime sleep tendency in preadolescents. In: Guilleminault, C, ed. Sleep and Its Disorders in Children. New York: Raven Press, 1987:43–52.

32. Karacan I, Anch M, Thornby JK, Okawa M, Williams RL. Longitudinal sleep patterns during pubertal growth: four-year follow-up. Pediatr Res 1975; 9:842–846.

33. Carskadon MA, Acebo, C, Labyak SE, Seifer R. Wake-dependent and circadian influences on reaction time, probed memory recall, and digit symbol substitution on adolescents. Sleep Res Online, 1999b; 2(suppl 1):598.

34. Carskadon MA, Acebo C, Labyak SE, Seifer R. Intrinsic circadian period of adolescent humans measured in conditions of forced desynchrony. Neurosci Lett 1999; 260:129–132.

35. Agnew HW, Webb WB, Williams RL. The first night effect: an EEG study of sleep. Psychophysiology 1966; 2:263–266.

36. Feinberg I, Koresko RL, Heller N. EEG sleep patterns as a function of normal and pathological aging in man. J Psychiatr Res 1967; 5:107–144.

37. Webb WB, Agnew HW. Measurement and characteristics of nocturnal sleep. In: Abt LE, Reiss BF, eds. Progress in Clinical Psychology, New York: Grune & Stratton, 1969:2–27.

38. Moses J, Lubin A, Naitoh P, Johnson LC. Reliability of sleep measures. Psychophysiology 1972; 9:78–82.

39. Feinberg I. Some observations of the reliability of REM variables. Psychophysiology 1974; 9:68–72.

40. Bixler EO, Kales A, Jacoby JA, Soldatos CR, Vela-Bueno A. Nocturnal sleep and wakefulness: effects of age and sex in normal sleepers. Int J Neurosci 1984; 23:3342.

41. Thoman EB, Korner A., Kraemer HC. Individual consistency in behavioral states in neonates. Dev Psychobiol 1976; 9:271-283.

42. Becker PT, Thoman EB. Organization of sleeping and waking states in infants: consistency across contexts. Physiol Behav 1983; 31:405–410.

43. Anders TF, Keener M. Developmental course of night-time sleep-wake patterns in full-term and premature infants during the first year of life. Sleep 1985; 8:173–192.

44. Sander LW, Stechler G, Burns P, Julia H. Early mother-infant interaction and 24–hour patterns of activity and sleep. J Am Acad Child Psychiatry 1970; 9:103–123.

45. Thoman EB, Whitney MP. Sleep states of infants monitored in the home: individual differences, developmental trends, and origins of diurnal cyclicity. Inf Behav Dev 1989; 12:59–75.

46. Thoman EB, Acebo C. Monitoring of sleep in neonates and young children. In: Ferber R, Kryger M, eds. Principles and Practices of Sleep Medicine in the Child. Philadelphia: Saunders, 1995:55–68.
47. Carskadon MA, Harvey K, Dement WC. Acute restriction of nocturnal sleep in children. Percept Motor Skills 1981a; 53:103–112.
48. Carskadon MA, Harvey K, Dement WC. Sleep loss in young adolescents. Sleep 1981b; 4:299–312.
49. Randazzo AC, Muehlbach MJ, Schweitzer PK, Walsh JK. Cognitive function following acute sleep restriction in children ages 10–14. Sleep 1998; 21:861-868.
50. Fallone G, Acebo C, Arnedt JT, Seifer R, Carskadon MA. Effects of acute sleep restriction on behavior, sustained attention, and response inhibition in children. Percept Motor Skills 2001; 93:213–229.
51. Sadeh A, Gruber R, Raviv A. The effects of sleep restriction and extension on school-age children: what a difference an hour makes. Child Dev 2003; 74:444–455.
52. Iglowstein I, Jenni OG, Molinari L, Largo RH. Sleep duration from infancy to adolescence: reference values and generational trends. Pediatrics 2003; 111:302–307.
53. Carskadon MA, Acebo C, Jenni OG. Regulation of adolescent sleep: implications for behavior. Ann NY Acad Sci 2004; 1021:276–291.
54. Borbely AA. A two process model of sleep regulation. Hum Neurobiol 1982; 1:195–204.
55. Daan S, Beersma DG, Borbely AA. Timing of human sleep: recovery process gated by a circadian pacemaker, Am J Physiol 1984; 246:R161-83.
56. Edgar DM, Dement WC, Fuller CA. Effect of SCN lesions on sleep in squirrel monkeys—evidence for opponent processes in sleep-wake regulation. J Neurosci 1993; 13:1065–1079.
57. Akerstedt T, Folkard S. Validation of the s and c components of the three-process model of alertness regulation. Sleep 1995; 18:1–6.
58. Edgar DM. In search of neurobiological mechanisms regulating sleep-wakefulness: an empirical and historical account of two opponent processes. Sleep Res Soc Bull 1995; 1:22–27.
59. Czeisler CA, Khalsa SBS. The human circadian timing system and sleep-wake regulation. In: Kryger MH, Roth, T, Dement WC, eds. Principles and Practice of Sleep Medicine, 3rd ed. Philadelphia: Saunders, 2000:353–375.
60. Van Dongen HPA, Dinges, DF. Circadian rhythms in fatigue, alertness, and performance. In Kryger MH, Roth T, Dement WC, eds. Principles and Practice of Sleep Medicine, 3rd ed Philadelphia: Saunders, 2000:391–399.
61. Carskadon MA, Acebo C. Regulation of sleepiness in adolescents: update, insights, and speculation. Sleep 2002; 25(6):606–614.
62. Strauch I, Meier B. Sleep need in adolescents: a longitudinal approach. Sleep 1988; 11(4):378–386.
63. Carskadon MA, Vieira C, Acebo C. Association between puberty and delayed phase preference. Sleep 1993; 16(3):258–262.
64. Gau SF, Soong WT. Sleep problems of junior high school students in Taipei. Sleep 1995; 18:667–673.
65. Wolfson AR, Carskadon MA. Sleep schedules and daytime functioning in adolescents. Child Dev 1998; 69:875–887.
66. Laberge L, Petit D, Simard C, Vitaro F, Tremblay RE, Montplaisir J. Development of sleep patterns in early adolescence, J Sleep Res 2001; 10:59–67.

67.  Gau SF, Soong WT. The transition of sleep-wake patterns in early adolescence. Sleep 2003; 26:449–454.
68.  Carskadon MA, Acebo C, Richardson GS, Tate BA, Seifer R. An approach to studying circadian rhythms of adolescent humans. J Biol Rhythms 1997; 12:278–289.
69.  Dijk D-J, Czeisler CA. Contribution of the circadian pacemaker and the sleep homeostat to sleep propensity, sleep structure, electroencephalographic slow waves and sleep spindle activity in humans. J Neurosci 1995; 15:3526–3538.
70.  Mosko S, Richard C, McKenna J. Infant arousals during mother-infant bed sharing: implications for infant sleep and sudden infant death syndrome research. Pediatrics 1997; 100:841–849.
71.  Weissbluth M, Davis AT, Poucher J. Night waking in 4 to 8–month-old infants. J Pediatr 1984; 104:477.
72.  Sadeh A, Raviv A, Gruber R. Sleep patterns and sleep disruptions in school-age children. Dev Psychol 2000; 36(3):291–301.
73.  Tynjala J, Kannas L, Valimaa R. How young Europeans sleep? Health Educ Res 1993; 8:69–80.
74.  Macgregor IDM, Balding JW. Bedtimes and family size in English schoolchildren. Ann of Hum Biol 1988; 15:435–441.
75.  Carskadon MA. Patterns of sleep and sleepiness in adolescents. Pediatrician 1990b; 17:5–12.
76.  Andrade MM, Silva-Benedito AA, Domenice EES, Arnhold IJP, Menna-Barreto LM. Sleep characteristics of adolescents: a longitudinal study. J Adolesc Health 1993; 14:401–406.
77.  Park YM, Matsumoto K, Shinkoda H, Nagashima H, Kang MJ, Seo YJ. Age and gender difference in habitual sleep-wake rhythm. Psychiatry Clin Neurosci 2001; 55:201–202.
78.  Carskadon MA, Orav EJ, Dement WC. Evolution of sleep and daytime sleepiness in adolescents. In C. Guilleminault C, Lugaresi E, eds. Sleep/Wake Disorders: Natural History, Epidemiology, and Long-Term Evolution. New York: Raven Press, 1983:201–216.
79.  Rugg-Gunn AJ, Hackett AF, Appleton DR, Eastoe JE. Bedtimes of 11 to 14–year-old children in north-east England. J of Biosoc Sci 1984; 16:291–297.
80.  Thorleifsdottir B, Bjornsson JK, Benediktsdottir B, Gislason T, Kristbjarnarson H. Sleep and sleep habits from childhood to young adulthood over a 10–year period. J Psychosom Res 2002; 53:529–537.
81.  Fukuda K, Ishihara K. Age-related changes of sleeping pattern during adolescence. Psychiatry Clin Neurosci 2001; 55(3):231–232.
82.  Carskadon MA. The second decade. In C. Guilleminault C. ed. Sleeping and Waking Disorders: Indications and Techniques. Menlo Park, CA: Addison-Wesley, 1982:99–125.
83.  Allen R. Social factors associated with the amount of school week sleep lag for seniors in an early starting suburban high school. Sleep Res 1992; 21:114.
84.  Wolfson AR, Acebo C, Fallone G, Carskadon MA. Actigraphically-estimated sleep patterns of middle school students. Sleep 2003 (suppl); 26:A126–127.
85.  Price VA, Coates TJ, Thoresen CE, Grinstead, OA. Prevalence and correlates of poor sleep among adolescents. Am J Dis Child 1978; 132:583–586.
86.  Nudel M. The schedule dilemma. Am School Board J 1993; 180(11):37–40.

87. Wolfson A. Bridging the gap between research and practice: what will adolescents' sleep/wake patterns look like in the 21st century? In: Carskadon MA, ed. Adolescent Sleep Patterns: Biological, Social, and Psychological Influences. New York: Cambridge University Press, 2002:198–219.

88. Szymczak JT, Jasinska M, Pawlak E, Swierzykowska M. Annual and weekly changes in the sleep-wake rhythm of school children. Sleep 1993; 16(5):433–435.

89. Epstein R, Chillag N, Lavie P. Starting times of school: effects of daytime functioning of fifth-grade children in Israel. Sleep 1998; 21:250–256.

90. Allen R, Mirabile J. Self-reported sleep-wake patterns for students during the school year from two different senior high schools. Sleep Res 1989; 18:132.

91. Carskadon M, Wolfson A, Acebo C, Tzischinsky O, Seifer R. Adolescent sleep patterns, circadian timing, and sleepiness at a transition to early school days. Sleep 1998; 21(8):871–881.

92. Wahlstrom K. Accommodating the sleep patterns of adolescents within current educational structures: an uncharted path. In Carskadon M, ed. Adolescent Sleep Patterns: Biological, Sociological, and Psychological Influences. Cambridge: Cambridge University Press, 2002:172–197.

93. Rosa RH. What can the study of work scheduling tell us about adolescent sleep? In: Carskadon MA, ed. Adolescent Sleep Patterns: Biological, Sociological, and Psychological Influences. Cambridge: Cambridge University Press, 2002:159–171.

94. Rosa RH, Harma M, Pulli K, Mulder M, Nasman O. Rescheduling a three-shift system at a steel rolling mill: effects of a 1–hour delay of shift starting times on sleep and alertness in younger and older workers. Occup Environ Med, 1996; 53:677–685.

95. Rosa RR, Bonnet MH. Performance and alertness on 8–hour and 12–hour rotating shifts at a natural gas utility, Ergonomics 1993; 36:1177–1193.

96. Carskadon MA. Adolescent sleepiness: increased risk in a high-risk population. Alcohol, Drugs Driving 1990a; 5/6:317–328.

97. Wolfson A, Dahl R, Trentacoste S. Sleep in children with behavioral and psychiatric disorders. In: Loughlin G, Carroll J, Marcus C, eds. Sleep and Breathing During Sleep in Children: A Developmental Approach. New York: Marcel Dekker, 2000:385–395.

98. Birmaher R, Ryan ND, Williamson DE, Brent DA, Kaufman J, Dahl RE, Perel J, Nelson B. Childhood and adolescent depression: a review of the past ten years, Part I. J Am Acad Child Adolesc Psychiatry 1996; 35 (11):1427–1439.

99. Choquet M, Kovess V, Poutignat N. Suicidal thoughts among adolescents: an intercultural approach. Adolescence 1993; 28:649–659.

100. Patten CA, Choi WS, Gillin JC, Pierce JP. Depressive symptoms and cigarette smoking predict development and persistence of sleep problems in U.S. adolescents. Pediatrics 2000; 106(2):1–17.

101. Corkum P, Tannock R, Moldofsky H. Sleep disturbance in children with attention-deficit/hyperactivity disorder. J Am Acad Child Adolesc Psychiatry 1998; 37:637–646.

102. Corkum P, Tannock R, Moldofsky H, Hogg-Johnson S, Humphries T. Actigraphy and parental ratings of sleep in children with attention-deficit/hyperactivity disorder (ADHD). Sleep 2001; 24:303–312.

103. Mindell JA, Owens JA. A Clinical Guide to Pediatric Sleep: Diagnosis and Management of Sleep Problems. Philadelphia: Lippincott Williams & Wilkins, 2003.

104. Poceta JS, Mitler MM, eds. Sleep Disorders: Diagnosis and Treatment. Totowa, NJ: Humana Press, 1998.
105. Ohayon MM, Roberts RE, Zully J, Smirne S, Priest RG. Prevalence and patterns of problematic sleep among older adolescents. J Am Acad Child Adolesc Psychiatry 2000; 39:1549–1556.
106. Morrison DN, McGee R, Stanton WR. Sleep problems in adolescence. J Am Acad Child and Adolesc Psychiatry 1992; 31(1):94–99.
107. Roberts RE, Roberts CR, Chen IG. Functioning of adolescents with symptoms disturbed sleep. J Youth Adolesc 2001; 30(1):1–18.
108. Roberts RE, Roberts CR, Chen IG. Impact of insomnia on future functioning of adolescents. J Psychos Res 2002; 53:561–569.
109. Garcia J, Rosen G, Mahowald M. Circadian rhythms and circadian rhythm disorders in children and adolescents. Semin Pediatr Neurol 2001; 8 (4):229–240.
110. Thorpy MJ, Korman E, Speilman AJ, Glovinsky PB. Delayed sleep phase syndrome in adolescents. J Adolesc Health Care 1988; 9(1):22–27.
111. Zammit, G.K. Delayed sleep phase syndrome and related conditions. In: Pressman MR, Orr WC, eds. Understanding Sleep: The Evaluation and Treatment of Sleep Disorders. Washington, DC: American Psychological Association (APA), 1997.
112. Fallone G, Owens JA, Deane J. Sleepiness in children and adolescents: clinical implications. Sleep Med Rev 2002; 6:287–306.
113. Stickgold R, Whidbee D, Schirmer B, Patel V, Hobson JA. Visual discrimination task improvement: a multi-step process occurring during sleep. J Cognit Neurosci 2000; 12(2):246–254.
114. Wolfson AR, Carskadon MA. Understanding adolescents' sleep patterns and school performance: a critical appraisal. Sleep Med Rev. In press.
115. Manber R, Bootzin RR, Acebo C, Carskadon MA. The effects of regularizing sleep-wake schedules on daytime sleepiness. Sleep 1996; 19(5):432–441.
116. Quine L. Severity of sleep problems in children with severe learning difficulties: description and correlates. J Commun Appl Soc Psychol 1992; 2(4):247–268.
117. Dahl RE, Carskadon, MA. Sleep in its disorders in adolescence. In: Ferber R, Kryger M, eds. Principles and Practice of Sleep Medicine in the Child. Philadelphia: Saunders, 1995:19–27.
118. Dahl RE, Holttum J, Trubnick L. A clinical picture of childhood and adolescent narcolepsy. J Am Acad Child Adolesc Psychiatry 1994; 33:834–841.
119. Guilleminault C, Winkle R, Korobkin R. Children and nocturnal snoring: evaluation of the effects of sleep related respiratory resistive load and daytime functioning. Eur J Pediatr 1982; 139:165–171.
120. Kataria S, Swanson MS, Trevathan GE. Persistence of sleep disturbances in preschool children. Pediatrics 1987; 110(4):642–646.
121. Fisher BE, Rinehart S. Stress, arousal, psychopathology and temperament: a multidimensional approach to sleep disturbance in children. Personal Individ Diff 1990; 11(5):431–438.
122. Wolfson AR, Tzischinsky O, Brown C, Darley C, Acebo C, Carskadon M. Sleep, behavior, and stress at the transition to senior high school. Sleep Res 1995; 24:115.
123. Aronen ET, Paavonen EJ, Fjallberg M, et al. Sleep and psychiatric symptoms in school-aged children. J Am Acad Adolesc Psychiatry 2000; 39 (4):502–508.
124. Spiegel K, Leproult R, Van Cauter E. Impace of sleep debt on metabolic and endocrine function. Lancet 1999; 354:1435–1439.

125. Vignau J, Bailly D, Duhamel A, Bervaecke P, Beuscart R, Collinet C. Epidemiological study of sleep quality and troubles in French secondary school adolescents. J Adolesc Health 1997; 21:343–350.

126. Pilcher JJ, Ginter DR, Sadowsky B. Sleep quality versus quantity: relationships between sleep and measures of health, well-being and sleepiness in college students. J Psychosom Res 1997; 42(6):583–596.

127. Liu X, Uchiyama M, Okawa M, Kurita, H. Prevalence and correlates of self-reported sleep problems among Chinese adolescents. Sleep 2000; 23:27–34.

128. Centers for Disease Control, Division of Injury Control. Childhood injuries in the United States. Am J Dis Child 1990; 144:626–646.

129. Castillo DN, Landen DD, Layne LA. Occupational injury deaths of 16– and 17–year-olds in the United States. Am J Public Health 1994; 84(4); 646–649.

130. Cowell JM, Marks BA. Health behavior in adolescents. In: Gochman DS, ed. Handbook of Health Behavior Research. III. Demography, Development, and Diversity, New York: Plenum Press, 1997.

131. Acebo C, Carskadon MA. Influence of irregular sleep patterns on waking behavior. In: Carskadon MA, ed. Adolescent Sleep Patterns: Biological, Social, and Psychological Influences. New York: Cambridge University Press, 2002:220–235.

132. National Research Council/Institute of Medicine. Sleep needs, patterns, and difficulties of adolescents: summary of a workshop. Washington, DC: National Academy Press, 2000.

133. Kumra V, Markoff BA. Who's smoking now? The epidemiology of tobacco use in the United States and abroad. Clin Chest Med 2000; 21(1):1–9.

134. Centers for Disease Control (CDC, January 28, 2000). Tobacco use among middle and high school students—United States, 1999. MMWR 2000; 49:49–53.

135. Phillips BA, Danner FJ. Cigarette smoking and sleep disturbance. Arch Intern Med 1995; 155:734–737.

136. Johnson EO, Breslau N. Sleep problems and substance use in adolescence. Drug Alcohol Depend 2001; 64:1–7.

137. Fallone G, Seifer R, Acebo C, Carskadon MA. Prolonged sleep restriction in 11- and 12-year-old children: effects on behavior, sleepiness, and mood. Sleep 2000; 23(suppl 2):A28.

138. Taylor D, Acebo C, Carskadon MA. MSLT across 36 hr of sleep loss in adolescents. Sleep 2003; 26:189.

139. Randazzo AC, Schweitzer PK, Walsh JK. Cognitive function following 3 nights of sleep restriction in children ages 10–14. Sleep 1998; 21:s249.

140. Copes K, Rosentswieg J. The effects of sleep deprivation upon motor performance of ninth grade students. J Sports Med 1972; 12:47–53.

# 9

## Pregnancy and Postpartum

**ERIKA GAYLOR AND RACHEL MANBER**

Stanford University, Stanford, California, U.S.A.

## I. Introduction

There is a growing interest in understanding how hormones affect mood and sleep. The last decade has evidenced great strides in researching women's health and specifically sleep issues during women's reproductive years. Nevertheless, there is still a paucity of data culled from well-designed and carefully controlled studies of women's sleep during pregnancy. This review summarizes the existing literature of how sleep continuity and sleep architecture change across the trimesters of pregnancy and factors that may contribute to these changes. It proceeds with a description of what is known about the prevalence of sleep disorders during pregnancy and pregnancy-related factors that may impact sleep disorders during pregnancy. This is followed by a discussion of the consequences of sleep deprivation during pregnancy for the mother and her fetus and issues related to the assessment and treatment of sleep disorders during pregnancy. We also discuss sleep and sleep deprivation during the first 6 months postpartum. We conclude with a discussion of critical issues and directions for future research.

## II. Changes in Sleep Associated with Pregnancy

### A. Sleep-Wake Patterns

The nature, prevalence, and etiology of disturbed sleep are influenced by the gestational stage of the pregnant woman. Overall, the most common nighttime symptom is awakenings and the most common daytime symptom is fatigue. Cross-sectional and longitudinal studies that use subjective (self-reported) and objective (laboratory and home polysomnography) measures of sleep continuity have consistently documented increased night waking during the first trimester relative to prepregnancy and nonpregnant women, and a further increase in night waking during the third trimester (1–4). Additionally, sleep efficiency is significantly reduced during the third trimester (3,4). In contrast, sleep continuity of pregnant women during the second trimester is not significantly altered compared to nonpregnant women.

Both hormonal and physical changes associated with pregnancy contribute to the documented decrease in sleep continuity. Although progesterone, which increases sharply during the first trimester of pregnancy and then more gradually thereafter, is a sedating agent (5–8), its central action appears to be offset by other factors. For example, progesterone's inhibitory effect on smooth muscle functioning leads to increased micturition and associated awakenings (9,10). The progressive increase of prolactin during pregnancy (11) may also contribute to decreased sleep continuity, as it was shown to increase sleep fragmentation in rats (12). In addition, to make room for the enlarging uterus, the diaphragm is constricted and the intestines and esophageal sphincter are displaced. These topological changes may contribute to the frequency and/or the duration of night awakenings by altering breathing during sleep (13), by causing reflux and heartburn, and by making it difficult to find a comfortable sleeping position. Leg cramps, leg pain (4), back pain (4,9), and increased fetal movement (14) further contribute to wakefulness after sleep onset.

Whereas increased night awakenings during pregnancy appears to be a consistent finding across studies, changes in total sleep time across pregnancy appear to vary with the method of measurement and study design and are, therefore, difficult to interpret. Cross-sectional surveys of pregnant women do not find a difference in self-reported total nocturnal sleep time between the three trimesters of pregnancy (1,15). In contrast, one longitudinal study, which followed women from prepregnancy to the postpartum period, found that total sleep time determined by home polysomnography increases during the first trimester and decreases during the third trimester when compared to prepregnancy (2).

### B. Sleep Architecture

Most polysomnographic (PSG) studies focus on the third trimester of pregnancy. Studies published in the past 10 years consistently report that percent REM sleep decreases during the third trimester compared to an age-matched control group

(4), compared to the same women earlier in pregnancy (16), and compared to the same women during postpartum (17), with some evidence that the decrease in REM sleep may already emerge during the second trimester (3).* There is also a consistent finding that the percent of slow-wave sleep (SWS) during the third trimester, which ranges between 5% and 10% of total sleep time, is markedly diminished compared to age-matched control groups (13–20%) (2,4,17,19–21), and in one study NREM stage 4 sleep was completely suppressed during the third trimester (22).† In addition, the third trimester is associated with an overall decrease in electroencephalographic (EEG) power density (3), increased prevalence of alpha-delta sleep (21), and increased percent of time spent in NREM stage 1 sleep (4), the lightest sleep stage.

The observed changes in sleep EEG during pregnancy may be impacted by hormonal changes. Prolactin, which increases during pregnancy, has been shown to suppress REM sleep (23). Progesterone administration induces a significant decrease in SWS (24) and in slow EEG frequency (7) and it has also been linked to a reduction in REM sleep (7,25). The effect of progesterone on REM sleep during pregnancy may be mediated by cortisol, which suppresses REM sleep (26), and is enhanced by progesterone (16). In addition to hormones, sleep fragmentation resulting from other pregnancy-related factors may directly contribute to the observed alteration in sleep stages during the third trimester of pregnancy, as it does in nonpregnant, mixed-gender samples (27).

Together, alteration in EEG patterns during pregnancy and subjective reports of increased night awakenings suggest that the third trimester of pregnancy may be associated with lower arousal thresholds. Lower arousal thresholds may be evolutionarily adaptive in that women with lower arousal thresholds will be less likely to sleep in any one position too long and may therefore reduce constriction of the fetus.

### C. Daytime Sleepiness and Fatigue

Fatigue is commonly experienced during pregnancy, beginning in the first trimester (28,29). Self-reported levels of fatigue are highest during the first trimester, decrease during the second trimester, and increase again during the third trimester (30). Daytime sleepiness is conceptually different from daytime fatigue. Whereas fatigue is usually assessed by measuring levels of energy, vigor, and vitality, daytime sleepiness is interpreted in the sleep research field as a high propensity to sleep onset. Similar to daytime fatigue, complaints of a problem with daytime sleepiness appear to be most prevalent during the first 10 weeks of

---

*In contrast, two earlier studies found increased percent REM sleep during the third trimester relative to the earlier trimesters of pregnancy (18,19).

†One exception to this body of data is a small study ($n = 5$) that reported increased SWS from the first to third trimester in a limited observation period (16).

pregnancy (27%), decrease during the next 20 weeks (11%), and increase again during the last 10 weeks of pregnancy (16%) (1). Consistent with the temporal pattern of changes in daytime fatigue and sleepiness, the first trimester of pregnancy is associated with the highest percentage of women taking daytime naps (between 46% and 61%) (1,31). In contrast, excessive daytime sleepiness, as measured by the Epworth Sleepiness Scale (32), does not change significantly across pregnancy (1). The Epworth Scale asks the individual to rate the probability that he or she will fall asleep in a variety of sleep-conducive situations. Epworth scores during pregnancy reflect a subclinical, moderate level of daytime sleepiness, with highest scores reported toward the end of the first trimester of pregnancy (1).

Factors that contribute to fatigue during pregnancy include disturbed or insufficient sleep, low levels of ferritin and hemoglobin (first trimester), and low levels of folic acid (third trimester) (29). During the first trimester, 70% of the variance in reported fatigue is explained by low prepregnancy ferritin and hemoglobin levels, sleep fragmentation, and young age (29). During the third trimester, increased level of fatigue is negatively correlated with levels of folic acid and with shortened nocturnal sleep (29).

A variety of factors may contribute to the moderate levels of daytime sleepiness reported during pregnancy. Although total nighttime sleep does not substantially decrease during pregnancy, sleep fragmentation does increase across trimesters. Sleep fragmentation has long been recognized as an important factor contributing to daytime sleepiness (33). Sources of sleep fragmentation during pregnancy include physical discomfort and micturition as well as an increased incidence of sleep-disordered breathing and leg movements, which are discussed in the following section. In addition, the hormonal milieu during the first trimester of pregnancy, including increases in progesterone and human chorionic gonadotropin, may directly contribute to daytime sleepiness (34,35).

## III.  Sleep Disorders in Pregnancy

### A.  Sleep and Breathing (See Also Chap. 5)

The effects of mechanical and biochemical changes associated with pregnancy on the waking respiratory system are most pronounced during the third trimester. As the uterus grows, the diaphragm elevates, leading to a decrease in respiratory reserve volume associated with a 20% reduction in daytime measures of functional residual capacity (FRC). In addition to lung restriction, pregnancy is associated with changes in mucosa, reduced pharyngeal dimension (36), nasal congestion, and rhinitis that may be attributed to increased levels of estrogen and increased blood volume during pregnancy (13,37,38). Although these changes can potentially compromise respiration during sleep (13), other changes in the respiration system act to protect against upper-airway occlusion. For example, there is a right shift of the oxyhemoglobin dissociation curve during pregnancy, which provides some compensation to the reduction in FRC. High progesterone levels associated with pregnancy also stimulate respiration centrally (39) and have excitatory effects on the genioglossus muscle, one of the major muscles responsible for dilation of the upper airway. In addition to its potential beneficial effects on respiration during pregnancy, progesterone's upregulation of the central respiratory drive might lead to instability of the respiratory control pathways and increased diaphragmatic effort that may induce upper airway collapse during sleep (40). The net effect of pregnancy-related changes on respiration, oxygenation, and associated sleep fragmentation during sleep is likely to vary across individuals.

In the absence of epidemiological data, the prevalence of sleep-disordered breathing (SDB) during pregnancy remains unknown. Three existing surveys of a total of approximately 1000 pregnant women indicate that the incidence of snoring is higher for pregnant women during the second half of pregnancy (12%–23%) than for age-matched nonpregnant controls (approximately 4%) (41–43). The documented increase in the incidence of snoring, mouth breathing, and awakening with choking sensations during pregnancy (1,43) suggests that the prevalence of sleep-disordered breathing, such as upper-airway resistance, might also be higher during late pregnancy than in nonpregnant age-matched controls.

It appears that obesity and large weight gain during pregnancy increase the risk of sleep apnea. Franklin and colleagues (43) found that pregnant women who are habitual snorers (nightly or almost every night) are more likely to report observed apnea than nonsnorers (11% vs. 2%) and that habitual snorers had larger prepregnancy weight and had more pronounced weight gain during pregnancy than nonsnorers (43).

Polysomnographic studies of disordered respiration during sleep in pregnant women are based on small samples. Integration of data from these small studies suggests that late pregnancy may be associated with a marginal increase in the respiratory disturbance index (RDI, number of abnormal breathing events per hour of sleep) (44) and in inspiratory-flow limitations (45). However, obstructive sleep apnea is not precipitated by normal pregnancy in the nonobese (40,46) or in individuals who are not otherwise predisposed to SDB. In contrast, obesity, which is a known risk factor for obstructive sleep apnea, is associated with an increased RDI during pregnancy, particularly during the second half of pregnancy (44). Since the first reports of obstructive sleep apnea in obese women during pregnancy and its potential impact on fetal growth (47), additional case reports of apnea during pregnancy have been published (48–55). The reported cases tend to be of obese women (50–53) or women who are otherwise predisposed to SDB [e.g., preexisting sleep-disordered breathing (50,56), abnormal upper airway anatomy (48), or other comorbid conditions (54,55,57)].

Perhaps the most clinically relevant respiratory parameter during pregnancy is the degree of oxygen desaturation and the potential impact of hypoxemia on the developing infant. Although basal $SaO_2$ during sleep of near-term pregnant women may be marginally lower than that of nonpregnant controls (58,59), the limited available data suggest that most nonobese pregnant women, even those with multiple pregnancies, preeclampsia, or snoring during pregnancy, do not appear to experience hypoxemia (39,41,45,60) and that the birth weight of infants born to women who snore is not different from the weight of infants born to mothers who do not snore (42). In contrast, most case reports of apnea during pregnancy, which involved obese women, were associated with compromised infant growth (55,61) that is commonly attributed to fetal hypoxemia. Similarly, Franklin and colleagues (43) found that mothers who were habitual snorers were more likely to be above recommended weight before pregnancy and were more likely to have infants who were small-for-gestational-age compared to mothers who were nonhabitual snorers. It is of note that even after controlling for weight, snoring during pregnancy remained a risk factor for infant growth retardation (43).

### B. Restless Legs and Periodic Limb Movements of Sleep (See Also Chap. 5)

Restless legs syndrome (RLS) is a movement disorder that is characterized by a crawling, burning, or aching sensation in the calves (sometimes in the thighs or feet) that emerges during rest, typically in the evening, and is accompanied by an irresistible urge to move the legs, which temporarily relieves the sensation. RLS is probably the most common movement disorder during pregnancy (62), and RLS associated with pregnancy is considered a secondary form of RLS, as opposed to the primary, or idiopathic, form of RLS. It is different from leg cramps, which are also known to increase during pregnancy and to cause arousals during sleep (63). RLS is often associated with difficulty initiating sleep. With increased number of awakenings after sleep onset during pregnancy, RLS can also prolong time awake after sleep onset, and it can, therefore, be a cause of sleep deprivation and fatigue during pregnancy. Prospective data suggest that the prevalence of RLS increases across the trimesters of pregnancy (1,64). Its overall estimated prevalence during pregnancy in cross-sectional studies is 10–20% (65–67), and it is much more prevalent in women who do not take folate supplements (80%) (68). For most women, RLS emerges during pregnancy and remits following delivery, but may reemerge in subsequent pregnancies (67). Compared with pregnant women who do not experience RLS during pregnancy, pregnant women who do experience RLS have lower ferritin and folate levels preconception (64). During the third trimester, when RLS is most prevalent, the number of nights in which RLS is experienced correlates negatively with serum folate levels (64). Although most pregnant women in Western societies take multivitamins that include iron and folate, symptomatic women with low levels of iron and folate might benefit from additional supplementation (64). Data on the prevalence of periodic limb movement of sleep (PLMS) is sparse. It is likely that PLMS is present in the majority of pregnant women with RLS, as it is in many nonpregnant individuals with RLS (69).

### C. Parasomnias

The incidence of parasomnias, associated with partial arousal from SWS, such as sleepwalking, decreases during pregnancy (1,70), most likely because of a decrease in SWS during pregnancy (2,4). However, because parasomnias that are related to confusional arousal from SWS increase during periods of sleep deprivation and during periods of increased stress, it is possible that some women with prepregnancy parasomnias may experience a worsening of symptoms. One case report of recurrence of sleepwalking during pregnancy in a woman with a history of childhood sleepwalking (71) is consistent with this cautionary comment.

Other parasomnias also appear to be impacted by the condition of pregnancy. The incidence of hypnagogic hallucinations and nightmares is also lower during pregnancy, particularly late in pregnancy, compared to prepregnancy (70), possibly because of the decrease in REM sleep in late pregnancy. The incidence of bruxism decreases and the incidence of nocturnal enuresis and sleep paralysis increases during pregnancy (70). Sleep paralysis, which occurs primarily during the transition between sleep and wakefulness, is higher during the second and third trimesters relative to pre-pregnancy (70) and relative to early pregnancy (1), probably because of increased sleep fragmentation.

### D. Psychophysiological Insomnia

Despite the ample documentation of the ubiquitous nature of frequent night waking during the latter part of pregnancy and during the first 3 months postpartum, there are no data on the prevalence of psychophysiological insomnia during pregnancy or postpartum. Although almost all women experience an increase in night waking during the third trimester (97%), less than 20% view their awakenings as problematic (1). Women who view their night awakenings as problematic may belong to a subgroup of individuals who experience difficulty settling back into sleep. Inferring from epidemiological studies, it appears that whereas pregnancy does not impact sleep-onset insomnia, it may increase the prevalence or severity of sleep-maintenance insomnia.

### E. Sleep in Pregnant Women with Current or Past History of Depression

Sleep disturbance is a common symptom of depression. Women who meet criteria for a major depressive episode during pregnancy are more likely to report a greater frequency of insomnia and somatic symptoms compared to pregnant nondepressed women (72). Even pregnant women who have a positive history of a mood disorder but are not currently symptomatic experience more disturbed sleep than pregnant women without a history of mood disorder (31). For example, women with a positive history of a mood disorder are more likely to have problems maintaining sleep, spend more time in bed, and have longer sleep times in early pregnancy, and subsequently experience a greater decrease in total sleep time from the first to the third trimester of pregnancy. There has not been a systematic study of sleep in pregnant depressed women. In an unpublished analysis of baseline data from 61 participants in an ongoing controlled treatment outcome study of pregnant women with a major depressive disorder (MDD), the second author (RM) found that the incidence of disturbed sleep in depressed pregnant women was significantly greater than the incidence reported in the literature for non-depressed pregnant women. For example, at average gestation week 20, 31% of depressed pregnant women reported difficulty falling asleep on at least 4 nights a week as compared with less than 1% in the healthy pregnant women sampled by Mindell and Jacobson (1). Moreover, in the same clinical sample, 30% of the women reported restless or disturbed sleep and an additional 61% reported difficulty returning to sleep in the middle of the night but less than 5% of healthy women of comparable gestation age surveyed by Mindell and Jacobson reported having a problem with frequent night awakenings (1). Early-morning awakening, a virtually nonexistent complaint in healthy pregnant women at average gestation week 20, was present in approximately 20% of the clinical sample of pregnant depressed women at the same average gestation week.

## IV.  Consequences of Sleep Deprivation

Sleep deprivation has a profound effect on adults' daily cognitive, psychological, and social functioning (27,73), but the impact of experimentally induced sleep deprivation during pregnancy has not been investigated. The potential consequences of poor sleep during pregnancy may, however, be inferred from studies of cognitive functioning during pregnancy. At least two studies have examined the validity of anecdotal complaints that women become more forgetful during pregnancy. These studies found that self-reported deficits in memory are positively correlated with self-reported sleep disturbance (74,75). In contrast, objective tests of memory are not correlated with self-reported sleep and memory during pregnancy (74–76). Interestingly, both pregnant and postpartum groups of women score lower on tests of working memory compared to age-matched controls although their scores are within the normal range of functioning.

Very little data exist on the impact of maternal sleep deprivation on the health and well-being of the developing fetus and eventual live newborn. There is some evidence that pregnant shift workers and resident physicians may have a higher rate of pregnancy complications (77), premature labor (78), and pregnancy-induced hypertension (79), but it is not clear whether sleep deprivation is the primary cause of these complications or if it is the stressful conditions of these women's work environments that increase the adverse outcomes. Furthermore, there is no relationship between subjective sleep quality and adverse pregnancy outcomes. In fact, women who worked full-time during pregnancy in jobs that did not require extended hours or overnight shifts did not differ from women who did not work during pregnancy in terms of the length of labor or the type of delivery (80). Further investigation into the impact of sleep deprivation during pregnancy on maternal well-being and on fetal outcomes is warranted.

## V.   Diagnosis and Treatment of Sleep Disorders in Pregnancy and Postpartum

### A.   Diagnosis

Sleep disorders are probably underdiagnosed during pregnancy. Women do not spontaneously report sleep disturbances because of (a) the transient nature of pregnancy, (b) the assumption that insomnia is part and parcel of being pregnant and therefore does not merit treatment, and/or (c) the wish to avoid ingesting hypnotic medications and the assumption that not much else can be done to improve sleep. Obstetricians and family physicians do not often specifically ask pregnant women about their sleep for some of the same reasons that women do not spontaneously report them. The main diagnostic challenges for sleep disorders during pregnancy are related to differentiating between common pregnancy symptoms, such as leg cramps, heartburn, and fatigue, and sleep disorders and sleep-disorder-related symptoms, such as restless legs, gastroesophageal reflux, and excessive daytime sleepiness. Although pregnancy is rarely a risk factor for moderate to severe sleep apnea (46), an assessment of SDB is warranted in pregnant women who are predisposed to disordered breathing during sleep, including obese women, women with very large weight gain, and women with excessive daytime sleepiness. In these cases, treatment of SDB, frequent fetal growth monitoring, and appropriate timing of delivery are likely to reduce infant growth restriction. Assessment of SDB in pregnant women with preeclampsia is also warranted because continuous positive airway pressure (CPAP) treatment of those with a positive diagnosis can reduce blood pressure during sleep (81).

### B.   Treatment

Pharmacological treatments of disturbed sleep during pregnancy and lactation remain beyond the scope of this chapter. The U.S. Food and Drug Administration classifies drugs into the following four categories: A: Controlled studies show no risk to fetus. B: Human trials demonstrate no risk to fetus, animal studies show some risk or no adequate human trials but animal studies demonstrate no risk to fetus. C: No human studies, but animal studies demonstrate fetal risk or are unavailable. D: Experimental or marketing information demonstrates fetal risk but possible benefits outweigh risk (82,83). For example, dopaminergic medications, which are used to treat RLS and PLMS, are contraindicated for lactating women because of the inhibitory action of dopamine on prolactin release, possibly interfering with lactation (84). In a study in the early 1970s, approximately 12% of women used a sleep aid at some point during the pregnancy (85); current usage of hypnotic medications during pregnancy is unknown.

General recommendations to improve maternal sleep, reduce sleep deprivation, and minimize maternal and fetal health risks are as follows: (a) Women should try to sleep on their left side and avoid sleeping in the supine position (86), particularly during the second half of pregnancy. Avoiding the supine position will ease the stress on the heart, will reduce constriction of the space available to the fetus, will reduce the pressure to the inferior vena cava that carries blood back to the heart from the feet and legs, and will improve respiration during sleep. The left side is preferred because it reduces pressure on the liver and it reduces the frequency of gastroesophageal reflux (87). (b) If symptoms of RLS are present, consider an evaluation of ferritin, hemoglobin, and folate levels and supplement when indicated. (c) Treat sleep-disordered breathing with CPAP. (d) Avoid staying in bed when unable to sleep. Instead, supplement nocturnal sleep with short (30–60 min) midafternoon naps. (e) Address anxiety-provoking issues to reduce overall level of arousal. For example, childbirth- and parenting-preparation classes may help alleviate a common source of anxiety during pregnancy. (f) Consider regular exercise. Pregnant women (gestation week 30) who exercise at least three times a week for at least 30 min have less insomnia and anxiety than pregnant women who do not exercise (88). (g) Treat psychophysiological insomnia with empirically supported cognitive behavioral therapy for insomnia (89).

## VI.  Postpartum Sleep Deprivation

Disturbed sleep and fatigue are common during the postpartum period (90,91). During the period immediately after delivery, sleep disruptions are impacted by physical discomfort (22,85,92), recovery from labor and delivery (90,91,93), endocrine changes (94), and medications used during delivery. Following this initial recovery period, the primary factors impacting maternal sleep are infant temperament, infant sleep pattern, parenting style (including method of feeding), family size, paternal involvement, and social support.

Longitudinal studies document that the first 6 months postpartum are associated with a substantial increase in time awake after sleep onset and a decrease in sleep efficiency relative to the last trimester of pregnancy, which itself was associated with elevated wake after sleep onset (WASO) compared to nonpregnant women (2,4,16,95–98). A gradual improvement in sleep continuity typically begins at 3-months postpartum and becomes more pronounced during the 6–12-month postpartum period (99). The pattern of consolidation in maternal sleep is closely tied to the sleep patterns and mode of feeding of their infants. For example, although breast-feeding mothers and bottle-feeding mothers do not differ in total nocturnal sleep time (100), breast-feeding mothers report more night awakenings (100,101) and more fatigue (100). Sleep fragmentation is even greater in breast-feeding women who are cosleeping with their infants compared to breast-feeding mothers whose infants sleep separately (102).

The persistent maternal sleep fragmentation and sleep deprivation during the initial postpartum months are associated with an alteration in maternal sleep architecture, including a marked increase in SWS (2,22,31) and an increased REM pressure (94), as evidenced by earlier REM onset. Whereas these changes are consistent with what is observed upon recovery from experimentally induced sleep disruption or sleep restriction (103,104), the percentage of REM sleep, which typically increases after sleep deprivation, remains unaltered during the initial 3 months postpartum (31). This is not surprising because polysomnographic studies of postpartum women do not assess recovery sleep, rather they simulate typical maternal sleep conditions, in which infants sleep in close proximity to their mothers, thus allowing continued REM deprivation. Both REM latency and the percent time spent in SWS normalize by 3 months postpartum and are comparable to those observed in the same women before pregnancy (2,102) and in age-matched nonpregnant women (102).

The impact of maternal postpartum sleep deprivation on the mother's daytime sleepiness and mood has not been studied extensively. There is evidence that maternal daytime sleepiness is prevalent throughout the first postpartum year. Many mothers report increased daytime sleepiness (105), napping (106,107), and fatigue (108,109), and there appears to be an association between overall sleep quality and daytime sleepiness (105).

There is also a strong association between the severity of infant sleep disturbance, the most common cause of sleep deprivation during the postpartum period, and maternal depressive symptoms. But the interpretation of this association is difficult. One interpretation is that maternal sleep deprivation caused by infant night waking may lead to, or exacerbate, anxiety and depression, especially when the mother is the primary nighttime caregiver (92,110). For example, Hiscock and Wake (111) found that only when mothers reported a diminished quality of their own sleep were the infants' sleep problem significantly correlated with postpartum depressive symptoms. Moreover, interventions to improve the infant's sleep and consequently, the mother's sleep, led to an improvement in maternal depressed mood (112–114). Although these intervention studies may suggest a causal influence of sleep deprivation on maternal distress, fatigue, and possibly depressive symptoms during the postpartum period, it is also possible that the intervention directly reduced maternal stress and improved maternal mood by facilitating the mother-infant relationship in general.

Alternatively, it is possible that maternal depressive symptoms contribute to the severity of their infant's sleep disturbance. For example, infants of depressed mothers may sleep poorly because they are distressed, not sufficiently active during the day, or receive insufficient environmental cues to entrain their circadian rhythms (115). In addition, the observed increase in sleep disturbance in infants of depressed mothers may simply reflect a reporting bias in that postpartum women with current or past MDD are awake during the night more than women without MDD (31) and might, therefore, be more aware of, and more likely to report, infant sleep disturbances than nondepressed mothers.

## VII.  Conclusions and Future Directions

The extant research indicates that the majority of pregnant women experience some level of sleep disturbance during their pregnancy, which is most pronounced during the first and third trimesters and least pronounced during the second trimester. The two most common sleep-related complaints of pregnant women are a decrease in sleep continuity and an increase in daytime fatigue. Sleep macroarchitecture is also altered during the third trimester, with a marked decrease in SWS and a small decrease in REM sleep. There is also evidence that RLS and PLMS increase during pregnancy, which may be caused by deficits in ferritin and/or folic acid. Snoring also increases during pregnancy but most nonobese pregnant women, including those with multiple pregnancies, preeclampsia, or snoring during pregnancy, do not appear to experience hypoxemia. In addition, pregnancy may further perturb sleep in some subgroups of pregnant women. For example, obese women experience elevation in RDI during pregnancy, particularly during the second half of pregnancy, and their infants are more likely to experience hypoxemia. Similarly, women who are depressed during pregnancy have more disturbed sleep than non-depressed pregnant women.

The etiologies of the observed sleep-related changes during pregnancy are not well understood. Factors such as hormonal, physical, and psychological changes have been implicated, but the complex relationships between these factors have not been sufficiently studied. Most of what we know of women's sleep during pregnancy comes from research conducted in the past decade. As we learn more, we also become more aware of what we do not yet understand and of the methodological challenges unique to the study of sleep during pregnancy and postpartum. We highlight below some directions for future research and hope that understanding these three domains may eventually facilitate the development of effective and acceptable treatments for insomnia and daytime fatigue during pregnancy and lactation.

To date, there has not been a systematic study of sleep maintenance insomnia during pregnancy. Whereas epidemiological studies clearly document increased night waking in the majority of pregnant women, it is not clear under what conditions night awakenings are prolonged and when sleep-continuity disturbances are associated with distress or with clinically meaningful daytime impairment.

The prevalence of daytime sleepiness and its impact on daily functioning during pregnancy and postpartum is not well understood. Although the extant research suggests moderate degrees of daytime sleepiness and fatigue, the impact of such deficits on the developing fetus are unknown and the potential efficacy of nutritional supplementation of ferritin and/or folic acid has not been systematically evaluated.

Finally, it is important to clarify the complex relationship between maternal sleep (sleep deprivation, sleep fragmentation, and sleepiness), maternal mood, and fetal/infant outcome during pregnancy and postpartum. Although many studies point to robust correlations, such a complex issue requires creative research methodology to tease apart the direct and indirect relationships.

## References

1. Mindell J, Jacobson BJ. Sleep disturbances during pregnancy. J Obstet Gynecol Neonatal Nurs 2000; 29:590–597.
2. Lee K, Zaffke ME, McEnany G. Parity and sleep patterns during and after pregnancy. Obstet Gynecol 2000; 95:14–18.
3. Brunner D, Munch M, Biederman K, Huch R, Huch A, Borbely A. Changes in sleep and sleep electroencephalogram during pregnancy. Sleep 1994; 17:576–582.
4. Hertz G, Fast A, Feinsilver, SH, Albertario CL, Schulman H, Fein AM. Sleep in normal late pregnancy. Sleep 1992; 15:246–251.
5. Freeman M, Crissman JK Jr, Louw GN, Butcher RL, Inskeep EK. Thermogenic action of progesterone in the rat. Endocrinology 1970; 86:717–720.
6. Heuser G, Ling GM, Kluver M. Sleep induction by progesterone in the pre-optic area in cats. Electroceph Clin Neurophysiol 1967; 22:122–127.
7. Lancel M, Faulhaber J, Holsboer F, Rupprecht R. Progesterone induces changes in sleep comparable to those of agonistic GABA (A) receptor modulators. Am J Physiol 1996; 271:E763–E772.
8. Little B, Matta RJ, Zahn TP. Physiological and psychological effects of progesterone in man. J Nerv Ment Dis 1974; 159:256–262.
9. Baratte-Beebe K, Lee K. Sources of midsleep awakenings in childbearing women. Clin Nurs Res 1999; 8.
10. Bassett J, Wolfson AR, Anwer U, Trentacoste S, McGurn K, Hoag A. Sleep/wake disruptions in the final weeks of pregnancy. Sleep 1998; 121:276.
11. Suzuki S, Dennerstein L, Greenwood KM, Armstrong SM, Sano T, Satohisa E. Melatonin and hormonal changes in disturbed sleep during late pregnancy. J Pineal Res 1993; 15:191–198.
12. Lin S, Arai AC, Espana RA, Berridge CW, Leslie FM, Huguenard JR, Vergnes M, Civelli O. Prolactin-releasing peptide (PrRP) promotes awakening and suppresses absence seizures. Neuroscience 2002; 114:229–238.
13. Kryger M, Roth T, Dement WC. Principles and Practice of Sleep Medicine. Philadelphia: Saunders, 2000.
14. Worth J, Onyeije CI, Ferber A, Pondo JS, Divon MY. The association between fetal and maternal sleep patterns in third-trimester pregnancies. Am J Obstet Gynecol 2002; 186:924–925.
15. Suzuki S, Dennerstein L, Greenwood KM, Armstrong SM, Satohisa E. Sleeping patterns during pregnancy in Japanese women. J Psychosom Obstet Gynecol 1994; 15:19–26.
16. Driver H, Shapiro CM. A longitudinal study of sleep stages in young women during pregnancy and postpartum. Sleep 1992; 15:449–453.
17. Anders T, Roffwarg HP. The relationship between infant and maternal sleep. Sleep 1968; 5:227–228.
18. Branchey M, Petre-Quadens O. A comparative study of sleep parameters during pregnancy. Acta Neurol Belg 1968; 68:453–459.

19. Petre-Quadens O, deBarsy AM, Devos J, Sfaello A. Sleep in pregnancy: evidence of foetal sleep characteristics. J Neurol Sci 1967; 4:600–605.

20. Hoppenbrouwers T, Hodgman JE, Berntsen I, Sterman MB, Harper RM. Sleep in women during the last trimester of pregnancy. Sleep Res 1979; 8:150.

21. Schorr S, Chawla A, Devidas M, Sullivan CA, Naef RW, Morrison JC. Sleep patterns in pregnancy: a longitudinal study of polysomnography recordings during pregnancy. J Perinatol 1998; 18:427–430.

22. Karacan I, Heine W, Agnew HW, Williams RL, Webb WB, Ross JJ. Characteristics of sleep patterns during late pregnancy and the postpartum periods. Am J Obstet Gynecol 1968; 101:579–586.

23. Spiegel K, Follenius M, Simon C, Saini J, Ehrhart J, Brandenberger G. Prolactin secretion and sleep. Sleep 1994; 17:20–27.

24. Friess E, Tagaya H, Trachsel L, Holsboer F, Rupprecht R. Progesterone-induced changes in sleep in male subjects. Am J Physiol 1997; 272:E885–E891.

25. Lancel M, Faulhaber J, Schiffelholz T, Romeo E, DiMichele F, Holsboer F, Rupprecht R. Allopregnanolone affects sleep in a benzodiazepine-like fashion. J Pharmacol Exp Ther 1997; 282:1213–1218.

26. Born J, Spath-Schwalbe E, Schwakenhofer H, Kern W, Fehm HL. Influences of corticotropin-releasing hormone, adrenocorticotropin, and cortisol on sleep in normal man. J Clin Endocrinol Metab 1989; 68:904–911.

27. Martin S, Wrath PK, Deary IJ, Douglas NJ. The effect of nonvisible sleep fragmentation on daytime function. Am J Respir Crit Care Med 1997; 155:1596–1601.

28. Behrenz K, Monga M. Fatigue in pregnancy: a comparative study. Am J Perinatol 1999; 16:185–188.

29. Lee K, Zaffke ME. Longitudinal changes in fatigue and energy during pregnancy and the postpartum period. J Obstet Gynecol Neonatal Nurs 1999; 28:183–191.

30. Lee K. Sleep and fatigue. Annu Rev Nurs Res 1999; 19:249–273.

31. Coble P, Reynolds CF, Kupfer DJ, Houck PR, Day NL, Giles DE. Childbearing in women with and without a history of affective disorder. II. Electroencephalographic sleep. Compr Psychiatry 1994; 35:215–224.

32. Johns M. A new method for measuring daytime sleepiness: the Epworth Sleepiness Scale. Sleep 1991; 14:540–545.

33. Stepanski EJ. The effect of sleep fragmentation on daytime function. Sleep 2002; 25:268–276.

34. Manber R, Armitage R. Sex, steroids, and sleep: a review. Sleep 1999; 22:540–555.

35. Toth P, Lukacs H, Hiatt ES, Reid KH, Iyer V, Rao CV. Administration of human chorionic gonadotropin affects sleep-wake phases and other associated behaviors in cycling female rats. Brain Res 1994; 654:181–190.

36. Pilkington S, Carli F, Dakin MJ, et al. Increase in Mallampati score during pregnancy. Br J Anaesth 1995; 74:638–642.

37. Elkus R, Popovich J Jr. Respiratory physiology in pregnancy. Clin Chest Med 1992; 13:555–565.

38. Mabry R. Rhinitis of pregnancy. South Med J 1986; 79:965–971.

39. Brownell L, West P, Kryger MH. Breathing during sleep in normal pregnant women. Am Rev Respir Dis 1986; 133:38–41.

40. Edwards N, Middleton PG, Blyton DM, Sullivan CE. Sleep disordered breathing and pregnancy. Thorax 2002; 57:555–558.

41. Guilleminault C, Querra-Salva M, Chowdhuri S, Poyares D. Normal pregnancy, daytime sleeping, snoring and blood pressure. Sleep Med 2000; 1:289–297.
42. Loube D, Poceta JS, Morales MC, Peacock MD, Mitler MM. Self-reported snoring in pregnancy: Association with fetal outcome. Chest 1996; 109:885–889.
43. Franklin K, Holmgren PA, Jonsson F, Poromaa N, Stenlund H, Svanborg E. Snoring, pregnancy-induced hypertension, and growth retardation of the fetus. Chest 2000; 117:137–141.
44. Maasilta P, Bachour A, Teramo K, Polo O, Laitinen LA. Sleep-related disordered breathing during pregnancy in obese women. Chest 2001; 120:1448–1454.
45. Connolly G, Razak ARA, Hayanga A, Russell A, McKenna P, McNicholas WT. Inspiratory flow limitation during sleep in pre-eclampsia: comparison with normal pregnancy and nonpregnant women. Eur Respir J 2001; 18:672–676.
46. Littner M, Brock BJ. Snoring in pregnancy: disease or not? Chest 1996; 109:859–861.
47. Joel-Cohen S, Schoenfeld A. Fetal response to periodic sleep apnea: a new syndrome in obstetrics. Eur J Obstet Gynecol Reprod Biol 1978; 8:77–81.
48. Conti M, Izzo V, Muggiasca ML, Tiengo M. Sleep apnoea syndrome in pregnancy: a case report. Eur J Anaesthesiol 1988; 5:151–154.
49. Kowall J, Clark G, Nino-Murcia G, Powell N. Precipitation of obstructive sleep apnea during pregnancy. Obstet Gynecol 1989; 74.
50. Charbonneau M, Falcone T, Cosio MG, Levy RD. Obstructive sleep apnea during pregnancy: therapy and implications for fetal health. Am Rev Respir Dis 1991; 144:461–463.
51. Sherer D, Caverly CB, Abramowicz JS. Severe obstructive sleep apnea and associated snoring documented during external tocography. Am J Obstet Gynecol 1991; 165:1300–1301.
52. Lefcourt L, Rodis JF. Obstructive slee apnea in pregnancy. Obstet Gynecol Surv 1996; 51:503–506.
53. Lewis D, Chesson AL, Edwards MS, Weeks JW, Adair CD. Obstructive sleep apnea during pregnancy resulting in pulmonary hypertension. South Med J 1998; 91:761–762.
54. Taibah K, Ahmed M, Baessa E, Saleem M, Rifai A, Al-arifi A. An unusual cause of obstructive sleep apnoea presenting during pregnancy. J Laryngol Otol 1998; 112:1189–1191.
55. Brain K, Thornton JG, Sarkar A, Johnson AOC. Obstructive sleep apnoea and fetal death: successful treatment with continuous positive airway pressure. Br J Obstet Gynecol 2001; 108:543–544.
56. Hastie S, Prowse K, Perks WH, Atkins J, Blunt VAW. Obstructive sleep apnoea during pregnancy requiring tracheostomy. Aust NZ J Obstet Gynaecol 1989; 29:365–367.
57. Pieters T, Amy JJ, Burrini D, Aubert G, Rodenstein DO, Collard Ph. Normal pregnancy in primary alveolar hypoventilation treated with nocturnal nasal intermittent positive pressure ventilation. Eur Respir J 1995; 8:1424–1427.
58. Feinsilver S, Hertz G. Respiration during sleep in pregnancy. Clin Chest Med 1992; 13:637–644.
59. Bourne T, Ogilvy AJ, Vickers R, Williamson K. Nocturnal hypoxaemia in late pregnancy. Br J Anaesth 1995; 75:678–682.

60. Nikkola E, Ekblad U, Ekhom E, Mikola H, Polo O. Sleep in multiple pregnancy: breathing patterns, oxygenation, and periodic leg movements. Am J Obstet Gynecol 1996; 174:1622–1625.
61. Schoenfeld A, Ovadia Y, Neri A, Freedman S. Obstructive sleep apnea (OSA)— implications in maternal-fetal medicine: a hypothesis. Med Hypoth 1989; 30:51–54.
62. Golbe L. Pregnancy and movement disorders. Neurol Clin 1994; 12:497–508.
63. Zib M, Lim L, Walters WAW. Symptoms during normal pregnancy: a prospective controlled study. Aust NZ J Obstet Gynaecol 1999; 39:401–410.
64. Lee K, Zaffke ME, Baratte-Beebe K. Restless legs syndrome and sleep disturbance during pregnancy: the role of folate and iron. J Wom Health Gender Med 2001; 10:335–341.
65. Ekbom K. Restless legs syndrome. Neurology 1960; 10:868–873.
66. Lang A. Akathisia and the restless legs syndrome. In: Jankovic J, Tolosa E, eds. Parkinson's Disease and Movement Disorders. Baltimore: Williams & Wilkins, 1993:399–418.
67. Goodman J, Brodie C, Ayida GA. Restless legs syndrome in pregnancy. Br Med J 1988; 297:1101–1102.
68. Botez M, Lambert B. Folate deficiency and restless legs syndrome in pregnancy. N Engl J Med 1977; 297:670–.
69. Montplaisir J, Boucher S, Poirer G, Lavigne G, Lapierre O, Lesperance P. Clinical, polysomnographic, and genetic characteristics of restless legs syndrome: a study of 133 patients diagnosed with new standard criteria. Mov Disord 1997; 12:61–65.
70. Hedman C, Pohjasvaara T, Tolonen U, Salmivaara A, Myllyla VV. Parasomnias decline during pregnancy. Acta Neurol Scand 2002; 105:209–214.
71. Berlin R. Sleepwalking disorder during pregnancy: a case report. Sleep 1988; 11:298–300.
72. Kelly R, Russo J, Katon W. Somatic complaints among pregnant women cared for in obstetrics: normal pregnancy or depressive and anxiety symptom amplification revisited? Gen Hosp Psychiatry 2001; 23:107–113.
73. Pilcher J, Huffcutt AI. Effects of sleep deprivation on performance: a metaanalysis. Sleep 1996; 19:318–326.
74. Casey P, Huntsdale C, Angus G, Janes C. Memory in pregnancy. II. Implicit, incidental, explicit, semantic, short-term, working and prospective memory in primigravid, multigravid, and postpartum women. J Psychosom Obstet Gynecol 1999; 20:158–164.
75. Janes C, Casey P, Huntsdale C, Angus G. Memory in pregnancy. I. Subjective experiences and objective assessment of implicit, explicit and working memory in primigravid and primiparous women. J Psychosom Obstet Gynecol 1999; 20:80–87.
76. Keenan P, Yaldoo DT, Stress ME, Fuerst DR, Ginsburg KA. Explicit memory in pregnant women. Am J Obstet Gynecol 1998; 179:731–737.
77. Nicholson P, D'Auria DAP. Shift work, health, the working time regulations and health assessments. Occup Med 1999; 49:127–137.
78. Osborn L, Harris DL, Reading JC, Prather MB. Outcome of pregnancies experienced during residency. J Fam Pract 1990; 31:618–622.
79. Phelan S. Pregnancy during residency. II. Obstetric complications. Obstet Gynecol 1988; 72:431–436.
80. Evans M, Dick MJ, Clark AS. Sleep during the week before labor: relationships to labor outcomes. Clin Nurs Res 1995; 4:238–252.

81. Edwards N, Blyton DM, Kirjavainen T, Kesby GJ, Sullivan CE. Nasal continuous positive airway pressure reduces sleep-induced blood pressure increments in preeclampsia. Am J Respir Crit Care Med 2000; 162:252–257.

82. Key to FDA-in-use pregnancy ratings. Physicians' Desk Reference. Montvale, NJ: Medical Economics Data Production Co, 1995.

83. Briggs GG, Freeman RK, Yaffe SJ. Drugs in Pregnancy and Lactation: A Reference Guide to Fetal and Neonatal Risk. Baltimore: Williams & Wilkins, 2001.

84. Chesson AJ, Wise M, Davila D, Johnson S, Littner M, Anders WM, Hartse K, Rafecas J. Practice parameters for the treatment of restless legs syndrome and periodic limb movement disorder. Sleep 1999; 22:961–968.

85. Schweiger M. Sleep disturbance in pregnancy. Am J Obstet Gynecol 1972; 114:879–882.

86. Ang C, Tan TH, Walters WAW, Wood C. Postural influence on maternal capillary oxygen and carbon dioxide tension. Br Med J 1969; 4:201–203.

87. Charan M, Katz PO. Gastroesophageal reflux disease in pregnancy. Curr Treat Options Gastro 2001; 4:73–81.

88. Goodwin A, Astbury J, McMeeken J. Body image and psychological well-being in pregnancy: a comparison of exercisers and non-exercisers. Aust NZ J Obstet Gynaecol 2000; 40:442–447.

89. Morin C, Culbert JP, Schwartz SM. Nonpharmacological interventions for insomnia: a meta-analysis of treatment efficacy. Am J Psychiatry 1994; 151:1172–1180.

90. Tribotti S, Lyons N, Blackburn S, Stein M, Withers J. Nursing diagnoses for the postpartum woman. J Obstet Gynecol Neonatal Nurs 1988; 17:410–416.

91. Troy N, Dalgas-Pelish P. The natural evolution of postpartum fatigue among a group of primiparous women. Clin Nurs Res 1997; 6:126–141.

92. Karacan I, Williams RL, Hursch CJ, McCaulley M, Heine MW. Some implications of the sleep patterns of pregnancy for postpartum emotional disturbances. Br J Psychiatry 1969; 115:929–935.

93. Thompson J, Roberts CL, Currie M, Ellwood DA. Prevalence and persistence of health problems after childbirth: associations with parity and method of birth. Birth 2002; 29:83–94.

94. Lee K, McEnany G, Zaffke ME. REM sleep and mood state in childbearing women: sleepy or weepy? Sleep 2000; 23:877–885.

95. Shinkoda H, Matsumoto K, Park,YM. Changes in sleep-wake cycle during the period from late pregnancy to puerperium identified through the wrist actigraph and sleep logs. Psychiatry Clin Neurosci 1999; 53:133–135.

96. Waters M, Lee KA. Differences between primigravidae and multigravidae mothers in sleep disturbances, fatigue, and functional status. J Nurse-Midwif 1996; 41:364–367.

97. Kang M, Matsumoto K, Shinkoda H, Mishima M, Seo YJ. Longitudinal study for sleep-wake behaviours of mothers from pre-partum to post-partum using actigraph and sleep logs. Psychiatry Clin Neurosci 2002; 56:251–252.

98. Nishihara K, Horiuchi S. Changes in sleep patterns of young women from late pregnancy to postpartum: relationships to their infants' movements. Percept Mot Skills 1998; 87:1043–1056.

99. Wolfson A, Anwer U. Sleep and affect in pregnancy and postpartum months, Annual meeting of the Northeast Sleep Society, Worcester, MA, 2000.

100. Quillin S. Infant and mother sleep patterns during 4th postpartum week. Issues Comp Ped Nurs 1997; 20:115–123.

101. Elias M, Nicolson NA, Bora C, Johnston J. Sleep/wake patterns of breast-fed infants in the first two years of life. Pediatrics 1986; 77:322–329.
102. Mosko S, Richard C, McKenna J. Maternal sleep and arousals during bedsharing with infants. Sleep 1997; 20:142–150.
103. Dement W, Greenberg S. Changes in total amount of stage 4 sleep as a function of partial sleep deprivation. Electroencephalogr Clin Neurophysiol 1966; 20:523–526.
104. Tilley A, Wilkinson RT. The effects of a restricted sleep regime on the composition of sleep and on performance. Psychophysiology 1984; 21:406–412.
105. Lee K, DeJoseph JF. Sleep disturbances, vitality, and fatigue among a select group of employed chidlbearing women. Birth 1992; 19:208–213.
106. Wolfson A, Crowley SJ, Anwer U, Bassett JL. Changes in sleep patterns and depressive symptoms in first-time mothers: last trimester to 1–year postpartum. Behav Sleep Med 2003; 1:54–67.
107. Swain A, O'Hara MW, Starr KR, Gorman LL. A prospective study of sleep, mood, and cognitive function in postpartum and nonpostpartum women. Obstet Gynecol 1997; 90:381–386.
108. Troy N. A comparison of fatigue and energy levels at 6 weeks and 14 and 19 months postpartum. Clin Nurs Res 1999; 8:135–152.
109. Campbell I. Postpartum sleep patterns of mother-baby pairs. Midwifery 1986; 2:193–201.
110. Errante J. Sleep deprivation or postpartum blues? Top Clin Nurs 1985; 6:9–18.
111. Hiscock H, Wake M. Infant sleep problems and postnatal depression: a community-based study. Pediatrics 2001; 107:1317–1322.
112. Armstrong K, Haeringen AR, Dadds MR, Cash R. Sleep deprivation or postnatal depression in later infancy: Separating the chicken from the egg. J Paediatr Child Health 1998; 34:260–262.
113. Leeson R Barour J, Ray KL, Warr R. management of infant sleep problem in a residential unit. Child Care Health Dev 1994; 20:89–100.
114. Hiscock H, Wake M. Randomised controlled trial of behavior infant sleep intervention to umprove infant sleep and maternal mood Br Med J 2002; 324:1–6.
115. Field T. The effects of mothers' physical and emotional unavailability on emotion regulation. Monogr Soc Res Child Dev 1994; 59:208–277.

# 10

## Epidemiological Health Impact

**DANIEL F. KRIPKE AND MATTHEW R. MARLER**

University of California–San Diego, La Jolla, California, U.S.A.

**EUGENIA E. CALLE**

American Cancer Society, Atlanta, Georgia, U.S.A.

## I.  Sleep Duration and Mortality Risk

In 1964, E. Cuyler Hammond presented preliminary findings of the American Cancer Society's Cancer Prevention Study I (CPSI), using early follow-ups (1). He noted that men who reported that they slept 7 hr had the lowest mortality in age groups from 45–49 to 85+ years. Both those men who reported that they slept 6 hr or less and those who reported that they slept 8 hr or more had higher mortality. Statistical reliability was self-evident from trend consistency among 17 of 18 groups studied. Results with 6-year follow-up of 1 million subjects of both sexes have expanded this result with control for several possibly confounding risk factors (2).

In the Cancer Prevention Study II (CPSII), a new prospective sample of 1.1 million participants aged 30–102 years was followed for 6 years (3). Similar to the prior results, reported sleep durations greater or less than 7 hr/night were associated with increased mortality after controlling for 32 risk factors. In CPSII, reported usual sleep of 6.5–7.4 hr had been coded as 7 hr, 7.5–8.4 hr as 8 hr, etc. In both CPSI and CPSII, the minimal mortality risk was found in the group reporting 1 hr less sleep than the mode of 8 hr. In the U-shaped relationship of mortality hazard to reported sleep duration, *long sleep was associated with more risk than short sleep.* This was both because there were more participants reporting sleep > 7 hr (46.3% women and 45.7% men) than those reporting sleep < 7 hr (20.2% and 19.1%, respectively), and because of a more rapidly increasing hazard curve > 7 hr sleep (3) (Fig. 1).

Additional smaller studies, some of them based on representative population samples, have also observed increased mortality associated with short and long sleep (4–14). Recent reports have further confirmed the U-shaped pattern with data from the Framingham Study and the Japan Collaborative Cohort Study (15,16). Important features of the Japanese collaborative study were confirmation that the minimum risk is at 7 hr for self-reported sleep duration and a control for depressive symptoms. There has been widespread and convincing replication of the epidemiological risks associated with reported short and long sleep. There has been no study that reliably contradicted the general findings of Dr. Hammond, though some studies with insufficient power have failed to replicate his findings.

In this discussion, we will present a reanalysis of the CPSII data, to further explore the influence of comorbid risk factors on the mortality associated with sleep duration. The risks associated with insomnia, shift work, and sleeping pills will also be examined.

## A. The Effects of Comorbidities

The question arises whether the association of sleep duration with mortality hazard could be an artifact of comorbidities, since so many diseases, disorders, and discomforts are associated with disturbed sleep. In our prior analysis of CPSII, we controlled as far as possible for the major risk factor data available from the CPSII questionnaires, to see if such extensive control for comorbidities would eliminate the significant associations of mortality hazard with sleep duration.

In Figure 1, the CPSII hazard ratios for sleep duration, derived from Cox proportional hazards survival models, are presented with controls only for gender, age, insomnia, and sleeping pill use. The hazard ratios are also presented (with confidence intervals) for models simultaneously controlling for 32 covariates and comorbidities, as described in our previous publication (3). Minor differences between Figure 1 and results previously reported were due to reediting of the data file and inclusion of those reporting 2–3 hr sleep as a single group, since too few reported 2 hr sleep for an accurate estimate. Also plotted are models restricting analysis to participants who were relatively healthy in the initial questionnaires, by considering only deaths taking place at least 1 year after entry into the study (to exclude those moribund at entry), and by eliminating individuals who had reported any cancer, heart disease, hypertension, stroke, chronic bronchitis, emphysema, asthma, or current illness (a "yes" answer to the question "are you sick at the present time?").

In Figure 1, it may be seen that controlling for the multiple comorbidities substantially reduced the hazard ratios related to sleep greater than 7 hr, and even more greatly reduced the hazard ratios associated with sleep less than 7 hr. Evidently, a higher proportion of deaths associated with short sleep could be attributed to comorbidities than deaths associated with long sleep. Further excluding those who died within the first year and excluding those who were not healthy

# WOMEN

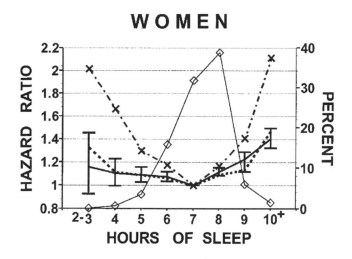

# MEN

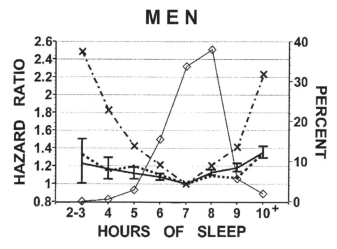

**Figure 1**   The relative 6-year mortality hazard ratios are shown for reported usual sleep hr from 2–3 hr/night to 10 or more hr/night, relative to 1.0 assigned to the hazard for 7 hr/night as the reference standard. The solid line with 95% confidence interval bars shows results from a 32-covariate Cox proportional hazards survival model, as reported previously (3). The dotted lines show data from models that excluded subjects who were not initially healthy, i.e., who died within the first year or whose questionnaires reported any cancer, heart disease, stroke, chronic bronchitis, emphysema, asthma, or current illness (a "yes" answer to the question "are you sick at the present time?"). The dot-dash lines with X symbols show models controlling only for age, insomnia, and use of sleeping pills. Data were from 635,317 women and 478,619 men. The thin solid lines with diamonds show the percent of subjects with each reported sleep duration (right axis).

at entry (instead of controlling for the same factors in the 32-covariate Cox proportional hazards models) made no consistent change in the hazard ratios. In summary, we were not able to account for all mortality associated with short and long sleep by controlling for other major risk factors. Association of sleep duration with mortality remained after maximal control for comorbidities.

### B.  The Question of Causality

We are not certain which comorbid risk factors cause mortality independent of sleep effects, and therefore, we cannot be certain whether we controlled too much or too little for comorbidities. For example, since short sleep or long sleep may cause a person to be "sick at present" or to get little exercise or to have heart disease (17), diabetes (18), etc., controlling for these possible mediating variables may have incorrectly minimized the hazards associated with sleep durations. This would be overcontrol. The hazard ratios for participants who were rather healthy at the time of the initial questionnaires were unlikely to be overcontrolled for initial illness. Since the 32-covariate models and the hazard ratios for initially healthy participants were similar, this similarity reduced concern that the 32-covariate models were overcontrolled. On the other hand, there may have been residual confounding processes that caused both short or long sleep and early death that we could not adequately control in the CPSII data set, either because available control variables did not adequately measure the confound or because the disease did not yet manifest itself. Depression, sleep apnea, and dysregulation of cytokines are plausible confounders that were not adequately controlled. It may be impossible to be confident that all conceivable confounds are adequately controlled in epidemiological studies of sleep.

The question of causality can only be fully resolved with controlled studies that randomly control sleep duration. For short sleep, controlled trials of long-term prescription of hypnotics or long-term use of sleep hygiene, etc., may help us understand the causal role of sleep. Similarly, for those with long sleep, controlled restriction of sleep or time-in-bed may help clarify the causal pathways.

An inverse correlation of sleep duration with longevity ($r = -0.52$) was found across 53 mammalian species, albeit these data are open to several interpretations (19). This interspecies comparison supports the hypothesis that long sleep may have an adverse causal effect on mortality, or conversely, that long wake may be life-preserving.

### C.  Confounding Variables

It is interesting to examine how control for various comorbid factors influences the mortality hazard associated with sleep durations. Comorbidities aside, in Cox proportional hazards models for each gender, controlling only for age and hours of sleep, the sample excess fractions (20) of deaths related to sleep durations other than 7 hr were 16.4% for women and 19.4% for men. These fractions are the percentage of observed deaths that would not have occurred in the 6-year follow-up, if those with all sleep durations had the same survival rates as those of the same age who slept 7 hr. In Table 1, we compare the sample excess fractions estimated similarly, controlling for one additional risk factor at a time. Table 1 shows that control for a report of being "sick at the present time" reduced by 3–4% the sample excess fraction related to sleep other than 7 hr. Control for exercise intensity reduced the fraction 2–3%. None of the other risk factors by itself could explain much of the total excess risk fraction for sleep durations. However, as previously reported (3), when all 32 available risk factors were entered into the model, these sample excess fractions of deaths were reduced to 6.3% for women and 5.3% for men. That is, of the mortality hazard associated with not sleeping about 7 hr, 62% of the hazard in women and 73% of the hazard in men could be attributed in the Cox models to a diverse combination of confounding comorbid factors. Although most of the mortality hazard associated with not sleeping 7 hr could be attributed to other factors, the remaining excess fraction was a serious portion of total sample deaths.

**Table 1** Excess Risk Fractions Associated with Sleep Hr by Covariates

| | Excess risk fractions | |
|---|---|---|
| Covariates | Women | Men |
| Age and sleep hours only | 0.164 | 0.194 |
| plus "sick at the present time" | 0.136 | 0.157 |
| plus exercise | 0.143 | 0.170 |
| plus diabetes | 0.153 | 0.186 |
| plus ever had heart disease | 0.153 | 0.179 |
| plus church frequency | 0.154 | 0.182 |
| plus fiber in diet | 0.156 | 0.191 |
| plus upsetting event (e.g., illness) | 0.156 | 0.181 |
| plus ever had stroke | 0.156 | 0.186 |
| plus occupation | 0.156 | 0.177 |
| plus pains in legs "when you walk" | 0.157 | 0.174 |
| plus ever had high blood pressure | 0.157 | 0.185 |
| plus education | 0.157 | 0.174 |
| plus insomnia | 0.158 | 0.187 |
| plus used blood pressure pills | 0.158 | 0.185 |
| plus used diuretics | 0.159 | 0.187 |
| plus race | 0.161 | 0.191 |
| plus sleeping pills | 0.162 | 0.190 |

The following covariates individually made no substantial changes in the excess risk fractions for men or women: race, fat in diet, body mass index, use of Tagamet, use of Valium, Librium, or Tylenol, ever had kidney disease, ever had bronchitis, marital status, and ever had cancer. Age was represented by a cubic polynomial.

## II. Long Sleep and Morbidity

Many people believe that sleep of 8 hr or more is necessary for optimal function and health, but this is not the case. Our University of California, San Diego group examined health-related quality of well-being in a representative sample of San Diego, from which objective home sleep recordings were obtained (21). There was no correlation of sleep duration with quality of well-being, a global measure of function. In college students, Pilcher and colleagues found that sleep quality (which was associated with psychological symptoms) was much more related to measures of health than was sleep quantity, which was not consistently related to the primary measures of health (22,23). It is interesting to note that cross-sectional and epidemiological studies have found that long sleepers have more psychopathology than short sleepers (24,25). In general, long sleepers appear more depressed and less energetic (26). In analysis of three large surveys, our group has found that those reporting longer-than-average sleep report some of the same complaints often associated with insomnia (3,27,28). Hartmann's classic studies described long sleepers as more depressed and anxious, but perhaps creative (24,29). Either long sleep or short sleep may be a symptom of depression, according to DSM-IV (30). In data from postmenopausal women, depressive symptoms seemed increased rather symmetrically among those with short and long sleep, as compared to those with average sleep (27).

Aeschbach's studies of a very small number of short and long sleepers showed that "short sleepers live under and tolerate higher homeostatic sleep pressure than long sleepers"; that is, short sleepers tend to go to sleep more rapidly and to sleep more deeply (31,32). Moreover, the long sleepers had more midsleep awakenings (poorer sleep efficiency). Numerous studies have found that daytime sleepiness is more closely associated with sleep fragmentation than with total sleep time (33,34), but excessive time in bed is one cause of such sleep fragmentation. This fragmentation is perhaps the quality most associated with dissatisfaction with sleep (33,35–37). Similarly, it has been reported that long sleepers actually have less slow-wave sleep than short sleepers (32,38), so reducing time in bed might improve the quality of sleep, in part, by increasing sleep homeostatic pressure.

The extent to which the *reported* long sleep in epidemiological studies represents above-average physiological sleep is unknown. There is evidence that the longer people spend in bed, the greater percentage of the time in bed they are awake; so their objective total sleep time may not be too prolonged. It is possible that reported long sleep largely represents spending an excessive time awake in bed (usually in the dark). This prolonged time in bed may be harmful (39,40).

## III. Short Sleep: Mortality and Morbidity

In CPSI and CPSII, the minimal mortality was observed 1 hr below the sample mode of 8 hr (approximately 1/2 hr below the median) (2,3). Increased mortality was observed among those reporting usual sleep 2 hr or more below the sample mode. In epidemiological studies, some excess mortality has been consistently associated with sleep of 6 hr or less (not fully attributable to comorbidities). After adjusting for comorbidities, although the hazard associated with 5 and 6 hr sleep was significantly greater than that associated with 7 hr, the hazard for those reporting 5 or 6 hr sleep remained in the lower half of hazard for the sample as a whole. The risk was above the median for the uncommon participants reporting sleep of less than 5 hr (0.8% of women and 0.7% of men). The one prospective sleep laboratory study available, which incorporated excellent control for depression and medical comorbidities, found a mortality ratio of 1.33 among those with sleep less than 6 hr, but the sample was small and the risk factor was not significant (41). In summary, the data indicate that sleep of 6 hr or less is associated with modest mortality risk, but the hazard for the population seems less than that of long sleep.

A creative series of studies found that young adult volunteers could reduce their habitual sleep from 8 hr to about 5 hr with almost undetectable effects on performance or mood, except for an increase in sleepiness (42,43). Such investigations should be repeated and expanded, to see if such sleep restriction is so free of morbid risk.

As noted earlier, epidemiological methods show little morbid impairment associated with shorter-than-average sleep. Among college students, those who sleep longer do not have higher grade-point averages—if anything, the reverse is true (44). Indeed, some studies have suggested that those with short sleep may often be optimistic, energetic, and productive, like the sterotypical hard-driving executive. For those with insomnia, sleep restriction may be a useful treatment, whereas for depression, sleep deprivation may produce dramatic benefit.

Contrasting with this perspective is a large, complex experimental literature demonstrating performance decrements among those subjected to acute experimental sleep deprivation. It is uncertain how relevant this literature may be to the issues of habitual sleep duration. For example, although many studies suggest that *acute* sleep loss increases driving accidents, acute sleep loss is often confounded with circadian effects of driving late at night, with substance abuse, and with risk-taking behaviors, e.g., the increased risk of young single men (45). Counter to intuition, some studies indicate that *habitual* sleep as short as 5 hr carries no excess driving risk (45,46). In the 32-covariate models of CPSII data, sleep duration did not predict total accident deaths among men (includes all accidents, not just driving). However, among women, 5 hr and 10+ hr sleep predicted increased accidents, but 3, 4, 6, or 9 hr sleep did not predict significantly increased risk compared to 7 hr; 8 hr predicted a significantly reduced risk ratio of 0.82. One study observed that long sleepers had the highest driving risk (47). With the partial exception of our limited study focusing on traffic violations (46), previous studies of driving risk lacked prospective representative sampling of subjects with varying habitual sleep durations, followed by objective assessment of the occurrence of accidents.

In summary, habitual sleep durations of 5–7 hr confer little mortality risk, and perhaps no substantial morbidity, although those with short sleep durations may fall asleep more rapidly and sleep more soundly.

## IV.  Insomnia (See Also Chap. 5)

The literature on insomnia is burdened by variations in definition and accuracy of ascertainment. Whereas insomnia is often equated with short sleep, many studies (including CPSI and CPSII) have shown that a large proportion of those individuals with sleep much shorter than average complain of no insomnia. However, many individuals who complain of insomnia (e.g., difficulty initiating or maintaining sleep) report sleep durations well within the normal range (48,49). Indeed, as mentioned, there is some increase in insomnia complaints among those reporting more than 8 hr sleep (3,27,28). The common polysomnographic criterion for insomnia of 6.5 hr total sleep time, which was accepted a generation ago, would today fall near the U.S. population median for weekdays (50,51). A long sleep latency and frequent awakenings within sleep seem better related to subjective distress than the actual duration of sleep, but even in these parameters, there is an enormous overlap between those who do and who do not complain of insomnia. Some studies attempt to isolate primary insomnia, by eliminating subjects whose insomnia can be attributed to underlying illnesses such as depression (the most common comorbidity), anxiety, sleep apnea, restless legs syndrome, circadian rhythm phase disorders, heart failure, cancer, arthritis, etc. Most epidemiological studies (such as CPSII) have been unable to make the distinction between primary and secondary insomnia.

In CPSII, in the 32-covariate models, reported insomnia was associated with risk ratios slightly but significantly less than 1.0, after controlling for sleep duration (3). A similar result was found in another study (52). This might imply a protective effect of insomnia. Similarly, insomnia did not predict total mortality when depression and other comorbidities were controlled in major Swedish studies (13,53). In general, studies that control well for comorbid factors do not find that insomnia predicts increased mortality independent of sleep duration and hypnotic drug use.

The question of insomnia effects on morbidity is more difficult. Since insomnia complaints are associated with depression, anxiety, neuroticism, and a wide variety of medical illnesses (44,49,54,55), it may be difficult to distinguish effects of insomnia from effects of the comorbid processes. In some cases, medications taken by insomniacs may be responsible for impairment. One attempt to assess disability related to insomnia found no association meeting Bonferroni criteria, after adjustment for age, gender, chronic disease, and major depression (56). It is possible that the trend for association would have been entirely eliminated had control been done for subthreshold depression, which was prevalent in the sample. Although sleep symptoms do predict future depression, they are less effective predictors than other symptoms that compose the incipient depressive syndrome (57). In some studies, insomniacs were found to be as alert as or more alert than controls and to perform as well (58). The question of distinguishing impairments attributable to insomnia from those attributable to comorbid processes may be unresolvable with epidemiological methods. Controlled studies of cognitive-behavioral treatment of insomnia may be useful to determine whether successful resolution of insomnia produces improved performance or function.

## V. Shift Work

Extensive studies have demonstrated that rotating shift workers and night workers have pervasive sleep disturbances and a variety of forms of morbidity (59–64). It is known that most people assigned to permanent night shifts sleep at night when off-duty, so they experience rotating schedules. Evidence for mortality associated with night work has been inconclusive, perhaps partly because workers might refuse night work when they become ill (65–67).

In CPSII, 5.9% of both women and men answered "yes" to the question "Do you work rotating shifts?" However, controlled for the other 32 covariates, working rotating shifts did not predict significant mortality hazard: the hazard ratios were 0.938 (0.860–1.022 95% CI) for women and 1.009 (0.953–1.068) for men. About 70% of men and 56% of women answered the question "What time of day do you start working?" Of these, 58% of women and 69% of men reported a start time of 7–8 A.M., which was chosen as the reference category in Cox models including the previously used 32 covariates plus rotating shift work and work start times. As shown in Figure 2, only five of the 22 work start times tested in women and men showed significantly elevated hazard ratios at a 95% confidence level, uncorrected for multiple testing. For women, significantly elevated hazard ratios were found at 1–2 A.M., 3–4 A.M., 9–10 A.M., and 11–12 A.M. For men, a significantly elevated hazard ratio was found only for 11 P.M.-midnight. To consider these findings reliable, we would like to see more consistency between the results for men and women than was observed. It would appear that working shifts starting at night has only modest effects on mortality risk, if any, but as reflected by the confidence intervals, too few night shift workers were observed to detect small increases in risk.

## VI. Sleeping Pill Effects

The question arises whether sleeping pills can be used to reduce the morbidity or mortality associated with short sleep by increasing sleep duration. Although many contemporary hypnotic drugs do increase polysomnographic sleep by 20–40 min in the first week or 2 of use, zaleplon "has not been shown to increase total sleep time or decrease the number of awakenings" (68). Zolpidem increased sleep for a few weeks but did not significantly improve polysomnographic sleep

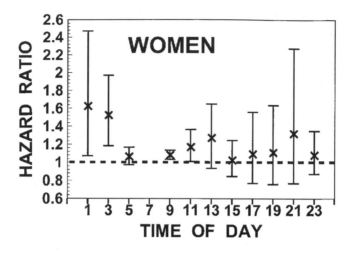

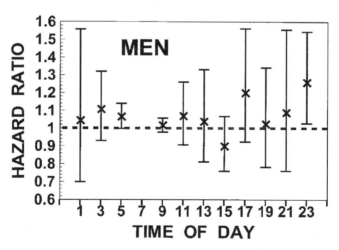

**Figure 2** Hazard ratios with 95% confidence intervals are shown for women and men versus the time of day when the subject started working (2 hr averaged). Thus, the bar over 1 represents work hr starting at 1–2 A.M.. The bar over 23 represents work starting from 11 P.M. to midnight. The reference category, work starting at 7–8 A.M., was arbitrarily assigned a relative hazard ratio of 1.0 (dotted line).

in the fifth week of usage at the recommended dosage (69). Likewise, zolpidem failed to significantly increase weekly sleep duration as compared to placebo beyond 4 weeks of intermittent use (70) and failed to significantly improve sleepiness, quality of life, cognition, or mood (71). A large number of studies have shown that contemporary hypnotics produce less impairment of daytime cognition and performance than older drugs with longer half-lives, but even with the most recently introduced hypnotics, there is more evidence for impairment than for improvement of daytime function (72).

CPSII found that habitual use of hypnotics was associated with less-than-average sleep (3), as has been shown in many other studies. A converse direction of causality has been assumed, but controlled evidence is lacking that any hypnotic can lengthen sleep over a period of years (73,74). CPSI found that people who reported taking sleeping pills had higher mortality, either with or without controlling for hr of sleep and insomnia (2). CPSII found significant hazard ratios associated with use of sleeping pills 30+ times/month (essentially nightly), 1.24 (1.12–1.38 95% CI) for women and 1.25 (1.14–1.38 95% CI) for men (3,75). Smaller but significant hazard ratios were associated with use of sleeping pills 1–29 times/month (median 3/month), 1.10 (1.03–1.17) for women and 1.15 (1.08–1.22) for men. Similar risk ratios have been observed in other studies that were smaller and had less power (11,13,76). Available evidence does not support the hypothesis that long-term use of sleeping pills could enhance survival.

## VII. Summary and Conclusions

Epidemiological studies indicate that habitual sleep 2 hr or more below the mode was associated with a very modest increase in mortality risk when comorbidities were controlled, but the greater risk was among those who sleep 8 hr or more. Little morbidity risk is associated with habitual sleep as short as 5 hr. More impairment may be associated with sleeping 9 hr or more. However, there has been relatively little study of those with long sleep. Little or no mortality risk may be attributable to insomnia or shift work. In terms of morbidity, it is difficult to determine how much disability associated with insomnia is attributable to depression or to other comorbid illness. The use of sleeping pills is certainly associated with excess mortality risk, but the association of sleeping pill use with morbidity may not be causal. Controlled trials are needed to determine whether any long-term intervention in sleep habits can prolong life or improve function.

There are two problems with an overemphasis on the dangers of sleep deprivation. First, it detracts from a focus on long sleep, which seems to be the greater problem. Second, fear of a short sleep length is one of the major cognitive factors that cause insomnia and the long-term use of sleeping pills. Publicity exaggerating the dangers of short sleep will tend to exacerbate the prevalence of insomnia and the misuse of hypnotics. Correcting the false belief that everybody needs 8 hr of sleep is an important element in treating insomnia (39,40). If we take a calm attitude toward habitual sleep of 5, 6, or 7 hr, it will benefit the public and reduce the burden of insomnia.

## Acknowledgments

Data were collected by the American Cancer Society. Data analyses were supported by the National Institutes of Health (AG15763, AG12364, HL61280).

## References

1. Hammond EC. Some preliminary findings on physical complaints from a prospective study of 1,064,004 men and women. Am J Public Health 1964; 54:11–24.
2. Kripke DF, Simons RN, Garfinkel L, Hammond EC. Short and long sleep and sleeping pills: is increased mortality associated? Arch Gen Psychiatry 1979; 36:103–116.
3. Kripke DF, Garfinkel L, Wingard DL, Klauber MR, Marler MR. Mortality associated with sleep duration and insomnia. Arch Gen Psychiatry 2002; 59:131–136.
4. Breslow L, Enstrom JE. Persistence of health habits and their relationship to mortality. Prev Med 1980; 9:469–483.
5. Wingard DL, Berkman LF, Brand RJ. A multivariate analysis of health practices: a nine year mortality follow-up of the Alameda County study. Am J Epidemiol 1979; 110:362.
6. Kaplan GA, Seeman TE, Cohen RD, Knudsen LP, Guralnik J. Mortality among the elderly in the Alameda county study: behavioral and demographic risk factors. Am J Public Health 1987; 77:307–312.
7. Chen D, Foley D. Prevalence of sleep disturbance and mortality in the U.S. population. Sleep Res 1994; 23:116.
8. Qureshi AI, Giles WH, Croft JB, Bliwise DL. Habitual sleep patterns and risk for stroke and coronary heart disease: a 10–year follow-up from NHANES I. Neurology 1997; 48:904–911.
9. Pollak CP, Perlick D, Linsner JP, Wenston J, Hsieh F. Sleep problems in the community elderly as predictors of death and nursing home placement. J Community Health 1990; 15(2):123–135.
10. Huppert FA, Whittington JE. Symptoms of psychological distress predict 7–year mortality. Psychol Med 1995; 25:1073–1086.
11. Kojima M, Wakai K, Kawamura T, Tamakoshi A, Aoki R, Lin Y, Nakayama T, Horibe H, Aoki N, Ohno Y. Sleep patterns and total mortality: a 12–year follow-up study in Japan. J Epidemiol 2000; 10(2):87–93.
12. Gale C, Martyn C. Larks and owls and health, wealth, and wisdom. Br Med J 1998; 317:1675–1677.
13. Mallon L, Broman J-E, Hetta J. Sleep complaints predict coronary artery disease mortality in males: a 12–year follow-up study of a middle-aged Swedish population. J Int Med 2002; 251:207–216.
14. Ayas NT, White DP, Manson JE, Stampfer MJ, Speizer FE, Malhotra A, Hu FB. A prospective study of sleep duration and coronary heart disease in women. Arch Intern Med 2003;163:205–209.

15. Patel SR, Ayas NT, Malhotra MR, White NP, Schernhammer ES, Speizer FE, Stampfer MJ, Hu FB. A prospective study of sleep duration and mortality risk in women. Sleep 2004; 27:440–444.
16. Tamakoshi A, Ohno Y, JACC Study Group. Self-reported sleep duration as a predictor of all-cause mortality; results from the JACC Study, Japan. Sleep 2004; 27:51–54.
17. Partinen M, Putkonen PTS, Kaprio J, Koskenvuo M, Hilakiui I. Sleep disorders in relation to coronary heart disease. Acta Med Scand 1982 (suppl); 660:69–83.
18. Spiegel K, Leproult R, Van Cauter E. Impact of sleep debt on metabolic and endocrine function. Lancet 1999; 354:1435–1439.
19. Zepelin H, Rechtschaffen A. Mammalian sleep, longevity, and energy metabolism. Brain Behav Evol 1974; 10:425–470.
20. Szklo M, Nieto FJ. Attributable risk. In: Epidemiology. Gaithersburg, MD: Aspen, 2000:98–105.
21. Jean-Louis G, Kripke DF, Ancoli-Israel S. Sleep and quality of well-being. Sleep 2000; 23(8):1115–1121.
22. Pilcher JJ, Ginter DR, Sadowsky B. Sleep quality versus sleep quantity: relationships between sleep and measures of health, well-being and sleepiness in colleges students. J Psychosom Res 1997; 42(6):583–596.
23. Pilcher JJ, Ott ES. The relationships between sleep and measures of health and well-being in college students: a repeated measures approach. Behav Med 1998; 23(4):170–178.
24. Hartmann E, Baekeland F, Zwilling GR. Psychological differences between long and short sleepers. Arch Gen Psychiatry 1972; 26:463–468.
25. Ford DE, Kamerow DB. Epidemiologic study of sleep disturbances and psychiatric disorders: an opportunity for prevention? JAMA 1989; 262(11):1479–1484.
26. Hicks RA. Normal Insomnia: Its Benefits and Its Costs. San Jose: San Jose State University, 1983.
27. Kripke DF, Brunner R, Freeman R, Hendrix S, Jackson RD, Masaki K, Carter RA. Sleep complaints of postmenopausal women. Clini J Women's Health 2001; 1(5):244–252.
28. Grandner MA, Kripke DF. Self-reported sleep complaints with long and short sleep: a nationally representative sample. Psychosom Med 2004; 66:239–241.
29. Hartmann E, Baekeland F, Zwilling G, Hoy P. Sleep need: how much sleep and what kind? Am J Psychiatry 1971; 127(8):1001–1008.
30. Task Force on DSM-IV. Diagnostic and Statistical Manual of Mental Disorders: DSM-IV. Washington, DC: American Psychiatric Association, 1994.
31. Aeschbach D, Postolache TT, Sher L, Matthews JR, Jackson Ma, Wehr TA. Evidence from the waking electroencephalogram that short sleepers live under higher homeostatic sleep pressure than long sleepers. Neuroscience 2001; 102(3):493–502.
32. Aeschbach D, Cajochen C, Landolt H, Borbely AA. Homeostatic sleep regulation in habitual short sleepers and long sleepers. Am J Physiol 1996; 270:R41–R53.
33. Stepanski E, Lamphere J, Badia P, Zorick F, Roth T. Sleep fragmentation and daytime sleepiness. Sleep 1984; 7(1):18–26.
34. Gillberg M. Sleepiness and its relation to the length, content, and continuity of sleep. J Sleep Res 1995; 4(S2):37–40.
35. Carskadon MA, Brown ED, Dement WC. Sleep fragmentation in the elderly: relationship to daytime sleep tendency. Neurobiol Aging 1982; 3:321–327.
36. Morin CM, Gramling SE. Sleep patterns and aging: comparison of older adults with and without insomnia complaints. Psychol Aging 1989; 4(3):290–294.

37. Keglund G, Akerstedt T. Objective components of individual differences in subjective sleep quality. J Sleep Res 1997; 6(4):217–220.

38. Benoit O, Foret J, Bouard G. The time course of slow wave sleep and REM sleep in habitual long and short sleepers: effect of prior wakefulness. Hum Neurobiol 1983; 2:91–96.

39. Edinger JD, Wohlgemuth WK, Radtke RA, Marsh GR, Quillian RE. Does cognitive-behavioral insomnia therapy alter dysfunctional beliefs about sleep? Sleep 2001; 24(5):591–599.

40. Morin CM, Hauri PJ, Espie CA, Spielman AJ, Buysse DJ, Bootzin RR. Nonpharmacologic treatment of chronic insomnia. Sleep 1999; 22(8):1134–1156.

41. Dew MA, Hoch CC, Buysse DJ, Monk T, Begley AE, Houck PR, et al. Healthy older adults' sleep predicts all-cause mortality at 4 to 19 years of followup. Psychosom Med. In press.

42. Mullaney DJ, Johnson LC, Naitoh P, Friedmann JK, Globus GG. Sleep during and after gradual sleep reduction. Psychophysiology 1977; 14(3):237–244.

43. Friedmann J, Globus G, Huntley A, Mullaney D, Naitoh P, Johnson L. Performance and mood during and after gradual sleep reduction. Psychophysiology 1977; 14(3):245–250.

44. Gray EK, Watson D. General and specific traits of personality and their relation to sleep and academic performance. J Personal 2002; 70(2):177–206.

45. Connor J, Norton R, Ameratunga S, Robinson E, Civil I, Dunn R, Bailey J, Jackson R. Driver sleepiness and risk of serious injury to car occupants: population based case control study. Br Med J 2002; 324(1125):1–5.

46. Kripke DF, Rex KM. Short sleepers are not at higher risk for driving accidents or other violations. Sleep 2002; 25(abstract Suppl):A284–A285.

47. Cummings P, Koepsell TD, Moffat JM, Rivara FP. Drowsiness, counter-measures to drowsiness, and the risk of a motor vehicle crash. Injury Prevent 2001; 7:194–199.

48. Edinger JD, Hoelscher TJ, Webb MD, Marsh GR, Radtke RA, Erwin CW. Polysomnographic assessment of DIMS: empirical evaluation of its diagnostic value. Sleep 1989; 12 (4):315–322.

49. Edinger JD, Fins AI, Glenn DM, Sullivan RJ, Jr., Bastian LA, Marsh GR, Dailey D, Hope TV, Young M, Shaw E, Vasilas D. Insomnia and the eye of the beholder: are there clinical markers of objective sleep disturbances among adults with and without insomnia complaints? J Consult Clin Psychol 2000; 68(4):586–593.

50. 2001 "Sleep in America" Poll. Washington: National Sleep Foundation, 2001.

51. Jean-Louis G, Kripke DF, Ancoli-Israel S, Klauber MR, Sepulveda RS. Sleep duration, illumination, and activity patterns in a population sample: effects of gender and ethnicity. Biol Psychiatry 2000; 47:921–927.

52. Foley DJ, Monjan AA, Brown SL, Simonsick EM, Wallace RB, Blazer DG. Sleep complaints among elderly persons: an epidemiologic study of three communities. Sleep 1995; 18(6):425–432.

53. Jensen E, Dehlin O, Hagberg B, Samuelsson G, Svensson T. Insomnia in an 80–year-old population: relationship to medical, psychological and social factors. J Sleep Res 1998; 7:183–189.

54. Vitiello MV, Moe KE, Prinz PN. Sleep complaints cosegregate with illness in older adults: clinical research informed by and informing epidemiological studies of sleep. J Psychosom Res 2002; 53:555–559.

55. Brabbins CJ, Dewey ME, Copeland RM, Davidson IA, McWilliam C, Saunders P, Sharma VK, Sullivan C. Insomnia in the elderly: prevalence, gender differences and relationships with morbidity and mortality. Int J Geriatr Psych 1993; 8:473–480.

56. Simon GE, VonKorff M. Prevalence, burden, and treatment of insomnia in primary care. Am J Psychiatry 1997; 154:1417–1423.
57. Roberts RE, Shema SJ, Kaplan GA, Strawbridge WJ. Sleep complaints and depression in an aging cohort: a prospective perspective. Am J Psychiatry 2000; 157:81–88.
58. Hauri PJ. Psychological and psychiatric issues in the etiopathogenesis of insomnia. Prim Care Compan J Clin Psychiatry 2002; 4(suppl 1):17–20.
59. Akerstedt T. Sleepiness as a consequence of shift work. Sleep 1988; 11(1):17–34.
60. Torsvall L, Akerstedt T. Sleepiness on the job: continuously measured EEG changes in train drivers. Electroencephalogr Clin Neurophysiol 1987; 66:502–511.
61. Alfredsson L, Akerstedt T, Mattsson M, Wilborg B. Self-reported health and well-being amongst night security guards: a comparison with the working population. Ergonomics 1991; 34(5):525–530.
62. Boggild H, Knutsson A. Shift work, risk factors and cardiovascular disease. Scand J Work Environ Health 1999; 25(2):85–99.
63. Gordon NP, Cleary PD, Parker CE, Czeisler CA. The prevalence and health impact of shiftwork. Am J Public Health 1986; 76(10):1225–1228.
64. Shift Work Committee. Opinion on night work and shift work. J Sci Labour 1979; 55:1–36.
65. McNamee R, Binks K, Jones S, Faulkner D, Slovak A, Cherry NM. Shiftwork and mortality from ischaemic heart disease. Occup Environ Med 1996; 53(6):367–373.
66. Boggild H, Suadicani P, Hein HO, Gyntelberg F. Shift work, social class, and ischaemic heart disease in middle aged and elderly men; a 22 year follow up in the Copenhagen male study. Occup Environ Med 1999; 56(9):640–645.
67. Schernhammer ES, Laden F, Speizer FE, Willett WC, Hunter DJ, Kawachi I, Colditz GA. Rotating night shifts and risk of breast cancer in women participating in the Nurses' Health Study. J Natl Cancer Inst 2001; 93(20):1563–1568.
68. Elan Pharmaceuticals. Sonata (zaleplon) Capsules. 11/26/2001. Philadelphia, Wyeth Laboratories.
69. Scharf MB, Roth T, Vogel GW, Walsh JK. A multicenter, placebo-controlled study evaluating zolpidem in the treatment of chronic insomnia. J Clin Psychiatry 1994; 55(5):192–199.
70. Walsh JK, Roth T, Jamieson A, Schweitzer PK, Scharf MB, Ware JC et al. Intermittent use of zolpidem for the treatment of primary insomnia. Sleep 2000; 23(suppl 2):A86.
71. Walsh JK. Zolpidem "as needed" for the treatment of primary insomnia: a double-blind placebo-controlled study. Sleep Med Rev 2002; 6(suppl 1):S7–S11.
72. Kripke DF. Chronic hypnotic use: deadly risks, doubtful benefit. Sleep Med Rev 2000; 4(1):5–20.
73. NIOM. Sleeping Pills, Insomnia, and Medical Practice. Washington, DC: National Academy of Sciences, 1979.
74. Committee on Halcion, IOM. Halcion: An Independent Assessment of Safety and Efficacy Data. Washington, DC: National Academy Press, 1997.
75. Kripke DF, Klauber MR, Wingard DL, Fell RL, Assmus JD, Garfinkel L. Mortality hazard associated with prescription hypnotics. Biol Psychiatry 1998; 43:687–693.
76. Allgulander C, Ljungberg L, Fisher LD. Long-term prognosis in addiction on sedative and hypnotic drugs analyzed with the Cox regression model. Acta Psychiatr Scand 1987; 75:521–531.

# 11

## Societal and Economic Impact of Sleep Loss and Sleepiness

**KIN YUEN**

Stanford University, Stanford, California, U.S.A.

**RITU DAVÉ**

Kaiser Permanente, Stockton Medical Center, Stockton, California, U.S.A.

**MARKKU PARTINEN**

University of Helsinki, Espoo, Finland, U.S.A.

## I. Introduction

The population, at large, has tolerated sleep deprivation during steadily progressive technological advancement since the Industrial Age. Thirty-three to thirty-nine percent of Americans surveyed have consistently obtained less than 6.9 hr of sleep per weekday (1). Men (6.7%) are more likely to sleep less during the weekday than women (7.0%) (1). As a result, 37% of 1010 adults surveyed reported that their daytime sleepiness interfered with their daily activities "a few days a month or more," and 16% reported up to "a few days per week or more."

The results of sleep deprivation have been linked to motor vehicle accidents, major industrial accidents such as the Exxon Valdez, and Three Mile Island, and the Space Shuttle Challenger disaster (2). The U.S. National Highway Traffic Safety Administration (NHTSA) in 1999 estimated that 56,000 police-reported crashes and 4% of all traffic crash fatalities (1550 cases) involved drowsiness and fatigue as principal causes (3). Sleepiness was a probable cause in about one third of all "fatal-to-driver" motor vehicle accidents involving commercial truck drivers (4).

## II.  Estimate of Total Cost of Accidents Related to Sleepiness

Damien Leger developed a special report for the National Commission on Sleep Disorders Research (NCSDR). He estimated that the total cost of accidents attributable to sleepiness in 1988 was between $43.15 billion and $56.02 billion dollars (5). He reported that in 1988, the costs of *all* motor vehicle accidents ($70.2 billion), work-related accidents ($47.1 billion), home-based accidents ($17.4 billion), and public accidents ($10.9 billion) were $143.4 billion. Any duplications between work-related and motor-vehicle accidents and home-based and motor-vehicle accidents were eliminated in the total by the author. Thus, the total amount was less than the sums.

Motor vehicle accidents in 1988 represented 49,000 deaths and 1,800,000 disabling injuries, producing a total cost of $70.2 billion. Included in this figure were lost wages based on the "human capital approach" of an estimate of a worker's earnings loss during disability or lifetime earnings in a fatality. Other costs included were medical expenses, insurance administration, and property damage from motor-vehicle accidents. To estimate the portion of motor-vehicle accidents related to sleepiness, Leger formulated two approaches to yield a lower and higher estimate of cost.

### A.  Cost of Motor-Vehicle Accidents Caused by Sleepiness

The lower estimate by Leger accounted for those vehicle accidents occurring during the maximum hours of sleepiness: 02:00–07:00 hr and 14:00–17:00 hr. For 1988, 36.1% of fatal accidents (17,689 deaths) and 41.6% of total accidents (resulting in 769,184 disabling injuries) occurred during the hours of maximum sleepiness. This yielded a cost of $29.2 billion.

According to the higher estimate, 54% of total vehicle accidents occurred at night, which represented 998,460 disabling injuries. Therefore, the total cost estimate was $37.9 billion.

### B.  Cost of Work-related Accidents Caused by Sleepiness

In 1988, the total cost of work-related accidents of $47.1 billion was based on 10,600 deaths and 1,800,000 disabling injuries. Included in the estimate of work-related accidents attributable to sleepiness were: (a) motor-vehicle accidents due to shift work and on-the-job motor vehicle accidents (35.0% of total work-related accidents), (b) falls during work caused by sleepiness or inattention (12.6%), and (c) water and transportation accidents (4.8%). Therefore, of all work-related accidents, about 52.5% might potentially be related to sleepiness and then, accounting for 5565 fatalities and 945,000 disabling injuries, resulted in a cost of $24.7 billion.

For the lower estimate, Leger assumed that the same proportion of injuries and fatalities resulted from maximum sleepiness-induced work-related accidents as in motor vehicle accidents. Thus, Leger estimated 41.6% of total accidents resulting in 393,120 disabling injuries and 36.1% of fatal accidents resulting in 2009 deaths, which generated a total cost of $10.3 billion. For the higher estimate, 54% of total accidents occurred at night, or 513,324 disabling injuries, which yielded a cost of $13.3 billion.

### C. Cost of Home-based Accidents Caused by Sleepiness

Falls represented 6500 of the 22,500 home-based accidental deaths, or 28.9% (982,600) of the 3,400,000 home-based disabling injuries. The cost of falls was 28.9% of $17.4 billion, or $5.03 billion. Again, Leger based the lower estimate of cost related to sleepiness at 41.6% of total home-based accidents resulting in 408,762 disabling injuries and 36.1% of total fatalities resulting in 2346 fatalities, yielding a cost of $2.09 billion. The higher estimate, again accounting for 54% of total accidents, yielded 530,604 disabling injuries and a total cost estimate of $2.72 billion.

### D. Costs of Public Accidents

Falls accounted for 4100 deaths, or 22.8% (524,400) of the 2,300,000 disabling injuries, or $2.5 billion of the $10.9 billion cost of accidents in public places. Using the lower cost estimate of 41.6% of total accidents (218,150 disabling injuries) that occurred at maximum hours of sleepiness and 36.1% of fatal accidents (1480 fatalities) accounted for a cost total of $1.04 billion. The higher estimate of 54% of total public accidents was due to nocturnal sleepiness, which yielded 283,176 disabling injuries at a total cost of $1.34 billion.

Therefore, the total estimated cost of accidents related to sleepiness was the sum total of all component costs. Thus, the lower estimate of cost related to sleepiness includes 1,907,072 disabling injuries and 24,318 fatalities, creating a cost of $43.15 billion in 1988. The higher estimate accounted for 2,474,430 disabling injuries, at a total cost of $56.02 billion (rounding would give a total of $43.2 billion and $55.9 billion, respectively).

Dr. Wilse Webb performed a different analysis from Leger's using the data of fatal and total motor-vehicle accidents as reported by the National Safety Council in 1988 (6). He proposed a conservative estimate of 1225 fatalities, 45,000 disabling injuries, and $1.75 billion in total cost from these accidents.

Webb argued against the inclusion of all accidents occurring between 7 P.M. and 7 A.M. as costs resulting from sleepiness. The inclusion of accidents occurring during the 2–5 P.M. period, he stated, neglected to account for other interactive factors "associated with exposure, sleep debt, alcohol and long or monotonous driving." He further refuted the inclusion of work-related accidents and home-based accidents as solely attributable to sleepiness. Work-related accidents, he argued, was accounted for by the total number of accidents. Of the home-based accidents associated with falls, 80% involved persons 65 years or older. Thus, he believed that physical disabilities rather than sleepiness would be the likely cause of these falls.

Webb cited data from the CARfile study of the U.S. Department of Transportation in 1985, which reported 1.4% of total accidents and 1.75% of fatal accidents were directly related to sleepiness (7). Lavie and Pollack studied 13,152 reports by the Israeli Police Department of hourly distribution of sleep-related motor vehicle accidents for 8 years, and found 390 injuries directly attributable to sleepiness (8). A special examiner at the scene assigned the reason for the accident. Lavie reported a highest yearly estimate of 1.0% motor vehicle accidents attributable to sleepiness (personal communication to Webb).

Therefore, Lavie proposed restricting the estimate of total accidents to the 2–6 A.M. period when 4.7% of the total vehicle accidents occurred. He added 1% of all car accidents to "circadian afternoon tendency or accidents by individuals with sleep disorders with a resultant severe daytime sleep demand" to the total car accidents.

Webb further delineated the interaction of alcohol consumption (apart from higher speed, younger drivers, and low traffic volume) and weather and lighting factors causing higher proportion of nighttime accidents, as reported in *Road Safety at Night* (9). He conservatively estimated only 33% of the 4.7%, or "1.56%," of nocturnal accidents were related to sleepiness. Adding the 1% derived from circadian factors yielded the total of 2.5% of all motor-vehicle accidents that could be attributable to sleepiness.

Leger, in response, reaffirmed his highest and lowest estimates cited earlier (5). He discussed the economic model that was used in the United States and Scandinavia that typically assigned responsibility to sleepiness or alcohol as binary. If an effect could be attributable to sleep, then responsibility was modeled as equal to 1; if not, then the responsibility was modeled as equal to 0. However, sleepiness was not ascribed as the sole cause of these motor vehicle accidents. Further research was strongly emphasized by both authors to delineate the role of sleepiness in car accidents.

Subsequently, the Council on Scientific Affairs of the American Medical Association (AMA) estimated that driver sleepiness "is a causative factor in 1% to 3% of all U.S. motor vehicle crashes" (10). The study also cited data from Knipling and Wang (11) that about 96% of sleep-related crashes involved passenger vehicle drivers and 3% involved drivers of large trucks. The databases used included the Transportation Research Information Service (TRIS) and Bibliographic Electronic Databases of Sleep (BEDS) from 1975 through 1997. Drivers deemed at high risk for sleep-related crashes were young drivers (aged 16–29 years), shift workers, drivers who used alcohol and other sedating drugs, drivers with sleep disorders, and commercial large-truck drivers. Federal Hours-of-Service Regulations and Truck Safety measures were introduced thereafter, and adopted by the AMA to help limit the human life and severe property loss.

As alluded to earlier, circadian factors have also been implicated as a contributing factor to traffic accidents. However, the interaction between circadian/homeostatic factors and sleep loss is complex and accident statistics often do not adequately capture the contribution of these important factors.

Despite this early glimpse of the effects of sleep loss, little is known of its full socioeconomic impact. First, ongoing research is beginning to illuminate the impact of sleep deprivation on neurocognitive behavior and other possible comorbidities. But the ramifications of sleep deprivation may not be known completely for years. Second, individuals subjected to the same degree of sleep deprivation often present with different manifestations and complaints of impairment. Given all the exciting advances in sleep medicine, newer tools to evaluate the sleep-deprived population undoubtedly will help clarify its true impact. Nonetheless, the existing literature has attempted to document the effects of sleep deprivation via sleep fragmentation and increased arousals caused by sleep disorders.

Of the 88 sleep disorders listed in the International Classification of Sleep Disorders (12), the better-known and more prevalent disorders are the obstructive sleep apnea syndrome, insomnia, restless legs syndrome/periodic limb movement disorder, and narcolepsy (see also Chap. 5).These sleep disorders are common, and are known to interfere with the quality of sleep; this chapter addresses the socioeconomic impact of these disorders.

The most common cause of excessive daytime sleepiness (EDS) is sleep deprivation. In a survey by Hublin et al. (13), up to one third of adults have sleepiness due to partial sleep deprivation and approximately 7% of middle-aged adults have EDS secondary to sleep disorders. Kapur et al. (14) found that in 6440 participants of the Sleep Heart Health study, there was an association between subjective complaints of daytime sleepiness, inadequate sleep time and insomnia, objective measures of sleep-disordered breathing, and an increase in health care utilization by a modified chronic disease score (CDS). The CDS score tabulated 1 year's pharmacy data based on the staff-HMO model at the Group Health Cooperative in Seattle, Washington. The subjects with the highest quartile of EDS as measured by the Epworth Sleepiness Scale (>11) had an 11% increase in health utilization as compared to the lowest quartile. Notably, however, subjects who did not have significant sleep-disordered breathing, but had feelings of sleepiness and fatigue, also demonstrated 18–20% higher health utilization. Thus, the socioeconomic impact from sleep disorders is likely associated with the effects of sleep fragmentation or sleep loss.

## III. Obstructive Sleep Apnea Syndrome

### A. Prevalence

Obstructive sleep apnea syndrome (OSAS) has been well reported to affect 4% of middle-aged men, and 2% of women aged 30–60 years (15). This prevalence rate is similar to that of asthma (16). Recent literature suggests a higher prevalence rate among minority groups and the elderly (2,17–22).

## B. Complications

### Motor-Vehicle Accidents

Long-haul truck drivers with OSAS were noted to have an increase in the rate of motor vehicle accidents (23). Findley et al. found a sevenfold greater rate of automobile accidents in 29 patients with OSAS compared with 35 subjects without sleep apnea, according to individual driving records from 1981 to 1985 kept by the Department of Motor Vehicles of the Commonwealth of Virginia (24). A subsequent collaborative study by Findley et al. and Masa in Spain reported that the 40 "habitually sleepy drivers had a 13-fold increased risk of having an automobile crash than the 23 control subjects, and there was a significantly higher prevalence of respiratory sleep disorders in the habitually sleepy subjects as compared to controls" (25). Teran-Santos reported that 102 subjects in Burgos or Santander, Spain, with an apnea-hypopnea index (AHI) >10 had an odds ratio of 6.3 for having a car accident as compared to 152 case-matched controls. Adjustments were made for alcohol consumption, body mass index (BMI), age, previous motor vehicle accidents, years of driving, use of sedative medications, visual acuity, and sleep schedule (26–28).

### Occupational Accidents

These type of accidents were also reported in Sweden (28). Of 704 consecutive patients and 580 age-matched controls, male heavy snorers were twice as likely to have occupational accidents as compared to age-matched controls, whereas female heavy snorers had a threefold increase compared to controls.

### End-Organ Complications

The prospective studies have also demonstrated an association between untreated moderate-to-severe levels of OSAS and hypertension, congestive heart failure, arrhythmias, myocardial infarction, pulmonary hypertension, cor pulmonale, and stroke after adjusting for confounding factors such as obesity (29–32). Preeclampsia and averse fetal outcome have recently been described (33–36).

### Neurocognitive Changes

Reduced concentration, memory, alertness, and task performance were noted in 841 subjects with an apnea-hypopnea index ≥ 5 (37). Depressive moods in patients with OSAS have been reported (38–40). Among children with learning difficulties, some are affected by undiagnosed sleep disorders. Gozal reported in 1998 on 297 first graders ranked at the bottom 10th percentile of academic performance who were screened with a questionnaire, a single night of pulse oximetry recording, and transcutaneous carbon dioxide for suspected OSAS (41). Fifty-four children (18.1%) were identified for intervention. The twenty-four children who underwent tonsillectomy and adenoidectomy showed improvements of their mean grades from 2.43 [0.17 standard error (SE)] to 2.87 (0.19 SEM) during the subsequent year. The 30 children in the control group whose parents elected no intervention showed no significant change in grades, 2.44 (0.13) to 2.46 (0.15).

### Quality-of-Life Effects

Akashiba et al. found that among 60 male patients with an AHI > 20/hr and oxygen saturation < 80%, OSAS patients had lower quality of life (QoL) on the Medical Outcomes Study Short-Form 36 (SF-36) as compared to 34 normal controls (42). This effect was again seen in the Sleep Heart Health Study of 5816 patients. Baldwin et al. further suggested that mild-to-moderate sleep-disordered breathing (SDB) was associated with lower scores in the vitality subscale of the SF-36, while severe SDB was "more broadly associated with poorer QoL" (43). Yang et al. showed a similar finding in a smaller sample size of 16 subjects and 46 controls (44). Furthermore, a higher divorce rate and higher level of irritability were found in patients with OSAS (45). Additionally, bed partners of snorers and patients with OSAS have been reported to exhibit more irritability and lower quality of life before treatment (46).

### Health-Care Utilization

Costs are often separated into direct and indirect costs. Direct costs typically consist of hospitalization costs, physician fees, laboratory fees, and costs of medical treatments/medications. Direct nonmedical costs can include costs of using transportation to and from the medical facility. Thus far, only direct costs have been estimated. Indirect/opportunity costs incurred with the death of a patient or while the individual is undergoing treatment are often expressed as days lost from work and reduced productivity. The so-called "intangible costs" are the monetary values of the results of pain and suffering.

Mostly, direct costs of health care utilization of OSAS patients have been reported. Indirect costs, productivity loss including sick days and costs of absenteeism, and costs of transportation have not yet been tabulated for OSAS.

The first published direct medical cost of sleep apnea was $275 million in 1990 by the National Commission on Sleep Disorders Research. (47). More recently, groups in Manitoba, Canada and Puget Sound, Washington published direct medical cost analyses. Health care utilization by children with OSAS has also been studied in Israel.

Ronald et al. analyzed the direct costs of physician claims and the number of hospital admissions for OSAS patients in the Canadian Manitoba governmental health agency database. They found that 181 patients (145 men, 36 women) with untreated OSAS were shown to utilize health care at twice the rate of controls up to 10 years before diagnosis (48). The most significant increase in physician claims was noted up to 3 years before diagnosis. The total physician claims were $686,365 (Canadian) with a mean of $3792/patient, whereas controls generated $356,376 with a mean of $1969/patient. OSAS patients had almost a two-fold increase in hospitalizations compared to controls over the 10-year period:

1118 nights (6.2/OSAS patient) and 676 nights (3.7/control patient). The total expenditure for the OSAS patients exceeded their controls by $771,989 ($1,804,365 for OSAS patients, and $1,032,376 for the controls) over 10 years prior to diagnosis.

The same group of investigators subsequently reported that the annual physician claims of 344 male OSAS patients and 1324 matched controls were significantly less at 2 years after diagnosis than the year before diagnosis: Canadian $174 (32.4 SE) versus $260 (35.7 SE), respectively. There were 499 less physician contacts, and 151 fewer ordered medical tests (electrocardiogram, radiological evaluations, hypothyroid screen, and lipid tests). Hospital stays also decreased from 1.27 (0.25 SE) days/patient/year at 1 year before diagnosis to 0.54 (0.14 SE) days/patient/year. Of the 344 subjects, 282 were "adhering" to continuous positive airway pressure (CPAP) treatment, and 62 were not. The treatment group's physician claims peaked 1 year before diagnosis, and soon began to decline after diagnosis. The treatment group's hospital stays also decreased from 1.25 (0.28 SE) days/patient/year at 1 year before diagnosis to 0.53 (0.14 SE) days/patient/year. The health care utilization of the nonadherent group remained high throughout the 5 years before diagnosis, and "this cost changed little over time" (49).

Kapur et al. also found a twofold increase in direct medical costs of 238 consecutive cases of moderate-to-severe SDB patients as compared to 476 age-, gender-, and body-mass-index (BMI)-matched controls at the Group Health Cooperative (GHC)-HMO model of Puget Sound, Washington (50). The mean annual medical cost was $2720 for OSAS cases prior to diagnosis, and $1384 for controls (1996 dollars). The mean annual costs in OSAS patients were higher than that found in primary-care patients with depressive and anxiety disorders ($2390) and much higher than that of primary-care patients without depressive and anxiety disorders ($1397). The OSAS subjects were further stratified by chronic disease score, and appeared to have a higher chronic disease burden compared to their controls 1 year before diagnosis. The medical costs were found to be directly related to the severity of OSAS after adjusting for age, gender, and obesity. Therefore, besides obesity as a possible confounder in increasing health care utilization, OSAS appeared to independently contribute to an increase in medical costs. Based on a previous published report of underdiagnosis of moderate-to-severe OSAS (51) and epidemiological data of OSAS prevalence in middle-aged adults, the authors estimated that $3.4 billion/year was attributable to untreated OSAS.

Pediatric OSAS patients demonstrated a similar pattern in Israel (52). Of 287 consecutive children with OSAS, there was at least a two fold increase in utilization of health care services compared to 149 controls 1 year before diagnosis. The high-cost contributors were hospital days, medications, and emergency-room visits. Subjects with untreated OSAS have many more sleepiness-related motor vehicle accidents as compared to a control group. However, the loss of productivity and opportunity loss have not yet been estimated for OSAS patients.

*Health Economic Evaluations*

For most health economic evaluations, which include cost-benefit, cost-effectiveness, and cost-utility analyses, one needs to choose a base-case scenario and the perspective of evaluation. Often, the societal perspective is adopted, but it can be from an individual's or a payer's perspective. The costs or benefits are valued in two approaches:

1. Human capital. This evaluates an intervention's effect on a patient's lifetime earnings. For example, a life saved at age 55 by an intervention = 10 years of expected earnings gained. Similarly, a life lost through an intervention or inaction can be evaluated the same way.
2. Willingness to pay. Patients are asked to value their own lives: How much are they willing to pay for a program that should reduce probability of death by a stated amount? An example of an application would be to estimate wage premiums to work in risky occupations.

Although these valuations of human life are used elsewhere, they have not been widely used in sleep medicine. Patient preference can also be measured in "utilities"—the degree of pleasure or satisfaction derived from the purchases of a product, i.e., the patient's preference for a certain health state or outcome of a treatment. Perfect health is assigned a value of 1, and death a value of 0. QoL instruments and recent work in utility measurements have made further advances in health economic evaluations.

Early work by Tousignant et al. found that nasal CPAP treatment of 19 patients with moderate-to-severe OSAS improved QoL (53). The mean utility before treatment was 0.63, and after treatment was 0.87. The annual treatment costs in Quebec, Canada included CPAP supplies, rental and maintenance costs for CPAP devices, and one-night polysomnography for diagnosis. Using Canadian life expectancy tables, the change in utilities and life expectancy yielded change in quality-adjusted life years (QALYs) based on treatment. Discounting costs at 5% in 1994 Canadian dollars, the cost per QALY gained was estimated at Canadian $3523–$9809. There were 3 patients who positively skewed the results. When these 3 patients were excluded, the cost for incremental QALY rose to $18,737. The authors concluded that CPAP treatment was cost-effective. For comparison, the incremental cost per QALY saved for lung transplant recipients was estimated to be $176,817 (54).

Chervin et al. performed a cost-utility study on three methods of diagnosing OSAS using preference values obtained by Tousignant et al. or by introspection (55). A more recent study in Europe found different sensitivities among the newer instruments as compared to utility models using the standard gamble approach (56). In a small pilot study of 30 patients with moderate-to-severe OSAS (mean AHI = 32.4) in the Stanford Sleep Disorders Clinic, we have similarly found improvements in SF-36 scores, but inconsistent utility improvements using visual analog scales as compared to the standard gamble approach (57).

Future research into the health economic burden of underdiagnosis and cost-effectiveness of treatment of OSAS, including other treatment modalities such as oral appliances and surgical procedures, will need to be actively pursued.

## IV.  Insomnia

### A.  Prevalence

The prevalence of chronic insomnia is estimated to be at 10% (2) based on different formats and definitions used in questionnaires. Between 30 to 50% of the general population were estimated to have insomnia of any duration or severity. In a survey of 1010 adults in 2002, the National Sleep Foundation found that 58% reported at least one of the following a few nights a week: "waking feeling unrefreshed, waking a lot during the night, difficulty falling asleep, and waking too early/not being able to get back to sleep." Of the respondents, 15% used either a prescription sleep medication (8%) and/or an over-the-counter (OTC) sleep aid (10%) to help them sleep at least a few nights a month for the past year. Furthermore, the prevalence of insomnia symptoms "generally increases with age, while the rates of sleep dissatisfaction and diagnoses have little variation with age" (58).

### B.  Complications

Mostly older data suggested daytime impairments similar to the obstructive sleep apnea syndrome. A Gallup poll in 1991 found subjects with insomnia complained more of lack of concentration, memory impairment, and difficulty enjoying family and social relationships compared to those without insomnia (59). The Gallup poll also found that 5% of insomniacs, compared to 2% without insomnia, reported a motor-vehicle crash related to fatigue at some time in their lives. Balter and Uhlenhuth in 1992 reported that insomniacs before treatment were more than four times as likely as controls to report a motor-vehicle accident or other serious accidents within the past year (60).

### C.  Direct Costs

Walsh and Engelhardt estimated the direct costs for insomnia in the United States to be $10.9 billion in 1990, whereas the National Commission on Sleep Disorders Research estimated the direct costs to be 15.4 billion in 1990 (61). Walsh and Engelhardt estimated in 1995 that the total direct costs increased to $13.9 billion. The costs were separated into health care services and substances used for insomnia.

Health care services included outpatient visits to physician, psychologist, social worker, sleep specialist, and mental health organization, as well as inpatient care and nursing-home care (when the primary reason for placement was the elders' sleep disturbance). The total health care services for 1995 were estimated at $13.9 billion, with nursing-home care as the major contributor to costs. Substances used for insomnia included prescription medications, nonprescription medications, alcohol, and melatonin. The total costs were estimated at $1.9 billion, with prescription medications and alcohol as the top contributors to costs.

Leger cited work from Weyerer and Dilling in 1991 (62,63), who had reported that insomniacs had about twice as many outpatient physician visits as good sleepers (12.9 vs. 5.2) in 1 year. Insomniacs were also more likely to have been hospitalized compared to good sleepers (21.9% vs. 12.2%, respectively).

### D.  Indirect Costs

#### Transportation

Walsh estimated in 1990 that transportation to and from health care providers generated 10 million visits; the estimated additional expense was $20 million at a minimum average cost of $2.00 per visit (61).

#### Loss of Productivity

In a 1992 report, adults who were described as having 7 or more nights of poor sleep per month missed 5.2 days of work per year more than persons who slept well. In 1991, Leigh surveyed 1308 workers, and found that insomnia, out of 37 variables, was the most predictive of absenteeism at work. Stoller estimated the loss of productivity to be $41.1 billion in 1998 (64). Lavie and Leger found that workplace accidents were two to seven times more common among insomniacs than good sleepers, respectively (63). Lower quality of health and health status has also been reported in patients with chronic insomnia (63). Surprisingly, there is a paucity of recent data further documenting the effects of insomnia. More systematic assessments similar to the progress made with the obstructive sleep apnea syndrome will help clarify the burden of insomnia and its economic and health effects.

### V.  Restless Legs Syndrome (RLS)

RLS is the subjective sensation of discomfort with a need or compulsion to move one's limb(s). Movement relieves the discomfort. Ekbom first reported this syndrome in 1960 (65). It affects about 5–15% of the general population, about 11–20% of pregnant women (12,66,67), 15–20% of uremic patients, and up to 30% of patients with rheumatoid arthritis. Allen and Earley reported a prevalence rate between 2.5 and 15% of the general population in 2001 (68). Phillips et al. found that 3% of the participants aged 18–29, 10% of those aged 30–79, and 19% of those aged 80 or more were experiencing restless legs 5 or more nights per month in the 1996 Kentucky Behavioral Risk Factor Surveillance Survey (69). It is highly prevalent in the elderly population; 10–35% of those over 65 years old are estimated to be affected by RLS (70). The association of RLS with iron deficiency anemia has been well described (65). In large kindreds, an autosomal dominant pattern of inheritance was seen (68). Desautels et al. reported the identification of a major susceptibility locus for RLS on chromosome 12q (71).

The links between RLS, difficulty initiating sleep, and its pathophysiology are being actively investigated. Symptoms of insomnia or fatigue are often reported by patients, as illustrated by the case presentation in the *New England Journal of Medicine* by Earley (72). Other symptoms cited by the author include "reduced concentration and memory, decreased motivation and drive, and depression and anxiety." Affected individuals often avoid activities that require prolonged sitting or immobilization such as long-distance traveling. Those affected by RLS were found to have a poorer general and mental health compared to those without RLS, by Phillips et al. (69). Those with RLS were 2.4 times more likely to self-report diminished general health, and experienced 5 additional days in poor mental health than those without.

Medications for treatment of RLS are available based on the level of distress and frequency of symptoms. Dopamine agonists, sedative-hypnotic medications, opiates, or anticonvulsants have been used for treatment. Nonetheless, it is suspected that RLS remains a disorder that is "unrecognized" and therefore "untreated." Although recent literature has began to report the social impact of RLS, its economic impact remains to be evaluated.

## VI. Periodic Limb Movement Disorder

Periodic limb movement "is characterized by periodic episodes of repetitive and highly stereotyped limb movements that occur during sleep" (12). It is reported to affect up to 34% of patients over age 60 years, and 1–15% of patients with insomnia. Movements are associated with partial awakening or arousals. Patients with isolated periodic limb movements in sleep (PLMS) without RLS may be asymptomatic.

Although PLMS is reported as "rare" in children, Chervin et al. found in 872 children aged 2–14 years that conduct problems (such as bullying and aggressive behavior) were more common among children with symptoms of sleep-disordered breathing, restless legs syndrome, and periodic leg movements in sleep (73). This suggested that assessment for sleep disorders might be beneficial in some children with behavioral problems. Future research will likely provide estimates as to how much PLMS contribute to the socioeconomic impact of sleep disruption in children and adults.

## VII. Narcolepsy

The prevalence of narcolepsy with cataplexy is 1 in 10,000 or 0.02% to 0.16% worldwide (69). Patients usually present with complaints of excessive daytime sleepiness before the onset of hypnogogic/hypnopompic hallucinations, sleep paralysis, sleep attacks, or cataplexy. Nocturnal sleep fragmentation is commonly found among individuals affected by narcolepsy. However, of those patients who have experienced cataplexy—unexpected loss of muscle tone during wakefulness—driving can present a challenge. There is a paucity of data reporting the number of motor vehicle accidents related to cataplexy or sleep attacks caused by narcolepsy before treatment.

The National Commission on Sleep Disorders Research published an estimated direct medical cost of narcolepsy as a minimum of $64.1 million in 1990 (47). The earlier literature reported that over 75% of 180 narcoleptic individuals in Canada as compared to age- and sex-matched controls had occupational problems. The narcolepsy group had statistically significant lower job performance, less promotions, lower earning capacity, more fear of or having more actual job loss, and higher disability insurance as compared to controls. Sixty-six percent of the narcoleptic patients fell asleep at the wheel, 67% had near or actual motor-vehicle accidents caused by drowsiness or falling asleep at the wheel, 29% experienced cataplexy while driving, and 12% had sleep paralysis while driving. Sleepiness or sleep-induced work or home accidents and smoking-related accidents were found in 49% of narcoleptics (74). In 1984, Broughton et al. compared (a) 60 patients with narcolepsy with cataplexy, (b) patients with temporal lobe seizures or primary generalized epilepsy, but without major organic pathology, and (c) age- and sex-matched controls (75). They discovered that narcoleptic patients had "poorer driving records, higher accident rates from smoking, and greater problems in planning recreation" than patients with epilepsy. The continuous excessive daytime sleepiness that persisted between "attacks" was noted to be the major contributor to psychosocial problems in narcoleptic patients, whereas epileptic patients were more "alert" between seizures.

Findley et al. compared 10 patients with narcolepsy before treatment against 10 age- and sex-matched volunteers using the Steer Clear system—a 30-min computer program simulating monotonous highway driving conditions with 780 obstacles. Narcoleptic patients, similar to untreated sleep apneic patients, had a statistically significant poorer performance as compared to controls (76). More recently, Leon-Munoz et al. in Spain studied 35 patients having narcolepsy with cataplexy between 1994 and 1998, and found that the narcoleptic group had a significantly higher number of accidents compared to 25 normal controls (77). Because of the fear of losing one's driver's license, some patients have chosen not to seek help, thus further compounding the risks to the individual and the public's safety.

Prior to the use of wakefulness-promoting agents, and in some pediatric patients, maintenance of wakefulness is dependent on stimulant medications and antidepressants. The safety of such medications during reproductive years and the risk of driving accidents without medication are typically handled during discussions between the prescribing practitioner and the patient. Irritability, anxiety, and erectile or ejaculatory dysfunction have been reported with these medications (78). The costs of newly approved medications for the treatment of narcolepsy, such as gamma hydroxybutyrate (GHB) and the wakefulness-promoting agent modafinil, despite partial medical insurance coverage, still remain prohibitive to some patients and their families.

## VIII.  Conclusions

Sleep disorders encompass a wide range of sleep disruption that may disturb patients or bed partners, ranging from easily observable events such as those associated with the obstructive sleep apnea syndrome to barely perceptible leg movements, as in the case of periodic limb movement disorder. The aging of the population will undoubtedly increase the propensity for insomnia. The young are not immune to the obstructive sleep apnea syndrome, restless legs, or periodic limb movements in sleep. With the limited amount of sleep that the working population allows itself, it is likely that the manifestations and effects of sleep deprivation will be substantially increased over the next decades. It is of paramount concern that further research into the neurocognitive impairment and socioeconomic effects of sleep deprivation continues. Thus, society-at-large will be able to better appreciate and understand the burden sleep loss carries in daily life.

## References

1.  Foundation NS. Sleep Am 2000–2003.
2.  Kryger M, Roth T, Dement W, eds. Principles and Practice of Sleep Medicine. 3rd ed. Philadelpia: Saunders, 2000.
3.  Drowsiness Driving and Automobile Crashes: NCSDR/NHTSA Expert Panel on Driver Fatigue and Sleepiness. 1999. (Accessed at www.nhtsa.gov/people/injury/drowsy_driving1/drowsy.html.)
4.  Board NTS. Factors That Affect Fatigue in Heavy Truck Accidents. Vol. 1. Analysis. Washington, DC: 1995.
5.  Leger D. The cost of sleep-related accidents: a report for the National Commission on Sleep Disorders Research. Sleep 1994; 17(1):84–93.
6.  Webb WB. The cost of sleep-related accidents: a reanalysis. Sleep 1995; 18(4):276–80.
7.  Transportation USDo. Report to the Senate Committee on Appropriations and the House Committee on Appropriations. Transportation-related research. CARfile study. Washington, DC; 1985.
8.  Lavie P WM, Pollack I. Frequency of sleep related accidents and hour of day. Sleep Res 1986; 15:275.
9.  Development OfEC-oa. Road Safety at Night. Paris: Organization for Economic Co-operation and Development; 1980.
10. Lyznicki JM, Doege TC, Davis RM, Williams MA. Sleepiness, driving, and motor vehicle crashes. Council on Scientific Affairs, American Medical Association. JAMA 1998; 279(23):1908–1913.

11. Knipling RR, Wang WJ. Crashes and Fatalities Related to Driver Drowsiness/ Fatigue. Washington, DC: Office of Crash Avoidance Research, US Department of Transportation, 1994.

12. Association ASD. The International Classification of Sleep Disorders: Revised Diagnostic and Coding Manual. Rochester, NY: American Sleep Disorders Association; 1997.

13. Hublin C, Kaprio J, Partinen M, Koskenvuo M. Insufficient sleep—a population-based study in adults. Sleep 2001; 24(4):392–400.

14. Kapur VK, Redline S, Nieto FJ, Young TB, Newman AB, Henderson JA. The relationship between chronically disrupted sleep and healthcare use. Sleep 2002; 25(3):289–296.

15. Young T, Palta M, Dempsey J, Skatrud J, Weber S, Badr S. The occurrence of sleep-disordered breathing among middle-aged adults. N Engl J Med 1993; 328(17):1230–1235.

16. MMWR Surveillance Summaries; 2002 March 29. Report No.: 51 (ss01).

17. Ancoli-Israel S, Kripke DF, Klauber MR, et al. Morbidity, mortality and sleep-disordered breathing in community dwelling elderly. Sleep 1996; 19(4):277–282.

18. Molho M, Shulimzon T, Benzaray S, Katz I. Importance of inspiratory load in the assessment of severity of airways obstruction and its correlation with $CO_2$ retention in chronic obstructive pulmonary disease. Am Rev Respir Dis 1993; 147(1):45–49.

19. Baum GL, Zwas T, Katz I, Roth Y. Changes in mucociliary clearance during acute exacerbations of asthma. Am Rev Respir Dis 1992; 145(1):237–238.

20. Katz I, Stradling J, Slutsky AS, Zamel N, Hoffstein V. Do patients with obstructive sleep apnea have thick necks? Am Rev Respir Dis 1990; 141(5 Pt 1):1228–1231.

21. Kripke D, Ancoli-Israel S., Klauber M. US population estimate for disordered sleep breathing: high rates in minority. Sleep Res 1995; 24:268.

22. Schmidt-Nowara WW, Coultas DB, Wiggins C, Skipper BE, Samet JM. Snoring in a Hispanic-American population: risk factors and association with hypertension and other morbidity. Arch Intern Med 1990; 150(3):597–601.

23. Stoohs RA, Guilleminault C, Itoi A, Dement WC. Traffic accidents in commercial long-haul truck drivers: the influence of sleep-disordered breathing and obesity. Sleep 1994; 17(7):619–623.

24. Findley LJ, Unverzagt ME, Suratt PM. Automobile accidents involving patients with obstructive sleep apnea. Am Rev Respir Dis 1988; 138(2):337–340.

25. Masa JF, Rubio M, Findley LJ. Habitually sleepy drivers have a high frequency of automobile crashes associated with respiratory disorders during sleep. Am J Respir Crit Care Med 2000; 162(4 Pt 1):1407–1412.

26. Teran-Santos J, Jimenez-Gomez A, Cordero-Guevara J. The association between sleep apnea and the risk of traffic accidents. Cooperative Group Burgos-Santander. N Engl J Med 1999; 340(11):847–851.

27. George CF. Reduction in motor vehicle collisions following treatment of sleep apnoea with nasal CPAP. Thorax 2001; 56(7):508–512.

28. Ulfberg J, Carter N, Edling C. Sleep-disordered breathing and occupational accidents. Scand J Work Environ Health 2000;26(3):237–242.

29. Bixler EO, Vgontzas AN, Lin HM, et al. Association of hypertension and sleep-disordered breathing. Arch Intern Med 2000; 160(15):2289–2295.

30.  Nieto FJ, Young TB, Lind BK, et al. Association of sleep-disordered breathing, sleep apnea, and hypertension in a large community-based study. Sleep Heart Health Study. JAMA 2000; 283(14):1829–1836.

31.  Peppard PE, Young T, Palta M, Skatrud J. Prospective study of the association between sleep-disordered breathing and hypertension. N Engl J Med 2000; 342(19):1378–1384.

32.  Partinen M, Jamieson A, Guilleminault C. Long-term outcome for obstructive sleep apnea syndrome patients: mortality. Chest 1988; 94(6):1200–1204.

33.  Edwards N, Blyton DM, Kirjavainen TT, Sullivan CE. Hemodynamic responses to obstructive respiratory events during sleep are augmented in women with preeclampsia. Am J Hypertens 2001; 14(11 pt 1):1090–1095.

34.  Connolly G, Razak AR, Hayanga A, Russell A, McKenna P, McNicholas WT. Inspiratory flow limitation during sleep in pre-eclampsia: comparison with normal pregnant and nonpregnant women. Eur Respir J 2001; 18(4):672–676.

35.  Maasilta P, Bachour A, Teramo K, Polo O, Laitinen LA. Sleep-related disordered breathing during pregnancy in obese women. Chest 2001; 120(5):1448–1454.

36.  Lefcourt LA, Rodis JF. Obstructive sleep apnea in pregnancy. Obstet Gynecol Surv 1996; 51(8):503–506.

37.  Kim HC, Young T, Matthews CG, Weber SM, Woodward AR, Palta M. Sleep-disordered breathing and neuropsychological deficits: a population-based study. Am J Respir Crit Care Med 1997; 156(6):1813–1819.

38.  Baran A, Richert AC. Obstructive sleep apnea and depression. CNS Spectrum 2003; 8(2):120–134.

39.  McMahon JP, Foresman BH, Chisholm RC. The influence of CPAP on the neurobehavioral performance of patients with obstructive sleep apnea hypopnea syndrome: a systematic review. Wmj 2003; 102(1):36–43.

40.  Means MK, Lichstein KL, Edinger JD, et al. Changes in depressive symptoms after continuous positive airway pressure treatment for obstructive sleep apnea. Sleep Breath 2003; 7(1):31–42.

41.  Gozal D. Sleep-disordered breathing and school performance in children. Pediatrics 1998; 102(3 Pt 1):616–620.

42.  Akashiba T, Kawahara S, Akahoshi T, et al. Relationship between quality of life and mood or depression in patients with severe obstructive sleep apnea syndrome. Chest 2002; 122(3):861–865.

43.  Baldwin CM, Griffith KA, Nieto FJ, O'Connor GT, Walsleben JA, Redline S. The association of sleep-disordered breathing and sleep symptoms with quality of life in the Sleep Heart Health Study. Sleep 2001; 24(1):96–105.

44.  Yang EH, Hla KM, McHorney CA, Havighurst T, Badr MS, Weber S. Sleep apnea and quality of life. Sleep 2000; 23(4):535–541.

45.  Wiegand L, Zwillich CW. Obstructive sleep apnea. Dis Month 1994; 40(4):197–252.

46.  McArdle N, Kingshott R, Engleman HM, Mackay TW, Douglas NJ. Partners of patients with sleep apnoea/hypopnoea syndrome: effect of CPAP treatment on sleep quality and quality of life. Thorax 2001; 56(7):513–518.

47.  Research NCoSD. National Commission on Sleep Disorders Research report. Executive Summary and executive report. Bethesda; 1993.

48.  Ronald J, Delaive K, Roos L, Manfreda J, Bahammam A, Kryger MH. Health care utilization in the 10 years prior to diagnosis in obstructive sleep apnea syndrome patients. Sleep 1999; 22(2):225–229.

49. Bahammam A, Delaive K, Ronald J, Manfreda J, Roos L, Kryger MH. Health care utilization in males with obstructive sleep apnea syndrome two years after diagnosis and treatment. Sleep 1999; 22(6):740–747.

50. Kapur V, Blough DK, Sandblom RE, et al. The medical cost of undiagnosed sleep apnea. Sleep 1999; 22(6):749–755.

51. Ohayon MM, Guilleminault C, Priest RG, Caulet M. Snoring and breathing pauses during sleep: telephone interview survey of a United Kingdom population sample. Br Med J 1997; 314(7084):860–863.

52. Reuveni H, Simon T, Tal A, Elhayany A, Tarasiuk A. Health care services utilization in children with obstructive sleep apnea syndrome. Pediatrics 2002; 110(1 pt 1):68–72.

53. Tousignant P, Cosio MG, Levy RD, Groome PA. Quality adjusted life years added by treatment of obstructive sleep apnea. Sleep 1994; 17(1):52–60.

54. Gross C, Savik K, Bolman RM, Hertz MI. Long-term health status and quality of life outcomes of lung transplant recipients. Chest 1995; 108:1587–1593.

55. Chervin RD, Murman DL, Malow BA, Totten V. Cost-utility of three approaches to the diagnosis of sleep apnea: polysomnography, home testing, and empirical therapy. Ann Intern Med 1999; 130(6):496–505.

56. Chakravorty I, Cayton RM, Szczepura A. Health utilities in evaluating intervention in the sleep apnoea/hypopnoea syndrome. Eur Respir J 2002; 20(5):1233–1238.

57. Yuen K, Goldstein M, Pelayo R, Guilleminault C. Prospective study of health-related quality of life in obstructive sleep apnea before and after treatment. Sleep 2001; 24(suppl):A284–285.

58. Ohayon MM. Epidemiology of insomnia: what we know and what we still need to learn. Sleep Med Rev 2002; 6(2):97–111.

59. Organization G. Sleep in America. Princeton, NJ: 1991.

60. Balter MB, Uhlenhuth EH. New epidemiologic findings about insomnia and its treatment. J Clin Psychiatry 1992; 53 (suppl):34–39; discussion 40–42.

61. Walsh JK, Engelhardt CL. The direct economic costs of insomnia in the United States for 1995. Sleep 1999; 22 (suppl 2):S386–393.

62. Weyerer S, Dilling H. Prevalence and treatment of insomnia in the community: results from the Upper Bavarian Field Study. Sleep 1991; 14(5):392–398.

63. Leger D. Public health and insomnia: economic impact. Sleep 2000; 23 (suppl 3):S69–76.

64. Stoller MK. Economic effects of insomnia. Clin Ther 1994; 16(5):873–897; discussion 54.

65. Ekbom KA. Restless legs syndrome. Neurology 1960; 10:868–873.

66. Goodman JD, Brodie C, Ayida GA. Restless leg syndrome in pregnancy. Br Med J 1988; 297(6656):1101–1102.

67. Lee KA, Zaffke ME, Baratte-Beebe K. Restless legs syndrome and sleep disturbance during pregnancy: the role of folate and iron. J Womens Health Gend Based Med 2001; 10(4):335–341.

68. Allen RP, Earley CJ. Restless legs syndrome: a review of clinical and pathophysiologic features. J Clin Neurophysiol 2001; 18(2):128–147.

69. Phillips B, Young T, Finn L, Asher K, Hening WA, Purvis C. Epidemiology of restless legs symptoms in adults. Arch Intern Med 2000; 160(14):2137–2141.

70. Milligan SA, Chesson AL. Restless legs syndrome in the older adult: diagnosis and management. Drugs Aging 2002; 19(10):741–751.

71. Desautels A, Turecki G, Montplaisir J, Sequeira A, Verner A, Rouleau GA. Identification of a major susceptibility locus for restless legs syndrome on chromosome 12q. Am J Hum Genet 2001; 69(6):1266–1270.

72. Earley CJ. Clinical practice: restless legs syndrome. N Engl J Med 2003; 348(21):2103–2109.

73. Chervin RD, Dillon JE, Archbold KH, Ruzicka DL. Conduct problems and symptoms of sleep disorders in children. J Am Acad Child Adolesc Psychiatry 2003; 42(2):201–208.

74. Broughton R, Ghanem Q, Hishikawa Y, Sugita Y, Nevsimalova S, Roth B. Life effects of narcolepsy in 180 patients from North America, Asia and Europe compared to matched controls. Can J Neurol Sci 1981; 8(4):299–304.

75. Broughton RJ, Guberman A, Roberts J. Comparison of the psychosocial effects of epilepsy and narcolepsy/cataplexy: a controlled study. Epilepsia 1984; 25(4):423–433.

76. Findley L, Unverzagt M, Guchu R, Fabrizio M, Buckner J, Suratt P. Vigilance and automobile accidents in patients with sleep apnea or narcolepsy. Chest 1995; 108(3):619–624.

77. Leon-Munoz L, de la Calzada MD, Guitart M. [Accidents prevalence in a group of patients with the narcolepsy- cataplexy syndrome]. Rev Neurol 2000; 30(6):596–598.

78. Douglas NJ. The psychosocial aspects of narcolepsy. Neurology 1998; 50(2; suppl 1):S27–30.

# 12

# General Occupational Implications of Round-the-Clock Operations

**MARK R. ROSEKIND, DAVID J. C. FLOWER, KEVIN B. GREGORY, AND W. EDWARD JUNG**

**Alertness Solutions, Cupertino, California, U.S.A.**

## I. Society's Evolution to Round-the-Clock Operations

Astronauts aboard the space shuttle sleep on average about 6.5 hr/day, although on the first and last days of a mission this can be as low as 5.7 hr (1,2). The flight controllers in the Mission Operations Directorate (MOD) who manage the shuttle flight on the ground are also averaging about 6.5 hr, except for those on the night shift (Orbit 3 ops) who sleep only about 6.1 hr/day (3). These findings parallel those of the general population in the United States, who are typically getting from 1 to 1.5 hr less sleep than physiologically required (4,5). Perhaps the astronauts on space shuttle missions and the flight controllers in MOD are not the "typical" examples used when portraying how sleep loss is experienced in occupational settings. However, they are excellent examples of how work requirements have significantly evolved in our society, far beyond our traditional concepts of work and shift schedules.

Historically, work was confined to daylight hours, that is until the industrial revolution provided the large-scale opportunity to expand the work day. With the availability of light and machines that do not require sleep, it became easier to work around the clock, which led to the now-common practice of shift work. Scheduling practices have evolved to provide a constant 24-hr workforce in many occupational settings. Although traditionally, "shift work" settings were generally found in manufacturing and assembly line operations where machines could be used for output around the clock, today, 24/7 occupational demand has evolved much further and is no longer restricted to the production environment.

Modern round-the-clock operations (RTC Ops) are now commonplace in almost every work setting, meeting continual 24/7 societal demands. In transportation, there is a need to fly airplanes; drive trucks, buses, and cars; and operate railways and ships around the clock as part of a global transportation system. Access to health care is available 24 hr/day, and includes everything from emergency medical services to laboratory work and surgery. Public safety requires law enforcement, fire fighting, and emergency medical services to provide around-the-clock assistance. In addition, military operations continue to be a 24/7 global activity. Consider how many other aspects of our modern 24/7 society have also evolved to continual operations. Communications, technology, and commerce (e.g., banking, trading) are cornerstones of modern society and require infrastructure and services to be available and functioning around the clock. Today, even "convenience" services such as gas stations and grocery stores are available any time of the day or night, but perhaps the Internet and the round-the-clock worldwide access that it provides is the epitome of the modern 24-hr society.

It is critical to consider how RTC Ops have moved far beyond the traditional view of shift work. Work schedules and occupational activities are no longer constrained or practiced in conventional ways. For example, historically, someone working a shift would generally be considered to be on days or nights or perhaps a rotating schedule. A modern view of RTC Ops expands this traditional view and perhaps the most inclusive definition of RTC Ops would involve anyone not working a "9-to-5" Monday-through-Friday schedule. This definition provides for traditional night work and rotating schedules but also acknowledges and expands the definition to include many diverse modern work practices. However, for completeness, RTC Ops must also be considered to include modern occupational practices that require time zone changes associated with travel, as these parallel the circadian disruption associated with irregular and altered schedules.

The world has evolved significantly, and with it, the need for RTC Ops to meet societal demands. Our traditional views, concepts, terminology, and data on shift work and occupational requirements no longer fully reflect the dramatic changes that are now commonplace in our society. Examining the role and effects of sleep loss in occupational settings requires an evolved definition that more accurately reflects the RTC Ops that pervade the modern workforce.

## II.  Sleep and Circadian Disruption Associated with RTC Ops

In 2000, the *Monthly Labor Review* reported 1997 data indicating that more than 25 million people in the United States worked variable hours, which accounted for about 28% of the U.S. workforce at the time (6). Using historical definitions, shift workers have been reported to work 400 more hours per year than those in more traditional 40 hr/week jobs (7). However, in many professions also, significant numbers of individuals work at different times of the day and night and 35% of nurses, for example, may be required to work at times other than a day shift (8). These data show that by traditional definitions, it is likely that about one third of the U.S. workforce is working some nonstandard or irregular schedule. Furthermore, expanding the definition as suggested above, such that RTC Ops most accurately represent modern work practices, would likely increase these numbers yet further.

The requirements for RTC Ops are important because they affect key physiological factors that have significant outcomes on alertness, safety, and performance. In this section, the physiological disruption associated with modern RTC Ops will be examined, common work-related practices described and how they create this physiological disruption, and finally, work activities in the "real world" are confronted by a multitude of challenges that can further exacerbate this physiological disruption. Some examples of these challenges also are discussed.

### A. Sleep and Circadian Factors

The 24/7 requirements of RTC Ops can affect both sleep and circadian rhythms. The scientific literature suggests that at least four core physiological factors can be affected by, or play a role in, work-related alertness, safety, and performance (9). These factors include sleep, continuous hours of wakefulness, circadian rhythms, and sleep disorders.

Sleep can be disrupted in two ways: acutely or through a cumulative sleep debt. Acute sleep loss will typically refer to the total amount of sleep an individual obtains in the 24-hr period prior to work. A work-related cumulative sleep debt can be calculated by adding the sleep loss acquired over days. This calculation should begin after an identified recovery period when an individual would have an opportunity to "zero out" any existing sleep debt. Sleep is a core physiological factor that affects waking alertness, safety, and performance and, as will be apparent, RTC Ops can affect sleep acutely and over time through a cumulative sleep debt.

The number of continuous hours of wakefulness creates another physiological disruption that can affect waking levels of alertness and performance and is usually associated with decreased sleep, either acute or cumulative. Classic definitions of fatigue involve "time on task" and translate directly to the physiological disruption associated with prolonged periods of wakefulness. This factor is also an example of the complex interactions among these core physiological variables. Sleep loss will often occur with periods of prolonged wakefulness where individuals are awake for a long time and have little sleep and this extended wakefulness is then also likely to extend through one of the windows of circadian low (e.g., natural daily/nightly periods of minimal alertness).

Circadian rhythms and time-of-day considerations therefore represent another of the core physiological factors that affect waking alertness, safety, and performance. RTC Ops can create circadian disruption through a variety of paths. The timing of work, for example at night, can create circadian disruption by forcing a pattern of night:work and day:sleep. At the extreme, this pattern can be the complete inverse of the natural human circadian programming of night:sleep and day:activity. Circadian disruption can also occur as a result of rotating shifts that continually provide mixed cues and patterns in conflict with natural internal circadian timing.

A further issue is the observation that individuals working night shifts never fully adapt to the altered circadian schedule (10). While it is commonly believed that consecutive nights of work lead to "adaptation," two main factors prevent the occurrence of adaptation. One is the morning exposure to light following a night work period, which maintains or resets the circadian clock to a day:wake and night:sleep pattern. The other factor is the typical practice of returning to a day:wake pattern on days off for social and other reasons. Both of these factors interfere with any significant circadian adjustment to night work.

Another circadian disruption not typically defined as associated with work is jet lag. Modern business activities often include transmeridian travel and the associated time zone changes can create both circadian and sleep disruptions. When considering the general occupational implications of sleep loss, travel is not usually acknowledged or appreciated for its effect on waking alertness, safety, and performance.

Finally, a wide range of sleep disorders have been demonstrated to affect waking function (11,12). Often, these are undiagnosed or misdiagnosed, and may affect an individual's performance and alertness without explicit knowledge of the underlying causal factor. An existing sleep disorder has the potential to create sleep loss and decrease waking function, which will be exacerbated further by work demands that lead to sleep loss and circadian disruption such as night work, travel across time zones and the need for periods of prolonged wakefulness.

RTC Ops can affect all of these physiological factors: acute sleep loss and cumulative sleep debt, hours of continuous wakefulness, circadian/time-of-day, and sleep disorders. Diverse work requirements lead inevitably to physiological disruptions and subsequent effects on waking alertness, safety, and performance.

### B. Work-Related Issues That Affect Sleep and Circadian Factors

The complexity of real-world operations presents a variety of work demands that can affect the physiological factors previously cited. Some examples of these common work-related issues provide insight to the sources of this complexity (Table 1).

Across many work settings, there is an increasing move to compress work time and schedules as a mechanism for obtaining more time off. As work settings

**Table 1** Work-Related Issues That Affect Sleep and Circadian Factors

- Compressed work time to obtain more time off
- Early start times
- Length of work days
- Day versus night work
- Changing day versus night work (direction/number of hours)
- Recovery sleep opportunities (predictable/protected)
- Consecutive work periods
- Predictability and stability of schedule
- Overtime (elective versus requirements)

create four 10 hr/day weeks or three 12 hr/day weeks, there is more time for social and family life. However, the condensed work schedule can create its own physiological disruption through a variety of mechanisms. Another common issue across modern work environments is the start time. The traditional "9-to-5" workday is often difficult to find in today's fast-paced society. It is not uncommon for the "work" to begin at 7 A.M. or even earlier in many settings and it will be clear that an early start time can infringe on the previous night's sleep and lead to an acute sleep loss. If individuals choose to engage in any activities prior to work this will further curtail their night's sleep. The length of the workday can also significantly affect the physiological factors identified. Society has moved from the historical "8-hr" workday to ones that last 10 or 12 hr and there are many circumstances where these longer days can be extended even further when individuals find themselves dealing with emergencies or working overtime. Inherent in the definition of RTC Ops is the requirement to have work activities or services available 24 hr/day. This requires both day and night work and in turn the physiological effect of circadian disruption and sleep loss. Related to this are the specifics of shift timing, and whether the shift in question is "permanent" or "rotating." Changing from day to night work (or vice versa) creates circadian disruption and associated factors include the direction of rotation and the number of hours that the schedule changes. One common shift-scheduling practice involves a "quick changeover," which is a backward rotation that involves a minimum rest period followed by another duty period. This can provide a compressed work schedule with more time off but provides a reduced sleep opportunity prior to the last duty in the cycle. One study found that workers obtained an average of only 5.1 hr of sleep during the 8 hr off between quick changes (13).

Inherent in RTC Ops is the associated sleep and circadian disruption that makes the opportunities for recovery sleep very important. Therefore, time off is an important scheduling issue to "zero out" any accumulated sleep debt and potentially stabilize any circadian disruption. It is critical that these recovery opportunities are both predictable and protected. Individuals working RTC Ops can plan for recovery sleep if the opportunity can be anticipated. Therefore, protecting the recovery opportunity from interruptions, whether work- or home-related, is critical. The number of consecutive work periods in turn is critical. The number of consecutive work periods that make up a "cycle," whether the schedule is compressed or not, can affect the total accumulated sleep debt or the extent of circadian disruption. Predictability and stability of schedules also can affect the other physiological factors under discussion.

Predictability provides an individual with the opportunity to plan, whether for work, recovery requirements, or home activities. When possible, schedule stability provides more consistent circadian cues and the opportunity to create individual patterns and habits that minimize the physiological disruptions. Modern work demands, especially 24/7 requirements, are often associated with overtime, which may be elective or on occasions required. Extending work has the potential to increase the continuous hours awake, be affected by circadian factors by working through a window of circadian low, and contribute to both acute sleep loss and a cumulative sleep debt. The timing and amount of overtime and whether it is elective or required, can all affect the level of physiological disruption.

### C.  Real-World Work Challenges That Affect These Physiological Factors

Many circumstances that occur in real-world work settings can further affect physiological factors. Some examples of these demonstrate the layers of complexity that are present when addressing these issues in actual operations. In health care, for example, continuity of care is often the rationale for extended work periods, sleep loss, and circadian disruption. In long-haul aviation operations there is the possibility of acute sleep loss due to time zone disruption, followed by a long-duty day for an international flight requiring extended hours of continuous wakefulness, and then a landing, which is of course the critical phase of the operation coming at the end of the "working day."

Scheduling practices, within an industry or company, can be affected by many different parameters. These practices may be developed to meet operational needs but then altered owing to business issues, economic circumstances, and negotiations among parties. The scheduling practices can also be significantly affected by regulatory requirements that may exist. Again, these regulatory requirements are also subject to diverse agendas and pressures. In any industry, the main consideration that drives regulatory structures is usually safety. However, they can, like scheduling practices, also be affected by other considerations. In addition, inherent in any regulatory scheme is a governmental and political process that must be engaged.

Commuting to and from work can significantly extend the workday and curtail available sleep time. Work in many metropolitan areas can involve long commutes as individuals travel in from outlying areas (14). Consider that a 30-min or 1-hr one-way commute time increases the "work day" by 1–2 hr. Combine this commute with an early start time and sleep can be shortened even further. Add to this circumstance an individual who conducts other activities before the start of the workday. For example, an individual might awaken at 4 A.M., prepare for work, address other home requirements, and then be on the road for a 1-hour commute to start the job by 7 A.M. To embellish this portrait further, this individual would have to be asleep by 8 P.M. to obtain 8 hr of sleep and, when arriving home after an 8-hr day at work, would have been awake for 12 hr and driven home during the afternoon window of circadian low. If this individual worked more than an 8-hr day, for whatever reason, then you can extend these figures accordingly to fully understand the potential risks to alertness, safety, and performance. This sort of example is by no means extreme in our modern society.

In any work setting there is the opportunity for unforeseen circumstances to occur. Weather, mechanical failures, emergency situations, etc. can all produce conditions that can create physiological disruption. This might come from a call to report unexpectedly or early to work, extending hours on the job, a road traffic accident that extends the 1-hr commute to 2 hr, or any one of an almost infinite array of possibilities.

Cultural attitudes and history in an organization can have direct effects on these physiological factors. Often overlooked, or at least minimized, is the corporate culture that can play a critical role in how or indeed whether these physiological considerations are addressed. Many scheduling practices have their roots extending over very long periods of time. It is quite common to hear the rationale for justifying historical training practices as "I trained with the same methods, schedule, ethos, etc., and so it's good enough for the new trainees." This corporate culture and attitude can impede opportunities to effectively address the physiological issues in RTC Ops and may contribute to potential risks. However, this avenue also offers opportunity, both near-term and into the future, as corporate culture can be a powerful force for change.

## III.   The Costs: Sleep Loss, Sleepiness, and Safety

RTC Ops demands disrupt sleep and circadian physiology with a variety of consequences. In this section, examples demonstrate how these consequences translate specifically into sleep loss, increased sleepiness, and decreased safety across a variety of representative work settings.

### A.   Sleep Loss

One clear outcome of the operational factors discussed thus far is that individuals lose sleep and can build a cumulative sleep debt. Examples of sleep loss experienced in transportation, health care, and public safety demonstrate how these actual operational demands can result in physiological disruption.

### B.   Sleep Loss in Transportation Operations (See Also Chap. 15)

RTC Ops clearly describe the requirements of the global transportation system. In one large study of commercial truck drivers, individuals obtained varying amounts of total sleep that was related both to the amount of off-duty time (opportunity) and time of day (15). Between 10-hr day shifts of driving, the drivers obtained 5.4 hr of sleep in the 10.7-hr off-duty period that was available. After a 13-hr day shift of driving, the drivers averaged 5.1 hr of total sleep in an 8.9-hr off-duty period. On a 10-hr rotating shift schedule, drivers obtained a total of 4.8 hr of sleep in the 8.7-hr off-duty period, and after a 13-hr night shift of driving, they obtained an average of 3.8 hr of sleep in the 8.6-hr off-duty period. Overall in this study, total sleep time averaged from just 3.8 to 5.4 hr and was reduced with less off-duty time and when driving at night or on rotating shifts.

In a Federal Railroad Administration study of train crews, the engineers averaged 4.6 hr of sleep during a 9.3 off-duty period and 6.1 hr of sleep during a 12-hr off-duty period (16). In another study, 60% of railroad engineers reported obtaining an average of 6 hr of sleep or less on days worked, with another 30% reporting an average of only 7 hr. Therefore, just 10% of the engineers reported an average of greater than 7 hr sleep or more on their days worked (17) although other work has shown that break duration and sleep onset time are the most predictive variables that determine sleep quantity in railroad crews (18).

National Aeronautics and Space Administration (NASA) studies of commercial airline pilots have involved a variety of methodologies examining total sleep time and cumulative sleep debt during actual trip schedules (19). One study of short-haul pilots found that they averaged 6.7 hr of sleep during their 12.5-hr layover period on a trip schedule. In a study of long-haul flight operations, pilots averaged 5.3 hr of sleep in their primary sleep period, though this was supplemented by napping to provide a 6.5-hr sleep total per 24 hr. This compared to their pretrip average sleep totals of 7.1 hr for their primary sleep period and 7.3 hr total per 24 hr. Overnight cargo freight pilots were found to average 4.6 hr of sleep for their primary sleep period and 6.3 hr of total sleep per 24 hr compared to their pretrip total of 7.5 hr. A study of North Sea helicopter pilots found that they averaged 6.4 hr of total sleep during a trip compared to a pretrip amount of 7.3 hr. Across these different flight environments and schedules, overall, 85% of pilots accumulated a sleep debt during their trips that ranged from only a few hours on some short-haul schedules to the equivalent of several days on long-haul trips.

Several studies have examined the total sleep times obtained by air traffic controllers (ATC) in different settings. In one Federal Aviation Administration (FAA) study of shift schedules, results showed that controllers averaged about 8 hr of sleep prior to an afternoon or midday shift (20) and about 7.5 hr of sleep before a day shift. The study also showed that controllers obtained a total of about 6.3 hr of sleep before an early-morning shift, about 4 hr before a midnight shift, and 4.6 hr after working a midnight shift. In a study conducted by the FAA's Civil Aeromedical Institute (CAMI) that also looked at shift patterns, controllers were found to average 5.1 hr of sleep prior to an early-morning shift when on a clockwise rotation and 5.5 hr when on a counterclockwise rotation (21). Prior to an afternoon shift, the controllers averaged 7.5 hr on the clockwise rotation and 7.9 hr on the counterclockwise rotation. Finally, in a U.S. Air Force study of ATC, results showed that controllers obtained an average of 5.4 hr of sleep after a day shift, 7.6 hr after a swing shift, and 6.3 hr after a night shift (22).

### C. Sleep Loss in Health Care Settings (See Also Chap. 18)

In one study involving nurses, individuals were found to average 6.9 hr of total sleep during the 11.5-hr off-duty period when working 12.5-hr shifts (23). In Alertness Solutions' surveys, health care workers have reported an average of 6.5 hr of sleep on days worked compared to an average of 7.8 hr sleep on days off. The issue of intern and resident work hours has become a highly visible topic of discussion and action within medicine (24,25). Generally, the focus has been on the issue of extended work hours, where typical work weeks are longer than 80 hr, with 100–120-hr weeks not uncommon for trainees (26,27). On-call periods can often extend from 24 to 36 hr and be associated with little or no sleep. Reduced total sleep times can also occur across different call schedules. One study of surgical residents found that they averaged 5–6 hr of sleep whether on-call every other, every third, or every fourth night (28). A survey of OB/GYN residents found that 71% reported less than 3 hr of sleep while on night call (29). Interestingly, as these physicians progressed through residency the hours on call declined and hours of sleep increased. In another study of OB/GYN residents, about 89% reported obtaining less than 4 hr of sleep when on-call (29). In a survey of California anesthesiologists, respondents reported an average of 4.8 hr of sleep when on-call compared to 7.2 hr of sleep when not on-call (30).

A study of attending physicians in an emergency department found that they obtained an average of 5.5 hr of sleep during the day after a night shift compared to an average of 8.3 hr of sleep at night after a day shift (31). In a follow-up intervention study conducted in the same emergency department, the group averaged 5.7 hr of sleep across the different conditions. Again, they obtained less sleep (5.2 hr) after night shifts compared to that after a day shift (6.3 hr) (32).

### D. Sleep Loss in Public Safety Settings

The data on the sleep duration of individuals in public safety occupations such as law enforcement and firefighting are relatively limited. However, because of the round-the-clock nature of their work, the data that are available all show substantial sleep loss. For example, in one study, police officers reported an average of 6.2 hr of sleep when on 8-hr shifts and 6.5 hr of sleep when on 12-hr shifts (33). In a more recent study, it was found that 53% of the officers surveyed averaged 6.5 hr of sleep or less (34).

In a study of firefighters on a rotating 8-hr shift schedule, it was found that they averaged significantly less sleep on the night shift (midnight to 8 A.M.) compared to those working day (8 A.M.–4 P.M.) or evening (4 P.M.–12 A.M.) shifts. Data from the middle day of a 2-week shift schedule showed that firefighters averaged about 5.1 hr of sleep when on the night shift compared to about 7.1 hr on the day shift and about 7.4 hr when on the evening shift (35).

In summary, across all of these examples, any type of "nonday" or "nonstandard" work schedule can result in an average total sleep time that is significantly below comparative baselines and demonstrates both the acute and cumulative sleep debt that results from RTC Ops.

### E.  Sleep Loss Leads to Sleepiness on the Job

Perhaps the most distinct, and obvious, outcome of sleep loss is sleepiness (36). The most natural outcome of sleep loss experienced as a consequence of work demands is sleepiness on the job. A significant number of shift workers, 60–70%, will report difficulty with sleep or sleepiness on the job (37) together with occurrences of falling asleep. An FAA study found that 48% of ATCs reported that "they often fall asleep unintentionally" (20). In a NASA survey examining fatigue in flight operations, 80% of regional pilots and 71% of corporate/business aviation pilots reported having nodded off in the cockpit during flight (38,39). In a field study conducted during actual long-haul flight operations using physiological measures, NASA documented 154 microevents (i.e., alpha or theta EEG and slow eye movements) in the last 90 min of a 9-hr flight that included descent and landing (40).

A study of daytime, nonshift industrial plant workers found that 23% complained of excessive sleepiness (41). A survey of New Zealand forest workers reported that 78% had experienced fatigue at least sometimes on the job, with near-miss injury events significantly more common among this group (42). Sleep complaints are more common in two- or three-shift work settings and with irregular schedules compared to day work, with sleepiness complaints ranging from 20 to 37% depending on the schedule (43). An Alertness Solutions' survey of health care workers found that 66% reported having nodded off while at work.

Anecdotally, as many as 80% of police officers report falling asleep once a week at night when at a stoplight (44). In one survey, 26% of police officers reported dozing off during daytime activities, while 41% of the officers working graveyard shift reported this (45). In this same survey, overall, 54% of police officers reported driving drowsy, rising to 68% of the graveyard shift officers.

In a laboratory-based study of sleepiness using the Multiple Sleep Latency Test (MSLT), hospital residents were found to be near the "twilight zone" following postcall (mean time to sleep of 5.5 min) (46). Perhaps most provocative was that their baseline (not on-call) level of sleepiness was not significantly different at 6.5 min. This demonstrated both the level of chronic sleep deprivation experienced (as reflected in the baseline condition) and the physiological level of sleepiness that can be expressed postcall. When the residents had the opportunity to increase their total sleep time, the extra sleep was associated with a significant improvement in alertness to within a normal range (12.8 min).

### F. Safety Consequences

The performance reductions and sleepiness associated with sleep loss and circadian disruption can lead to incidents and accidents. These accidents have led to significant societal tragedies, such as the Exxon Valdez grounding, Three Mile Island nuclear accident, and Space Shuttle Challenger explosion. Safety risks have been found in every mode of transportation and most shift work settings have identified incidents and accidents due to fatigue and there are a variety of sources that describe the impact of fatigue, sleep loss, and circadian disruption (1,4,47–50). These resources provide extensive coverage of these issues, though a few examples are useful. In one study, 41% percent of medical trainees reported having made an error due to fatigue (30). In a survey study of New Zealand anesthetists, 86% reported having made fatigue-related errors (51). In a study of more than 500 daytime industrial plant workers, those with complaints of excessive sleepiness had in excess of a twofold higher risk of sustaining an occupational injury (41). Almost all of those with excessive sleepiness (96%) reported this propensity for the past 2 years and over half (56%) had experienced it over the past 10 years. In a prospective study of snoring and excessive sleepiness, over a 10-year period those with both snoring and excessive sleepiness at baseline were at an increased risk of occupational accidents with an adjusted odds ratio of 2.2 (52). In surveys of health care workers conducted by Alertness Solutions, 17% of respondents reported worsening of a patient's condition owing to fatigue and 27% reported injuring themselves on the job related to being tired.

An increasingly visible, yet still underacknowledged, personal safety issue relates to drowsy driving. Often-cited official statistics estimate that 100,000 crashes, 71,000 injuries, and 1550 fatalities annually are fatigue-related (53). However, in a consensus statement by a group of experts, it was estimated that fatigue may contribute to up to 20% of all transportation accidents (54). Based on this estimate, there could be 1.2 million crashes in the United States related to fatigue, sleep loss, and circadian disruption. National Sleep Foundation poll data found 51% of respondents report having driven drowsy in the past year and 17% reported that they have nodded off behind the wheel (5). Alertness Solutions' surveys in actual work settings (e.g., corporate fleets) have found 88% reported driving drowsy in the past year, over 20% nodded off, and 14% reported an actual near-miss or accident owing to fatigue. In its surveys of health care workers, Alertness Solutions found that 39% of respondents reported nodding off while driving to or from work and 39% also reported a near-miss or accident related to being tired. These data about driving while tired (DWT), especially those that are occupationally related, appear to be a clear extension of the sleepiness reported while on the job.

## IV.  The Solutions

### A.  Complexity Precludes a Magic Bullet

The data are extensive and clearly demonstrate that RTC Ops create sleep loss
and circadian disruption that lead to reduced alertness, performance, and safety.
However, organizations and individuals confront five significant challenges when
attempting to address these issues (Table 2). First, there is tremendous diversity
among operational requirements. Even within specific work settings, the individual job activities are often quite different. For example, in aviation, short-haul,
long-haul, overnight cargo, helicopter, and regional flight operations may all
involve flying but each uses different equipment and requires distinct work
demands. Second, there are individual differences among the human operators in
a variety of factors. Physiological differences exist, for example, in sleep need
and in other factors such as age, experience, and training. Third, the physiological processes involved in sleep and circadian rhythms are quite complex. There is
an extensive scientific literature on these physiological factors and yet, there are
also gaps in this knowledge base as they apply to operational settings. Fourth, as
previously mentioned, history is often a formidable challenge to change, and historical practices, policies, and attitudes create the foundation of a corporate culture that may be difficult or slow to evolve. Fifth, economics can be one of the
most significant challenges confronted and in RTC Ops settings, cost/benefit
analyses and "bottom-line" concerns (not necessarily real data) can delay or stop
progress before there is even exploration of possible change opportunities.

When effectively addressed, these five challenges can lead to opportunity
and change or they can represent barriers that slow or prevent progress on these
issues. Taken together, they demonstrate why there will not be a simple or single
solution to effectively manage sleep loss and fatigue in occupational settings.
Acknowledging these five challenges explains why a "one-size-fits-all" approach
cannot be expected to address the complexity represented by these issues.
Organizations and individuals would like the "solution" to be easy, straightforward, quick, and at no cost—unfortunately, there is no magic bullet.

Consideration of the complexity represented by these challenges provides
an understanding of three important aspects of the physiological disruption discussed. One issue, as mentioned, is that the complexity precludes a simple solution. Another is that this complexity explains why it is sometimes difficult to

**Table 2**  Challenges to Change

- Diverse operational requirements
- Individual differences
- Complex physiological processes
- History
- Economics

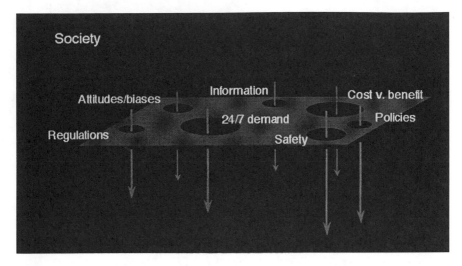

**Figure 1**   ARM model: risk factors associated with society.

quantify or identify sleep-loss and fatigue-related performance decrements, incidents, and accidents. Third, the complexity also means that a conceptual approach is required to effectively manage the sleep loss and fatigue issues in RTC Ops.

Figures 1–5 display a conceptual framework that can be used to consider the second and third issues raised above. The role of sleep loss, circadian disruption, and fatigue in reducing alertness, performance, and safety is often underes-

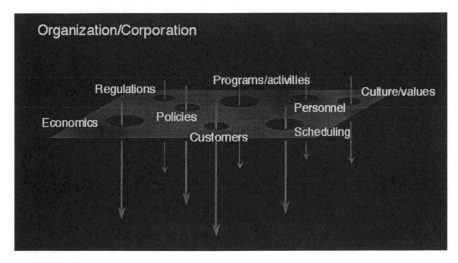

**Figure 2**   ARM model: risk factors associated with organizations or corporations.

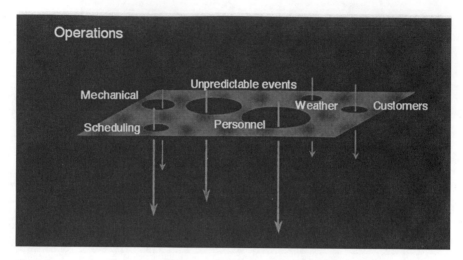

**Figure 3** ARM model: risk factors associated with operational demands.

timated, partly owing to the complexity described. Consider the following Alertness Risk Management (ARM) model, based on Reason (55), and extended to address sleep, circadian, and alertness issues.

Figures 1 through 4 portray some of the societal, organizational, operational, and individual issues associated with managing alertness. Each level identifies only some example issues and factors that can affect sleep loss, circadian

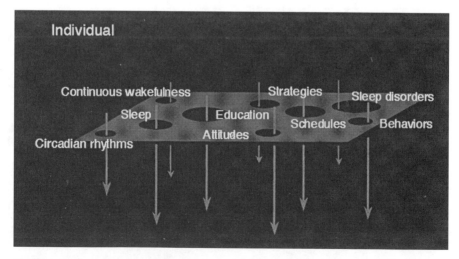

**Figure 4** ARM model: risk factors associated with the individual operator.

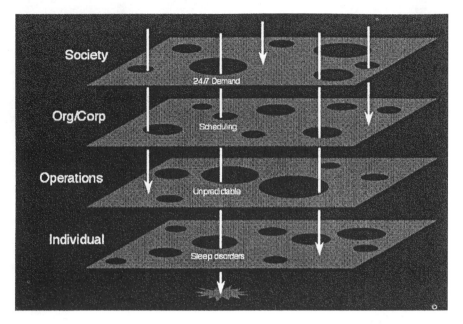

**Figure 5** ARM model: an accident or incident can occur when the risk factors "line up."

disruption, and their outcomes and demonstrates the complexity of these issues even at one level of the model.

Figure 5 illustrates the interaction of these different levels. Based on Reason's model, it explains that there are a number of significant and inherent risks in the system, and when the "holes line up," an incident or accident can occur.

### B. The Complexity Requires a Comprehensive Approach

This ARM model provides the conceptual basis for the use of a comprehensive approach to effectively address sleep loss and circadian disruption in RTC Ops. Given the complexity, five challenges described, and no magic-bullet solutions, a comprehensive Alertness Management Program (AMP) that acknowledges all of these provides the greatest opportunity for change (56–58). Such a program should involve at least the following five components: (a) education, (b) strategies, (c) scheduling, (d) healthy sleep, and (e) policies and scientific foundation. Each will be briefly described.

#### Education

Education creates the critical foundation for all other AMP activities. The educational component should include accurate, scientifically valid information on, at a minimum, the basics of sleep and circadian rhythms, and the risks associated with their disruption. A model Alertness Management educational module is available from the NASA Fatigue Countermeasures Group (http://human-factors.arc.nasa.gov/zteam/) and has been transferred to diverse operational settings through train-the-trainer workshops and modified to address specific flight environments such as regional and general aviation flight activities. A survey of NASA workshop participants found that the module was well received, useful, and led to some type of change in 58% of respondents' organizations (59). It is important that the educational component of an AMP be visible, be integrated into ongoing organizational activities, and be updated as appropriate.

### Strategies

A variety of alertness strategies or fatigue countermeasures can be used by individuals and organizations to improve alertness and performance in RTC Ops settings (57,60). This component of the AMP involves identifying alertness strategies suitable for the specific operational environment, educating individuals on their effective use, and providing appropriate organizational support where needed. Two examples of well-studied and effective strategies are planned naps and caffeine (40,61–63).

### Scheduling

Easily the most complex and contentious component of an AMP addresses scheduling practices. Scheduling issues epitomize the five challenges previously discussed and touch such diverse issues as quality-of-life concerns, economics for both the organization and individual operator, and contractual or regulatory requirements. At a minimum, this component can involve an analysis of vulnerabilities created by the current scheduling practices in an organization. This could start with an examination of the physiological factors previously identified and the work-related issues outlined in Table 1. Another level of activity could involve the development of scheduling alternatives that would address any of the identified vulnerabilities. Finally, actual implementation of proposed scheduling changes intended to improve current practices would provide the optimal benefit.

### Healthy Sleep

A variety of known sleep disorders have been documented to affect waking function. Sleep apnea is one example that can degrade waking alertness and performance and has been shown to increase risk for car accidents (64,65). Healthy sleep activities could range from informational materials to actual diagnostic screening of individuals in safety-sensitive positions.

### Policies and Scientific Foundation

Where appropriate, organizational policies should be established to provide explicit guidelines on relevant AMP issues. Such policies demonstrate clear support for AMP activities and create boundaries for all parties. This component of an AMP also emphasizes that all activities and information should be based on accurate and valid scientific information.

## V. Opportunity for Change

Humans were not physiologically designed to function 24/7 owing to our basic need for sleep and the intrinsic circadian pacemaker. It is therefore unlikely that sleep loss, circadian disruption, and fatigue can be eliminated from around-the-clock activities and it is clear that ignoring or underestimating the consequences related to sleep loss and circadian disruption in RTC Ops has resulted in significant, sometimes tragic, costs.

Scientific research and operational experience have clearly shown that there are effective approaches that can be used to reduce fatigue-related risks and improve alertness and performance. Using a comprehensive Alertness Management Program approach acknowledges the complexity of these issues, while offering specific actions that can improve the current situation. It is critical that actions be initiated now, wherever possible, at both the organizational and individual level, to address these identified risks. The immediate and near-term actions should be considered as only the initial steps in a long-term plan for change that will involve further individual, operational, organizational, and societal evolution. It is likely that RTC Ops will continue to increase to meet greater 24/7 global demands in the future, and therefore, these issues and risks will themselves continue to grow. Addressing the problem now, using a comprehensive Alertness Management Program approach, offers the opportunity to obtain benefits in current operating practices and creates a foundation for evolutionary change that integrates these advantages into the future.

## Acknowledgments

Our appreciation to Colette Staump, Elizabeth Co, and Reid Blank for important contributions to this manuscript and ongoing activities.

## References

1. Dinges DF. An overview of sleepiness and accidents. J Sleep Res 1995; 4:4–14.
2. Santy PA, Kapanka H, Davis JR, Stewart DF. Analysis of sleep on shuttle missions. Aviat Space Environ Med 1988; 59:1094–1097.
3. Kelly SM, Rosekind MR, Dinges DF, Miller DL, Gillen KA, Gregory KB, Aguilar RD, Smith RM. Flight controller alertness and performance during spaceflight shift-work operations. Hum Perf Extrem Environ 1998; 3:100–106.
4. Wake Up America: A National Sleep Alert. Executive Summary and Executive Report. Washington, DC: National Commission on Sleep Disorders Research, 1993.
5. Sleep in America Poll. Washington, DC: National Sleep Foundation, 2002.

6. Beers TM. Flexible schedules and shift work: replacing the "9-to-5" workday? Monthly Labor Rev 2000: 33–40.

7. Coleman RM. Shiftwork scheduling for the 1990's. Personnel (American Management Association), 1989.

8. Coffey LC, Skipper JK Jr, Jung FD. Nurses and shift work: effects on job performance and job-related stress. J Adv Nurs 1988; 13:245–254.

9. Rosekind MR, Gregory KB, Miller DL, Co EL, Lebacqz JV. Analysis of crew fatigue factors in AIA Guantanamo Bay aviation accident. In: Aircraft Accident Report: Uncontrollled Collision with Terrain, American International Airways flight 808, Douglas DC-8, N814CK, U.S. Naval Air Station, Guantanamo Bay, Cuba, August 18, 1993 (NTSB/AAR-94/04). Washington, DC: National Transportation Safety Board, 1994.

10. Akerstedt T. Work hours, sleepiness and the underlying mechanisms. J Sleep Res 1995; 4:15–22.

11. Thorpy MJ. Classification of sleep disorders. In: Kryger MH, Roth T, Dement WC, eds. Principles and Practice of Sleep Medicine. Philadelphia: Saunders, 2000:547–557.

12. Partinen M, Hublin C. Epidemiology of sleep disorders. In: Kryger MH, Roth T, Dement WC, eds. Principles and Practice of Sleep Medicine. Philadelphia: Saunders, 2000:558–579.

13. Totterdell P, Folkard S. The effects of changing from a weekly rotating to a rapidly rotating shift schedule. In: Costa G, ed. Shiftwork: Health, Sleep, and Performance. 1990.

14. Bowles S. Grab your coffee for an earlier morning rush. USA Today. McLean, VA: May 13, 1999:1A-2A.

15. Mitler MM, Miller JC, Lipsitz JJ, Walsh JK, Wylie CD. The sleep of long-haul truck drivers. N Engl J Med 1997; 337:755–761.

16. Thomas GR, Raslear TG, Kuehn GI. The Effects of Work Schedule on Train Handling Performance and Sleep of Locomotive Engineers: A Simulator Study. Washington, DC: Federal Railroad Administration., 1997.

17. Moore-Ede M, Mitchell RE, Heitmann A, Trutschel U, Aguirre A, Hajarnavis H. CANALERT '95—Alertness Assurance in the Canadian Railways. Appendices C, D, E, F. Cambridge, MA: Circadian Technologies, 1996.

18. Pilcher JJ, Coplen MK. Predictive models of sleep duration in irregular work/rest cycles [abstract]. Sleep 1999; 22(suppl 1):S140–S141.

19. Crew factors in flight operations: the Initial NASA-Ames Field Studies on Fatigue. Aviat Space Environ Med 1998; 69(9 suppl).

20. FAA Air Traffic Control Shiftwork Survey Results. Alexandria, VA: Human Resources Research Organization, 2001.

21. Cruz C, Detwiler C, Nesthus T, Boquet A. A Laboratory Comparison of Clockwise and Counter-clockwise Rapidly Rotating Shift Schedules, Part I. Sleep. Oklahoma City: Civil Aerospace Medical Institute, Federal Aviation Administration, 2002.

22. Luna TD, French J, Mitcha JL. A study of USAF air traffic controller shiftwork: sleep, fatigue, activity, and mood analyses. Aviat Space Environ Med 1997; 68:18–23.

23. Mills ME, Arnold B, Wood CM. Core-12: a controlled study of the impact of 12–hour scheduling. Nurs Res 1983; 32:356–361.

24. Gaba DM, Howard SK. Patient safety: fatigue among clinicians and the safety of patients. N Engl J Med 2002; 347:1249–1255.
25. Veasey S, Rosen R, Barzansky B, Rosen I, Owens J. Sleep loss and fatigue in residency training: a reappraisal. JAMA 2002; 288:1116–1124.
26. Daugherty SR, Baldwin DC Jr, Rowley BD. Learning, satisfaction, and mistreatment during medical internship: a national survey of working conditions. JAMA 1998; 279:1194–1199.
27. Schwartz RJ, Dubrow TJ, Rosso RF, Williams RA, Butler JA, Wilson SE. Guidelines for surgical residents' working hours: intent vs reality. Arch Surg 1992; 127:778–782; discussion 782–773.
28. Sawyer RG, Tribble CG, Newberg DS, Pruett TL, Minasi JS. Intern call schedules and their relationship to sleep, operating room participation, stress, and satisfaction. Surgery 1999; 126:337–342.
29. Defoe DM, Power ML, Holzman GB, Carpentieri A, Schulkin J. Long hours and little sleep: work schedules of residents in obstetrics and gynecology. Obstet Gynecol 2001; 97:1015–1018.
30. Gaba DM, Howard SK, Jump B. Production pressure in the work environment: California anesthesiologists' attitudes and experiences. Anesthesiology 1994; 81:488–500.
31. Smith-Coggins R, Rosekind MR, Hurd S, Buccino KR. Relationship of day versus night sleep to physician performance and mood. Ann Emerg Med 1994; 24:928–934.
32. Smith-Coggins R, Rosekind MR, Buccino KR, Dinges DF, Moser RP. Rotating shiftwork schedules: can we enhance physician adaptation to night shifts? Acad Emerg Med 1997; 4:951–961.
33. Peacock B, Glube R, Miller M, Clune P. Police officers' responses to 8 and 12 hour shift schedules. Ergonomics 1983; 26:479–493.
34. Vila B. Tired Cops: The Importance of Managing Police Fatigue. Washington, DC: Police Executive Research Forum, 2000
35. Paley MJ, Tepas DI. Fatigue and the shiftworker: firefighters working on a rotating shift schedule. Hum Factors 1994; 36:269–284.
36. Roehrs T, Carskadon MA, Dement WC, Roth T. Daytime sleepiness and alertness. In: Kryger MH, Roth T, Dement WC, eds. Principles and Practice of Sleep Medicine. Philadelphia: Saunders, 2000:43–52.
37. Akerstedt T, Torsvall L. Shift work: shift-dependent well-being and individual differences. Ergonomics 1981; 24:265–273.
38. Rosekind MR, Co EL, Gregory KB, Miller DL. Crew Factors in Flight Operations. XIII. A Survey of Fatigue Factors in Corporate/Executive Aviation Operations NASA Technical Memorandum #2000–209610. Moffett Field, CA: NASA Ames Research Center, 2000.
39. Co EL, Gregory KB, Johnson MJ, Rosekind MR. Crew Factors in Flight Operations. XI. A Survey of Fatigue Factors in Regional Airline Operations NASA Technical Memorandum #208799. Moffett Field, CA: NASA Ames Research Center, 1999.
40. Rosekind MR, Graeber RC, Dinges DF, Connell LJ, Rountree MS, Spinweber CL, Gillen KA. Crew Factors in Flight Operations. IX. Effects of Planned Cockpit Rest on Crew Performance and Alertness in Long-Haul Operations. NASA Technical Memorandum #108839. Moffett Field, CA: NASA, 1994.
41. Melamed S, Oksenberg A. Excessive daytime sleepiness and risk of occupational injuries in non-shift daytime workers. Sleep 2002; 25:315–322.

42. Lilley R, Feyer AM, Kirk P, Gander P. A survey of forest workers in New Zealand: do hours of work, rest, and recovery play a role in accidents and injury? J Safety Res 2002; 33:53–71.

43. Harma M, Tenkanen L, Sjoblom T, Alikoski T, Heinsalmi P. Combined effects of shift work and life-style on the prevalence of insomnia, sleep deprivation and day-time sleepiness. Scand J Work Environ Health 1998; 24:300–307.

44. Stanford Sleep Center, Why Should We Care About Sleep? pamphlet. Stanford, CA: Stanford Sleep Disorders Center, 1994.

45. Cochrane G. The effects of sleep deprivation. FBI Law Enforce Bull 2001; 70:22–25.

46. Howard SK, Gaba DM, Rosekind MR, Zarcone VP. The risks and implications of excessive daytime sleepiness in resident physicians. Acad Med 2002; 77:1019–1025.

47. Mitler MM, Carskadon MA, Czeisler CA, Dement WC, Dinges DF, Graeber RC. Catastrophes, sleep, and public policy: consensus report. Sleep 1988; 11:100–109.

48. Lauber JK, Kayten PJ. Sleepiness, circadian dysrhythmia, and fatigue in transportation system accidents. Sleep 1988; 11:503–512.

49. Mitler MM, Dement WC, Dinges DF. Sleep medicine, public policy, and public health. In: Kryger MH, Roth T, Dement WC, eds. Principles and Practice of Sleep Medicine. Philadelphia: Saunders, 2000:580–588.

50. Rosekind MR, Neri DF, Dinges DF. From Laboratory to Flightdeck: Promoting Operational Alertness, Fatigue and Duty Time Limitations—An International Review, London, UK, Sept 16, 1997. The Royal Aeronautical Society.

51. Gander PH, Merry A, Millar MM, Weller J. Hours of work and fatigue-related error: a survey of New Zealand anaesthetists. Anaesth Intens Care 2000; 28:178–183.

52. Lindberg E, Carter N, Gislason T, Janson C. Role of snoring and daytime sleepiness in occupational accidents. Am J Respir Crit Care Med 2001; 164:2031–2035.

53. Knipling R, Wang S. Revised Estimates of the U.S. Drowsy Driver Crash Problem Size Based on the General Estimates System Case Reviews, the 39th Annual Proceedings of the Association for the Advancement of Automotive Medicine, Chicago, IL, October 16–18, 1995.

54. Akerstedt T. Consensus statement: fatigue and accidents in transport operations. J Sleep Res 2000; 9:395.

55. Reason J. Human Error. New York: Cambridge University Press, 1990.

56. Rosekind MR, Gander PH, Gregory KB, Smith RM, Miller DL, Oyung R, Webbon LL, Johnson JM. Managing fatigue in operational settings. 2. An integrated approach. Behav Med 1996; 21:166–170.

57. Rosekind MR, Boyd JN, Gregory KB, Glotzbach SF, Blank RC. Alertness management in 24/7 settings: lessons from aviation. Occup Med 2002; 17:247–259.

58. Howard SK, Rosekind MR, Katz JD, Berry AJ. Fatigue in anesthesia: implications and strategies for patient and provider safety. Anesthesiology 2002; 97:1281–1294.

59. Rosekind MR, Neri DF, Gregory KB, Mallis MM, Bowman SL, Oyung RL. A NASA Education and Training Module on Alertness Management: A Survey of Implementation and Application [abstract]. Sleep 2001; 24 (suppl):A415.

60. Rosekind MR, Gander PH, Gregory KB, Smith RM, Miller DL, Oyung R, Webbon LL, Johnson JM. Managing fatigue in operational settings. 1. Physiological considerations and countermeasures. Behav Med 1996; 21:157–165.

61. Rosekind MR, Smith RM, Miller DL, Co EL, Gregory KB, Webbon LL, Gander PH, Lebacqz JV. Alertness management: strategic naps in operational settings. J Sleep Res 1995; 4:62–66.

62. Dinges DF, Broughton RJ. Sleep and Alertnes : Chronobiological, Behavioral, and Medical Aspects of Napping. New York: Raven Press, 1989.
63. Institute of Medicine (U.S.). Committee on Military Nutrition. Caffeine for the Sustainment of Mental Task Performance: Formulations for Military Operations. Washington, DC: National Academy Press, 2001.
64. Committee of the Assembly on Respiratory Neurobiology and Sleep ATS. Sleep apnea, sleepiness, and driving risk. Am J Respir Crit Care Med 1994; 150:1463–1473.
65. Findley LJ, Fabrizio M, Thommi G, Suratt PM. Severity of sleep apnea and automobile crashes. N Engl J Med 1989; 320:868–869.

# 13

## Impact on Self-reported Sleepiness, Performance, Effort, and Motivation

**JUNE J. PILCHER AND HEATHER N. ODLE-DUSSEAU**
Clemson University, Clemson, South Carolina, U.S.A.

## I.  Introduction

Sleep deprivation commonly occurs in a variety of situations in modern society. Shift work, especially night work, often results in chronic partial sleep deprivation. Furthermore, some segments of modern society, such as high-school and college students, voluntarily deprive themselves of sleep due to work, school, and social obligations (1,2). In addition, some segments of the population in such jobs as emergency services, medical care, and the military experience total sleep deprivation of 24 hr or more on a regular basis (3). In spite of the prevalence of partial and total sleep deprivation in our society, however, there remain many unanswered questions about the effects of sleep deprivation on human functioning.

Many studies have examined the effects of sleep deprivation on performance (e.g., Refs. 4–10). Narrative reviews of these and many other sleep deprivation studies have concluded that sleep deprivation negatively affects performance but that the extent of the decrement depends on the type of performance task, the length of the task, and the rate at which the task must be completed (11–14). Furthermore, two meta-analytic reviews examining the effect of sleep deprivation on performance resulted in similar conclusions (15,16).

Unfortunately, the effects of sleep deprivation on subjective experiences or verbal reports are much less well understood. The potential effect of sleep deprivation on subjective reports is an important consideration in the field. An individual's subjective assessment of the effects of sleep deprivation provides insight into that individual's knowledge of his or her limits under sleep deprivation conditions, which could, in turn, impact the individual's effort or decision-making capability. For example, shift workers who often live under partial sleep deprivation conditions, and at times total sleep deprivation conditions, must constantly assess their ability to function adequately to carry out their work. This self-assessment could in turn impact the decision-making process where the worker chooses to engage in relatively safe behavior or relatively unsafe behavior while on the job. In other words, if a worker accurately recognizes that his performance is decreased, the worker may logically reduce risk-taking behaviors on the job and thus decrease the likelihood of an accident. On the other hand, if a worker overestimates the effect of sleep deprivation on his performance, he may choose to operate slower or less efficiently in an effort to compensate when no compensation may actually be necessary.

Although a variety of self-report methods have been developed for and used in research in other areas such as memory, decision making, educational psychology, instruction, and clinical psychology (17,18), they have yet to be fully implemented in research on sleep deprivation. The purpose of this chapter is to examine the literature on verbal reports in sleep deprivation and to discuss future directions of research in the sleep deprivation field using verbal reports.

## II. Subjective Sleepiness

Perhaps the most common type of verbal report used in sleep deprivation studies is a measure of subjective sleepiness. Subjective sleepiness is generally assessed by self-report scales (see also Chap. 1), such as the Stanford Sleepiness Scale (19), the Epworth Sleepiness Scale (20), visual analog scales (21), and the vigor and fatigue subscales on the Profile of Mood States (POMS; Educational and Industrial Testing Service, San Diego, CA). These measures have been used in studies on the effects of sleep deprivation (22–25), shift work (26–28), and sleep disorders (29,30).

Assessing subjective sleepiness is an important issue in our 24/7 society. For instance, workers frequently have to rely on their internal assessment of sleepiness when making decisions about whether they are alert enough to work an extra shift or drive a little further before stopping. Often the subjective feeling of sleepiness may be one of the first cues that a worker has that he or she can no longer function on the job in a safe manner. Obviously this type of self-assessment can have profound safety implications in real-world settings.

A number of studies have investigated subjective sleepiness under sleep deprivation conditions. A study on the effects of partial sleep deprivation found that subjective sleepiness increased as the sleep deprivation period progressed across 5 consecutive days (31). Other studies have also found that sleepiness increased during different lengths of sleep deprivation and varied by time of day, with greater sleepiness reported at night (32). A similar time-of-day effect on subjective sleepiness has been shown in real-work conditions, such as in locomotive engineers, many of whom work under on-call work schedules (33).

Subjective sleepiness has also been studied as a potential predictor of task performance when sleep-deprived. Glenville and Broughton (34) reported that subjective sleepiness was significantly correlated with performance on tasks that produced deficits under sleep deprivation conditions. A follow-up study indicated that sleepiness was correlated more strongly with reaction time, the task that showed the greatest decrement under sleep deprivation (31). Based on these results, the authors concluded that subjective sleepiness may best predict performance for those tasks that result in considerably reduced performance efficiency. In contrast, another set of studies found that subjective ratings of sleepiness were only marginally related to performance (35,36). In an effort to contribute to this issue, Gillberg and colleagues (23) completed a study that examined the relationship between sleepiness and performance but specifically controlled for factors they felt could influence sleepiness, such as prior sleep duration and circadian phase. They found that subjective sleepiness was correlated with performance on a vigilance task.

The data summarized here indicate that, as would be expected, subjective sleepiness is related to the amount of sleep loss. The relationship of subjective sleepiness to performance under sleep deprivation conditions, however, is less well understood. This is especially true when considering that much of the recent research on examining subjective sleepiness and performance has been completed on vigilance-type tasks. Work-related tasks involve a much wider range of tasks, of which vigilance may be only one small part. Research investigating the relationships between subjective sleepiness and a variety of tasks ranging from simple reaction time to more complex cognitive tasks and decision-making tasks is still needed.

## III. Self-monitoring Performance

The relationship between subjective sleepiness and performance is only one method of examining potential relationships between how individuals perceive the effects of sleep deprivation on their ability to function. Another method is to examine how capable sleep-deprived individuals are of self-monitoring their level of performance. As with subjective sleepiness, the ability to accurately monitor performance under sleep-deprived conditions is an important issue for many workers in our society. Unfortunately, few studies have addressed this particular topic.

Historically, the literature examining self-monitoring of performance has led to two areas of research. One line of research has examined confidence in rating and judgment accuracy in response to performance on different types of tasks (e.g., Refs. 37,38). The second line of research has focused on the relationship between confidence assessment of performance and actual performance (39,40).

This second line of research is a type of calibration research (41), where participants complete a task multiple times, provide an assessment of how well they did, and provide a rating of how certain they feel of their judgment.

Although much of the research in the sleep deprivation field on self-monitoring performance has not specifically addressed the issue in regard to these two methodological approaches, the methods used can be classified into the two categories. Some studies have examined self-monitoring of performance on a task after a period of sleep deprivation while others have examined self-monitoring of performance on repeated tasks during the sleep deprivation period. However, the results from these studies were inconsistent. For example, one study asked doctors to answer a series of medically related questions after a night of on-call duty and after each question had them rate how certain they were that their answer was correct (42). This study concluded that although the doctors performed worse, they could accurately assess their performance. Similarly, another study indicated that sleep-deprived persons reported lower confidence in their incorrect responses to cognitive reasoning tasks (43). Dorrian and colleagues (44) asked sleep-deprived individuals to assess their performance on six different tasks that were repeated during the sleep deprivation period and found that self-ratings of performance were moderately to highly correlated with actual performance. In another study, college students were kept awake for one night and then asked to complete a complex linguistic task and assess their performance (45). This study concluded that the students performed worse, but overestimated their performance on the task. In contrast, two other studies examining self-monitoring of performance on tasks repeated during the night concluded that the individuals could accurately assess their performance ability (46,47).

One possible explanation for the different conclusions from these studies could be that some studies used a one-time performance assessment while others used a repeated performance assessment. However, this does not account for all differences since some studies used the same basic method, yet found different results. Another explanation could be the type of tasks used. Studies in the calibration research area have found that subjects have the tendency to overestimate their performance on difficult tasks but underestimate their performance on simple tasks, a phenomenon called the calibration difficulty effect (48,49). Although research in the sleep deprivation field has not specifically addressed the calibration difficulty effect, it is possible that it could apply to the reported results. For example, the tasks completed by the doctors (42) ranged in difficulty so that they could have been overestimating their performance on some tasks and underestimating their performance on others. The college students (45) completed a task that was cognitively challenging and, according to the calibration difficulty effect, should have overestimated their performance. Dorrian and colleagues (44) used several fairly simple vigilance and reaction time tasks and a more difficult grammatical reasoning task. Thus, it is possible that the type of task used was related to the strength of the correlation between self-rated performance and actual performance reported in their study.

Another aspect of self-monitoring performance while sleep-deprived is the ability to anticipate performance through prospective estimates in addition to correctly assessing performance through retrospective self-monitoring. Dorrian and colleagues (44) addressed this issue in their study and found moderate correlations between predicted performance scores and actual performance scores. However, they noted that the posttest self-ratings were better related to actual performance than the pretest ratings.

Unfortunately, few studies have examined the effect of sleep deprivation on self-monitoring of performance ability. Many questions still need to be addressed in this area. One potential research question involves whether the type of task is related to the ability to monitor performance. This could be particularly important when applying research results to a work setting in that many work settings require a wide range of tasks, some that may be quite easy and some that may require quick but complex judgment calls. Another potential research area is how and when performance is required. In other words, *is performance assessed during the sleep deprivation period to simulate a night shift or is performance assessed the next day to simulate performance during the day after sleep deprivation the previous night?* Finally, another area of research that has not been well investigated is the ability of a sleep-deprived individual to accurately predict his/her ability to perform a task, something that all workers must do on a regular basis while on the job.

## IV.  Subjective Effort

Another variable that can impact the effect of sleep deprivation on performance is the amount of effort that the individual devotes to completing the task. A number of researchers have speculated that sleep deprivation negatively affects performance largely through "resource limiting" (11,50) in that the sleep-deprived individuals may decrease their effort to perform as sleep deprivation progresses. Some researchers have supported the supposition that sleep deprivation can negatively affect the willingness of the subject to put forth the effort necessary to successfully complete a task (51). In contrast, other researchers have proposed that sleep-deprived individuals may actually realize that their performance is decremented and may increase their effort to compensate (44). Thus, the relationship between sleep deprivation and effort on task is another important component of understanding how sleep deprivation affects our ability to perform.

One means of examining the effect of sleep deprivation on effort is to ask sleep-deprived individuals to estimate how much effort they put into a task that they just completed. Although several sleep deprivation studies have used this approach, the results remains unclear. Some studies have reported decreased performance but increased effort on cognitive tasks (45), while other studies have seen an increased effort associated with no change in performance (52,53). Yet another study examining effort on cognitive tasks found no change in reported effort (54). Studies have also examined effort in relation to physical performance after sleep deprivation and have reported an increase in subjective effort (55,56).

Another means that researchers have used to examine effort is to allow individuals to choose between high-effort and low-effort tasks (57,58). Unfortunately, only a few studies have examined the effect of sleep deprivation on effort in this manner and compared the results to subjective effort. One study examining the effect of sleep deprivation on a chosen amount of exercise reported that exercise level was the same in sleep-deprived and non-sleep-deprived conditions but that self-reported effort in the sleep-deprived conditions was increased (59). In contrast, another study allowed individuals to match perceived effort when sleep-deprived with perceived effort after normal sleep conditions by increasing the incline on a treadmill and found that there was no change in the physical requirements chosen between the two conditions (60). A study by Legg and Haslam (61) reported similar results. They used an industrial repetitive lifting task to determine the chosen maximum lifting load under normal sleep and sleep deprivation conditions and concluded that there was no difference. In one study that allowed sleep-deprived individuals to choose complexity levels on a cognitive task (62), the participants chose less-demanding problems than individuals with no sleep loss but reported similar levels of subjective effort.

Although some research has been devoted to the relationship between performance and subjective effort in sleep-deprived individuals, many questions remain unanswered. More studies are needed that examine self-report effort on a variety of tasks to better understand how effort and sleep deprivation may interact in the typical work environment. In addition, more studies are needed that provide sleep-deprived individuals the chance to choose what tasks to complete, a situation that is common in many work settings. Results from studies such as these would allow for greater applicability from the basic research to the applied setting.

## V.  Subjective Motivation

An area of research in the sleep deprivation field that is closely tied in with effort to perform well is motivation. The more sleep-deprived individuals become, it seems intuitively obvious that they will be less fully committed to performing well on tasks, particularly demanding tasks (63). However, this disinclination to perform can be overcome, at least to some extent, through external sources of motivation.

One means of encouraging motivation is to provide information about performance while completing a task, what is known as knowledge of results. Wilkinson (64) was one of the first researchers to point out the positive effect of knowledge of results on performance. More recent studies have also supported the positive effect of knowledge of results on performance in sleep deprivation conditions (65,66). Offering other types of external sources of motivation has also proven to have a positive effect on performance under sleep deprivation conditions. For example, Horne and Pettitt (67) offered a significant monetary reward for correct responses and found that participants were capable of maintaining baseline performance levels for up to 36 hr of sleep deprivation.

Of interest for this chapter, however, is the ability of individuals to accurately assess their internal state of motivation during sleep deprivation conditions. Unfortunately, research in the sleep deprivation field has not yet addressed this issue. It would seem that questions assessing individuals' motivation to complete a task might be related to, yet different from, their subjective assessment of effort. Future studies could be designed to investigate the relationship between sleep deprivation and motivation to complete a task and the relationship of motivation to subjective effort.

## VI. Conclusions

Although the effects of sleep deprivation have been investigated quite thoroughly over the years, some aspects of sleep deprivation are not well understood. Some of the least-well-understood effects of sleep deprivation are the subjective aspects that have been summarized in this chapter. Although some research has been completed on topics such as subjective sleepiness, there remain quite a number of questions to be addressed especially in areas concerning performance when sleep-deprived. More research is needed on how subjective assessments of sleepiness are related to performance and on effort and motivation when sleep-deprived. Additional research is also needed to address the ability of sleep-deprived individuals to predict their performance before completing a task as well as estimate their performance after completing a task. Although these types of self-assessment questions can be difficult to answer because of the very nature of self-reported data, they are nonetheless worthy of well-thought-out and well designed research projects.

## References

1. Carskadon MA, Orav EJ, Dement WC. Evolution of sleep and daytime sleepiness in adolescents. In: Guilleminault C, Lugaresi E, eds. Sleep/Wake Disorders: Natural History, Epidemiology, and Long-term Evolutions. New York: Raven Press, 1983:201–216.
2. Pilcher JJ, Ott ES. The relationships between sleep and measures of health and well-being in college students: a repeated measures approach. Behavioral Medi 1998; 23:170–178.
3. Harrison Y, Horne JA. One night of sleep loss impairs innovative thinking and flexible decision making. Organizat Behav Hum Decis Process 1999; 78:128–145.
4. Buck L. Sleep loss effects on movement time. Ergonomics 1975; 18:415–425.

5.  Haslam DR. Sleep deprivation and naps. Behav Res Met Instrum Compu 1985; 17:46–54.
6.  Horne JA. Sleep loss and "divergent" thinking ability. Sleep 1988; 11:528–536.
7.  Jacques CHM, Lynch JC, Samkoff JS. The effects of sleep loss on cognitive performance of resident physicians. Fam Pract 1990; 30:223–229.
8.  Linde L, Bergstrom M. The effect of one night without sleep on problem-solving and immediate recall. Psychol Res 1992; 54:127–136.
9.  Symons JD, Bell DG, Pope J, VanHelder T, Myles WS. Electromechanical response times and muscle strength after sleep deprivation. Can J Sport Sci 1988; 13:225–230.
10. Webb WB. A further analysis of age and sleep deprivation effects. Psychophysiology 1985; 22:156–161.
11. Johnson LC. Sleep deprivation and performance. In: Webb WB, ed. Biological Rhythms, Sleep, and Performance. Chichester, U.K.: Wiley, 1982:111–141.
12. Krueger GP. Sustained work, fatigue, sleep loss and performance: A review of the issues. Work Stress 1989; 3:129–141.
13. Samkoff JS, Jacques CHM. a review of studies concerning effects of sleep deprivation and fatigue on residents' performance. Acad Med 1991; 66:687–693.
14. VanHelder T, Radomski MW. Sleep deprivation and the effect on exercise performance. Sports Med 1989; 7:235–247.
15. Koslowsky M, Babkoff H. Meta-analysis of the relationship between total sleep deprivation and performance. Chronobiol Int 1992; 9:132–136.
16. Pilcher JJ, Huffcutt AI. Effects of sleep deprivation on performance: a meta-analysis. Sleep 1996; 19:318–326.
17. Ericsson KA, Simon HA. Verbal reports as data. Psychol Rev 1980; 87:215–251.
18. Ericsson KA, Simon HA. Protocol Analysis: Verbal Reports as Data. Cambridge, MA: MIT Press, 1993.
19. Hoddes E, Zarcone V, Smythe H, Phillips R, Dement WC. Quantification of sleepiness: a new approach. Psychophysiology 1973; 10:431–436.
20. Johns MW. A new method for measuring daytime sleepiness: the Epworth Sleepiness Scale. Sleep 1991; 14:540–549.
21. Monk TH. A visual analogue scale technique to measure global vigor and affect. Psychiatry Res 1989; 27:89–99.
22. Dinges DF, Whitehouse WG, Orne EC, Orne MT. The benefits of a nap during prolonged work and wakefulness. Work Stress 1988; 2:139–153.
23. Gillberg M, Kecklund G, Akerstedt T. Relations between performance and subjective ratings of sleepiness during a night awake. Sleep 1994; 17:236–241.
24. Johnson S. How sleepy are practicing physicians? A field trial of the Epworth Sleepiness Scale. Sleep Res 1997; 26:671.
25. Reynolds CF, Kupfer DJ, Hoch CC, Stack JA, Houck PR, Berman SR. Sleep deprivation in healthy elderly men and women: effects on mood and on sleep during recovery. Sleep 1986; 9:492–501.
26. Bohle P, Tilley AJ. Predicting mood changes on night shift. Ergonomics 1993; 36:125–133.
27. Nicholson AN, Stone BM, Borland RG, Spencer MB. Adaptation to irregularity of rest and activity. Aviat Space Environ Med 1984; 55:102–112.
28. Paley M, Tepas DI. Fatigue and the shiftworker: firefighters working on a rotating shift schedule. Hum Factors 1994; 36:269–284.

29. Chervin RD, Aldrich MS, Pickett R, Guilleminault C. Comparison of the results of the Epworth Sleepiness Scale and the Multiple Sleep Latency Test. J Psychosom Res.1997; 42:145–155.

30. Lichstein KL, Wilson, NM, Noe SL, Aguillard RN, Bellur SN. Daytime sleepiness in insomnia: behavioral, biological, and subjective indices. Sleep 1994; 17:693–702.

31. Herscovitch J, Broughton R. Sensitivity of the Stanford Sleepiness Scale to the effects of cumulative partial sleep deprivation and recovery oversleeping. Sleep 1981; 4:83–92.

32. Mikulincer M, Babkoff H, Caspy T, Sing H. The effects of 72 hours of sleep loss on psychological variables. Br J Psychol 1989; 80:145–162.

33. Pilcher JJ, Teichman HM, Popkin SM, Hildebrand KR, Coplen MK. Effect of day length on sleep habits and subjective on-duty alertness in irregular work schedules. Transport Res Rec. In press.

34. Glenville M, Broughton R. Reliability of the Stanford Sleepiness Scale compared to short duration performance tests and the Wilkinson Auditory Vigilance task. In: Passouant P, Oswald I, eds. Pharmacology of the States of Alertness. Oxford: Pergamon, 1979:235–244.

35. Johnson LC, Spinweber CL, Gomez SA, Matteson LT. Daytime sleepiness, performance, mood, nocturnal sleep: the effect of benzodiazepine and caffeine on their relationship. Sleep 1990; 13:121–135.

36. Johnson LC, Freeman CR, Spinweber CL, Gomez SA. Subjective and objective measures of sleepiness: the effect of benzodiazepine and caffeine on their relationship. Psychophysiology 1991; 28:65–71.

37. Link SW. The Wave Theory of Difference and Similarity. Hillsdale, NJ: L. Erlbaum, 1992.

38. Petrusic WM. Semantic congruity effects and theories of the comparison process. J Exp Psychol Hum Perc Perf 1992; 18:962–986.

39. Gigerenzer G, Hoffrage U, Kleinbölting H. Probabilistic mental models: a Brunswikian theory of confidence. Psychol Rev 1991; 98:506–528.

40. Griffin D, Tversky A. The weighing of evidence and the determinants of confidence. Cog Psychol, 1992; 24:411–435.

41. Keren G. Calibration and probability judgments: conceptual and methodological issues. Acta Psychol 1991; 77:217–273.

42. Lewis KE, Blagrove M, Ebden P. Sleep deprivation and junior doctors' performance and confidence. Postgrad Med J 2002; 78:85–88.

43. Blagrove M, Akehurst L. Effects of sleep loss on confidence-accuracy relationships for reasoning and eyewitness memory. J Exp Psychol Appl, 2000; 6:59–73.

44. Dorrian J, Lamond N, Dawson D. The ability to self-monitor performance when fatigued. J Sleep Res 2000; 9:137–144.

45. Pilcher JJ, Walters AS. How sleep deprivation affects psychological variables related to college students' cognitive performance. J Am College Health 1997; 46:121–126.

46. Baranski JV, Pigeau RA. Self-monitoring cognitive performance during sleep deprivation: effects of modafinil, *d*-amphetamine and placebo. J Sleep Res 1997; 6:84–91.

47. Baranski JV, Pigeau RA, Angus RG. On the ability to self-monitor cognitive performance during sleep deprivation: A calibration study. J Sleep Res 1994; 3:36–44.

48. Lichtenstein S, Fischhoff B. Do those who know more also know more about how much they know? The calibration of probability judgments. Org Beh Hum Perf 1977; 20:159–183.

49.  Griffin D, Tversky A. The weighing of evidence and the determinants of confidence. Cog Psychol 1992; 24:411–435.
50.  Meddis, R. Cognitive dysfunction following loss of sleep. In: Burton E, ed. The Pathology and Psychology of Cognition. London: Methuen, 1982:225–252.
51.  Horne JA. Why We Sleep. New York: Oxford University Press, 1988.
52.  Chelette TL, Albery WB, Esken RL, Tripp LD. Female exposure to high g: performance of simulated flight after 24 hours of sleep deprivation. Aviat Space Environ Med 1998; 69:862–868.
53.  Hockey GRJ, Wastell DG, Sauer J. Effects of sleep deprivation and user interface on complex performance: a multilevel analysis of compensatory control. Hum Factors 1998; 40:233–253.
54.  Drummond SPA; Brown GG, Gillin JC, Stricker JL, Wong, EC, Buxton RB. Altered brain response to verbal learning following sleep deprivation. Nature 2000; 403:655–657.
55.  Martin B. Effects of sleep deprivation on tolerance of prolonged exercise. Eur J Appl Physiol 1981; 47:345–354.
56.  Rodgers CD, Paterson DH, Cunningham DA, Noble EG, Pettigrew FP, Myles WS, Taylor AW. Sleep deprivation: effects on work capacity, self-paced walking, contractile properties and perceived exertion. Sleep 1995; 18:30–38.
57.  Holding DH. Fatigue. In: Hockey GRJ, ed. Stress and Fatigue in Human Performance, Chichester: Wiley, 1983:145–168.
58.  Beck RC. Motivation. Englewood Cliffs, NJ: Prentice Hall, 1990.
59.  Soule R, Goldman R. Pacing of intermittent work during 31 hours. Med Sci Sports 1973; 5:128–131.
60.  Martin B, Haney R. Self-selected exercise intensity is unchanged by sleep loss. Eur J Appl Physiol 1982; 49:79–86.
61.  Legg SJ, Haslam DR. Effect of sleep deprivation on self-selected workload. Ergonomics 1984; 27:389–396.
62.  Engle-Friedman M, Riela S, Golan R, Ventuneac AM, Davis CM, Jefferson AD, Major D. The effect of sleep loss on next day effort. J Sleep Res 2003; 12:113–124.
63.  Mikulincer M, Babkoff H, Caspy T, Sing H. The effects of 72 hours of sleep loss on psychological variables. Br J Psych 1989; 80:145–162.
64.  Wilkinson R. Interaction of lack of sleep with knowledge of results, repeated testing and individual differences. J Exp Psychol 1961; 62:263–271.
65.  Steyvers FJJM. The influence of sleep deprivation and knowledge of results on perceptual encoding. Acta Psychol 1987, 66:173–187.
66.  Steyvers FJJM, Gaillard AWK. The effects of sleep deprivation and incentives on human performance. Psychol Res 1993; 55:64–70.
67.  Horne JA, Pettitt AN. High incentive on vigilance performance during 72 hours of total sleep deprivation. Acta Psychol 1985; 58:123–139.

# 14

## Driving Performance

**PIERRE PHILIP AND JACQUES TAILLARD**

Clinique du Sommeil Chu Bordeaux, Bordeaux, France

## I. Introduction

Traffic is rapidly increasing in all developed countries. In 1998, road traffic injuries were globally estimated to be then ninth leading cause of loss of healthy life and are projected to become the third leading cause by 2020 (1). This increase is associated with a major concern about safety from the traffic authorities. Several risk factors are now well identified (i.e., alcohol, speed) but sleepiness is still a concern in many countries.

If excessive somnolence at the wheel is thought to be an important cause of accidents in modern societies, the most important ways that sleepiness contributes to these accidents are still poorly understood. Sleepiness can be related to behavioral, pathological or pharmacological causes. This chapter will describe successive epidemiological studies that first highlighted the problem of sleepiness and driving. We will then consider the different methods developed by researchers to quantify driving impairment. The relationship between sleep schedules, organic sleep disorders, central nervous system drugs, and accidents will be reviewed. Finally, the impact of treatment in patients and the impact of countermeasures in healthy subjects on driving skills will be disclosed.

## II.  Epidemiology of Sleepiness Among the General Population and the Impact on Traffic Accidents

Chronic excessive daytime somnolence affects between 5 and 15% of the general population (2,3). Because of the potential risk of accidents related to excessive sleepiness or fatigue at the wheel, researchers have conducted studies to try to identify the prevalence of accidents due to one of these two factors. According to the populations studied or the methodology of the studies, the frequencies of sleep-related or fatigue-related accidents vary between 1 and 25%. This huge range highlights the difficulty of clearly identifying the causality of road accidents.

We will review several representative studies reflecting the prevalence of sleep-related accidents in Europe and United States. In the United States, Pack et al. (4) did a study utilizing the database at the Highway Safety Research Center at the University of North Carolina that is based on the uniform crash-reporting system in that state. Over the years 1990–1992, inclusive, there were 4333 crashes in which the driver was judged to be asleep but not intoxicated. The crashes were primarily of the drive-off-the-road type (78% of the total) and took place at higher speeds (62% in excess of 50 mph). The fatality rate was of similar magnitude to that of alcohol-related crashes with fatalities in 1.4% of such crashes (alcohol-related crashes had fatalities in 2.1%). The crashes primarily occurred at two times in a 24-hr period, during the nighttime period of increased sleepiness (midnight–7:00 A.M.) and during the midafternoon "siesta" time of increased sleepiness (3:00 P.M.). These crashes predominantly occurred in young people; 55% of these were individuals 25 years of age or younger, with a peak age of occurrence at age 20 years.

Horne and Reyner in England (5) considered single-car accidents where external factors (i.e., road, weather, or mechanical condition) could not explain the occurrence of accidents. They then asked the police forces to identify signs of reaction (brake or skid marks) from the drivers on the road and asked the drivers if they were sleepy at the wheel at the time of the accident. Sixteen percent of road accidents and 20% of highway accidents appeared to be related to sleepiness at the wheel. These accidents occurred more frequently at night and in the middle of the afternoon, and mainly affected young drivers.

In France, we performed a similar study (6) on a much larger database ($n$ = 67,671 single-car accidents). After eliminating possible confounding variables, we found that about 10% of these accidents were related to fatigue at the wheel. Here again, driving at night was a major risk factor for fatigue-related accidents. In Norway, Sagberg (7) also performed a study on traffic accidents. About 29,600 Norwegian accident-involved drivers received a questionnaire about the last accident reported to their insurance company. About 9200 drivers (31%) returned the questionnaire. Sleep or drowsiness was a contributing factor in 3.9% of all accidents, as reported by drivers who were at fault for the accident. This factor was strongly overrepresented in nighttime accidents (18.6%), running-off-the-road accidents (8.3%), accidents after driving more than 150 km on one trip (8.1%), and personal-injury accidents (7.3%).

Connor et al. (8) did an elegant controlled-group study in New Zealand to explore the relationship between sleepiness at the wheel and risk of traffic accidents. A total of 571 drivers involved in accidents where at least one occupant was admitted to the hospital or killed ("injury crash") and 588 car drivers recruited while driving on public roads (controls), representative of all time spent driving in the study region during the study period, were recruited for this study. The results showed that 19% of the total accidents could be explained by sleepiness at the wheel, driving at night, or suffering from sleep deprivation.

One could reasonably believe that complaining of chronic daytime somnolence is a major risk for traffic accidents. Surprisingly, studies on patients suffering from chronic daytime somnolence (9,10) failed to find a link between the risk of traffic accidents and sleepiness measured on a behavioral scale (i.e., Epworth Sleepiness Scale). This could be explained by the fact that subjective questionnaires do not correlate with objective measures of daytime vigilance (11). Another possible explanation could be that sleepiness is dangerous only when perceived during "at risk" activities.

Studies on apneic subjects (12,13) have shown that chronic subjective daytime somnolence is not responsible for traffic accidents but sleepiness at the wheel while driving is responsible for traffic accidents. These findings confirm the importance of behavioral somnolence and justify the responsibility of this symptom in the occurrence of an accident.

Few studies have explored the link between objective measures of somnolence and risk of accidents. Young et al. looked at the relationship between risk of traffic accidents and daytime somnolence as measured by the Multiple Sleep Latency Test (14). In this study, a positive correlation between daytime somnolence and traffic accidents was found only in men suffering from sleep-related breathing disorders. This result could be explained by the fact that men have a higher exposure to traffic accidents than women because of longer distance driven or increased risk taking. Another possibility is that objective measurement refers only to a short period of time (9 A.M.–5 P.M.) and that in real life, additive sleep deprivation can negatively influence the level of vigilance of apneic drivers. Unfortunately, the study of Young et al. did not investigate the sleep hygiene of the apneic drivers in the 24 hr before the accidents.

## III. How to Measure Driving Skills and the Impact of Sleepiness on Driving

Driving is a complex task that requires vigilance, attention, visual skills, and motor coordination. Accidents are also multicausal and involve behavioral and environmental factors (e.g., weather, mechanical, road conditions). Evaluating driving skills is therefore always difficult.

Driving simulators have been used in many conditions to test drivers. Simulation implies an absence of danger and frequently decreases external feedback. Most basic driving simulators in fact refer more to the measure of reaction time or divided attention. Findley et al. created a test called Steer Clear (15). This test is based on a computer program simulating a long and monotonous highway drive that presents 780 obstacles in 30 min. Hack et al. (16) used a simulated steering performance over 30-min "drives," which quantifies the standard deviation (SD) of road position, the deterioration in SD across the drive, the length of drive before "crashing," and the number of off-road events. The reaction times to peripheral target stimuli during the drive are also measured in this divided-attention task. We used a similar task to compare the performance of drivers involved in a nonprofessional long-distance journey and a control group. In this task, lateral deviations from the center of the road were a parameter that was significantly affected by the fatigue generated by the trip. Some sophisticated simulators reproduce 180° of display and road vibrations through suspended real vehicles, which increases the cognitive feedback to the drivers. Nevertheless the absence of risk probably still affects the motivation of drivers to perform.

Real driving conditions are supposed to give the most accurate information on driving ability. This methodology of testing was initially developed to test the effects of drugs on driving (17–20). The usual methodology refers to a driving test on a quiet freeway in a car equipped with a video to quantify the lateral deviations during driving. Instrumentation attached to the driving wheel record the response of the driver during the drive. Other more sophisticated experiments recorded the ability of the driver to maintain a safe distance between the driver's car and a leading vehicle (21). Real-driving experiments also suffer limitations. Even if a co-driver permanently monitors the safety of the drive, the most severe patients cannot be tested for safety reasons. The interference with the external traffic requires also the selection of driving segments where research assistants can safely monitor other cars.

## IV. Sleep-Wake Schedules, Driving Management, and Traffic Accidents

### A. Sleep-Wake Schedules and Driving Management

Until the mid '90s, no study demonstrated the main factors responsible for sleep-related accidents. We questioned, apart from organic sleep disorders, whether modifications of the sleep-wake schedules could be responsible for sleepiness at the wheel. Studying large populations of drivers (22,23), we demonstrated that long-distance driving was frequently associated with sleep curtailment. Our first study (22), performed on a freeway rest stop area in 1993, showed that 50% of drivers ($n = 567$ drivers) reduced their sleep duration in the 24 hr before departure for a long-distance journey. Ten percent of drivers had no sleep in the 24 hr before the interview. These stunning results could have been explained by a selected sample of exhausted drivers we recruited at a rest area. Therefore, we decided to run a larger study in partnership with the highway patrol to confirm our results. We randomly stopped 2196 automobile drivers at a freeway tollbooth. Fifty percent of the drivers decreased their total sleep time in the 24 hr before the interview compared with their regular self-reported sleep time; 12.5% presented a sleep debt > 180 min and 2.7% presented a sleep debt > 300 min. Figure 1 shows the relationship between sleep deprivation and duration of driving. Being young, commuting to work, driving long distances, starting the trip at night, being an "evening" person, being a long sleeper during the week, and sleeping-in on the weekend were risk factors significantly associated with sleep debt. After identifying the problem of sleep deprivation among drivers we performed electroencephalographic (EEG) recordings on these drivers to evaluate their level of sleepiness during the stops (24). Compared to a control group, our sleep-deprived drivers showed a very altered level of vigilance.

Sleep deprivation affects not only automobile drivers but also many truck drivers. In a study of professional U.S. truck drivers, Mitler et al. (25) recorded the EEG of 20 drivers on four different work schedules. This study demonstrated a mean duration of sleep of 4.78 hr in a 5-day period. Fifty-six percent of drivers presented at least 6 noncontinuous min of EEG-recorded sleep during the driving

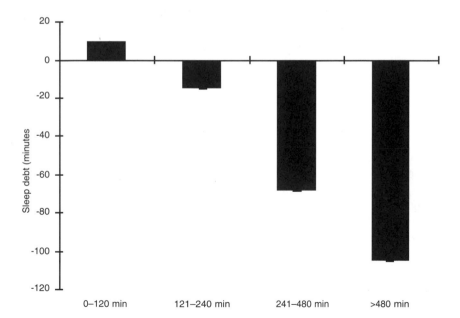

**Figure 1** Relationship between the sleep debt in the 24 hr before the interview and the duration of driving.

sessions. The vast majority of these microsleep episodes occurred during the late night and early morning.

We conducted a study on 227 professional European drivers interviewed at a rest area (26). The drivers were found to have a fairly consistent total nocturnal sleep time during their work week, but on the last night at home prior to the new work week there was an abrupt earlier wake-up time associated with a decrease in nocturnal sleep time. The results showed that 12.3% of the drivers had slept less than 6 hr in the 24 hr prior to the interview and 17.1% of the drivers had been awake more than 16 hr. These results confirm those of Mitler et al., and suggest that an improvement of driving regulations is required to increase professional drivers' safety.

### B.  Accidents

In 1995, a study by the National Transportation Safety Board on fatal accidents in professional trucks drivers (27) showed that the mean duration of sleep among drivers was below 6 hr of sleep in the last 24 hr before the accident. Connor et al. (8) showed that sleepiness at the wheel increased the risk of causing a traffic accident by 8.2-fold. Sleeping less than 5 hr in the 24 hr before the accident and driving between 2 and 5 A.M. were also significant risk factors for accidents [odds ratio (OR) = 2.7 and OR = 5.6, respectively].

### V.  Sleep Disorders and Traffic Accidents

Many studies looked at traffic accidents among patients suffering from sleep disorders. It is worth noting that these studies, for the vast majority, used cohorts of patients and had very little or no connections with police forces. It is therefore very hard to get information on the nature of the accident (sleep-related) or even the degree of responsibility of the driver.

In the late '80s, Findley et al. (28) published a study on a small population of apneic patients compared to controls (29 apneics vs. 35 controls). A higher risk of traffic accidents was found among patients suffering from sleep-related breathing disorders compared to the controls.

In the early '90s, Haraldsson et al. (29) published an elegant and well-designed study that showed that untreated apneics had a higher single-car accident rate than controls. A questionnaire was addressed to 140 patients with and 142 controls without symptoms associated with the obstructive sleep apnea syndrome (OSAS). Seventy-three of the patients had a complete triad of OSAS-associated symptoms. The ratio of drivers being involved in one or more combined-car accidents was similar for patients and control drivers, but for single-car accidents the ratio was about 7 times higher for patients with a complete triad of symptoms of OSAS compared to controls ($p < 0.001$). When corrected for mileage driven, the total number of single-car accidents was almost 12 times higher among patients with sleep spells while driving, compared to controls ($p <$

0.001). In Germany, Cassel et al. (30) at the same time showed that apneic patients diagnosed by clinical interview and polysomnography were frequently involved in sleep-related accidents (30).

In the United States in 1996, Wu and Yan-Go (31) also reported a higher accident rate in patients with OSAS. The best predictors for car accidents were falling asleep at the wheel and driving past destinations. This driving risk appeared so important that the American Thoracic Society published recommendations about driving safety among apneic subjects (32).

Stoohs et al. (33) performed an integrated analysis of recordings of sleep-related breathing disorders and self-reported automotive and company-recorded automotive accidents in 90 commercial long-haul truck drivers (see also Chap. 15). Truck drivers with sleep-disordered breathing had a twofold higher accident rate per mile than drivers without sleep-disordered breathing. Accident frequency was not dependent on the severity of the sleep-related breathing disorder.

Teran-Santos et al. (10) published a case-control study on the risk of car accidents among apneic subjects. The case patients were 102 drivers who received emergency treatment at hospitals, after highway traffic accidents. The controls were 152 patients randomly selected from primary-care centers and matched with case patients for age and sex. As compared to those without OSAS, patients with an apnea-hypopnea index (AHI) of 10 or higher had an odds ratio of 6.3 (95% confidence interval, 2.4–16.2) for having a traffic accident. This relation remained significant after adjustment for potential confounders, such as alcohol consumption, visual-refraction disorders, body mass index, years of driving, age, history with respect to traffic accidents, use of medications causing drowsiness, and sleep schedule.

George and Smiley (34) published complementary data on the relationship between the AHI and the risk of accidents. In this study on 460 apneic patients, only the most severe patients (AHI > 30) presented with an accident risk factor higher than controls.

All of these studies confirm the risk of traffic accidents for apneic patients. Sleepiness at the wheel is obviously a main symptom to investigate in conjunction with the severity of the disease (AHI > 30).

Subjective (e.g., Epworth Sleepiness Scale) and objective [e.g., Multiple Sleep Latency Test (MSLT)] daytime somnolence quantification does not seem to provide valuable information on patients' risks. This could be explained by the fact that sleep-related accidents occur at certain times when behavioral and chronobiological factors play an important role. Medical and legal issues could nevertheless require an objective test, such as the Maintenance of Wakefulness Test (MWT), to confirm that treated apneic patients present a normal level of vigilance.

Narcolepsy is a major pathology responsible for excessive daytime somnolence, and it has also been studied as a risk factor for traffic accidents. Aldrich (35) showed that narcoleptic patients presented a higher risk of sleep-related accidents than apneic subjects. Here again, the MSLT did not correlate with the rate of accidents among sleepy patients. However, the number of patients in the study with MSLTs was quite limited (46 apneics, 22 narcoleptics, 17 with other causes of excessive daytime somnolence), which could explain the lack of power of the study. It is worth noting that in all sleep pathologies, victims of accidents presented sleep latencies lower than controls. The results of Aldrich are in line with those of Young et al. (14), confirming that further studies on bigger samples, with the MWT as a measure of somnolence, and documentation of the cause of the accident would probably better help us to understand the relationship between daytime somnolence and accidents.

Although periodic limb movement disorder (PLMD) and restless legs syndrome (RLS) are frequent pathologies (36,37) that may induce daytime somnolence, almost no studies exist on the risk of accidents among these patients. Of 26 subjects suffering from PLMD or RLS, Aldrich (35) reported 4 subjects who were involved in traffic accidents, but it is very hard to conclude from these figures the risk attributed to these pathologies.

Obviously, sleep disorders are a major cause of traffic accidents because of their prevalence but also because of their danger (high-risk ratio of death and injury). If OSAS is a well-covered field, other diseases such as narcolepsy and hypersomnias are not as frequently investigated. This could be explained by the low prevalence and therefore the limited public-health impact of accidents generated by these patients. We strongly believe that research must be conducted in this field to provide better information on the driving aptitude of these patients.

Quite surprisingly, although PLMD and RLS are very frequent disorders that are known to induce daytime somnolence, no real study has been conducted on the accident risk of these patients. Here again, more information is necessary, especially regarding driving aptitude before and after treatment.

## VI.  Central Nervous System Drugs, Sedation, and Driving

Drugs affecting the central nervous system (CNS) have been incriminated in the occurrence of traffic accidents (see also Chaps. 20 and 27). In 1977, Garriott et al. (38) published a study investigating the incidence of alcohol and drugs in fatal accidents. Blood samples obtained at autopsy or at the time of hospital admission were analyzed for the presence of drugs and alcohol. The minor tranquilizer diazepam accounted for over half of all positive drug findings, while barbiturates, antihistamines, methaqualone, propoxyphene, and pentazocine were each detected in more than one instance. Similar results were published 2 years later by Skegg et al. (39), showing that drivers taking benzodiazepines had an odds ratio for severe road accidents of 4.9 compared to controls.

Hemmelgarn et al. (40) showed that in older subjects only the long-acting benzodiazepines represented a danger. Short-acting benzodiazepines presented no risk for traffic accidents. Leveille et al. (41) found that benzodiazepines and antihistamines moderately increased the risk of accidents in older drivers. Nevertheless, cyclic antidepressant and opioid analgesics significantly amplified the risk of accidents. In a survey on a large population ($n = 318,994$ subjects) Neutel confirmed the risk of taking benzodiazepines. Analysis showed an odds ratio (OR) of 3.9 (1.9–8.3) for persons taking benzodiazepine hypnotics and an OR of 2.5 (1.2–5.2) for those taking benzodiazepine anxiolytics, with regard to hospitalization due to traffic accidents within 4 weeks after the prescription was filled. Within 2 weeks after the prescription was filled, the ORs had risen to 6.5 (1.9–22.4) for hypnotics and 5.6 (1.7–18.4) for anxiolytics. After 1 week, the ORs were even higher (9.1 and 13.5), but the confidence limits were wide. The highest-risk groups were the youngest age group (20–39 years old) and men. This study highlighted the significant risk of sleep-inducing pills. Because of the design of the study the authors did not manage to get information on the time of the accidents and last intake of the hypnotic drugs.

Studies (42–44) showed that patients treated with antiparkinsonian drugs suffer from sleep attacks. These attacks were responsible for traffic accidents (45); modafinil can efficiently counterbalance this symptom in patients suffering from Parkinson's disease (46).

All of these studies show that potentially sleep-inducing drugs represent a major risk in terms of traffic accidents. Pharmaceutical characteristics (short-acting vs. long-acting), duration of prescription, and age seem to have a major influence on the risk of accidents. Since some evidence already supports physicians' carefulness when prescribing CNS drugs to drivers, further studies need to be performed to know the type of accidents (sleep-related or not, daytime or nighttime) associated with pharmaceutical class, and the impact of the time of drug ingestion on the risk of accidents.

## VII.   The Impact of Treatment of Sleep Disorders on Accident Risk

As described previously, sleep disorders can be related to an increase in traffic accidents. It seems reasonable to believe that the treatment of these disorders will decrease the risk of accident.

In 1992, Haraldsson et al. (47) showed that uvulopalatopharyngoplasty significantly decreased the rate of traffic accidents in snorers compared to controls. In France, Krieger et al. (48) showed on a cohort of 893 apneic patients that continuous positive airway pressure (CPAP) decreased the number of traffic accidents. This study on a large number of patients did not integrate the usual risk factors such as driving exposure, but opened the way toward posttreatment evaluation of the patients. George (49) demonstrated that 3 years of CPAP treatment removed the risk of motor vehicle accidents in apneic subjects compared to controls having a similar driving exposure.

Very little work, as yet, has been done regarding the effects of alerting substances on traffic accidents. Even though several studies have shown an increased risk of traffic accidents in narcoleptic patients, no study has proven the efficacy of drugs such as modafinil or methamphetamine in reducing the accident rate in narcoleptic patients.

## VIII. Conclusions

Sleepiness at the wheel, related to behavior or pathologies, is no longer a risk to be neglected by drivers and physicians. A vast majority of these accidents can be avoided by respecting the simple rules of sleep hygiene. Avoiding sleep deprivation before departure or driving in the middle of the night can decrease the rate of traffic accidents in the general population by 19% (8).

Many patients also have a high risk for traffic accidents and do not necessarily address this problem with their physicians. When exploring sleepy patients, the routine investigation should include questions about sleepiness at the wheel, the need to stop driving because of sleepiness, and whether the patient has been a victim of a sleep-related accident.

After treatment, physicians should evaluate the ability of patients to drive without suffering from sleepiness. If physicians question treatment efficacy, an objective evaluation of the ability to stay awake should be performed, especially for professional drivers who cannot escape the risk of falling asleep at the wheel.

## References

1. Ghaffar A, Hyder AA, Bishai D, Morrow RH. Interventions for control of road traffic injuries: review of effectiveness literature. J Pak Med Assoc 2002; 52:69–73.
2. Ohayon MM, Caulet M, Philip P, Guilleminault C, Priest RG. How sleep and mental disorders are related to complaints of daytime sleepiness. Arch Intern Med 1997; 157:2645–2652.
3. Philip P, Taillard J, Niedhammer I, Guilleminault C, Bioulac B. Is there a link between subjective daytime somnolence and sickness absenteeism? A study in a working population. J Sleep Res 2001; 10:111-115.
4. Pack AI, Pack AM, Rodgman E, Cucchiara A, Dinges DF, Schwab CW. Characteristics of crashes attributed to the driver having fallen asleep. Accid Anal Prev 1995; 27:769–775.
5. Horne JA, Reyner LA. Sleep related vehicle accidents. Br Med J 1995; 310:565–567.
6. Philip P, Vervialle F, Le Breton P, Taillard J, Horne JA. Fatigue, alcohol, and serious road crashes in France: factorial study of national data. Br Med J 2001; 322:829–830.
7. Sagberg F. Road accidents caused by drivers falling asleep. Accid Anal Prev 1999; 31:639–649.
8. Connor J, Norton R, Ameratunga S, et al. Driver sleepiness and risk of serious injury to car occupants: population based case control study. Br Med J 2002; 324:1125.
9. Barbe, Pericas J, Munoz A, Findley L, Anto JM, Agusti AG. Automobile accidents in patients with sleep apnea syndrome: an epidemiological and mechanistic study. Am J Respir Crit Care Med 1998; 158:18–22.

10. Teran-Santos J, Jimenez-Gomez A, Cordero-Guevara J. The association between sleep apnea and the risk of traffic accidents. Cooperative Group Burgos-Santander. N Engl J Med March 18, 1999; 340.

11. Chervin RD, Aldrich MS. The Epworth Sleepiness Scale may not reflect objective measures of sleepiness or sleep apnea. Neurology 1999; 52:125–131.

12. Masa JF, Rubio M, Findley LJ. Habitually sleepy drivers have a high frequency of automobile crashes associated with respiratory disorders during sleep. Am J Respir Crit Care Med 2000; 162:1407–1412.

13. Lloberes P, Levy G, Descals C, et al. Self-reported sleepiness while driving as a risk factor for traffic accidents in patients with obstructive sleep apnoea syndrome and in non-apnoeic snorers. Respir Med 2000; 94:971-976.

14. Young T, Blustein J, Finn L, Palta M. Sleep-disordered breathing and motor vehicle accidents in a population-based sample of employed adults. Sleep 1997; 20:608–613.

15. Findley L, Unverzagt M, Guchu R, Fabrizio M, Buckner J, Suratt P. Vigilance and automobile accidents in patients with sleep apnea or narcolepsy. Chest 1995; 108:619–624.

16. Hack MA, Choi SJ, Vijayapalan P, Davies RJ, Stradling JR. Comparison of the effects of sleep deprivation, alcohol and obstructive sleep apnoea (OSA) on simulated steering performance. Respir Med 2001; 95:594–601.

17. Brookhuis KA, Volkerts ER, O'Hanlon JF. Repeated dose effects of lormetazepam and flurazepam upon driving performance. Eur J Clin Pharmacol 1990; 39:83–87.

18. Brookhuis KA, de Waard D. The use of psychophysiology to assess driver status. Ergonomics 1993; 36:1099–110.

19. Brookhuis KA, de Vries G, de Waard D. The effects of mobile telephoning on driving performance. Accid Anal Prev 1991; 23:309–316.

20. Ramaekers JG, van Veggel LM, O'Hanlon JF. A cross-study comparison of the effects of moclobemide and brofaromine on actual driving performance and estimated sleep. Clin Neuropharmacol 1994; 17 (suppl 1):S9–18.

21. Brookhuis KA, De Vries G, De Waard D. Acute and subchronic effects of the H1-histamine receptor antagonist ebastine in 10, 20 and 30 mg dose, and triprolidine 10 mg on car driving performance. Br J Clin Pharmacol 1993; 36:67–70.

22. Philip P, Ghorayeb I, Stoohs R, et al. Determinants of sleepiness in automobile drivers. J Psychosom Res 1996; 41:279–288.

23. Philip P, Taillard J, Guilleminault C, Quera Salva MA, Bioulac B, Ohayon M. Long distance driving and self-induced sleep deprivation among automobile drivers. Sleep 1999; 22:475–480.

24. Philip P, Ghorayeb I, Leger D, et al. Objective measurement of sleepiness in summer vacation long-distance drivers. Electroencephalogr Clin Neurophysiol 1997; 102:383–389.

25. Mitler MM, Miller JC, Lipsitz JJ, Walsh JK, Wylie CD. The sleep of long-haul truck drivers. N Engl J Med 1997; 337:755–761.

26. P. Philip JT, D. Léger, K. Diefenbach, T. Akerstedt, B. Bioulac, C. Guilleminault. Work and rest sleep schedules of 227 European truck drivers. Sleep Med 2003 In press.

27. NTSB. Factors that affect fatigue in heavy truck accidents. Safety study NTSB/SS 95/01. Washington, DC.: National Transportation Safety Board, 1995.

28. Findley LJ, Unverzagt ME, Suratt PM. Automobile accidents involving patients with obstructive sleep apnea. Am Rev Respir Dis 1988; 138:337–340.

29. Haraldsson PO, Carenfelt C, Diderichsen F, Nygren A, Tingvall C. Clinical symptoms of sleep apnea syndrome and automobile accidents. ORL J Otorhinolaryngol Relat Spec 1990; 52:57–62.
30. Cassel W, Ploch T, Peter JH, von Wichert P. [Risk of accidents in patients with nocturnal respiration disorders]. Pneumologie 1991; 45 (suppl 1):271-275.
31. Wu H, Yan-Go F. Self-reported automobile accidents involving patients with obstructive sleep apnea. Neurology 1996; 46:1254–1257.
32. Sleep apnea, sleepiness, and driving risk. American Thoracic Society. Am J Respir Crit Care Med 1994; 150:1463–1473.
33. Stoohs RA, Bingham LA, Itoi A, Guilleminault C, Dement WC. Sleep and sleep-disordered breathing in commercial long-haul truck drivers. Chest 1995; 107:1275–1282.
34. George CF, Smiley A. Sleep apnea and automobile crashes. Sleep 1999; 22:790–795.
35. Aldrich MS. Automobile accidents in patients with sleep disorders. Sleep 1989; 12:487–494.
36. Ohayon MM, Roth T. Prevalence of restless legs syndrome and periodic limb movement disorder in the general population. J Psychosom Res 2002; 53:547–554.
37. Odin P, Mrowka M, Shing M. Restless legs syndrome. Eur J Neurol 2002; 9 Suppl 3:59–67.
38. Garriott JC, DiMaio VJ, Zumwalt RE, Petty CS. Incidence of drugs and alcohol in fatally injured motor vehicle drivers. J Forens Sci 1977; 22:383–389.
39. Skegg DC, Richards SM, Doll R. Minor tranquillisers and road accidents. Br Med J 1979; 1:917–919.
40. Hemmelgarn B, Suissa S, Huang A, Boivin JF, Pinard G. Benzodiazepine use and the risk of motor vehicle crash in the elderly. JAMA 1997; 278:27–31.
41. Leveille SG, Buchner DM, Koepsell TD, McCloskey LW, Wolf ME, Wagner EH. Psychoactive medications and injurious motor vehicle collisions involving older drivers. Epidemiology 1994; 5:591-598.
42. Frucht S, Rogers JD, Greene PE, Gordon MF, Fahn S. Falling asleep at the wheel: motor vehicle mishaps in persons taking pramipexole and ropinirole. Neurology 1999; 52:1908–1910.
43. Larsen JP, Tandberg E. Sleep disorders in patients with Parkinson's disease: epidemiology and management. CNS Drugs 2001; 15:267–275.
44. Miranda M, Diaz V, Venegas P, Villagra R. [Sleepiness attacks while driving: adverse effects of new antiparkinson drugs]. Rev Med Chil 2001; 129:585–586.
45. Ferreira JJ, Galitzky M, Montastruc JL, Rascol O. Sleep attacks and Parkinson's disease treatment. Lancet 2000; 355:1333–1334.
46. Montastruc JL, Rascol O. Modafinil and pramipexole-associated somnolence. Mov Disord 2001; 16:783–784.
47. Haraldsson PO, Carenfelt C, Tingvall C. Sleep apnea syndrome symptoms and automobile driving in a general population. J Clin Epidemiol 1992; 45:821-825.
48. Krieger J, Meslier N, Lebrun T, et al. Accidents in obstructive sleep apnea patients treated with nasal continuous positive airway pressure: a prospective study. The Working Group ANTADIR, Paris and CRESGE, Lille, France. Association Nationale de Traitement a Domicile des Insuffisants Respiratoires. Chest 1997; 112:1561-1566.
49. George CF. Reduction in motor vehicle collisions following treatment of sleep apnoea with nasal CPAP. Thorax 2001; 56:508–512.

# 15

## Commercial and Public Transportation Impact

**RICCARDO STOOHS**

Dortmund Sleep Disorders Center, Dortmund, Germany

## I. Introduction

Commercial and public transportation have become an integral part of Western societies ensuring that the flow of goods to consumers is uninterrupted. In Germany, for example, commercial trucking has drastically increased since 1993 when freight tariffs were deregulated. As a result, there has been a marked shift from rail transportation to trucking. A 60% increase in trucking transportation is expected by 2015 (1). Despite a reduction in overall weight of goods transported by trucking in 2001 in Germany, the ratio of distance per weight transported is steadily increasing (2).

Commercial and public transportation heavily relies on human operators. There is growing evidence that sleep loss may play a large role in transportation accidents. A committee formed at the 1986 meeting of the Association of Professional Sleep Societies found that numerous performance failures leading to catastrophic events occur most often at times of day coincident with the temporal patterns of brain processes associated with sleep (3). In addition, an investigation in the Netherlands showed that the highest accident rate in public transit accidents occurred in bus drivers who began an early work shift (4). An assessment of the impact of sleep loss in commercial and public transportation is therefore needed.

To better understand the impact of sleep loss in transportation, I will discuss the current evidence evaluating the relationship between safety and sleep loss in road, rail, air, and marine transportation.

## II. Factors Responsible for Accidents Attributed to Sleep Loss

Investigations have shown that sleep loss has a significant impact on vehicular accidents. The temporal distribution of single-vehicle accidents within the 24-hr cycle is important (5–8). Vehicle operators are most susceptible to fatigue-induced crashes in the early-morning hours. Recent data published by the Federal Motor Carrier Safety Administration show that 32% of all fatal large-truck accidents occurred at night with 16.4% between 12 A.M. and 6 A.M. and that 17% of all fatal large-truck crashes were single-vehicle accidents (9). Thus, it is not surprising that data from the largest over-the-road study involving commercial motor vehicle drivers in the United States concluded that the strongest factor influencing driver fatigue and alertness was the time of day. Video observation of the drivers' ($n = 80$) faces indicated that signs of drowsiness were markedly greater during nighttime driving. It was also shown that the drivers with less time asleep during their last sleep period were more likely to fall asleep during the middle of the night than the middle of the day (10). The importance of hours-of-work was demonstrated by Hamelin, who found that accident risk doubles when hours-of-work exceed the 11-hr limit (11).

## III. The Impact of Sleep Loss in Commercial and Public Transportation

### A. Surface Transportation

*Road Commercial Transportation*

In 1990, the National Transportation Safety Board (NTSB) completed a study of 182 fatal-to-the-driver truck accidents to investigate the probable cause of the accidents. While the study was designed under the assumption that most fatal heavy truck crashes may be related to alcohol and other drugs, it was found that the most frequently determined probable cause was fatigue (12). A 1993 analysis of the Fatal Accident Report System (FARS) also suggested that truck driver fatigue is a contributing factor in about 30% of heavy truck accidents.

The NTSB then initiated a study of 113 single-vehicle heavy-truck accidents in which the driver survived. Information about the 96-hr period prior to the crash was collected from 107 drivers. The analysis concluded that 58% of the accidents were fatigue-related. Eighteen percent of the drivers admitted having fallen asleep while driving (13). These data were not based on anecdotal driver reports but on a multivariate analysis of a predefined set of factors, including measures of the drivers' duty, sleep times, rest times, road conditions, and weather conditions. The most critical factors in predicting fatigue-related accidents were the duration of the sleep period prior to the accident, the amount of sleep in the past 24-hr cycle, and the presence of split sleep patterns, i.e., daily sleep period split in two or more sections. Drivers participating in this study had an average of 2.5 hr shorter sleep period prior to the accident than drivers involved in non-fatigue-related accidents (5.5 vs. 8.0 hr). Overall, they also had 2.4 hr less sleep in the 24-hr period prior to the accident than drivers with non-fatigue-related accidents (6.9 vs. 9.3 hr). Interestingly, the data also suggest that there may be a relationship between driver compensation and fatigue-related truck accidents. Truck drivers in the United States are paid by the mile driven; this payment system is illegal in Europe. The results of experimental studies point in the same direction. A laboratory investigation of commercial driver sleep schedules was conducted in 66 drivers by Balkin and colleagues (14). They were monitored under varying bed times: 3, 5, 7, or 9 hr. The results showed that even a short reduction in the amount of average sleep leads to a measurable drop in performance measured as reaction time. The group with the lowest time in bed for 7 nights did not fully recover even after 3 consecutive nights of recovery sleep (14).

### Road Public Transportation

It is logical that some or all contributing factors arising from driver fatigue in commercial trucking may also be applicable to the sector of public transportation. In 2001, the Federal Motor Carrier Safety Administration (FMSCA) reported a total of 331 fatalities involving buses in the United States. Although fewer data are available on the impact of sleep loss and driver fatigue in public transportation, several reports suggest that fatigue may also play a considerable role.

Several motor-coach accidents have prompted the NTSB in the past to conduct a thorough investigation into accidents where fatigue may have played a role. In 1997, the NTSB investigated the crash of a 47-passenger motor coach in Burnt Cabines, Pennsylvania, which traveled off the road and crashed into the back of a parked tractor–semi trailer killing the bus driver and six passengers. The accident occurred at 4:05 A.M. The investigators concluded that an irregular 4-day work-rest cycle with sleep during the daytime, aggravated by a known complaint of insomnia by the driver, were contributing factors to the accident (15). Two additional bus accidents prompted an investigation of motor-coach issues (16) involving driver fatigue as a significant contributor to the fatal accidents. It was concluded that inverted duty-sleep periods (1997 Rite-Way accident in Stony Creek) caused the bus driver to fall asleep and run off the road. Inverted duty-sleep schedules were defined as driving schedules calling for a period of rest on one day while scheduling a driving period during the same time on the following day.

### Railroad

In 1990, for the first time, human factors were identified as the most common cause of railroad accidents. The NTSB reviewed data from the Federal Railroad Administration (FRA) for the period 1990–1999 and concluded that in "only" 18 cases a causal or contributing factor to the incident was the operator falling asleep. However, this is thought to be an underestimate of the true contribution of fatigue to railroad accidents (17). A 1985 NTSB report concluded that railroad crews are subjected to the most unpredictable work/rest cycles in the transportation industry with a high level of duty start time variability (18). This is also true for work/rest cycles of railroad crews in Europe. A U.S. investigation found that more human factors contributed to railroad accidents between 2 A.M. and 6 A.M. than in any other 4-hr segment of the 24-hr cycle (19). A study of 198 locomotive engineers revealed that one third of them work in duty/rest cycles shorter than 24 hr. This is associated with a report of less overall sleep and reduced sleep quality (20).

As with other modes of transportation, numerous investigative reports have found that falling asleep while on duty has caused railroad accidents. These include the 1997 collision of two Union Pacific Railroad trains in Delia, Kansas on July 2, 1997 and the collision of two Union Pacific Railroad trains near Navasota, Texas on October 29, 1997 where the combination of sleepiness and alcohol intake may have contributed to the accident. A more recent accident killing two engineers of an oncoming train occurred in an area near Clarkston, Michigan on November 15, 2001. Both the engineer and train conductor of the train that caused the collision had previously diagnosed but untreated obstructive sleep apnea syndrome and fell asleep around 6 A.M. Their medical condition was not listed in their company's medical record. While the primary feature of obstructive sleep apnea syndrome on sleep structure is sleep fragmentation and not necessarily sleep loss, this incident highlights the fact that medical conditions leading to alteration of normal sleep can adversely influence performance.

### B. Aviation

### Air Traffic Controllers (ATCs) (See Also Chap. 12)

Fatigue in commercial and public air transportation can have catastrophic consequences as a result of ATC, pilot, and potentially aircraft maintenance engineer failure. For ATCs, the potential dangers from shift work should receive most of the attention because it can cause a significant sleep debt, reduced alertness, and poor performance. This problem is particularly important during night shifts (21,22) where ATCs have reported increased sleepiness compared to the day shift and at the beginning of early-morning shifts (23–25). Similar to sleep periods of pilots on duty (later in this chapter) studies have shown that unintentional sleep episodes can also occur in ATCs (26). This was demonstrated using actigraph recordings in nine U.S. Air Force ATCs indicating significantly more sleep on the night shift compared to day shift. This does not mean that there are no problems associated with the day shift. ATCs do not necessarily try to recuperate lost sleep by going to bed earlier after working on an early-morning shift. Data from a study released in 1996 showed that five consecutive daytime sleeps imbedded in shift work schedules result in a total loss of 10 hr of sleep. A comparison of day and evening sleep showed that more sleep was lost during evening sleep than during day sleep (27), possibly a result of the clock-dependent alerting function.

### Aircraft Maintenance Engineers (AMEs)

For AMEs the situation is even worse. In January 2002, Rhodes and Associates published an assessment of AMEs' hours-of-work for the Transportation Development Centre Transport of Canada. It concluded that AMEs are working an average of 50 hr/week, many extending 12-hr shifts, or working additional 12-hr shifts on days off (28). The study was based on questionnaires from 1209 AMEs and interviews of 12 AMEs. Study results showed that long working periods with very few days off for recovery are customary. AMEs from the airlines working extended night shifts (longer than 12 hr) indicated significantly more fatigue during these shifts. Twenty-five to thirty-eight percent of airline AMEs reported having nodded off at the wheel, and 9–12% had actually fallen asleep at the wheel. AME napping is forbidden at major airlines, although unplanned naps are not uncommon at airlines and general aviation facilities.

### Flight Crew (See Also Chap. 12)

The problem of sleep loss in flight crews, namely pilots, is twofold. Sleep loss can be induced both by individual hours of service and by jet lag—which can be compared to the impact of shift work. With respect to flight operations, sleep loss—often referred to as fatigue—can have catastrophic consequences. This fundamental problem may be as old as the history of flying itself. During his transatlantic flight, Charles Lindbergh used his thumbs to pry open eyelids heavy with sleepiness. He later reported "ghostly presences" of others in the cockpit. The occurrence of hallucinations in severe sleepiness is common and was reported by many long-haul truck drivers who participated in a field study conducted in Utah and published in 1994 (29). A recent investigation demonstrated that inverted duty-sleep periods are of specific concern to public transportation; this has been addressed in a study involving flight personnel (30).

Much of today's understanding of the contributing factors and consequences of fatigue in the field of aviation comes from research that has been conducted by the National Aeronautics and Space Administration (NASA) Ames Research Center over the past 20 years. Early field studies documented the existence of fatigue in flight operations. The results obtained from laboratory and field studies demonstrated that fatigue plays a major role in flight operations. This applies to short-haul operations where crew members have less sleep on trips, an increased difficulty falling asleep, and the subjective sensation of lighter and less restful sleep (31). Sleep loss and circadian rhythm disturbance from long-haul flights have been identified as major causes of fatigue in public and commercial flight operations. Although short-haul operations do not have to cope with the consequences of traveling across multiple time zones, they are characterized by long duty periods, multiple flight segments, and relatively long periods on the ground. Since it has been demonstrated that the most vulnerable flight phases are takeoff and landing (32), multiple flights during one duty period may pose an increased risk for reduced performance and increased fatigue (33). It has also been shown that overall sleep time is decreased on short-haul trip nights compared to pretrip nights. This phenomenon was partly due to the fact that short-haul operators had to report earlier for duty. This loss in overall sleep time may accumulate during the trip and lead to sleepiness and performance impairment on duty (34). Early trip onset also has recently been documented to have a detrimental effect on performance and wakefulness in automobile drivers (35). It is not surprising that crew members consumed 1.5 times more caffeine during the trip than on pretrip days. Consumption of this stimulant together with reduced sleep time, and difficulties falling asleep on pretrip days, may explain the increased amount of alcohol ingestion during trips, used as help to wind down. Together, sleep loss and late-afternoon alcohol intake will have additive effects on daytime sleepiness the following day (36).

Operational demands in long-haul operations across multiple time zones are different from those in short-haul operations. Duty cycles and layover periods are much longer. In addition, multiple time zones are crossed, desynchronizing the 24-hr rhythm to which the circadian clock is synchronized. Sleep episodes on trips and total sleep within 24 hr are shorter than under pretrip conditions (37). Sleep patterns in long-haul crews show a split pattern with more than one episode of sleep within the 24-hr rhythm. During an 8-day long-haul trip to London 33% of crew members accumulated a cumulative sleep debt of 16 hr (37). Although no safety-related incidents occurred during the observational studies, experimental studies have shown that a cumulative sleep debt this large is associated with reduced performance and shortened sleep onset times in Multiple Sleep Latency Tests (MSLTs) (34,38). Adverse effects on sleep and performance in long-haul flight crew crossing multiple time zones are more pronounced when the direction of the trip is eastward than westward (39). Age may also play a role. Long-haul crew members are often older than crew members in the other operations. They tend to be morning type, an observation consistent with the effect of aging on morningness/eveningness and the notion that morning types have more difficulty adapting to changes in circadian timing (40). Logbooks and observations in cockpits have shown that pilots are sometimes asleep in their cockpit seats (41). Objective evidence of cockpit sleep also comes from in-flight monitoring of electroencephalography (EEG) showing that microsleep (longer than 5 sec) can be a feature of fatigue in long-haul operations during landing (42).

As with other modes of transportation, evidence for fatigue-related accidents in aviation exists. In 1993, the NTSB concluded in its report regarding the loss of a Douglas DC-8 at Guantanamo Bay, Cuba that the impaired judgement, decision-making, and flying abilities of the captain and flight crew attributable to the effects of fatigue led to the accident (43). In an NTSB safety study of U.S. major carrier accidents involving flight crew from 1978 to 1990, it was concluded: "Half the captains for whom data were available had been awake for more than 12 hr prior to their accidents. Half the first officers had been awake for more than 11 hr. Crews comprising captains and first officers whose time since awake was above the median for their crew position, made more errors overall, and made significantly more procedural and tactical decision errors" (32).

### C. Marine

The nature of marine pilot work is characterized by irregular work schedules where the entire 24-hr cycle is part of the schedule (44). Thus, roughly 50% of a marine pilot's workload falls into the night period. Rest periods are often far from home so that they need to be spent in hotels. Duty/rest periods are very variable and largely depend on the nature of the specific operation, the region in which those operations are carried out, and the company's system of assigning pilots to the task.

In 1996, a report was issued determining that 16% of critical vessel casualties and 33% of personnel injury casualties in U.S. coastal waters during the second half of 1995 had some fatigue contribution (45). Investigations of marine accidents have revealed that a single factor rarely causes an accident. Instead, a chain of events or decisions that lead to the accident causes the accident (46). Based on the analysis of duty/rest cycles, sleep loss is an important contributor to fatigue in maritime personnel. A survey of health, stress, and fatigue of Australian seafarers determined that 31% of pilots had an average of less than 4 hr sleep per day, while 65% had between 4–6 hr of sleep per day. Subjective perception of sleep quality showed that more than 50% of pilots in that study rated their sleep as fair, poor, or very poor. This finding was in sharp contrast to more than 75% of pilots sleeping between 7 and 8 hr in off-duty periods, with sleep quality ratings between good and very good (47).

The grounding of the tank ship Exxon Valdez in March 1989 highlights the extent of the damage that can result from catastrophic events involving fatigue or a combination of fatigue and alcohol intoxication. In this accident, a combination of alcohol intoxication (master) and fatigue (third mate) (48) caused the ship to run aground on Bligh Reef of Prince William Sound spilling 11.2 million gallons of crude oil. While the loss of the tank ship and cargo was estimated at about $30 million, the cost for the cleanup and reimbursements amounted to over $2 billion.

## IV. Current Hours-of-Service Regulations

Each of the different transportation modes in the United States has regulations specifying maximum on-duty times and rest periods. Some of the regulations remain unchanged while others have been continuously updated. Regulations for motor-carrier operations were enacted in 1937 and virtually no changes have been made since. The Railroad Hours of Service Act from 1907 was revised in 1969, 1976, and again in 1988.

Aviation limits were addressed in the Civil Aeronautics Act of 1938 and the Federal Aviation Act of 1958. In 1985, domestic flight limitations and some commuter limitations were updated.

The work-hour regulations for marine operators are specified in Title 46 *United States Code* (U.S.C.) 8104 and date back to the early part of the twentieth century. In 1997, work-hour regulations from the *Standards for Training, Certification, and Watchkeeping* of the International Maritime Organization became effective, requiring a minimum 10-hr rest period during any 24-hr period. The work and rest provisions for American and European operators in the various modes are summarized in Tables 1 and 2, respectively. The regulations for aviation, highway, and some marine vessel types impose weekly work and rest limits. Only the aviation mode has monthly and annual limits as well. The maximum number of hours an employee of each mode is permitted to work in the course of a 30-day period is shown in Table 1. A commercial pilot may fly up to 100 hr/month; a truck driver may be on duty up to about 260 hr/month; licensed individuals on an ocean-going vessel or coastwise vessel of not more than 100 gross tons (GT) may operate up to 360 hr/month when at sea; and locomotive engineers may operate a train up to 432 hr/month.

**Table 1**   U.S. Hours of Service Regulations for the Different Transportation Modes (49)

---

**US—Motor Carrier (49 CFR Part 395)**
- Drivers may drive for 10 hr or be on duty for 15 hr.
- Drivers must have 8 consecutive hr off following a 10/15 hr on-duty period.
- If drivers use a sleeper berth, they may split the 8–hr period into two periods as long as neither period is less than 2 hr.
- Drivers may not exceed 70 hr in 8 days, if the carrier operates 7 days a week.
- Drivers may not exceed 60 hr in 7 days if the carrier does not operate every day of the week.

**US—Rail (49 U.S.C. 211; 49 CFR Part 228)**
- Maximum duty limit of 12 hr.
- Must be off-duty for 10 consecutive hr, after working 12 consecutive hr or off 8 consecutive hr if worked less than 12 consecutive hr.
- Time spent in transportation (deadheading) to duty assignment counts toward on-duty time.
- Time deadheading from duty assignment does not count toward on-duty or off-duty time.

*Continued*

**Table 1**   Continued

### US—Aviation (14 CFR Part 121; 14 CFR Part 135)

- Pilots flying domestic Part 121 operations may fly up to 30 hr/week, 100 hr/month, and 1,000 hr/year.
- Pilots flying domestic Part 135 operations may fly up to 34 hr/week, 120 hr/month, and 1,200 hr/year.
- If the scheduled flight time is less than 8 hr, the minimum rest period in the 24 hr preceding the scheduled completion of the flight segment is 9 hr. This time may be reduced to 8 hr if the following rest period, to begin no later than 24 hr after the commencement of the reduced rest period, is increased to 10 hr.
- If the scheduled flight time is 8–9 hr, the minimum rest period in the 24 hr preceding the scheduled completion of the flight segment is 10 hr. This time may be reduced to 8 hr if the following rest period, to begin no later than 24 hr after the commencement of the reduced rest period, is increased to 11 hr.
- If the scheduled flight time is equal to or greater than 9 hr, the minimum rest period in the 24 hr preceding the scheduled completion of the flight segment is 11 hr. This time may be reduced to 9 hr if the following rest period, to begin no later than 24 hr after the commencement of the reduced rest period, is increased to 12 hr.

### US—Marine (46 U.S.C. 8104; 46 CFR Parts 15.705, 15.710, and 15.1111)

- Hours-of-service or watch requirements vary depending on type of vessel.
- An officer must be off duty for at least 6 hr within the 12 hr immediately before leaving port before taking charge of the deck watch on a vessel when leaving port.
- On an oceangoing or coastwise vessel of not more than 100 gross tons (GT), a licensed individual may not work more than 9 of 24 hr when in port or more than 12 of 24 hr at sea, except in an emergency.
- On a towing vessel operating on the Great Lakes, harbors of the Great Lakes, and connecting or tributary waters between Gary, Indiana; Duluth, Minnesota; Niagara Falls, New York; and Ogdensburg, New York, a licensed individual or seaman in the deck or engine department may not work more than 8 hr in one day, except in an emergency.
- On a merchant vessel of more than 100 GT, the licensed individual shall be divided into three watches and shall be kept on duty successively to perform ordinary work incident to the operation and management of the vessel.
- On a towing vessel, an offshore supply vessel, or a barge that is engaged on a voyage of less than 600 miles, the licensed individual and crewmembers may be divided, when at sea, into two watches.
- On a fish-processing vessel, the licensed individuals and deck crew shall be divided into three watches. However, if the vessel entered into service before January 1, 1988, and is more than 1,600 GT, or entered into service after December 31, 1987, and has more than 16 individuals on board primarily employed in the preparation of fish or fish products, then the licensed individuals and deck crew shall be divided into two watches.

*Continued*

**Table 1** Continued

- On a tanker, a licensed individual or seaman may not work more than 15 hr in any 24–hr period or more than 36 hr in any 72–hr period, except in an emergency or a drill.
- On a fish tender vessel of not more than 500 GT engaged in the Aleutian trade, the licensed individuals and crew members shall be divided into at least three watches. However, if the vessel operated in that trade before September 8, 1990, or was purchased to be used in that trade before September 8, 1990, and entered into that trade before June 1, 1992, the licensed individuals and crew members may be divided into two watches.
- On a vessel used only to respond to a discharge of oil or a hazardous substance, the licensed individuals and crew members may be divided into two watches when the vessel is engaged in operation less than 112 hr.
- On a towing vessel operating in the Great Lakes, harbors, or connecting or tributary waters or a merchant marine vessel of more than 100 GT, a seaman may not work alternately in the deck and engine compartments, or be required to work in the engine department if engaged for deck department duty or required to work in the deck department if engaged for engine department duty. A seaman cannot be required to do unnecessary work on Sundays, New Year's Day, July 4, Labor Day, Thanksgiving Day, or Christmas Day, when the vessel is in safe harbor. When a vessel is in safe harbor, 8 hr is a day's work.
- Officers in charge of a navigational or engineering watch on board any vessel that operates beyond the boundary line shall receive a minimum of 10 hr rest in any 24–hr period. The hr of rest may be divided into no more than two periods, of which one must be at least 6 hr in length. The hr of rest do not need to be maintained in an emergency. The hr of rest may be reduced to 6 hr if no reduction extends beyond 2 days and not less than 70 hr of rest are provided in each 7–day period.

## V.  Conclusions

Twenty-four-hour operations in the field of public and commercial transportation will automatically place operators at risk for sleep loss. This sleep loss mainly stems from a disruption of circadian biological rhythms due to the nature of the service around the clock. While human operator failure cannot be avoided entirely, precautions must be taken to minimize the risk of accidents due to fatigue.

Numerous accidents that have occurred under the influence of operator fatigue have been documented by institutions such as the National Transportation Safety Board in the United States. Some of these accidents have been described earlier in this chapter. As a result of these incidences extensive research has been conducted to address the factors involved in human operator fatigue. Federal institutions in the United States and Canada primarily commissioned this research.

**Table 2** European hours of Service Regulations for the Different Transportation Modes (50)

**EU—Surface: Road and Rail VO (EWG) Nr. 3820/85**
- Time on driving duty between 2 rest periods may not be longer than 9 hr and can be extended to 10 hr no more than 2 times per week.
- After a maximum of 6 driving duty periods a rest period of 45 hr must follow.
- Total driving duty may not exceed 90 hr in 2 weeks.
- After a driving duty of 4.5 hr a break of at least 45 minutes has to be taken unless the driver starts a rest period.
- These breaks can be substituted by 15 min breaks if they are taken during the driving duty.
- During these breaks the driver may not engage in other than driving-work-related tasks.
- These breaks may not be applied to rest periods.
- Within a 24–hr period the driver has to take a rest period of 11 contiguous hr which can be reduced to no less than 9 hr for a maximum of 3 times per week.
- Rest time lost in reduced rest periods must be substituted by the end of the next week.
- Rest periods may be taken in a vehicle with sleeper berth if the vehicle is not in motion.
- To ensure the safety in commercial and public transportation paid compensation for drivers may not be based on mileage driven or on the amount of goods transported.

**EU—Marine 2000/34/EG**
- Generally maximum daily hr-of-work of 8 hr.
- The maximum number of daily hr-of-work may not exceed 14 hr within a 24–hr period and 72 hr in 1 week (7 days).
- Rest periods may not be shorter than 10 hr within one 24–hr cycle and 77 hr within 1 week (7 days).
- Rest periods may not be split into more than 2 periods.
- One rest period must have at least a duration of 6 hr. If 2 periods are chosen they must occur in a time frame of no longer than 14 hr.
- 24 hr of rest per week and rest during holidays.
- Paid vacation of at least 4 weeks/year.

**EU—Aviation Amendment of (EEC) No 3922/91**
- Pilots may fly up to 60 hr/week, 190 hr in any 28 consecutive days, and 900 cumulative block hr (time from takeoff to engine halt) per year.
- The maximum basic daily flying duty period is 13 hr.
- The maximum daily flying duty period can be extended by up to 1 hr.
- Extensions are not allowed for a basic flying duty period of 6 sectors or more.
- When a flight duty period with extension starts in the period 22:00–04:59 hr the operator will limit the flying duty period to 11.45 hr.
- The Window of Circadian Low (WOCL) is the period between 02:00 hr and 05:59 hr. Within a band of 3 time zones the WOCL refers to home base time. Beyond these 3 time zones the WOCL refers to home base time for the first 48 hr after departure from home base time zone, and to local time thereafter.
- The minimum rest that must be provided before undertaking a flight duty period starting at base shall be at least as long as the preceding flight duty period or 12 hr, whichever is the greater.

In Europe, little or no work has been officially commissioned to investigate underlying factors for human operator fatigue. Consequently, for many years new laws have been implemented in the United States and Canada to reduce the risk of fatigue-related catastrophes, while outdated regulations are still in effect in Europe. Therefore, it is not surprising that the latest implementation of hours-of-service regulations for European pilots, A5-0263/2002 (50), has been heavily opposed by the European Cockpit Association.

Based on extensive research in the field of performance and sleep loss, the only effective countermeasure to fatigue is sleep. Hours-of-service regulations have to take this fact into account and be tailored around it. Adequate rest periods with sleep are far more efficient to combat fatigue than tasks examining fitness for duty. About 25 years ago in his doctoral thesis J. H. Peter demonstrated that trained professionals could adapt to a paced secondary task enforcing wakefulness while being drowsy (51). The concept of sleep as a countermeasure against fatigue has been implemented in long-haul flights of U.S. pilots. Rosekind et al. demonstrated that napping during long-haul flights is a proven measure to reduce microsleep episodes during the most vulnerable in-flight task of landing (42).

In aviation much consideration has been given to the maximum duration of duty periods. In Europe the amendment A5-0263/2002, which has recently been passed by the European Parliament, determines a maximum duty period of 14 hr for pilots. Therefore, the European Cockpit Association has argued that this maximum allowable period together with the mandated rest times may constitute a recipe for cumulative sleep debt. This suspicion is supported by the work of Hamelin, who found that accident risk doubles when duty periods exceed 11 hr. Thus, this new EU regulation is weaker in its potential to prevent pilot fatigue than the old UK regulation.

Hours-of-service regulations differ for the various modes of transportations. While in the United States commercial truck drivers may be on driving duty for 10 hr (9 hr in Europe), commercial pilots may be on flying duty for up to 14 hr in Europe. This disparity does not make sense and therefore it can be concluded that hours-of-service regulations for the different modes of transportation are not based on the same principles of factors leading to fatigue. Overall duty period length may also be influenced by operator compensation. In any field, compensation should not be based on distance traveled. Public and commercial operators should not be tempted or rewarded for sleep loss. In Europe, this problem has been identified where compensation for distance traveled is illegal.

Furthermore, rest is poorly defined. As stated earlier, sleep is the only effective countermeasure to fatigue/sleepiness. Rest needs to be redefined explicitly as sleep although it may be difficult to enforce.

Accident data show a strong influence of time-of-day factors. Thus, hours-of-service regulations cannot be based only on the overall length of the duty period. Instead, they must include a careful consideration of the positioning of the duty period within the 24-hr cycle. In addition, inverted duty-sleep periods need to be avoided. If operators are to work during their usual period of sleep, enough lead time must be given to minimize the risk of sleep loss.

Finally, sleep disorders per se can have the same outcome on operator performance as sleep loss or alcohol intoxication. It does not make sense that commercial truck drivers must be screened for arterial hypertension but not for obstructive sleep apnea syndrome. The need for general screening of commercial and public operators for obstructive sleep apnea syndrome is highlighted by the fatal train accident in Clarkston, Michigan on November 15, 2001, in which the engineer's untreated and conductor's insufficiently treated sleep apnea were determined as the probable primary cause of the accident.

## References

1. Bundesministerium für Verkehr, Bau und Wohnungswesen. Daten und Fakten— Mobilität und Verkehr, 2002:6.
2. Bundesamt für Güterverkehr. Marktbeobachtung Güterverkehr. Jahresbericht 2001, 2002:4.
3. Mitler M et al. Catastrophes, sleep, and public policy: consensus report. Sleep 1988; 11:100–109.
4. Pokorny MLl, Blom DHJ, van Leeuwen P, van Nooten WN. Shift sequences, Duration of rest periods, and accident risk of bus drivers. Hum Factors 1987; 29:73–81.
5. Lavie P, Wollman M, Pollack I. Frequency of sleep related traffic accidents and hour of the day. Sleep Res, 1986; 15:275.
6. Lin T-D, Jovanis PP, Yang C-Z. Time of day models of motor carrier accident risk. Transport Res Rec 1467 1994: 1–8.
7. Pack AI, Pack AM, Rodgman E, Cucchiara A, Dinges DF, Schwab C.W. Characteristics of crashes attributed to the driver having fallen asleep. Accid Anal Prev 1995; 27: 769–775.
8. Philip P, Vervialle F, Le Breton P, Taillard J, Horne JA. Fatigue, alcohol and serious road crashes in France: factorial study of national data. Br Med J 2001; 322: 829–830.
9. Federal Motor Carrier Safety Administration. Large Truck Crash Facts. FMCSA-Ri-02-003, 2002: 34, 29.
10. Mitler MM, Miller JC, Lipsitz JJ, Walsh JK, Wylie CD. The sleep of long-haul truck drivers. N Engl J Med 1997; 337: 765–761.
11. Hamelin P. Lorry driver's time habits in work and their involvement in traffic accidents. Ergonomics 1987; 30:1323–1333.
12. National Transportation Safety Board. Fatigue, alcohol, other drugs, and medical factors in fatal-to-the-driver heavy truck crashes. Safety Study NTSB/SS-90/01 Washington, DC: NTSB, 1990.
13. National Transportation Safety Board. Factors that affect fatigue in heavy truck accidents. Vol 1: Analysis. Safety Study NTSB/SS-95/01. Washington, DC: NTSB, 1995.
14. Balkin T, Thorne D, Sing H, Thomas M, Redmond D, Wesensten N, Williams J, Hall S, Belenky G. Effects of sleep schedules on commercial motor vehicle driver performance. Department of Transportation Federal Motor Carrier Safety Administration, Washington. Technical Report DOT-MC-00-133. 2000.

15. National Transportation Safety Board. Greyhound run-off-the-road Accident, burnt cabins, Pennsylvania, June 20, 1998. Highway Accident Report NTSB/HAR-00/01. Washington, DC: NTSB, 2000.

16. National Transportation Safety Board. Selective motorcoach issues. Highway Special Investigation Report NTSB/SIR-99/01. Washington, DC. NTSB, 1999.

17. National Transportation Safety Board. Evaluation of U.S. Department of Transportation efforts in the 1990s to address operator fatigue. Safety Report NTSB/SR-99/01. Washington, DC: NTSB, 1999.

18. National Transportation Safety Board. Head on collision of Burlington Northern Railroad Freight Trains Extra 6714 West and Extra 7820 East Wiggins, Colorado, April 13. NTSB Report: RAR-85-041984. 1985. Washington, DC: NTSB,

19. U.S. General Accounting Office. Railroad safety: engineer work shift length and schedule variability. Report No: GAO/RCED-92–133, 1992.

20. Pilcher JJ, Coplen MK. Work/rest cycles in railroad operations: effects of shorter-than 24-hour shift work schedules and on-call schedules on sleep. Ergonomics 2000; 43:573–588.

21. Cruz C, Della Rocco P. Investigation of sleep patterns among air traffic control specialists as a function of time off between shifts in rapidly rotating work schedules. Proceedings of the Eighth International Symposium on Aviation Psychology, 2, 974–979, Ohio State University, Columbus, OH, April 24–27, 1995.

22. Rhodes W, Szlapetis I, Hahn K, Heslegrave R, Ujimoto KV. A study of the impact of shiftwork and overtime on air traffic controllers. Phase I. Determining appropriate research tools and issues. Final report TP 12257E, Transportation Development Centre, Transport Canada, 1994.

23. Luna TD. Air traffic controller shiftwork: What are the implications for aviation safety? A review. Aviat, Space Environ Med 1997; 68:69–79.

24. Luna T, French J, Mitcha J. A study of USAF air traffic controller shiftwork: sleep, fatigue, activity, and mood analyses. Aviat, Space Environ Med 1997; 68:18–23.

25. Costa G. Fatigue and biological rhythms. In Garland DJ, Wise JA, and Hopkin V, eds. Handbook of Aviation Human Factors. Mahwah, NJ: Lawrence Erlbaum Associates, 1999: 235–255.

26. Luna TD, French J, Mitcha JL, Neville KJ. Forward rapid rotation shiftwork in USAF air traffic controllers: sleep, activity, fatigue and mood analyses. Interim report AL/CF-TR-1994-0156, Armstrong Laboratory, Crews Systems Directorate, Brooks Air Force Base, TX 78235-5104.

27. Rhodes W, Heslegrave R, Ujimoto KV, et al. Impact of shiftwork and overtime on air traffic controllers. Phase II. Analysis of shift schedule effects on sleep, performance, physiology and social issues. Final report TP 12816E, Transportation Development Centre, Transport Canada, 1996.

28. Rhodes and Associates. Assessment of Aircraft Maintenance Engineers (AMEs) hours of work. Phase I. Final report TP 13875E, Transportation Development Centre, Transport Canada, 2002.

29. Stoohs RA, Guilleminault C, Itoi A, Dement WC. Traffic accidents in commercial long-haul truck drivers: the influence of sleep-disordered breathing and obesity. Sleep 1994; 17:619–623.

30. Lyman EG, Orlady HW. Fatigue and associated performance decrements in air transport operations, NASA Ames Research Centre, Battelle Columbus Laboratories, ASRS Office, 1981.

31. Gander PH, Gregory KB, Graeber RC, Connell LJ, Miller DL, Rosekind MR. Flight crew fatigue. II. Short-haul fixed-wing air transport operations. Aviat Space Environ Med 1998; 69(9,suppl.):B8–B15.

32. National Transportation Safety Board. A review of flightcrew-involved major accidents of U.S. air carriers, 1978 through 1990. NTSB Safety Study SS-94/01. Springfield, VA: National Technical Information Service, 1994.

33. Harris WC, Sachau D, Hanis SC, Allen R. The relationship between working conditions and commercial pilot fatigue development. Proceedings of the Human Factors and Ergonomics Society 2001:185–188.

34. Carskadon MA, Dement WC. Cumulative effects of sleep restriction on daytime sleepiness. Psychophysiology 1981; 18:107–13.

35. Philip P, Ghorayeb I, Stoohs R, Menny JC, Dabadie P, Bioulac B, Guilleminault C. Determinants of sleepiness in automobile drivers. J Psychosom Res 1996; 41(3):279–288.

36. Landolt HP, Roth C, Dijk DJ, Borbely AA. Late-afternoon ethanol intake affects nocturnal sleep and the sleep EEG in middle-aged men. J Clin Psychopharmacol 1996; 16:428–436.

37. Gander PH, Rosekind MR, Gregory KB. Flight crew fatigue. VI. A synthesis. Aviat Space Environ Med 1998; 69(9, suppl.):B49–B60.

38. Dinges DF, Pack F, Williams K, Gillen KA, Powell JW, Ott GE, Aptowicz C, Pack AI. Cumulative sleepiness, mood disturbance, and psychomotor vigilance performance decrements during a week of sleep restricted to 4–5 hours per night. Sleep 1997; 20:267.

39. Gander PH, Gregory KB, Miller DL, Graeber RC, Connell LJ, Rosekind MR. flight crew fatigue. V. Long-haul air transport operations. Aviat Space Environ Med 1998; 69(9, suppl.):B37–B48.

40. Gander PH, Nguyen D, Rosekind MR, Connel LJ. Age, circadian rhythms, and sleep loss in flight crews. Aviat Space Environ Med 1993; 64:189–195.

41. Graeber RC. Aircrew fatigue and circadian rhythmicity. In: Weiner EL, Nagel DC, eds. Human Factors in Aviation. New York: Academic Press, 1988: 305–344.

42. Rosekind MR, Graeber RC, Dinges DF, Connell LJ, Rountree MS, Spinweber CL, Gillen KA. crew factors in flight operations. IX. Effects of planned cockpit rest on crew performance and alertness in long haul operations (NASA Technical Memorandum 108839). Moffett Field, CA: NASA Ames Research Center, 1994.

43. National Transportation Safety Board. Uncontrolled collision with terrain American International Airways Flight 808, Douglas DC-8-61, N814CK U.S. Naval Air Station Guantanamo Bay, Cuba August 18, 1993. NTSB Report: AAR-94-04, 1994.

44. Shipley P, Cook TC. Human factors studies of the working hours of Uk ship's pilots. Part 2. A survey of work-scheduling problems and their social consequences. Appli Ergonom 1980; 11:151–159.

45. McCallum MC, Raby M, Rothblum AM. Procedures for investigating and reporting human factors and fatigue contributions to marine casualties, Report No. CG-D-09–97, National Technical Information Service, Springfield, VA, 1996.

46. Wagenaar WA, Groeneweg J. Accidents at sea: multiple causes and impossible consequences. Int. J. Man-Machine Stud 1987; 27:587–598.

47. Parker AW, Hubinger L, Green S, Sargent L, Boyd R. A survey of the health, stress and fatigue of australian seafarers. Australian Maritime Safety Authority, Canberra, 1997.

48.  National Transportation Safety Board. Grounding of U.S. tankship Exxon Valdez on Bligh Reef, Prince William Sound near Valdez, AK March 24, 1989. NTSB Report: MAR-90–04, 1990.

49.  National Transportation Safety Board. Evaluation of U.S. Department of Transportation Efforts in the 1990s to address operator fatigue safety report NTSB/SR-99/01, 1999.

50.  Simpson, B. Report on the amended proposal for a European Parliament and Council regulation amending Council Regulation (EEC) No 3922/91 on the harmonisation of technical requirements and administrative procedures in the field of civil aviation (COM(2002) 30–C5-0047/2002–2000/0069(COD)). Committee on Regional Policy, Transport and Tourism. European Parliament, 2002.

51.  Peter JH, Cassel W, Ehrig B, Faust M, Fuchs E, Langanke P, Meinzer K, Pfaff U. Occupational performance of a paced secondary task under conditions of sensory deprivation. II. The influence of professional training. Eur J Appl Physiol Occup Physiol 1990; 60:315–320.

# 16

## Military Operational Effectiveness

**GREGORY BELENKY, THOMAS J. BALKIN, AND
NANCY J. WESENSTEN**

**Walter Reed Army Institute of Research, Silver Spring, Maryland, U.S.A.**

### I.  Introduction

Success in combat operations depends on effective mental as well as physical performance at all levels of command and control. Effective performance depends on
speed of responding and attention to context. Take, for example, the crew of an
M-1 tank, and in particular consider the tank commander. An M-1 tank has a crew
of four, the commander, the gunner, the driver, and the loader. The tank commander's responsibilities in combat include (a) maneuvering his tank (through
verbal commands to his driver) in relation to and in support of other friendly combat elements (tanks, fighting vehicles, dismounted infantry) while taking tactical
advantage of the terrain for position and concealment; (b) locating (acquiring)
possible targets and identifying them as friend or foe; (c) passing a target identified as foe to the gunner and ensuring that the gunner sees the same thing he sees;
and (d) repeating the cycle. The gunner's responsibilities include receiving the
identified target from the commander, slewing the tank turret to point toward the
target, measuring the range to the target, setting the elevation of the tank gun, and
firing at the target. The driver drives. The loader loads rounds into the tank gun.

---

The views expressed herein are those of the authors and do not necessarily represent
those of the Department of the Army or Department of Defense.

As a practical matter, the tank crew's overall success depends on the speed and accuracy of the tank commander. As long as the commander sees the enemy tank or fighting vehicle before the enemy sees him, he and his crew can usually destroy the enemy. This is termed "staying inside the enemy's decision loop." If the enemy sees him first then the outcome is likely to be catastrophic for him and his crew. Speed is of the essence. Also, crucial is the accuracy of the friend/foe determination to prevent friendly-fire casualties. Identification of friend or foe is highly contextual and depends on what the Army calls "situational awareness." Situational awareness is highly complex and depends on an accurate understanding of the moment-to-moment dynamics of the fire and maneuver of the particular battle.

An excellent example in which this process went well comes from the Battle of the 73rd Easting during the 1990–91 Gulf War. In this battle, outnumbered elements of the Second Armored Cavalry Regiment (2ACR) destroyed an Iraqi brigade yet suffered no casualties themselves (1). The Institute for Defense Analysis (IDA) developed a computer-based simulation of the Battle of the 73rd Easting and conducted counterfactual analyses. In a series of iterations, IDA changed various parameters of interest in the simulation and refought the battle. In most instances the outcome was still victory; however, almost any change in battle parameters resulted in American casualties (and in some instances, high American casualties). These counterfactual analyses suggest that the elements of the 2ACR found a singularly casualty-free path through the time and space of the battle. They appear to have done this (and won their lopsided victory) by skillfully adapting their superior technology *on-the-fly* to exploit Iraqi errors. The Battle of the 73rd Easting provides a case history illustrating the importance of cognitive readiness (operationally defined as the skillful application of technology in real time to exploit opportunities as they emerge) to successful operational outcome and the adaptability and flexibility desirable in future Army units. It is an example of intelligence as efficient search and of a decentralized group adopting a common mental model of what constitutes a successful outcome and working in parallel to achieve this outcome. The ability to implement such *Auftragstaktik* (tasks tactics) depends on highly complex mental operations— cognitive integration at the highest levels. This integration is the purview of higher cortical areas, particularly the prefrontal cortex.

Sleep deprivation and sleep restriction impair cognitive performance (2,3), including general speed of responding and complex mental operations, particularly the ability to anticipate, plan, and maintain good situational awareness. Our functional brain-imaging studies, measuring regional brain glucose uptake by positron emission tomography (PET) and fluoro-deoxy-glucose (FDG), show that 24 hr of total sleep deprivation reduces brain activity by 6% with further, larger deactivations (12–14%) in the prefrontal cortex, the parietal association cortices, and the thalamus (4)—those brain areas responsible for complex, higher-order thinking and processing (anticipation, planning, attention, and situational awareness). Other, complementary, brain-imaging studies show that the same brain areas most impaired during prolonged waking are also deactivated to the greatest degree during sleep (5,6), suggesting that these regions have a greater need for sleep-mediated recuperation. These findings are consistent with the results of our debriefings of friendly fire incidents during the 1990-91 Gulf War (7). These debriefings indicated friendly-fire incidents resulted from the simultaneous *loss* of situational awareness (orientation to the battlefield and hence of the ability to distinguish friend from foe), a complex, presumably prefrontal, cognitive ability, and the *preservation* of the ability to put crosshairs on suspected targets and send rounds accurately downrange (a simple mental task with less prefrontal cortical involvement). Thus, sleep deprivation impairs cognitive performance by decreasing global and regional brain activation, and this impairment appears to map onto performance failures in operational settings. For well-equipped, well-trained, well-motivated soldiers in cohesive units with good morale, sleep becomes a salient factor in sustaining cognitive readiness.

Combat is a subset of a broad array of military and civilian operational settings. In its most abstract form, an operational setting is one in which the accurate and timely performance by the human being is critical to a successful outcome. In the operational setting, the "person-in-the-decision-loop" must make a correct (and usually reasonably complex) judgment within a set time limit or the system will fail. This definition clearly applies to a host of contexts both within the military and in the broader civilian community, e.g., aviation, ground transportation, power and communication grid management, and medicine. Sleep deprivation/restriction degrade operational performance.

## II. Sleep in Military Operations

Owing to the industrialization of warfare, the development and application of night vision, and information-based technologies, military operations are conducted around the clock, and the norm for military personnel, operationally deployed, is chronic, mild-to-moderate sleep restriction, termed continuous operations (defined as >4 hr and ≤7 hr sleep/24 hr), punctuated by episodes of more severe sleep restriction or acute total sleep deprivation, termed sustained operations (defined as ≤4 hr sleep/24 hr) [see U.S. Army Field Manuals FM 6-22.5 *Combat Stress* and FM 22-51 *Leader's Manual for Combat Stress Control*; both available on the World Wide Web—http://www.globalsecurity.org/military/library/policy/army/fm/ (accessed February 2003)]. The same developments leading to 24-hr operations also devolve greater and greater responsibilities to lower and lower levels (echelons) of command and control. There are few jobs in the current Army that do not involve a significant cognitive component. The problem of sustaining operational performance is the problem of sustaining cognitive function in personnel in continuous and sustained operations.

Subsets of the military operational community differ in their relative doctrinal emphasis on continuous versus sustained operations. The special operations units in all three services (U.S. Army, U.S. Navy, and U.S. Air Force) and the U.S. Air Force long-range bomber community focus on the problems of sustained operations. The Marine Corps and the conventional U.S. Army units focus on the problems of continuous operations. In all three services, the reality, whatever the relative doctrinal emphasis, is continuous operations punctuated by periods of sustained operations—chronic mild-to-moderate sleep restriction with superimposed periods of total sleep deprivation or severe sleep restriction. This reality is combined with the need to sustain optimal cognitive performance at all levels of command and control.

Until recently, it has been assumed that the performance effects of chronic sleep restriction were a milder version of the effects of acute, total sleep deprivation and that recovery from both was rapid once normal amounts of sleep were restored. Results from a study recently completed in our laboratory suggest that this may not be the case.

In a sleep dose-response study (3,8) we examined the effects of three conditions of sleep restriction [3, 5, or 7 hr time in bed (TIB)] and one condition of sleep augmentation (9 hr TIB) on performance over 7 days and during the subsequent 3 days of recovery (all groups = 8 hr TIB). These sleep dose-response effects were compared against the training/baseline period in which all groups were allowed 8 hr TIB.

In this study, there was a clear sleep-dose-dependent response during the sleep restriction period. For moderate sleep restriction (7-hr TIB and 5-hr TIB groups), performance (as measured by speed on the psychomotor vigilance task [PVT]) degraded over the first few days of the restriction period and then appeared to stabilize. For severe sleep restriction (3-hr TIB group), performance continued to degrade across the entire period of sleep restriction. Together, these patterns of (a) continuously declining performance during the experimental phase in the 3-hr TIB group and (b) a leveling-off of performance in the 5- and 7-hr TIB groups at dose-dependently reduced levels suggest that there exists a critical threshold sleep duration, somewhere around 4 hr of total sleep time—below this threshold, a homeostatic equilibrium between the alertness/performance-decrementing effects of extended wakefulness and the alertness/performance-restoring effects of the subsequent (shortened) sleep period cannot be established. The stabilization of performance with moderate sleep restriction contrasts with the continued, linear decline in performance seen in severe sleep restriction and acute, total sleep deprivation (Fig. 1).

In the recovery period, the 3-hr TIB group showed an improvement in performance after the first night of recovery (8 hr TIB) sleep, reaching the level of the 5- and 7-hr TIB groups. The 5- and 7-hr groups showed no improvement in performance over the 3 days of recovery, remaining at the level of stable but lower performance they had reached toward the end of the sleep restriction period. This stabilization of performance (in the 5- and 7-hr TIB group) during the sleep restriction period and the failure to return to baseline in all sleep-restricted groups (3-, 5-, and 7-hr TIB groups) suggest that the brain attempts to adjust to sleep

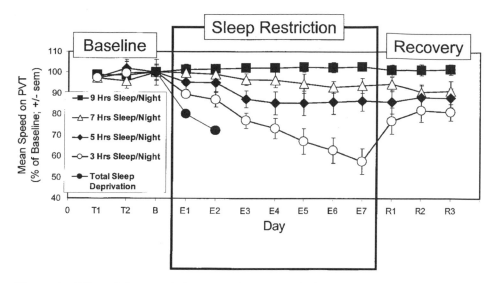

**Figure 1** Effect of sleep restriction on performance and subsequent recovery. (Adapted from Belenky et al. 2003.)

restriction by capping brain operational capacity and that this adaptation takes time (days) to undo, delaying recovery (Fig. 1). This is in contrast to the linear decline and rapid recovery seen in acute, total sleep deprivation and suggests that acute, total sleep deprivation and chronic sleep restriction have different behavioral consequences both during the actual deprivation/restriction period and once normal amounts of sleep are restored.

These data suggest that it is possible, over the longer term, to adjust to moderate levels of sleep restriction to achieve stable, albeit lower, levels of performance. These results, combined with the findings that many Americans sleep less than the recommended 8 hr/night, suggest that it is common to trade off daytime performance for extra time awake. In strictly economic terms, a lower rate of production sustained over a longer period of time may lead to greater aggregate production.

The pattern of adaptation to chronic sleep restriction punctuated with acute, total sleep deprivation and rapid recovery from the latter may yield the types of changes in performance depicted in Fig. 2. Across the three armed services, in combat operations and in training for combat operations, severe total sleep deprivation is rare. Much more common for all is chronic, moderate sleep restriction at levels that would be expected to produce stable, albeit degraded performance.

Results from our unpublished field studies (in which wrist-worn actigraphs were used to record sleep/wake history) conducted at the National Training Center (NTC), the U.S. Army's desert warfare training center in the high desert of Southern California, indicate that the higher the rank and the higher the echelon of command and control, the less the sleep obtained over the 14 days of the

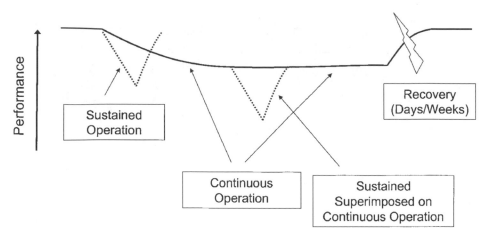

**Figure 2**   Continuous and sustained operations.

typical NTC rotation (Fig. 3). At brigade and battalion levels of command and control and at the rank of Colonel (COL)/Lieutenant Colonel (LTC), the degree of sleep restriction is sufficient to impair cognitive performance over the first few days of the exercise with subsequent stabilization in performance at a lower-than-baseline level. Again, it would be expected that once normal amounts of sleep were restored, recovery would take days. Our observations of NTC rotations suggest that periods of acute, total sleep deprivation and severe sleep restriction do punctuate the chronic, moderate sleep restriction that characterizes the 14-day exercise, and that these periods exacerbate the already-degraded performance of command and control elements. We observed one commander passively accept capture by the opposing force and another commander charge with his command directly into the rising sun when the planned direction of attack was due west. Both of these officers were competent and well regarded, but sleep-loss-induced degradation of critical cognitive abilities did them in.

It is important to bear in mind that in the friendly-fire incidents we debriefed in the 1990–91 Gulf War, in our observations of sleep deprivation/ restriction performance degradation at the NTC, and in examples of sleep deprivation performance degradation from other venues (e.g., the 1993 DC-8 crash in Guantanamo Bay, Cuba; Ref. 9), accidents, errors, and catastrophes occurred when personnel were sleep-deprived but, by behavioral criteria, awake. This is consistent with our findings of (a) performance degradation and decreased brain activation (as measured by PET/FDG) in subjects 24-hr sleep deprived but who were awake by polysomnographic criteria during task performance and FDG uptake (4), and (b) sleep-dose-dependent degradation in PVT performance, regardless of whether we evaluated mean speed, lapses, or fastest 10% of responses (3). These suggest that there is considerable degradation in perform-

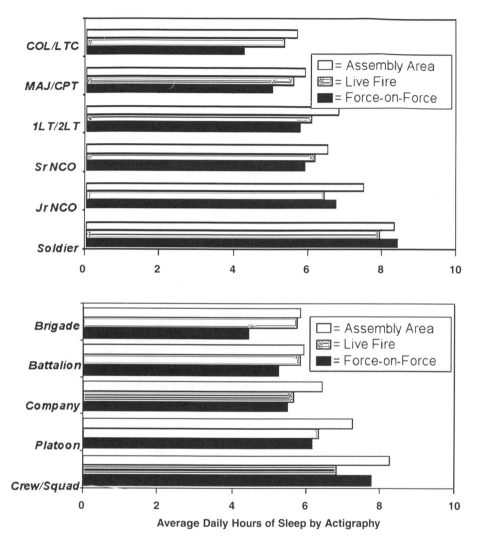

**Figure 3** Sleep by echelon and rank at NTC.

ance independent of lapses in attention or overt episodes of sleep. Going further, there are clear anecdotal examples (e.g., Ref. 9) of impaired performance from sleep deprivation despite high levels of arousal and the apparent subjective sense of exerting great effort in task performance.

Combining these anecdotal observations with our findings of selectively greater deactivation in the prefrontal cortex when compared to the whole brain in sleep deprivation (4), a picture emerges of conscientious application of effort to task performance but a gradual shift from perseverance (trying a succession of possible solutions until one is successful) to perseveration (repeated application of the same failed solution) in progressive sleep deprivation/restriction. An excellent example of this is the captain of the DC-8 in the 1993 Guantanamo Bay crash perseverating on finding the strobe light marking Cuban airspace and failing to fly the aircraft (Co-Pilot: "Do you think you are going to make this?" Captain: "Yeah . . . if I can catch the strobe light"); this perseveration was coupled with apparent, intense subjective effort (Captain: "I got it, back off") (9).

The U.S. Army is developing a Warfighter Physiologic Status Monitor (WPSM), which will consist of sensors and software for real-time biomedical measurement and status assessment of all soldiers in an operational setting. The WPSM will be integrated into the soldier computer, which in turn will be linked through a wireless local area network to the global command, control, and communication (C3) system to enable web-centric, information warfare. One component of the WPSM is the sleep management system, implemented in the form of a wrist-worn Sleep Watch (discussed in Sec. III.B).

Commanders manage many different quantities to sustain their soldiers, e.g., food, water, fuel, ammunition. Thus, for example, effective management of fuel requires that the commander know (a) how much is on hand and (b) what the expected rate of consumption is, based on the anticipated mission profile. Given these two pieces of information the commander can plan for intelligent resupply of fuel to sustain mission performance. From an operational perspective, it is worthwhile to consider sleep as an item of logistic resupply. As with fuel, commanders must know how much sleep they and their soldiers have been getting and how long this will sustain their performance in their anticipated mission. The sleep management system will provide commanders with objective measures of sleep, quantitative predictions of performance, and integrated recommendations for pharmacological and nonpharmacological (behavioral) interventions to sustain performance.

## III. Components of a Deployable Sleep Management System

Central elements of the sleep management system are the means to objectively quantify sleep/wake time under operational conditions and the means of estimating cognitive performance/effectiveness based on this information, i.e., a mathematical model to predict performance based on sleep/wake history. Information from these two components serves as the basis for specific doctrine and doctrine-implemented-in-software recommendations for optimizing sleep and cognitive readiness during combat and other operational deployments. These recommendations stem from additional elements of the sleep management system, including (a) pharmacological countermeasures—stimulants to temporarily restore and sustain cognitive performance when no sleep is possible or sleep inducers to facilitate recuperative sleep with no subsequent performance decrements; and (b) non-pharmacological countermeasures for long-term sustainment of personnel. A final element of the sleep management system is on-line, real-time monitoring of cognitive performance to warn the soldier and the soldier's chain of command of an imminent failure in cognitive readiness. These five elements are discussed below with examples of their implementation.

### A. Quantifying Sleep/Wake Under Operational Conditions

The objective quantification of sleep under operational conditions must occur under more demanding constraints than those in laboratory or even field studies: the recording device must be lightweight (not adding to the soldier's load), portable, unobtrusive, have low-power consumption, be suitable for continuous wear, and be durable under extreme environmental conditions. We have developed an application-specific integrated circuit (ASIC)-based sleep/activity monitor (actigraph) that meets these criteria. Actigraphs are preferable to other methods of recording sleep/wake history in the operational environment because they objectively and accurately measure and record sleep/wake history (unlike sleep diaries) and because they do so unobtrusively, with no required maintenance for weeks or even months at a time (unlike standard polysomnographic techniques). They require nothing more of the soldier than that the device be worn. Actigraphs have been field-tested in the U.S. Army Ranger School (Fig. 4), the U.S. Army's National Training Center (the Army's desert warfare training center in the high

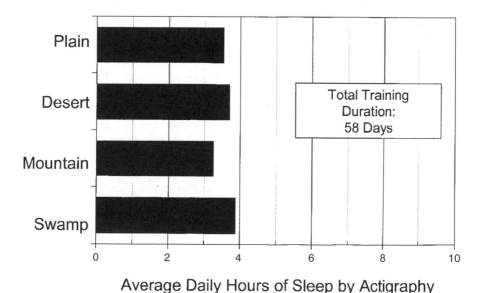

**Average Daily Hours of Sleep by Actigraphy**

**Figure 4** Sleep during Ranger training.

desert of Southern California) (Fig. 3), and Operation Desert Storm during the 1990–91Gulf War. For a review of actigraphy see Sadeh and Acebo (10).

### B.  Cognitive Readiness Prediction from Sleep/Wake History

Reliably and objectively recording sleep/wake history is important for managing sleep. However, without a means of quantifying how far the current supply of sleep will take the soldier in terms of cognitive readiness and operational performance, the utility of the sleep measurement itself is limited (11). As U.S. Army Gen. Max Thurman said, when we showed him an early version of our actigraph, "I do not care how much they sleep; I want to know how well they will perform." Thus, a second and crucial element for the sleep management system is the means for predicting cognitive readiness/performance on the basis of the actigraphically recorded sleep/wake history. Under most circumstances, a cognitive readiness prediction would not be used to make a "Go/No Go" decision since in most military and some civilian operations, "No Go" is not feasible. Rather, the prediction could be used to optimize operational deployment, to decide who among the personnel available should be sent into action first (Fig. 5). As an example, consider a situation in which four of six available units are needed for an upcoming operation, and that the members of three of these units are, in aggregate, well rested, whereas members of the other three are in various stages of recovery from previous missions. Other things being equal, the three well-rested units would be tasked with the first phase of the operational mission, along with whichever of the remaining, still-recovering units was in the best relative condition (which could be determined by the model—comparing how much sleep had been lost during the prior mission, how much sleep had been made up since the end of the mission, how long it had been since the past recovery sleep period, etc.). In addition, countermeasures (see below) might be recommended to enhance this fourth unit's readiness level, with the model specifying when and at what doses these countermeasures should be administered to optimize performance during the mission. The point of this example is that the ability to measure sleep and to predict performance provide commanders with the tools and data they need to make informed decisions relating to cognitive readiness, and to take this factor into account in much the same way as other factors are considered, e.g., experience, training, immediate past operational history, and supplies of other consumables that are normally included in operational planning.

No absolute line of demarcation divides "acceptable" and "unacceptable" levels of predicted cognitive readiness—such a demarcation would necessarily be task- or occupation-specific and would likely encompass a range or band of acceptable values. For example, the level and range of cognitive readiness acceptable for the commander making tactical decisions would likely be higher and narrower than those for the soldier loading ammunition. In operational planning, decisions are often based on judgments regarding which unit or units are best able to accomplish the mission. Sleep/wake history and attendant performance prediction are an additional factor to consider when assessing relative individual and unit readiness.

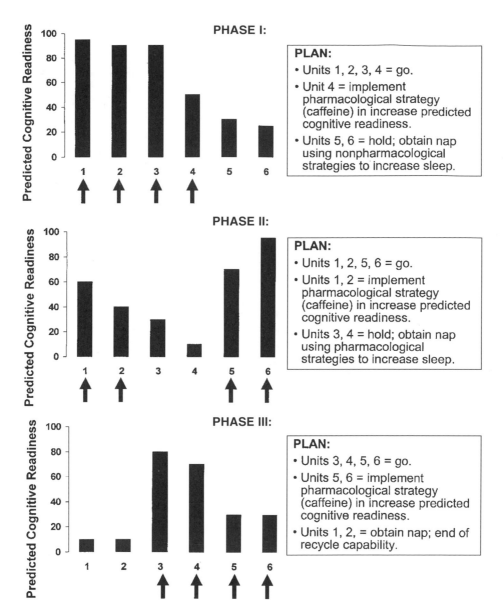

**Figure 5** Optimizing operational deployment.

Existing mathematical models predicting cognitive readiness/performance from sleep/wake history are based on the interaction of three factors. These factors are sleep homeostasis, circadian rhythm, and sleep inertia (12). Three-factor models successfully predict performance effects of acute, total sleep deprivation and performance during recovery. They do not predict well the effects of sleep restriction on performance and performance during recovery from sleep restriction (3,13–16). In addition, there are substantial individual differences in tolerance to sleep deprivation/restriction (Fig. 6) as measured by speed (1/RT) on the psychomotor vigilance task (PVT). Both the issue of accurately predicting the effects of sleep restriction on performance and recovery and the issue of individualizing the model to a particular person remain areas for further research and development.

Our current version of the Sleep Watch contains an ASIC-based actigraph, a central processing unit, random access memory, and software implementations of a sleep-scoring algorithm and a performance prediction model that uses as input the sleep/wake history from the sleep-scoring algorithm. All components are integrated into a wrist-worn device. The Sleep Watch and its output—activity counts, sleep/wake scoring, and performance prediction—can be seen in Fig. 7. The next iteration of the Sleep Watch will include all the functionality noted above, plus the functionality of a standard sports watch. It will be a true wristwatch replacement. Future iterations will include a wireless connection (wireless body-local area network) to the WPSM and soldier-worn computer—which in turn will link the device and the information it contains to unit- and higher-echelon-communications systems to inform commanders of the biomedical status of their soldiers for the purpose of operational planning.

## C. Pharmacological Countermeasures

Because past, current, and projected military operations call for episodic sustained operations with little or no opportunity to sleep for several days, pharmacological countermeasures have been—and will continue to be—important

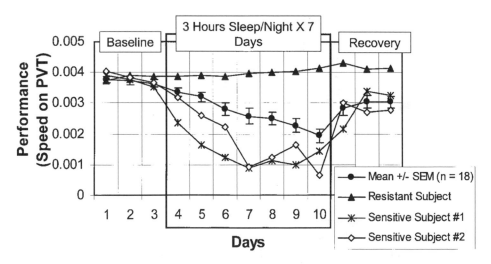

**Figure 6**  Variation between individuals in resistance and sensitivity to sleep restriction.

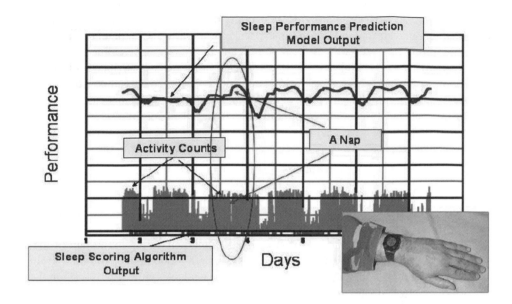

**Figure 7** The Sleep Watch in action: actigraph + sleep/wake scoring algorithm + performance prediction model.

elements of a sleep management system. Two basic strategies should be available for pharmacologically enhancing cognitive readiness in the operational environment: (a) directly but temporarily-enhancing cognitive readiness with wake-promoting agents (stimulants) when operational exigencies preclude sleep; and (b) indirectly enhancing cognitive readiness by optimizing sleep with sleep-inducing agents when the opportunity to obtain at least some sleep is available but the ability to sleep is diminished by circadian and/or environmental factors.

Pharmacological agents with these effects are available. However, guidance for their use is inadequate. For pharmacological agents to be used effectively, they need to be integrated into the doctrine and practice of sleep management, and built into the software of the sleep management system. Thus, for example, recommendations for use of a stimulant drug could be based on individual and unit sleep/wake history, likely duration of the upcoming mission, likely intercalated opportunities for sleep, and the known trade-offs between sleep, naps, and drugs in terms of their aggregate effect in sustaining performance.

*Wake-promoting Agents (Stimulants) (See Also Chap. 20)*

For military operations, the ideal wake-promoting agent would restore cognitive readiness to well-rested levels with few side effects (to include minimal interference with recovery sleep once an opportunity to sleep became available and minimal rebound sleepiness). Of the many wake-promoting agents potentially available for military use, two have had significant use: (a) *d*-amphetamine (the "gold standard" in terms of stimulant effectiveness, it is currently prescribed for a small number of operators—e.g., U.S. Air Force pilots—and used only under strict control); and (b) caffeine (because of its wide availability and status as a noncontrolled substance, it is already commonly used, albeit informally, to maintain alertness and cognitive readiness in a wide range of operational environments). Although the performance-enhancing effects of *d*-amphetamine in the operational environment have been well established (as described in Refs. 17–19), it is unlikely that its use in military operations will ever be widespread because it is available only by prescription and is a controlled substance. Caffeine, in doses ranging from 300 to 600 mg, restores cognitive performance and objective alertness to well-rested levels during total sleep deprivation (20,21). Higher doses are required with greater amounts of sleep deprivation and during the trough of the circadian phase in cognitive performance, i.e., 0600-1000 hours. However, even at higher doses, caffeine is relatively safe. It is available without prescription, is a non-controlled substance that is well tolerated, and it causes few side effects (22). Caffeine is now available in a variety of formulations including chewing gum (23). However, both *d*-amphetamine and caffeine can interfere with recovery sleep should the opportunity for sleep become available before the drug has cleared (24,25).

Many other stimulant agents are potentially available for use in the operational environment, e.g., modafinil, methylphenidate, pemoline, and nicotine. Modafinil has been considered for military operations because of claims that this substance may actually reduce the need for sleep. Modafinil is indicated for treating the excessive daytime sleepiness associated with the sleep disorder narcolepsy. We have compared the efficacy of modafinil (100, 200, or 400 mg) to that of caffeine (600 mg) for restoring cognitive performance and alertness after 41.5 hr of continuous wakefulness (21). Modafinil 200 and 400 mg significantly improved objective alertness and response speed on a psychomotor vigilance test (PVT) relative to placebo, and effects were comparable to those obtained with caffeine 600 mg (Fig. 8). As was found for caffeine, modafinil's performance-enhancing effects were especially salient during the circadian nadir in performance (06:00–10:00 hr), which lagged the circadian nadir in temperature by approximately 2 hr (21). Few instances of adverse subjective side effects (e.g., nausea, heart pounding) were reported. Therefore, in this study, it was concluded that modafinil was effective for restoring cognitive readiness and objective alertness during moderate sleep deprivation. However, modafinil was not significantly more effective than caffeine 600 mg, and its side effect profile was no more favorable than that of caffeine 600 mg. Claims that modafinil reduces the need for recovery sleep have not been substantiated. Because modafinil is a controlled substance like amphetamine, it is unlikely that modafinil use will be widespread in the military (although like *d*-ampheta-

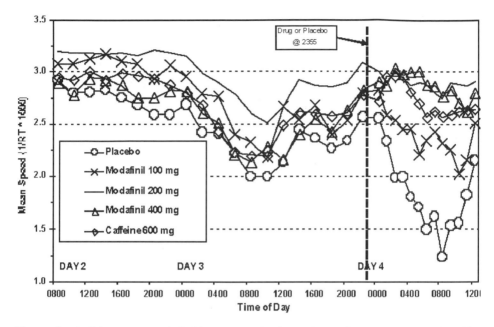

**Figure 8** Caffeine versus modafinil in sleep deprivation (Adapted from Wesensten et al, 2002.)

mine it may be available to certain special populations under the direction of a field or flight surgeon). Thus, caffeine remains the current stimulant of choice for temporarily restoring cognitive readiness during continuous and sustained military operations.

### Sleep-Inducing Agents

One reason why sleep tends to be inadequate during continuous operations is that even when they are sleep-deprived, commanders and soldiers are not always able to take full advantage of emergent opportunities to sleep. Their only opportunity for sleep may occur during the ascending phase of the circadian alertness rhythm, or the sleep environment may not be conducive because of noise, light, commotion, etc. It is under these operational circumstances that pharmacological enhancement of sleep may be useful.

For operational use, the ideal sleep-inducing agent would increase recuperative sleep time (via rapid onset and possibly short duration of action) without resulting in impaired cognitive readiness upon awakening. Benzodiazepine (BZ) receptor agonists such as triazolam and zolpidem induce sleep under operational conditions (daytime sleep under simulated troop transport conditions in otherwise well-rested subjects—Refs. 26–28). However, sleep-inducing agents also impair cognitive performance (in particular, acquisition of new memories) at their peak sleep-inducing effects (26–28). Effective sleep-inducing agents are available only by prescription and are controlled substances, thus limiting their fieldability (29). An alternative strategy involves blocking triazolam- and zolpidem-induced performance deficits with another agent when rapid return to operational status is necessary. Attempts to reverse the effects of sleep-inducing agents with stimulants such as caffeine have met with little success (30). However, flumazenil (a BZ receptor antagonist indicated for reversing BZ sedation and BZ overdose) is extremely effective. In one study we found that flumazenil completely reversed triazolam's and zolpidem's memory-impairing effects (Fig. 9) (31). Unlike caffeine, flumazenil is not a stimulant and is ineffective for restoring cognitive performance during sleep deprivation (32). The development of a dual-drug system (i.e., zolpidem or triazolam to induce sleep followed by flumazenil for rapid awakening and readiness restoration) for use in inducing recuperative sleep during long-range deployments by air would constitute a significant step forward in developing pharmacological tools for use in sleep management. Flumazenil is currently only available in an intravenous formulation. A fieldable dual-drug system would require that flumazenil be administered orally or in some other noninvasive way.

Melatonin is not currently recommended for enhancing sleep or adjusting to shift work because the factors (dose, timing, level of extant sleep debt) governing melatonin's effects have yet to be clearly elucidated—and, until then, a simplified doctrine applicable for military use is not possible. Although it has

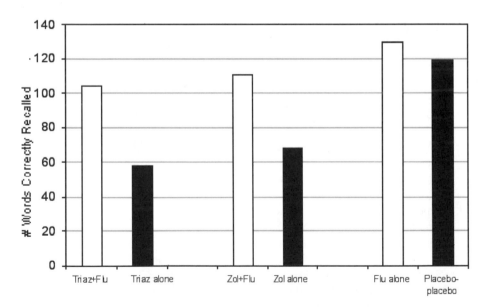

**Figure 9** Reversing triazolam triazolam (Triaz) effects with flumazenil (Flu). (Adapted from Wesensten et al., 1995b.)

been suggested that melatonin speeds adjustment of some physiological parameters to new time zones (33), with few exceptions (34) there is no evidence that melatonin improves cognitive readiness and performance.

Issues that are unique to the operational environment in general (and military operations in particular) regarding the use of sleep-inducing agents are highlighted by two field studies. First, in a study of the 18th Airborne Corps deployed as part of the Army's annual Operation Bright Star field exercise from the Eastern United States to Egypt, 68 soldiers received either triazolam 0.5 mg or placebo on the first leg (from the United States to Germany) of their flight to the Middle East. Despite several laboratory studies in which it was shown that triazolam 0.5 mg induces sleep (26–28), in this field study triazolam 0.5 mg failed to improve actigraphically recorded in-flight sleep (35). This negative finding was probably due to a lack of control over the cabin environment, which included an in-flight hot meal service that (a) commenced 3 hr after soldiers had taken the drug or placebo (ideally, it would have started prior to, or immediately after, drug administration, or box lunches passed out at the beginning of the flight); and (b) lasted well over 2 hr (during which time no one was able to sleep as trays of food were being passed continuously up and down the line of soldiers sitting in their webbed seats side by side with their backs to the sides of the aircraft). This field study highlighted one possible contraindication for use of sleep-inducing agents during deployment, that is, how likely is it that soldiers will not have an opportunity to sleep undisturbed by events requiring action on their part?

Another field study highlights other risks attendant to the use of sleep-inducing agents in the field. In an unpublished field study we conducted at Ft. Lewis, Washington, nine Ranger rifle platoons were evaluated during exercises in which they were sleeping in the open in subfreezing temperatures but otherwise with no disruptions. They received triazolam 0.5, 0.25, or placebo just before an actigraphically recorded 4-hr nighttime sleep period. Triazolam 0.5 and 0.25 mg substantially improved sleep—however, triazolam also caused some soldiers to fall asleep (often bareheaded and wearing only T-shirts and undershorts) before they had zipped themselves into their sleeping bags. We observed soldiers sound asleep and shivering, half in and half out of their sleeping bags—and only with great difficulty were we able to arouse them sufficiently to get them into their sleeping bags and get them zipped up. When sleep-inducing agents are administered in the field (i.e., in other than climate-controlled conditions), precautions must be taken to ensure that a "designated sleep manager" is on hand to monitor soldiers for safety.

### D.  Nonpharmacological Countermeasures

The principal nonpharmacological countermeasures that have been shown to have consistent beneficial effects on cognitive performance are (a) napping (36,37; see also Chap. 22), and (b) behavioral measures to protect sleep.

Substantial benefit can be realized from even a short nap—in an unpublished comparison of cognitive performance data from two separate sleep deprivation studies conducted at our laboratory, we found that after 72 hr awake, individuals who were allowed only 30 min/day to sleep (a total of 1.5 hr sleep across 72 hr) performed nearly 25% better than subjects who obtained no sleep at all (Fig. 10). The daily 30-min nap was extremely "efficient" (consolidated); subjects spent nearly the entire nap time in stages 2, slow-wave sleep, or rapid-eye-movement (REM) sleep and almost no time awake or in stage 1 sleep. Naps of similar or longer durations have also been found to improve performance and alertness (38–41). Work by Dinges et al. (Dinges, personal communication, 2002) indicates that moderate-duration napping appears to be more effective for sustaining performance than low-to-moderate dosages of stimulant drugs; and combining the two (naps and stimulants) appears even more advantageous. For military operations, our recommendation is to "nap early, nap often." This straightforward rule is easily applied in any operational setting.

Nonpharmacological strategies to protect sleep increase the likelihood that sleep will actually occur during naps or other designated sleep periods. These measures include (a) timing the sleep period for the early morning or early afternoon, and (b) protecting the sleep environment from noise, light, and other disruptions either by isolating the sleeper or by using earplugs, sleep masks, eye patches, or constant "white noise" (42).

A variety of other nonpharmacological strategies for increasing alertness and cognitive readiness have been proposed and shown to be ineffective.

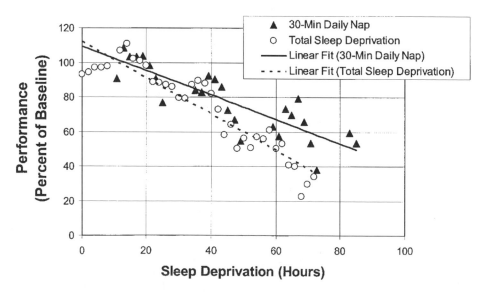

**Figure 10**   Thirty-minute daily nap versus total sleep deprivation.

Ineffective measures include exposure to cold air, loud sounds such as music, and brief bouts of physical exercise (43; see also Chap. 21). Although these strategies temporarily improve feelings of alertness, they have no lasting effect on mental operations—particularly compared to wake-promoting agents such as caffeine—and thus are not recommended for use during military operations. The inherent danger in such strategies is that since they may improve subjective feelings of alertness without actually improving objective cognitive performance, they might instill in the operator a false impression of improved capacity to perform.

Finally, there is what can be best termed a folk belief, held by a number of military personnel, that high motivation as well as the excitement and adrenaline produced by a high-operational tempo can keep soldiers performing even in the face of severe sleep restriction/deprivation. However, motivation has been shown to be ineffective in sustaining performance (44; see also Chap. 21). Anecdotal accounts of combat indicate that the effects of adrenaline release are short-lived and are followed by extreme fatigue and sleepiness (45).

### E.  On-line, Real-time Monitoring of Cognitive Performance

Performance prediction based on sleep/wake history provides an estimate of current cognitive readiness (see above). At this point in its development, the predictive model is "one-size fits-all" and no provision is made for individual differences in response to sleep deprivation/restriction. Thus, though at the group level predictions are good, there can be a considerable mismatch between any given individual's actual performance and his or her predicted performance based on sleep/wake history. In addition, the model predicts average performance over an interval and does not predict the normal moment-to-moment fluctuations in alertness. The solution is to monitor cognitive performance in real time. For use in the operational environment, a cognitive performance monitor must be unobtrusive—ideally such monitoring would derive from or be embedded in the soldier's ongoing task. Multiple objectives could be achieved with on-line, real-time monitoring, including (a) verification/validation of the cognitive readiness prediction; (b) adaptation of the cognitive readiness prediction to individual soldiers by taking into account individual differences in sensitivity/resistance to continuous or sustained operations; and (c) warning the soldier and the soldier's chain of command of an imminent failure in cognitive performance.

### IV.  Guidance and Doctrine for Sleep Management System Implementation

A vital component of any sleep management system is guidance and doctrine for its implementation. Ideally, such information would (a) be built into the sleep management system's software; (b) be automatically triggered by the combination of sleep/wake history, performance prediction, and projected mission requirements; and (c) generate specific recommendations for pharmacological countermeasures, napping strategies, etc. In practice, guidance/doctrine could also take the form of a designated sleep manager (as mentioned above) to ensure that scheduling of individual-level (e.g., living quarters, daylight exposure), unit-level (e.g., training/meal/briefing schedules), and materiel-level (e.g., equipment maintenance, refueling) mission-supporting activities are optimized to protect sleep.

### V.  The Sleep Management System in Action: A Projection to the Year 2012

It is August 2012. An American expeditionary force is deploying to contain aggression by a disciplined, well-equipped, technologically sophisticated, and well-led force in Southwest Asia. The Americans are deploying by air after 5 days of preparation during which there was little opportunity for sleep. All personnel are wearing the Warfighter Physiological Status Monitor (WPSM) including the sensors and software of the sleep management system. Sleep management system software located with command and control elements at all echelons periodically interrogates, through a local area radio-frequency network, the sleep/activity monitor of each soldier's personnel status monitor, generating reports on sleep obtained and predicting effects on cognitive readiness. The integrated sleep management system, including hardware, software, modular integration into the personnel status monitor, pharmacological agents to assist in managing the sleep/wake cycle, on-line/real-time cognitive readiness monitoring, and appropriate doctrine, had been introduced into the American armed forces 2 years earlier. Reports generated by the sleep management system indicate that, on average, most personnel had managed to obtain 4.5 hr of broken sleep each night over the last 5 nights while higher echelons of command and control managed to obtain only 3.5 hr of sleep each night. The sleep management system predicts that cognitive readiness by all echelons will be below optimum. On the basis of current intelligence, commanders are anticipating immediate engagement with the enemy upon insertion. Given mission requirements, optimum cognitive readiness is essential. The sleep management system predicts that 6 continuous hr of sleep for all personnel will improve cognitive readiness and increase the probability of a successful operation.

Lead elements are now only 2–3 hr from take-off. As suggested by the sleep management system software, commanders elect to implement the sleep-induction/rapid-reawakening system for all soldiers once they are airborne. This consists of two pills, orally administered, given sequentially. The first, a sleep inducer, is administered prior to the sleep period to induce sleep. The second, an antidote to the sleep inducer, is administered at the end of the sleep interval to restore full alertness and cognitive readiness. Once airborne, soldiers take their sleep inducer. Light levels, noise, and commotion are kept to a minimum during the sleep period. After 6.5 hr of sleep, the soldiers are awakened. Immediately, they take their antidote. Within 20 min all personnel are fully alert. They are refreshed from their sleep. Their thinking is clear and rapid. Their motivation is high. They are ready for combat. A query to the sleep management system indicates that personnel obtained an average of 5.5 hr sleep during the in-flight sleep period. Factoring in this additional sleep, the sleep management system predicts individual and unit cognitive readiness on arrival to be near-optimal, a substantial improvement over presleep, preflight estimates.

Enemy resistance to the insertion of the expeditionary force is suppressed. The buildup in-theater continues. The alertness and cognitive performance of critical command and control personnel are continually monitored by the on-line, real-time alertness monitoring system. Forty-eight hours into the operation, the expeditionary force comes under pressure as the enemy launches all its forces in a coordinated counterattack. Commanders expect a brief but intense period of sustained operations. At this point, again in accordance with sleep management system-suggested interventions, commanders elect to implement short-term stimulant use to enhance the alertness of personnel at all positions and help ensure adequate performance over the ensuing 10–12 hr. The counterattack is repulsed; the operation proceeds as planned. Commanders continue to use the sleep management system to manage the sleep/wake cycle to optimize cognitive readiness. Two weeks into the operation, organized enemy action ceases. The first phase of the operation concludes successfully with minimal casualties from enemy action and no losses from accident or friendly fire.

## VI. Summary

Sleep sustains cognitive readiness—the sum of mental abilities necessary for effective combat performance. Sleep is as important to combat operations as the proverbial beans and bullets. Like food, water, fuel, ammunition, and other consumables, sleep must be considered an item of logistic resupply. To manage sleep, commanders must know how much sleep they and their men have been getting and how long and how well this sleep will sustain them in their proposed operational profile. Then they can plan for timely resupply. A deployable sleep management system will provide commanders with effective tools for managing sleep to maximize individual and unit cognitive readiness. The sleep management system in development by the U.S. Army includes: (a) a means to objectively and unobtrusively record and score sleep/wake to determine the sleep/wake history of individual soldiers under operational conditions; (b) a mathematical model which uses the sleep/wake history to provide soldiers and their commanders with a prediction of their cognitive readiness; (c) pharmacological tools to maintain or restore cognitive readiness, e.g., stimulants and sleep-inducing medications, and guidance for their use; (d) nonpharmacological tools to maintain and restore cognitive readiness, e.g., napping, timing of main sleep periods, and behavioral interventions to protect the integrity of sleep; and (e) a means to monitor cognitive performance in real time to inform and individualize model predictions, and to provide moment-to-moment assessment of cognitive readiness. The sleep management system for the soldier will be incorporated into a broader suite of biomedical sensors and software, the Warfighter Physiological Status Monitor (WPSM), and integrated into the soldier computer, the basic element of web-enabled warfare.

## References

1.  Biddle S. Victory misunderstood: what the gulf war tells us about the future of conflict. Int Secur 1996; *21*(2):139–141.
2.  Harrison Y, Horne JA. The impact of sleep deprivation on decision making: a review. J Exp Psychol Appl 2000; *6*(3), 236–49.
3.  Belenky G, Wesensten NJ, Thorne DR, Thomas ML, Sing HC, Redmond DP, Russo BM, Balkin TJ Patterns of performance degradation and restoration during sleep restriction and subsequent recovery: a sleep dose-response study. J Sleep Res 2003; 12:1–13.
4.  Thomas M, Sing H, Belenky G, Holcomb H, Mayberg H, Dannals R, Wagner H, Thorne DR, Popp K, Rowland L, Welsh A, Balwinski S, Redmond D. Neural basis of alertness and cognitive performance impairments during sleepiness. I. Effects of 24h of sleep deprivation on waking human regional brain activity. J Sleep Res 2000; *9:*335–352.
5.  Braun AR, Balkin TJ, Wesensten NJ, Carson RE, Varga M, Baldwin P, Selbie S, Belenky G, Herscovitch P. Regional cerebral blood flow throughout the sleep-wake cycle: an H2(15)O positron emission tomography study. Brain 1997; *120*:1173–1197.
6.  Balkin TJ, Braun AR, Wesensten NJ, Jeffries K, Varga M, Baldwin P, Belenky G, Herscovitch P. The process of awakening: a PET study of regional brain activity patterns mediating the re-establishment of alertness and consciousness. Brain 2002; *125*: 2308–2319.
7.  Belenky G, Martin JA, Marcy, SC. Debriefings and battle reconstructions following combat. In: *The Gulf War and Mental Health: A Comprehensive Guide.* Martin J. A., Sparacino L, Belenky G, eds., Westport, CT: Praeger:, 1996:105–114.
8.  Balkin T, Thorne D, Sing H, Thomas M, Redmond D, Wesensten N, Williams J, Hall S, Belenky G. *Effects of Sleep Schedules on Commercial Driver Performance.* DOT-MC-00-133, Washington, CD: US Department of Transportation, Federal Motor Carrier Safety Administration; 2000.
9.  NTSB *Aircraft Accident Report (PB94-910406, NTSB/AAR-94/04): Uncontrolled Collision with Terrain, American International Airways, Flight 808, Douglas DC-8-61, N814CK, U.S. Naval Air Station, Guantanamo Bay, Cuba, August 18,1993,*Washington, DC: National Transportation Safety Board (NTSB); 1994 (available on the World Wide Web—*http://olias.arc.nasa.gov/zteam/PDF_pubs/ G_Bay/GuantanamoBay.pdf*—accessed February 2003).
10.  Sadeh A, Acebo C. The role of actigraphy in sleep medicine. Sleep Med Revi, 2002; *6:*113–124.
11.  Dinges DF, Achermann P. Commentary: future considerations for models of human neurobehavioral function. J Biol Rhythms 1999; *14:*598–601.

12. Akerstedt T, Folkard S. The three-process model of alertness and its extension to performance, sleep latency, and sleep length. Chronobiol Int 1997; *14*:115–23.

13. Hursh SR, Redmond DP, Johnson ML, Thorne DR, Belenky G, Balkin TJ, Storm WF, Miller JC, Eddy DR. Fatigue models for applied research in warfighting. Aviat Space Environ Med. *In press.*

14. Neri DF, Friedl KE, Foster RE, Ahlers S, Mallis MM, Larkin W, Popkin S, Reifman J, Dinges DF, Van Dongen HPA, Ritzer DR, Vigneulle RM. An overview of fatigue and performance modeling. Aviat Space Environ Med. *In press.*

15. Van Dongen HPA, Dinges DF. Chronic partial sleep deprivation data point to a novel process regulating waking behavioural alertness. Sleep 2002; *11*(suppl 1):232.

16. Van Dongen HPA, Shah AD, de Brunier AB, Dinges DF. Behavioural alertness and the two-process model of sleep regulation during chronic partial sleep deprivation. Sleep 2002, *11*(suppl 1):233.

17. Caldwell JA, Caldwell JL. An in-flight investigation of the efficacy of dextroamphetamine for sustaining helicopter pilot performance. Aviat Space Environ Med. 1997a; *68:*1073–1080.

18. Caldwell JA, Caldwell JL, Smythe NK, Hall KK. A double-blind, placebo-controlled investigation of the efficacy of modafinil for sustaining the alertness and performance of aviators: a helicopter simulator study. Psychopharmacology 2000; *150*:272–282.

19. Newhouse PA, Belenky G., Thomas M., Thorne D, Sing HC, Fertig J. The effects of *d*-amphetamine on arousal, cognition, and mood after prolonged total sleep deprivation. Neuropsychopharmacology 1989; *2:*153–164.

20. Penetar DM, McCann UD, Thorne D, Schelling A., Galinski C, Sing H, Thomas M, Belenky G. Caffeine reversal of sleep deprivation effects on alertness and mood. Psychopharmacology 1993; *112*:359–365.

21. Wesensten NJ, Belenky G, Kautz MA, Thorne DR, Reichardt RM, Balkin TJ Maintaining alertness and performance during sleep deprivation: modafinil versus caffeine. Psychopharmacology 2002; *159:*238–247.

22. Dews P, Grice HC, Neims A, Wilson J, Wurtman R. Report of Fourth International Caffeine Workshop, Athens, 1982. Food and Chemical Toxicology 1984, *22:*163–169.

23. Kamimori GH, Karyekar CS, Otterstetter R, Cox DS, Balkin TJ, Belenky GL, Eddington ND. The rate of absorption and relative bioavailability of caffeine administered in chewing gum versus capsules to normal healthy volunteers. Int J Pharmacol 2002; *234:* 159–167.

24. Penetar DM, Sing H, Thorne D, Thomas M, Fertig J, Schelling A, Sealock J, Newhouse PA, Belenky G. Amphetamine effects on recovery sleep following total sleep deprivation. Hum Psychopharmacol 1991; *6:*319–323.

25. Caldwell JA, Caldwell JL. Recovery sleep and performance following sleep deprivation with dextroamphetamine. J Sleep Res 1997b; *6:*92–101.

26. O'Donnell VM, Balkin TJ, Andrade JR, Simon LM, Kamimori GH, Redmond DP, Belenky G. Effects of triazolam on sleep and performance in a model of transient insomnia. Hum Perform 1988; *1:*145–160.

27. Balkin TJ, O'Donnell VM, Wesensten NJ, McCann UD, Belenky G. Comparison of the daytime sleep and performance effects of zolpidem versus triazolam. Psychopharmacology 1992; *107:*83–88.

28.  Wesensten NJ, Balkin TJ, Belenky G. Effects of daytime administration of zolpidem versus triazolam on memory. Eur J Clin Pharmacol 1995a; *48:*115–122.

29.  Caldwell JA, Caldwell JL. Comparison of the effects of zolpidem-induced prophylactic naps to placebo naps and forced rest periods in prolonged work schedules. Sleep 1998; *21*(1):79–90.

30.  Mattila MJ, Vainio P, Nurminen ML, Vanakoski J, Seppala T. Midazolam 12 mg is moderately counteracted by 250 mg caffeine in man. Int J Clin Pharmacol Ther 2000; *38:*581–587.

31.  Wesensten NJ, Balkin TJ, Davis HQ, Belenky G. Reversal of triazolam- and zolpidem-induced memory impairment by flumazenil. Psychopharmacology 1995b; *121:*242–249.

32.  Wesensten NJ, Balkin TJ, Belenky G. Is the benzodiazepine antagonist flumazenil intrinsically alerting? (abstr) Sleep Res 1996; *25:*74.

33.  Takahashi T, Sasaki M, Itoh H, Yamadera W, Ozone M, Obuchi K, Hayashida K, Matsunaga N, Sano H. Melatonin alleviates jet lag symptoms caused by an 11-hour eastward flight. Psychiatry Clin Neurosci 2002; *56:*301–302.

34.  Comperatore CA, Lieberman HR, Kirby AW, Adams B, Crowley JS. Melatonin efficacy in aviation missions requiring rapid deployment and night operations. Aviat Space Environ Med. 1996; *67:*520–524.

35.  Penetar DM, Belenky G, Garrigan JJ, Redmond DP. Triazolam impairs learning and fails to improve sleep in a long-range aerial deployment. Aviat. Space Environ Med. 1989; *60:*594–598.

36.  Purnell MT, Feyer AM, Herbison GP. The impact of a nap opportunity during the night shift on the performance and alertness of 12-h shift workers. J Sleep Res 2002; *11:*219–227.

37.  Tietzel AJ, Lack LC. The recuperative value of brief and ultra-brief naps on alertness and cognitive performance. J Sleep Res 2002; *11:*213–218.

38.  Bonnet MH, Arand DL. The use of prophylactic naps and caffeine to maintain performance during a continuous operation. Ergonomics 1994; *37:*1009–1020.

39.  Bonnet MH, Arand DL. Consolidated and distributed nap schedules and performance. J Sleep Res 1995; *4*(2):71–77.

40.  Dinges DF, Orne MT, Whitehouse WG, Orne EC Temporal placement of a nap for alertness: contributions of circadian phase and prior wakefulness. Sleep 1987; *10*(4):313–29.

41.  Sallinen M, Harma M, Akerstedt T, Rosa R, Lillqvist O. Promoting alertness with a short nap during a night shift. J Sleep Res 1998; *7*(4):240–247.

42.  Comperatore CA, Caldwell JA, Caldwell JL. *Leader's Guide to Crew Endurance*; U.S. Army Aeromedical Research Laboratory and U.S. Army Safety Center: Fort Rucker, AL, 1997 (available on the World Wide Web—http://safety.army.mil/pages/pov/arac/crewend.pdf (accessed February 2003).

43.  Reyner LA, Horne JA. Evaluation of "in-car" countermeasures to sleepiness: cold air and radio. Sleep 1998; *21,*46–50.

44.  Horne JA, Anderson NR, Wilkinson RT. Effects of sleep deprivation on signal detection measures of vigilance: implications for sleep function. Sleep 1983; *6*(4):347–58.

45.  Marshall SLA. *Night Drop: The American Airborne Invasion of Normandy*; New York: Little Brown

# 17

## Athletic Performance

**ROGER S. SMITH**

Stanford University Sleep, Stanford, California, U.S.A.

**THOMAS P. REILLY**

Liverpool John Moores University, Liverpool, England

> *In strength of lift both subjects lose quite regularly and seriously,*
> *but regain nearly all after sleep.*
>
> —Patrick GTW, Gilbert JA.
> September, 1896

## I. Introduction

Athletes have been searching for performance advantages for more than 2700 years (2). Athletic performance advantages are gaining importance as the margin of victory narrows and the financial rewards of victory increase. Sleep deprivation has rather significant adverse effects on general human performance measures. Therefore, a precise understanding of the effects of sleep deprivation on athletic performance may prove to be of great value to athletes.

Unfortunately, at least three research protocol features are needed to define the effects of sleep deprivation on athletic performance with any accuracy. (a) The research protocol should isolate the homeostatic from the circadian components as the two so frequently confound each other (3,4). (b) The protocol should include a meaningful competitive event to decrease the chance of motivational confounds and reduce the distortion inherent in extrapolating pieces to a whole (i.e., anaerobic capacity of the quadriceps muscle does not necessarily predict World Cup victory). (c) Finally, the protocol should effectively reduce the myriad of confounding variables associated with sports such as home field advantage, weather, injuries, field conditions, and so on.

If these research design features had been mandatory, this chapter would be exceedingly short. Thankfully, undaunted researchers have collected a substantial amount of data that, when pressed against the filter of scientific rigor, yields at least indirect evidence. Still, there are times when indirect evidence is quite ample and convincing (e.g., Einstein's Theory of Special and General Relativity).

Athletic performance includes not only the competitive event itself, but also optimal training and avoidance of injuries prior to and during the event. Therefore, in addition to reviewing the effects of sleep deprivation on athletic performance measures, this chapter will also examine similar observations on athletic training and injuries.

## II. Sleep Deprivation and Athletic Performance

In an effort to illustrate an essential point, the following oversimplification is required. Athletes can be studied in the field relative to their actual performance or in the laboratory relative to their predicted performance. Field studies more accurately reflect the entire performance whereas laboratory studies more precisely measure individual aspects of performance. Both have their respective advantages and disadvantages.

### A. Field Studies

Relatively few studies have examined the effects of sleep deprivation on athletic performance in the field and even fewer are associated with a meaningful competitive event. Therefore, indirect evidence from military research and subjective reports from elite athletes participating in ultraendurance races will also be reviewed.

The Race Across America (RAAM) is an all-out 2900-mile solo bicycle race across the United States. Unlike the Tour de France, there are no programmed stops or rest periods. The winner typically rides across the entire country in 8 days. Smith et al. (5) studied a total of seven athletes over 3 years and reported that the winners averaged approximately 2 hr of sleep per day. It was concluded that some athletes have the remarkable ability to perform and win ultraendurance races in the face of severe sleep deprivation.

This conclusion has also been supported by many other ultraendurance races. For example, the Eco-Challenge requires teams to cover hundreds of miles over various terrain in extremes of weather conditions. The first team to cross the finish line wins. Sleep, like many other physical needs, is constantly being prioritized for optimal performance. In the 2002 race, the winning team completed the course in approximately 170 hr during which time the team members slept a mere 17 hr. This represented an increase in percentage sleep time compared to their 2001 Eco-Challenge race during which the team leader developed extreme physical and cognitive fatigue collectively known by these athletes as "the sleep monster." Their sleep strategy was reprioritized in 2002 to "no more than 30 hr without sleep" from the 2001 strategy of "sleep only if you absolutely have to" because of their impairment in performance after 50–60 hr of sleep deprivation in the 2001 race (Nathan Fa'avae, personal communication, 2002).

Ultraendurance races like RAAM and the Eco-Challenge exemplify the classic question in sleep deprivation research on athletes, *"At what point does sleep deprivation become detrimental to athletic performance?"* It is a question of probability rather than possibility. For the moment, the answer appears to vary greatly.

Edinger et al. (6) followed two adult men during a 146-hr tennis match. Both subjects were allowed 4–5 hours of sleep per night. From prematch to post-match, a decline was noted in memory and perceptual-motor coding (Digit Symbol Substitution Test). Over the course of the match both players reported increasing fatigue. Injuries were more common in one subject who also developed intermittent disorientation on day 6.

Reilly and Walsh (7) monitored two teams playing five-a-side football indoors for 91.8 hr. A rest period of 5 min was permitted every 50 min. Throughout this study spontaneous work rate varied in a circadian fashion in-phase with the body temperature curve. This rhythm was superimposed on a deteriorating trend in work rate indicative of fatigue. Increased lapses of attention and delays in reaction times were more pronounced than trends in physical measures such as grip strength, which was highly resistant to the influence of sleep loss. The impairment in mental performance was evident after only one night. In other studies, a decline in a 60-min vigilance task (relevant to sailing) and a 10-min choice reaction time test (relevant to driving) is usually noted after a single night of sleep loss (8).

Several field studies of sleep deprivation and athletes involve sailing races. Ellen MacArthur, a competitor in the 2001 Vendee Globe 25,000-mile solo sailing race, practiced the cluster-napping technique acquired through the prerace program of alertness management suggested by Dr. Claudio Stampi (BBC news, Feb. 21, 2001). The duration of sleep varied with environmental conditions, and was generally supported by daytime naps. This strategy entails breaking up a long sleep into shorter naps of about 25–40 min each, making quick checks on equipment and weather conditions when awake, and then immediately resuming sleep. Her average sleep time per nap was 36 min, with an approximate average total sleep time per day of 5.5 hr over the 94 days of the race. She clocked the fastest time ever for a woman racing in the Vendee Globe and very nearly won placing second overall.

Bennet (9) investigated 19 solo sailors racing across 3000 miles of the Atlantic. Most competitors woke themselves at intervals to check heading or weather and make adjustments. One sailor woke himself every 30 min day and night for the 38 days. The degree of sleep deprivation and mean sleep times resulting from this significant sleep fragmentation were not reported in the study. Errors were especially common during adverse external events such as having problems with the boat. Visual, auditory, and olfactory illusions or hallucinations were noted by a few of the participants.

Reilly and George (10) investigated the etiology of these disturbances in thinking and perceptual processes. They observed 10 footballers playing five-a-side indoors for 71 hr and found evidence suggesting that *b*-phenylethylamine, a naturally occurring brain amine, may play a role in the cycles of unusual behavior and mood during prolonged sleep loss. The concentrations of the free amine measured in urine increased with each day, superimposed on a circadian rhythm. Despite the occasionally bizarre behavioral symptoms, the grip strength of these subjects also remained relatively stable over the 3 days, once values were corrected for a circadian rhythm.

Subjective states were also monitored regularly in the footballers over the 71 hr. The data in Figure 1a illustrate how anxiety increased with successive nights of sleep deprivation. The influence of a circadian subharmonic in the observations is also obvious. Unprepared reaction time, recorded on each participant regularly through the entire period, deteriorated in phase with subjective states (Fig. 1b). Prolonged gaps in attention, when the subject failed to respond at all to the visual stimulus, were excluded from the data.

In an attempt to approximate competitive sport conditions, Sinnerton and Reilly (11) focused on swimming performance and on restricted nightly sleep. Eight swimmers were tested in a 50-m pool on 4 consecutive days, morning (06:30 hr) and evening (17:30 hr), under conditions of normal sleep and under partial sleep deprivation (2.5 hr sleep a night). Measurements included grip and back strength, lung function (vital capacity, forced expiratory volume in 1 sec), resting heart rate, and mood states. Swimming performances over four trials at 50 m and one trial at 400 m were also measured. No decrements were noted with sleep deprivation either in back or grip strength, lung function, or swim times, although these variables demonstrated an effect of time of day. Sleep loss affected mood states, increasing depression, tension, confusion, fatigue, and anger while decreasing vigor significantly. The data were interpreted as supporting Horne's (12) brain restitution theory of sleep, suggesting that the primary need for sleep is located in nerve cells rather than in other biological tissues.

International travel is a common precipitant of sleep deprivation in athletes. Smith et al. (13) followed 12 Olympic athletes prior to, during, and after their flight from Korea to the Atlanta XXVI Olympic Games (10 time zones). Approximately half of the athletes experienced a significant increase in daytime sleepiness (Epworth Sleepiness Scale Scores) and most experienced fatigue, although nearly all athletes maintained the same total sleep time (sleep logs) regardless of location or proximity to the date of travel. This foreshadows the importance of circadian confounds discussed below.

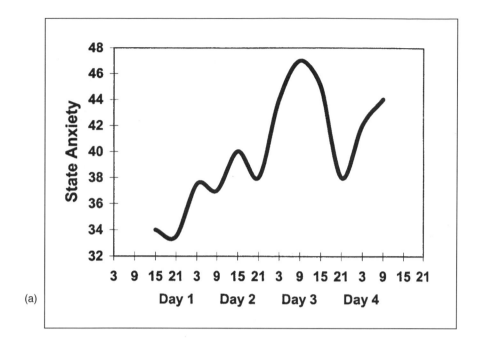

(a)

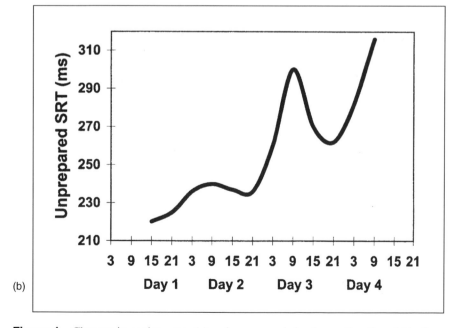

(b)

**Figure 1** Changes in anxiety state (a) and unprepared simple reaction time (b) in five-a-side players over 71 hr without any sleep. The data show a trend with time of sleep deprivation and a time-of-day effect. (Adapted from Ref. 10.)

Guezennec et al. (14) studied 27 male soldiers participating in a 5-day combat course of heavy and continuous physical activity (energy expenditure was estimated to exceed 21 megajoules [MJ]/day) with less than 4 hr of sleep per solar day. The soldiers were randomly assigned to three groups, receiving 7.6 MJ/day (low intake), 13.4 MJ/day (medium intake), or 17.6 MJ/day (high intake). Maximal oxygen uptake ($\dot{V}O_{2\ max}$) and anaerobic performances were measured before and after the combat course. While the soldiers on the medium- and high-energy intakes maintained their performance measures, those on the low-energy intake displayed a significant decline in $\dot{V}O_{2\ max}$ (8%) and in anaerobic power (14%). The observations suggest that only a severe energy deficit leads to decreased performance capability over 5 days of reduced sleep combined with heavy physical activity. They point also to the adverse consequences of large energy deficits when activity must be sustained over many days and with reduced sleep.

In a broadly similar study of military personnel conducted over 4 days of sustained activity in which only 2 hr sleep was allowed daily, soldiers were deemed to be ineffective at the end (15). This conclusion was based on performance in a 1-km assault course, a shooting test, and a 3-km run. In this case, provision of a high-energy diet failed to offset the impairments. The declines may have been a fatigue effect rather than attributable to sleep loss per se, since others have reported that soldiers deprived of sleep for 2–3 nights but not physically fatigued were able to perform highly demanding tasks at the same work rate as fresh troops (16).

How et al. (17) studied naval seamen who were totally deprived of sleep over 72 hr. After 36 hr there were pronounced falls in performance requiring cognitive, vigilance, psychomotor, and, to a smaller extent, physical functions. Greater effects were observed in tests that involved cognition, speed, and precision and smaller effects were noted in routine tasks that entailed close manual movement. In all cases, performances showed a diurnal rhythm and a strong correlation with self-reported sleepiness. Although the research was directed toward naval personnel, the observations have relevance also to competitive long-distance sailors.

The increased mental drive necessary to maintain performance was apparent in another study of military recruits kept awake for 3 successive nights (18). An increase in fatigue was accompanied by a decline in rifle-shooting accuracy, both reflecting circadian rhythmicity over which the deteriorating trend was superimposed. There was a clear rhythm in circulating noradrenaline whose peak increased on each of the 3 days of sleep deprivation.

In conclusion, field studies are limited in number and precision. High variance in study design no doubt contributes to inconsistencies in findings. Perhaps the best evidence for athletic performance decrement secondary to significant sleep deprivation is the complete absence of any study that has deliberately deprived elite athletes of sleep prior to a meaningful competitive event. There have been ample opportunities, but apparently no volunteers.

## B.  Laboratory Studies

A single reliably predictive laboratory measure of athletic performance does not yet exist. As a result, for practical application to athletes, findings in laboratory studies are extrapolated to competitive conditions. As extrapolation can be misleading, many studies employ only the most commonly used laboratory performance measures such as maximal oxygen uptake ($\dot{V}O_{2\,max}$), anaerobic power and capacity, endurance, time to exhaustion, perceived exertion, reaction time, etc.

Measurable decreases in $\dot{V}O_{2\,max}$ after various degrees of sleep deprivation have been noted in several studies (19–24). Plyley et al. (20), in a simple crossover study design ($n = 12$, sleep debt = 64 hr), showed a small but significant decrease in $\dot{V}O_{2\,max}$ while ensuring maximal effort with a plateau in $\dot{V}O_2$ indicating $\dot{V}O_{2\,max}$. The decrease in $\dot{V}O_{2\,max}$ was seen with and without intermittent treadmill walking during the sleep deprivation period which suggests that moderate activity is not the reason for the decrease in $\dot{V}O_{2\,max}$. Chen ($n = 15$, sleep debt = 30 hr) observed decreased maximal exercise performance with decreased maximal heart rate, peak $O_2$ consumption, peak $\dot{V}CO_2$, and reduced time to exhaustion (21).

Other studies have shown no change in $\dot{V}O_{2\,max}$ after various degrees of sleep deprivation (25–31). Horne and Pettitt (25) found no change at 40, 60, and 80% $\dot{V}O_{2\,max}$ ($n = 7$, sleep debt = 72 hr). They noted that work capacity was also unchanged with sleep loss. However, their study used physically untrained subjects and $\dot{V}O_{2\,max}$ was estimated from submaximal heart rates. Martin and Gaddis (26) utilized a cycle ergometer with different loads but examined only 25, 50, and 75% $\dot{V}O_{2\,max}$, and subjects were allowed caffeine ($n = 6$, sleep debt = 30 hr). McMurray and Brown (27) showed no change in responses to exercise at 80% $\dot{V}O_{2\,max}$ but the slow component of recovery (3–15 min) showed significant increases in oxygen uptake ($n = 5$, sleep debt = 24 hr). They speculated an attenuation in the recovery process but offered no suggestion of the mechanism responsible. Goodman et al. (29) demonstrated no effect on maximal oxygen uptake determined on a cycle ergometer but they allowed potentially unsupervised 10–20-min breaks every 1.5–2 hr ($n = 12$, sleep debt = 60 hr). Mougin et al. (30) allowed subjects only 4 hr of sleep on one night and found no change in $\dot{V}O_{2\,max}$, peak power, mean power, or peak velocity the following day ($n = 8$, sleep debt = partial).

Looking further into the $\dot{V}O_{2\,max}$ data yields some insight but still no definitive conclusion. There seems to be no necessary impairment in maximal oxygen uptake after 1 night's partial (25) or complete (26) sleep loss or 3 consecutive nights of partial sleep deprivation (32). The main difficulty is getting the compliance of subjects to exercise to voluntary exhaustion with evidence that the criteria for attaining $\dot{V}O_{2\,max}$ have been applied. Plyley et al. (20) reported that $\dot{V}O_{2\,max}$ was reduced with deprived sleep, suggesting a shortened time to exhaustion and an impaired endurance capability. Mougin et al. (23) supported these observations, also reporting a higher lactate accumulation as well as reduced $\dot{V}O_{2\,max}$ after partial sleep loss. There was no drop in the maximal exercise intensity at which the peak $\dot{V}O_2$ was attained. These latter findings raise questions about the potential confounding influence of nutritional support (if any) during the periods of deprived sleep, since only moderate alterations to macronutrient intake can affect blood lactate responses to exercise (33). A question remains about the relative contribution of aerobic and anaerobic energy sources to performance in such progressive incremental tests.

A reduction in $\dot{V}O_{2\,max}$ without a decrease in the total work performed might reflect a shift from aerobic to anaerobic energy. Hill et al. (34) examined the effect of total sleep deprivation on the contributions of the aerobic and anaerobic systems to the performance of all-out exercise. For 3 days after 1 sleepless night, neither men nor women showed a decrease in the amount of work performed in short all-out bouts of exercise on a cycle ergometer. Although there was a tendency toward a reduction in $\dot{V}O_{2\,max}$ which failed to reach statistical significance, the contributions of the anaerobic and aerobic energy systems to the high-intensity exercise were unaffected by the sleep deprivation. Mougin et al. (22) measured seven endurance athletes on a cycle ergometer and suggested that even a partial night's sleep loss may impair aerobic pathways.

Similar to the $\dot{V}O_{2\,max}$ findings, muscular power has been found to be decreased (32,35–37) and to be unchanged (34,36) after various degrees of sleep deprivation. As with $\dot{V}O_{2\,max}$, much of the result depends on the study design. Takeuchi et al. (36) discovered differential effects in the same study. After 64 hr of sleep deprivation, vertical jump was reduced 5%, slow-knee-extension torque was reduced 20% but grip strength and peak torque leg extension were unchanged.

Endurance and time to exhaustion are also important components of athletic performance. Decreases in either measure were observed in several studies (19,21,38–42). Holland (38) noted a 10% reduction in work performed during all-out cycle ergometer exercise after 24 hr of sleep deprivation. Brodan and Kuhn (39) evaluated subjects ($n = 7$, sleep debt = 120 hr) with the Harvard step test (reflects cardiorespiratory endurance and recovery) and revealed adaptation during the test but impaired recovery. Martin (41) utilized treadmill testing at 80% $\dot{V}O_{2\,max}$ and found decreased time to exhaustion, increased perceived exertion, and increased minute ventilation ($n = 8$, sleep debt = 36 hr). Martin and Chen (42) revealed a 20% reduction in time to exhaustion after 50 hr of sleep deprivation. Decreased time to exhaustion after 30 hr of sleep deprivation has been demonstrated even when subjects were allowed caffeine intake (21).

Nevertheless, there are studies showing no change in endurance and time to exhaustion (29,32,35,43). The degree of sleep restriction in studies showing no change in endurance has ranged from only a few hours each night up to 60 hr of total sleep deprivation. These findings may have something to tell about the commitment of the participants to engage in endurance exercise. In a study of one participant exercising nonstop for 100 hr, performance was at a fixed energy expenditure (alternating every 20 min between cycling, walking at 5 km/hr and rowing on an ergometer). It was possible to maintain exercise without desisting but visual hallucinations became increasingly common with successive nights (44).

Making the situation even more complex, Chen (21) observed the dissociation of physiological correlates of maximal performance and endurance. One night of sleep deprivation produced decreases in resting values of heart rate, catecholamines, and blood pH whereas minute ventilation and $\dot{V}CO_2$ were increased. Maximal exercise performance was reduced by sleeplessness, and reflected also by decreases in maximal heart rate and peak values for $\dot{V}O_2$ and $\dot{V}CO_2$. There was no significant effect on exercise performance at 75% $W_{max}$ (maximal power output), raising doubts about the voluntary exhaustion required in the progressive incremental test to record maximal physiological variables.

In an elaborate research design, Reilly and Deykin (32) investigated the effects of partial sleep deprivation on a battery of psychomotor, physical working capacity, and subjective-state tests in a group of trained men over 3 nights of sleep loss and a single night of subsequent recovery sleep. A novel feature of the study was the measurement of various performance tasks concomitant with running on a treadmill at 10 km/hr to investigate the effects of exercise as an antidote to sleep loss. In summarizing their observations, Reilly and Deykin concluded that gross motor functions including muscle strength, lung power, and endurance running on a treadmill can remain unaffected by 3 nights of severely restricted sleep. Decrements occurred in a range of psychomotor functions, the majority of which were evident after only 1 night of reduced sleep. Exercise had a beneficial effect on arousal after sleep loss, providing an obvious temporary antidote to counteract falls in mental concentration. All functions monitored were restored to normal after a full night of recovery sleep.

Several elements of performance show more consistent results. Reaction time is characteristically lengthened after sleep deprivation and this result appears to include both physically well trained and untrained subjects (32,45–47). Perceived exertion is increased after sleep deprivation of 30–64 hr (19,20,26,28,31,41). Heart rate, especially peak heart rate, tends to be lower after sleep deprivation, suggestive of an alteration in autonomic drive (21,26,43).

In conclusion, laboratory studies examining sleep deprivation effects on athletic measures are prevalent but results are mixed and require significant extrapolation for application to competitive sport performance. With the exception of the heart rate data (which may prove advantageous to athletes involved in shooting and archery sports), all of these studies showed either no change or significant impairment of performance measures after sleep deprivation. Given this body of evidence, it is highly unlikely any athlete or coach will preferentially choose the sleep-deprived state prior to a meaningful competitive event.

## III. Sleep Deprivation and Athletic Training

### A. Overtraining Syndrome

The physiological similarities between sleep deprivation and the overtraining syndrome (OTS) are not surprising. Simply put, both are due to an imbalance between activity and rest. OTS has been described as one of the most feared complications in competitive athletes (48). OTS is defined as an imbalance between training and recovery, or exercise and exercise capacity, resulting in a sports-specific decrease in performance and disturbance in mood state. Underperformance secondary to OTS can persist despite a period of recovery lasting weeks to months (49,50). The interaction between sleep deprivation and OTS has not been formally investigated but some research suggests a link.

For example, Lehmann et al. (51) reviewed overtraining in endurance athletes. They examined the literature for cardiopulmonary, blood-chemical, neuroendocrine, and muscular markers of OTS. Likewise, Urhausen and Kindermann (48) in a more recent review, also examined the available tools for diagnosing OTS, such as hormone assays, metabolic markers, immunological parameters, and respiratory-exchange ratios. Although there are no singularly reliable predictive measures of OTS, some typical abnormalities are present. These abnormalities share some similarities with those found after sleep deprivation, such as impaired autonomic, immune, metabolic, hypothalamic, and neurochemical function (49,52–57). The overlap of physiological abnormalities found after sleep deprivation and in the OTS suggests a possible common pathway.

Additionally, Urhausen and Kindermann's 2002 extensive review revealed that one of the four best tools for predicting OTS was a report of sleep disturbances (48). This agreed with previous investigations by Hooper et al. (58). They discovered athletes' ratings of sleep at midseason predicted the staleness score (i.e., overtraining) before the deterioration in performance became apparent several weeks later in the season. As an aside, it is possible to reflect at this point on the high prevalence of increased ratings of perceived exertion by athletes during sleep deprivation (19,20,26,28,41). Perhaps it represents an inherent protective mechanism against the damage of OTS as sleep deprivation progresses.

### B.   Optimal Training Load

Evidence describing the impairment of $\dot{V}O_{2\,max}$, anaerobic power, and endurance secondary to various degrees of sleep deprivation is noted above. These adverse effects may be relevant to training as well. Wilson et al. (59) studied three different training modalities and found that the experimental group that trained with the load that maximized mechanical power garnered the greatest enhancement of dynamic athletic performance with significant ($p < .05$) improvement in most tests. If sleep deprivation limits maximal power, it limits maximal load and therefore limits development of dynamic athletic performance.

Further evidence of the importance of maximizing power and endurance during training is incorporated in the official position statement of the American College of Sports Medicine regarding progression models in resistance training (60). It is clear throughout the pronouncement that optimal characteristics of strength-specific programs include maximal loading, repetitive sets, and then 2–10% increases in load upon successful completion of each new load level. This same general recommendation was made at the U.S. Olympic Committee (USOC) Human Performance Summit in 2000 on Power and Speed (61) and in other articles (62–65).

Training loads may be considered cognitive in addition to physical. Cognitive training is dependent upon learning, which, in turn, has often been linked to sleep (66,67). Evidence supports a role for sleep in the consolidation of general learning and memory tasks (66) as well as more specific sequential motor tasks and motor skill memory, including a reduction in error rates (67). A 20% increase in motor speed without loss of accuracy has been noted after a night of sleep compared to no sleep (68). High-level cognitive and sensory processing and cognitive throughput, a measure of processing speed, are adversely affected by sleep deprivation (69–71). Clearly, these skills are essential in training for team sports and performances that rely on decision making and strategy.

While athletes may be able to overcome the adverse effects of sleep loss in single all-out efforts, they may be unable or unwilling to maintain a high level of performance in repeated exercise bouts such as those that occur in extended training sessions. Reilly and Piercy (37) focused on weight-lifting tasks, using typical weight-training exercise as maximal lifts and a psychophysical approach toward assessing repeated submaximal efforts. There was no significant effect of sleep loss on performance of maximal biceps curl but a significant effect was noted on maximal bench press, leg press, and dead lift. Trend analysis indicated decreased performance in submaximal lifts for all four tasks: the deterioration was significant after the second night of sleep loss. These changes are evident in the perception of effort—whether rated for breathing, muscles or general—as indicated by the responses to biceps curl (Fig. 2a) and dead lift (Fig. 2b). Results indicate that submaximal lifting tasks are more affected by sleep loss than are maximal efforts, particularly for the first 2 nights of successive sleep restriction. The observations highlighted that the greatest impairments were found the later in the protocol that the lifts were performed, indicating a cumulative fatigue effect accruing during the training session due to sleep loss (Fig. 3).

## C. Doping

Ergogenic aids purport to increase energy production and efficiency and improve athletic training and performance. One article estimated that 1–3 million athletes in the United States have used anabolic steroids (72). Recombinant human growth hormone is one of the most popular performance enhancing drugs used by athletes (73,74). Androstenedione use in baseball players is commonly cited by the news media. The list goes on. Given the potential benefits and extremely low apparent risk, it will be interesting to see whether athletes ever view optimal sleep as a natural doping agent. Alternatively, they may be more likely to use central-nervous-system stimulants to counteract effects of sleep loss.

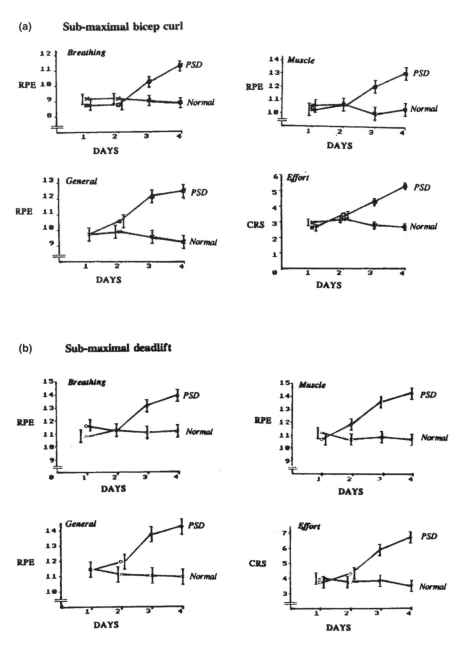

**Figure 2**  Perceived exertion (RPE) during sustained biceps curl (a) and deadlift (b), rated for breathing, muscle, and general whole-body feeling. The CRS scale refers to category ratio. Day 1 indicates a baseline day after a normal sleep, and PSD refers to partial sleep deprivation. (From Ref. 37.)

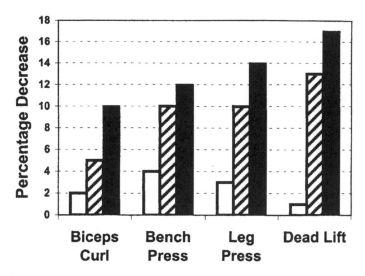

**Figure 3**  Percentage decreases in weight lifted, compared to baseline, over 4 days of partial sleep deprivation. White—day 2; black and white—day 3; black—day 4. (Adapted from Ref. 37.)

## IV.  Sleep Deprivation and Athletic Injuries

Athletic injuries impair performance, prolong training and, at worst, end careers or even lives. Avoiding injury is critical to athletic performance, except in those extremely rare examples where the adversity of injury propels an athlete beyond even his/her own personal best. Sleep deprivation is commonly cited as a precipitating or causal factor in accidents and injuries (see Chaps. 10, 12, 14, and 15). It is therefore curious to discover that there is essentially no scientific research on sleep deprivation and athletic injury. Lund (75) followed 12 volleyball players over 61 hr of sleep deprivation. There were 29 minor injuries, which seemed elevated, but there was no control group for comparison.

Military studies do not involve athletes although they may provide a close approximation given the degree of physical exertion and relative good health/fitness associated with this population. Burgess (76) recorded injuries to cadets from 1994 to 1997 and identified four main causes of injury, one of which was lack of sleep. Miser et al. (77) followed 471 Rangers during Operation Just Cause (December 1989–January 1990) and found an astounding 35% casualty rate. They also discovered that the majority of these soldiers went into battle with little sleep. Most injuries were musculoskeletal in nature (e.g., sprains). Salter et al. (78) performed an in-depth investigation of sleep-related injuries in the U.S. Army between 1984 and 1991. However, these injuries were due to sleeping in the wrong place, at the wrong time and, for example, being accidentally run over by machinery. One interesting aside in the research was that the average duration of the last sleep period prior to the accident occurring was only 5.1 hr. Perhaps the error in judging a "safe" place to sleep was due in part to sleep deprivation.

Illness is not considered injury, but it shares similar adverse effects on athletic training and performance. It is doubtful any athlete would choose to have the flu during competition. Sleep deprivation and human immune function has been extensively researched and reviewed (79). Significant detrimental effects on immune function have been demonstrated after both complete and partial sleep deprivation (56,79). The interactions are complex. Some sleep deprivation and strenuous exercise may even enhance certain aspects of immune function (80). This represents yet another area of much-anticipated research and potential impairment to athletic performance.

At least one study examining athletic injuries cited the importance of appropriate rest periods and even noted increases in injuries when appropriate rest was less likely to occur (81). Others do not even mention the confounds of sleep and rest (82,83). In a PubMed search on injuries and sports (August 2002), only 4 of 14,529 articles listed had any information directly related to sleep.

## V.  Discussion

Approximately 2300 years ago Sun Tzu wrote *The Art of War* and described the importance of avoiding fatigue in military conflict (84). Over 100 years ago, Patrick and Gilbert published research findings of significant changes in muscular strength after sleep deprivation (1). Every human seems to have an intuitive sense that, at some point, sleep is required to reverse the deterioration of performance due to sleep deprivation. Yet there remain the contradictory findings reviewed in this chapter. Here are a few thoughts about this conundrum.

First, the circadian and homeostatic drives of sleep must be separated to accurately examine the effects of either. Although the forced desynchrony protocol (3,4) accomplishes this goal, no study to our knowledge has utilized this technique in athletes. Nearly all studies reviewed herein tested subjects during the day (sleep deprivation durations of 24, 30, 36, 50, 60, 72, and 120 hr), which may have significantly skewed the results. Circadian rhythms have been demonstrated in anaerobic power and capacity, reaction time, speed, accuracy, etc., with many showing a peak in the late afternoon, and early evening and a nadir in the very-early-morning hours (85–90). Fluctuation in measured performance can range 5–10% throughout the 24-hr period (87). Precise conclusions cannot be drawn in the face of this continued confound. Compared to homeostatic physiology, circadian rhythm physiology may hold greater athletic performance enhancement potential, and may be more practically applied to athletes (91).

Complete sleep deprivation is difficult to verify without objective measurement. Only one study employed polysomnograms to assess sleep and that involved partial sleep deprivation (92). Most studies used the honor system or third-party observers to verify sleep deprivation. This may be a fatal flaw as ultrashort sleep strategies, microsleeps, and napping temper the effects of sleep deprivation (93–95; see also Chap. 22). The imprecision of ensuring sleep deprivation in these studies on athletes is highlighted by research demonstrating dose-response relationships between sleep deprivation and human vigilance/alertness, which have been described with less than 8 hr variance in sleep loss (96).

Contradictory findings are bound to occur when study protocols differ so dramatically. For example, level of fitness has ranged from physically untrained subjects (25) to elite athletes (13,91). The type of sport also varied widely, from sailing (9) to weight lifting (37). Perhaps most poignantly, the duration of sleep deprivation ranged from 1 night of partial deprivation (30) to 120 hr of complete sleep loss (39).

In other studies of sleep deprivation the adverse effects on general human performance were dependent upon time-on-task. Duration of testing was often only a few minutes in the athletic performance tests reviewed. Cognitive performance is particularly sensitive to time-on-task testing after sleep deprivation. No study has directly examined cognitive athletic performance, let alone across various time frames. Results of Reilly and Piercy (37) suggest time-on-task is an important differentiator both physically and cognitively.

Notwithstanding, sleep deprivation tends to have greater adverse effects on the older adult. With the exception of one protocol (40), all of these studies were limited to young adults, which creates potential inaccuracies when extrapolating to the youth soccer league or the aging baby boomer who runs marathons. Optimal performance is important to athletes of all ages and abilities.

Other variables abundantly contribute to disagreement and inconsistencies among the data collected (Table 1). For example, during field studies confounds

**Table 1** Effects of Sleep Loss on Athletic Performance May Depend on a Host of Factors

- Circadian phase
- Degree of sleep deprivation
- Motivation
- Physical/cognitive ratio of task/sport
- Duration of task/sport
- Complexity of task/sport
- Degree of exertion
- Level of fitness
- Interindividual differences
- Intraindividual differences
- Body temperature
- Pharmacological compounds (caffeine)
- Type/stage of sleep deprivation
- Napping
- Energy deficit
- Environmental stress
- Previous experience
- Gender
- Age

such as home field advantage, weather, injuries, playing-surface conditions, etc. are clearly present. Data variance originates from significant interindividual and even intraindividual differences in gross mechanical efficiency (25) and an athlete's response to sleep disturbances (13,41,97). Male and female athletes may be differentially affected by sleep deprivation (29,34,47). Caffeine, which has cognitive alerting effects and some possible ergogenic effects as well (98), was allowed in some studies but not in others. Increased body temperature has been shown to correlate with improved performance and alertness (99). Subjects cannot easily be blinded to their own sleep deprivation. Exercise itself may have a disruptive effect on the sleep period after the exercise depending on its intensity (100–102) and thereby act as an additional confound. In studies of partial sleep deprivation, the researcher is frustrated by the reality that there is no effective placebo.

Performance effects may also depend on the particular sleep stage that is being deprived (68). In addition, and as originally noted in rat studies, the measured adverse effect of sleep deprivation may be in part due to the act and method of sleep depriving the animal rather than the sleep deprivation itself (54). Finally, nearly all studies reviewed herein utilized small numbers of subjects, which invites inconsistency when comparing data or applying the findings to larger populations.

Laboratory testing has fewer confounds but is often less accurately reflective of actual event performance. Field testing during a competitive event has many more confounds, yet captures the all-important aspects of maximal effort and pure applicability. Study designs incorporating the strengths of each approach (91) will likely bring greater clarity to the fundamental question *"At what point does sleep deprivation become detrimental to athletic performance?"*

## VI.  Conclusions

Athletes are evidently capable of tolerating tortuous degrees of sleep deprivation and physical exertion during meaningful competitive events. They are also bound by the limits of human physiology, including those of sleep, as fully described in this chapter.

Both partial and complete sleep deprivation have plausible adverse effects on athletic performance, training, and injuries. Research conclusions range widely from no effects to very significant effects, with the absence of any study describing beneficial effects after sleep deprivation. Therefore, an optimal sleep strategy clearly represents a potential performance advantage for athletes.

### References

1.    Patrick GTW, Gilbert JA. On the effects of loss of sleep. Psycholo Rev 1896; 3:469–483.

2.  Minetti AE, Ardigo LP. Biomechanics: Halteres used in ancient Olympic long jump. Nature 2002;420:141–142.
3.  Czeisler CA, Duffy JF, Shanahan TL, Brown EN, Mitchell JF, Rimmer DW, Rhonda JM, Silva EJ, Allan JS, Emens JS, Dijk DJ, Kronauer RE. Stability, precision, and near-24-hour period of the human circadian pacemaker. Science 1999; 284:2177–2181.
4.  Dijk DJ, Duffy JF, Czeisler CA. Circadian and sleep/wake dependent aspects of subjective alertness and cognitive performance. J Sleep Res 1992; 1:112–117.
5.  Smith RS, Walsh J, Dement WC. Sleep deprivation and the Race Across America (abstr). Sleep 1998; 22(S1):303.
6.  Edinger JD, Marsh GR, McCall WV, Erwin CW, Lininger AW, Daytime functioning and nighttime sleep before, during, and after a 146-hour tennis match. Sleep 1990; 13:526–532.
7.  Reilly T, Walsh TJ. Physiological, psychological and performance measures during an endurance record for 5-a-side soccer play. Bri J Sports Med 1981; 15:122–128.
8.  Colquhoun WP. Biological Rhythms and Human Performance. New York: Academic Press, 1971.
9.  Bennet G. Medical and psychological problems in the 1972 singlehanded transatlantic yacht race. Lancet 1973; 2(7832):747–754.
10. Reilly T, George A. Urinary phenythylamine levels during three days of indoor soccer play. J Sports Sci 1983; 1:70.
11. Sinnerton SA, Reilly T. Effects of sleep loss and time of day in swimmers. In: MacLaren D, Reilly T, Lees A, eds. Biomechanics and Medicine in Swimming. Swimming Science IV. 1992:399–405.
12. Horne JA. Why We Sleep. Oxford: Oxford University Press, 1988.
13. Smith RS, Yang CK, Kim BH. Jet lag and the Atlanta Olympic Games (abstr). Sleep Res 1997; 26:754.
14. Guezennec CY, Satabin P, Legrend H, Bigard AX. Physical performance and metabolic changes induced by combined prolonged exercise and different energy intake in humans. Eur J Appli Physiol 1994; 68:525–530.
15. Rognum TO, Vartdel F, Rodahl K, Opstad PK, Knudson-Baes O, Kindt E, Withey WR. Physical and mental performance of soldiers during prolonged heavy exercise combined with sleep deprivation. Ergonomics 1986; 29:859–867.
16. Myles WS Romer TT. Self-paced work in sleep deprived subjects. Ergonomics 1987; 30:1175–1184.
17. How JM, Foo SC, Low E, Wong TM, Vijayan A, Siew MG, Kanapathy R. Effect of total sleep deprivation on performance of naval seamen: Total sleep deprivation on performance. Ann Acad Med 1994;23: 669–675.
18. Froberg JE, Karlsson CG, Levi L, Lidberg L. Circadian rhythms of catecholamine excretion, shooting range performance and self-ratings of fatigue during sleep deprivation. Biol Psychol 1975; 2:175–188.
19. Bond V, Balkissoon B, Franks BD, Brwnlow R, Caprarola M, Bartley D, Banks M. Effects of sleep deprivation on performance during submaximal and maximal exercise. J Sports Med 1986; 26:169–174.
20. Plyley MJ, Shepard RJ, Davis GM, Goode RC. Sleep deprivation and cardiorespiratory function—influence of intermittent submaximal exercise. Eur J Appl Physiol 1987; 56:338–344.

21.  Chen HI. Effects of 30-h sleep loss on cardiorespiratory functions at rest and in exercise. Med Sci Sports Exerc 1991; 23:193–198.

22.  Mougin F, Davenne D, Simon-Rigaud ML, Renaud A,Garnier A, Magnin P. Disturbance of sports performance after partial sleep deprivation. CR Seances Soc Biol Fil 1989; 183:461–466.

23.  Mougin F, Simon-Rigaud ML, Davenne D, Renaud A, Garnier A, Kantelip JP, Magnin P. Effects of sleep disturbances on subsequent physical performance. Eur J Appl Physiol Occup Physiol 1991; 63:77–82.

24.  Martin BJ. Sleep loss and subsequent exercise performance. Acta Physiol Scand 1988; 133(suppl):28–32.

25.  Horne JA, Pettitt AN. Sleep deprivation and the physiological response to exercise under steady state conditions in untrained subjects. Sleep 1984; 7:168–179.

26.  Martin BJ, Gaddis GM. Exercise after sleep deprivation. Med Sci Sports Exerc 1981; 13:220–223.

27.  McMurray RG, Brown CF. The effect of sleep loss on high intensity exercise and recovery. Aviat Space Environ Med 1984;55: 1031–1035.

28.  Symons JD, Vanhelder T, Myles WS. Physical performance and physiological responses following 60 hours of sleep deprivation. Med Sci Sports Exerc 1988; 20:374–380.

29.  Goodman J, Radomshi M, Hart L, Plyley M, Shephard RJ. Maximal aerobic exercise following prolonged sleep deprivation. Int J Sports Med 1989; 10:419–423.

30.  Mougin F, Bourdin H, Simon-Rigaud ML, Didier JM, Toubin G, Kantelip JP. Effects of a selective sleep deprivation on subsequent anaerobic performance. Int J Sports Med 1996; 17:115–119.

31.  VanHelder T, Radomski MW. Sleep deprivation and the effect on exercise performance. Sports Med 1989; 7:235–247.

32.  Reilly T, Deykin T. Effects of partial sleep loss on subjective states, psychomotor and physical performance tests. J Hum Move Stud 1983; 9:157–170.

33.  Reilly T, Woodbridge V. Effects of moderate dietary manipulation on swim performance and on blood lactate—swimming velocity curves. Int J Sports Med 1999; 20:93–97.

34.  Hill DW, Borden DO, Darnaby KM, Hendricks DN. Aerobic and anaerobic contributions to exhaustive high intensity exercise after sleep deprivation. J Sports Sci 1994; 12:455–461.

35.  Bulbulian R, Heaney JH, Leake CN, Sucec AA, Sjoholm NT. The effect of sleep deprivation and exercise load on isokinetic strenght and endurance. Eur J Appl Physiol 1996; 73:273–277.

36.  Takeuchi L, Davis EM, Plyley M, Goode R, Shephard RJ. Sleep deprivation, chronic exercise and muscular performance. Ergonomics 1985; 28:591–601.

37.  Reilly T, Piercy M. The effect of partial sleep deprivation on weight-lifting performance. Ergonomics 1994; 37:107–115.

38.  Holland GJ. Effects of limited sleep deprivation on performacnce of selected motor tasks. Res Q 1968; 39:285–294.

39.  Brodan V, Kuhn E. Physical performance in man during sleep deprivation. J Sports Med 1967; 7:28–30.

40.  Copes K, Rosentswieg J. The effects of sleep deprivation upon motor performance of ninth-grade students. J Sports Med Phys Fitness 1972; 12:47–53.

41. Martin BJ. Effect of sleep deprivation on tolerance of prolonged exercise. Eur J Appl Physiol 1981; 47:345–354.
42. Martin BJ, Chen H. Sleep loss and the sympathoadrenal response to exercise. Med Sci Sports Exerc 1984; 16:56–59.
43. Pickett GF, Morris AF. Effects of acute sleep and food deprivation on total body response time and cardiovascular performance. J Sports Med 1975; 15:49–56.
44. Thomas V, Reilly T. Circulatory, psychological and performance variables during 100 hours of paced continuous exercise under conditions of controlled energy intake and work output. J Hum Move Stud 1995; 1:149–155.
45. Dinges DF, Pack F, Williams K, Gillen KA, Powell JW, Ott GE, Aptowicz C, Pack AI. Cumulative sleepiness, mood disturbance, and psychomotor vigilance performance decrements during a week of sleep restriction to 4–5 hours per night. Sleep 1997; 20:267–277.
46. Powell NB, Schechtman KB, Riley RW, Li K, Troell R, Guilleminault C. The road to danger: the comparative risks of driving while sleepy. Laryngoscope 2001; 111:887–93.
47. Reilly T, Hales AJ. Effects of partial sleep deprivation on performance measures in females. In: Megaw ED, ed. Contemporary Ergonomics: Proceedings of the Ergonomics Society's Annual Conference. London: Taylor & Francis, 1988:505–515.
48. Urhausen A, Kindermann W. Diagnosis of overtraining: what tools do we have? Sports Med 2002; 32:95–102.
49. Lehmann M, Foster C, Dickhuth HH, Gastmann U. Autonomic imbalance hypothesis and overtraining syndrome. Med Sci Sports Exerc 1998; 30:1140–1145.
50. Fry RW, Morton AR, Keast D. Overtraining in athletes. Sports Med 1991; 12:32–65.
51. Lehmann M, Foster C, Keul J. Overtraining in endurance athletes: a brief review. Med Sci Sports Exerc 1993;25:854–862.
52. MacKinnon LT. Special feature for the Olympics: effects of exercise on the immune system: overtraining effects on immunity and performance in athletes. Immunol Cell Biol 2000; 78:502–509.
53. Krueger JM, Obal FJ, Fang J, Kubota T, Taishi P. The role of cytokines in physiological sleep regulation. Ann NY Acad Sci 2001; 933:211–221.
54. Rechtschaffen A, Bergmann BM, Everson CA, Kushida CA, Gilliland MA. Sleep deprivation in the rat. X. Integration and discussion of the findings. Sleep 1989; 12:68–87.
55. Kato M, Phillips BG, Sigurgsson G, Narkiewicz K, Pesek CA, Somers VK. Effects of sleep deprivation on neural circulatory control. Hypertension 2000; 35:1173–1175.
56. Rogers NL, Szuba MP, Staab JP, Evans DL, Dinges DF. Neuroimmunologic aspects of sleep and sleep loss. Semin Clin Neuropsychiatry 2001; 6:295–307.
57. Mougin F, Bourdin H, Simon-Rigaud ML, Nguyen NU, Kantelip JP, Davenne D. Hormonal responses to exercise after partial sleep deprivation and after a hypnotic drug-induced sleep. J Sports Sci 2001; 19:89–97.
58. Hooper SL, Traeger-Mackinnon L, Howard A, Gordon RD, Bachmann AW. Markers for monitoring overtraining and recovery. Med Sci Sports Exerc 1995; 27:106–112.

59. Wilson GJ, Newton RU, Murphy AJ, Humphries BJ. The optimal training load for the development of dynamic athletic performance. Med Sci Sports Exerc 1993; 25:1279–1286.

60. Kraemer WJ, Adams K, Cafarelli E, Dudley GA, Dooly C, Feigenbaum GA, Fleck SJ, Franklin B, Fry AC, Hoffman JR, Newton RU, Potteiger J, Stone MH, Ratamess NA, Triplett-McBride T. Progression models in resistance training for healthy adults. Med Sci Sports Exerc 2002; 34:364–380.

61. Skinner J, Lawson E, Hoffman J, Newton R, Chrosslian D, Kramer B, Turin J, Dudley G, Fleck S. Power and speed: getting faster, jumping higher, being stronger. Human Performance Summit, USOC/ACSM.Indianapolis, Indiana, June 4, 2000.

62. Foster C, Daines E, Hector L, Snyder AC, Welsh R. Athletic performance in relation to training load. Wisc Med J 1996; 95:370–374.

63. Cronin J, McNair PJ, Marshall RN. Developing explosive power: a comparison of technique and training. J Sci Med Sport 2001; 4:59–70.

64. Hostler D, Crill MT, Hagerman FC, Staron RS. The effectiveness of 0.5–lb increments in progressive resistance exercise. J Strength Cond Res 2001; 15:86–91.

65. McBride JM, Triplett-McBride T, Davie A, Newton RU. The effect of heavy vs. light load jump squats on the development of strenght, power and speed. J Strength Cond Res 2002; 16:75–82.

66. Stickgold R, Hobson JA, Fosse R, Fosse M. Sleep, learning and dreams: off-line memory reprocessing. Science 2001; 294:1052–1057.

67. Fischer S, Hallschmid M, Elsner AL, Born J. Sleep forms memory for finger skills. Proc Natl Acad Sci USA 2002; 99:11987–11991.

68. Walker MP, Brakefield T, Morgan A, Hobson JA, Stickgold R. Practice with sleep makes perfect: sleep-dependent motor skill learning. Neuron 2002; 35:205–211.

69. Thomas M, Sing H, Belenky G, Holcomb H, Mayberg H, Dannals R, Wagner H, Thorne D, Popp K, Rowland L, Welsh A, Balwinski S, Redmond D. Neural basis of alertness and cognitive performance impairments during sleepiness. I. Effects of 24 h of sleep deprivation on waking human regional brain activity. J Sleep Res 2000; 9:335–352.

70. Monk TH, Carrier J. Speed of mental processing in the middle of the night. Sleep 1997; 20:399–401.

71. Jewett ME, Kronauer RE. Interactive mathematical models of subjective alertness and cognitive throughput in humans. J Biol Rhythms 1999; 14:588–601.

72. Silver MD. Use of ergogenic aids by athletes. J Am Acad Orthop Surg 2001; 9:61–70.

73. Bidlingmaier M, Wu Z, Strasburger CJ. Doping with growth hormone. J Pediatr Endocrinol Metab 2001; 14:1077–1083.

74. Jenkins PJ. Growth hormone and exercise: physiology, use and abuse. Growth Horm IGF Res 2001; 11 (suppl):S71–77.

75. Lund PM. Marathon volleyball: changes after 61 hours play. Br J Sports Med 1985;19:228–229.

76. Burgess JE. Analysis of Y listings and medical discharges of officer cadets at RMAS from January 1994 to May 1997, with actions to prevent injuries. JR Army Med Corps 1998; 144:152–155.

77. Miser WF, Doukas WC, Lillegard WA. Injuries and illnesses incurred by an army ranger unit during Operation Just Cause. Mil Med 1995; 160:373–380.

78. Salter CA, Crowley JS, Allan LW. Sleep-related injuries in the US Army, 1984–1991. Mil Med 1993; 158:782–785.
79. Dinges DF, Douglas SD, Hamarman S, Zaugg L, Kapoor S. Sleep deprivation and human immune function. Adv Neuroimmunol 1995; 5:97–110.
80. Boyum A, Wiik P, Gustavsson E, Veiby OP, Reseland J, Haugen AH, Opstad PK. The effect of strenuous exercise, caloric deficiency and sleep deprivation on white blood cells, plasma immunoglobulins and cytokines. Scand J Immunol 1996; 43:228–235.
81. Sands WA, Shultz BB, Newman AP. Women's gymnastics injuries, a 5–year study. Am J Sports Med 1993; 21:271–276.
82. Knapik JJ, Jones BH, Bauman CL, Harris JM. Strength, flexibility and athletic injuries. Sports Med 1992; 14:277–288.
83. Caine D, Cochrane B, Caine C, Zemper E. An epidemiologic investigation of injuries affecting young competitive female gymnasts. Am J Sports Med 1989; 17:811–820.
84. Griffith SB. Sun Tzu, The Art of War. Oxford: Oxford University Press, 1963.
85. Winget CM, DeRoshia CW, Holly DC. Circadian rhythms and athletic performance. Med Sci Sports Exerc 1985; 17:498–516.
86. Shephard RJ. Circadian rhythms and the athlete. Can J Sport Sci 1991; 16:5–6.
87. Hill DW, Smith JC. Circadian rhythm in anerobic power and capacity. Can J Sports Sci 1991; 16:30–32.
88. Baxter C, Reilly T. Influence of time of day on all-out swimming. Br J Sports Med 1983; 17:122–127.
89. Smith RS, Jamieson M, Dement WC. A comparison of peak performance, competition, and training times in elite athletes (abstr). Sleep Res 1996; 25:574.
90. Callard D, Gauthier A, Maffiuletti N, Davenne D, Van Hoecke J. Circadian fluctuations in the muscular efficiency of athletes: with sleep versus sleep deprivation. J Soc Biol 2000; 194:165–169.
91. Smith RS, Guilleminault C, Efron B. Circadian advantage and peak athletic performance in the National Football League. Sleep 1997; 20:362–365.
92. Mougin F, Simon-Rigaud ML, Davenne D, Bourdin H, Guilland JC, Kantelip JP, Magnin P. Tolerance to exertion after sleep reduction and after taking a hypnotic: zolpidem. Arch Int Physiol Biochim Biophys 1992; 100:255–262.
93. Koslowsky M, Babkoff H. Meta-analysis of the relationship between total sleep deprivation and performance. Chronobiol Int 1992; 9:132–136.
94. Reilly T, Atkinson G, Waterhouse, J. Chronobiology and physical performance. In: Garrett WE Jr, Kirkendall DT, eds. Exercise and Sport Science. Philadelphia: Lippincott Williams & Wilkins, 2000:351–372.
95. Rosekind MR, Smith RM, Miller DL, Co EL, Gregory KB, Webbon LL, Gander PH, Lebacqz JV. Alertness management: strategic naps in operational settings. J Sleep Res 1995; 4:62–66.
96. Jewett ME, Dijk DJ, Kronauer RE, Dinges DF. Dose-respose relationship between sleep deprivation and human psychomotor vigilance and subjective alertness. Sleep 1999; 22:171–179.
97. Meney I, Waterhouse J, Atkinson G, Reilly T, Davenne D. The effect of one night's sleep deprivation on the temperature, mood, and physical performance in subjects with different amounts of habitual physical acivity. Chronobiol Int 1998; 15:349–363.

98.  Graham TE. Caffeine and exercise: metabolism, endurance and performance. Sports Med 2001; 31:785–807.
99.  Wright KP Jr, Hull JT, Czeisler CA. Relationship between alertness, performance and body temperature in humans. Am J Physiol Regul Integr Comp Physiol 2002 (epub ahead of print).
100.  Driver HS, Rogers GG, Mitchell D, Borrow SJ, Allen M, Luus HG, Shapiro CM. Prolonged endurance exercise and sleep disruption. Med Sci Sports Exerc 1994; 26:903–907.
101.  Browman CP. Sleep following sustained exercise. Psychophysiology 1980; 17:577–580.
102.  Shapiro CM. Sleep and the athlete. Br J Sports Med 1981; 15:51–55.

# 18

# Medical Resident/Physician Performance

**JUDITH A. OWENS**

**Rhode Island Hospital, Providence, Rhode Island, U.S.A.**

*I always had a prior theory that when you look up all the old sixties research, how do you brainwash someone? You sleep deprive them. That's number one, two, and three. Sleep deprive them. You feed them bad food and you repeat things over and over again. It's like, that kind of covers residency*

—Surgical resident, 2001

## I. Introduction

It is clear that acute and chronic sleep loss, whether partial or complete, substantially impairs physical, cognitive, and emotional functioning. Memory, vigilance, mental processing of complex information, and decision-making skills represent only a few of the cognitive domains integral to adequate performance of daily tasks that are negatively impacted upon by inadequate sleep. In addition, substantial evidence suggests that the detrimental effects on performance resulting from even modest amounts of sleep loss over time, or "sleep debt," may be cumulative. Equal consideration must also be given to the influence of human circadian physiology, which dictates both that wakefulness and alertness are for the most part at optimal levels during daylight hours, and that sleep propensity is maximized at night. It follows that the increase in sleepiness and fatigue levels and decline in waking function that are the outcomes of the failure to adhere to this need for both appropriately timed and adequate amounts of sleep are particularly relevant in the context of occupational settings.

Yet, these considerations stand in stark contrast to the fact that modern society increasingly measures performance and productivity on a 24-hr basis. The need for round-the-clock operations in many spheres, including manufacturing, transportation, and health care, often takes precedence over the basic physiological principles governing sleep and wakefulness, at times with devastating results. As a result of several highly publicized fatigue-related accidents, and of the increased recognition of the repercussions of prolonged work hours and shift work, both the level of scientific inquiry and the magnitude of public awareness and concern regarding the issue of sleep loss and fatigue in the workplace have significantly increased.

However, despite the fact that few areas of human performance have greater impact on life and death outcomes than physician training and education, the issue of work-related sleep loss and fatigue in the medical profession, particularly during residency training when many would consider both the risks and the stakes to be highest, has until recently received less attention. The health care professions have been slow to acknowledge that physicians and other health care workers are themselves governed by these same circadian rhythms and homeostatic influences, and, as a result, may be compromised in the performance of their professional duties. In particular, the long continuous shifts, reduced opportunities for sleep, and minimal recuperation time traditionally experienced by medical students and house staff during training, and frequently by physicians in practice as well, are likely to impact on their work, health, and well-being, and on the quality of their educational experience. In light of recent advances in circadian and sleep biology, these traditional practices have begun to raise important questions regarding the effects of sleep loss and fatigue on learning, on patient safety and medical errors, and on trainees' lives.

## II. Historical Context

It should be emphasized that to a large extent, progress in addressing the issue of sleep loss and fatigue in medical training has been hampered both by the absence of a coordinated and comprehensive body of research, and by the potential political, professional, and economic repercussions of any proposed systemwide changes in current practice. Despite the fact that substantial empirical evidence has accumulated regarding the effects of sleep loss in general on human performance in the laboratory setting and in other occupational settings, the specific evidence linking fatigue with performance deficits during medical training, as discussed below, is not only relatively sparse, but also less consistent across studies. Furthermore, it is necessary to view the existing empirical data on sleep and fatigue in medical training within the historical, political, and scientific context in which they have evolved, to fully understand the implications of these findings.

In particular, two separate but related series of developments have converged over the past 15 years to provide the impetus for what is clearly now a heightened interest in this issue. The first development was increasing pressure in the past several years from medical student and resident groups to institute state and federal regulation of work hours as the primary strategy to address sleep loss and fatigue in residents. Although the Accreditation Council for Graduate Medical Education (ACGME), which accredits training programs in the medical specialties through its Residency Review Committees (RRCs), currently requires all institutions that sponsor residency programs to monitor the duty hours of residents, the individual RRCs have varied in their standards related to work hours and programs typically have not lost accreditation solely for work hour violations (1). In September 2001, however, the ACGME charged its Work Group on Resident Duty Hours and the Learning Environment with developing a set of recommendations regarding common requirements for resident duty hours across accredited programs in all medical specialties. These recommendations, which include an 80-hr work week, continuous duty hours limited to 24 hr, and 1 day in 7 free of patient duties, were published in June 2002 and went into effect in every residency program in the United States on July 1, 2003 (2). National medical education organizations have also publicly supported revision of policies on resident work hours; for example, in October 2001 the Association of American Medical Colleges (AAMC) specified that resident physicians should be scheduled for no more than 80 duty hr/week and no more than 24 consecutive duty hr (3).

There have also been attempts to introduce legislation on this issue on the statewide level, although New York is the only state to date that has enacted legislation related to resident work hours. This action evolved from the 1989 recommendations of the Bell Commission, a task force established by the New York State Commissioner of Health to investigate the death of a young woman named Libby Zion at a New York City teaching hospital in 1988. The Bell Commission concluded that trainee fatigue, as well as inadequate supervision, contributed to the adverse outcome in the Zion case, and subsequently recommended limiting trainees to 80 hr on duty per week (averaged over a 4-week period) and 24 consecutive hospital duty hr (4). Reports of widespread violations of the New York regulations and concern about the ability of medical education and professional organizations to enforce compliance with RRC work hour standards eventually helped to prompt the filing of a petition with the Occupational Health and Safety Administration (OSHA) by several trainee groups in the spring of 2001 (5). This petition alleged that excessive work hours were harmful to resident physician health, and requested that OSHA limit work hours to 80/week and limit work shifts to a maximum of 24 hr. Similar requirements were subsequently incorporated into bills introduced in the House of Representatives (H.R. 3236) by Representative John Conyers and in the Senate (S. 2614) by Senator Jon Corzine in 2001–02. This legislation would require hospitals, as a condition for participation in Medicare, to limit resident work hours to 80/week and shifts to 24 hr (for an excellent summary of the similarities and differences among proposed work hour regulations, see Ref. 1).

At the same time that these political developments were occurring, public interest in the issue of sleep loss and fatigue in medical training was galvanized by the National Academy of Sciences Institute of Medicine report *To Err is Human* released in the spring of 2000 (6). This report estimated that as many as 98,000 patients die each year as a result of medical errors occurring in hospitals, and stressed the need to investigate and address human factors that are potentially involved in violations of patient safety, such as sleep deprivation. As a result of the report, a committee was appointed by the Institute of Medicine, which recommended the establishment of a federally funded center for patient safety, and additional federal dollars were allocated to address issues related to preventing medical errors.

Political pressure and public concern alone, however, could not form the basis for a rational and informed discussion of the issue of sleep and fatigue in medical training without the addition of a third element, namely, an expanded understanding of the science of sleep loss and fatigue. The existence of supporting data from research regarding the effects of sleep loss and fatigue in laboratory studies of animals and humans (7–13), from field studies in other occupations, and from studies directly addressing residency training is obviously critical to the formulation of an empirically based approach to this issue. Given this premise, then, *what conclusions may be reasonably drawn from the body of research on this topic that has been conducted in the last several decades?*

## III. Overview of the Literature: Impact of Sleep Loss and Fatigue in Medical Training

The consequences related to sleep loss and shift work in physicians in training, like those in any occupational setting, are potentially broad in scope and are likely to occur in a number of domains. They include personal and family consequences (mood disturbances, increased stress, adverse health consequences, negative effects on personal relationships, increased potential for alcohol and substance abuse, and increased risk of motor vehicle crashes); negative effects on cognitive and neurobehavioral functioning (attention, reaction time, vigilance, memory, as well as motivation); impact on the performance of professional duties (including procedures such as intravenous insertion, cognitive tasks such as electrocardiogram [EKG] interpretation, and patient-related behavior such as communication skills); and implications for the quality of medical education (decreased retention of information, impaired information processing, and decreased motivation to learn). Finally, the net impact of potential deficits related to sleep loss and fatigue in residency training on the quality of patient care and on commission of errors in the hospital setting is of particular concern in this era of increasing accountability in health care.

To date, there are over 50 studies in the literature on sleep loss and fatigue in medical training, including 33 performance studies (14–47) that have examined specific effects on a variety of different performance and performance-related measures. These outcome variables may be broadly categorized as effects on neurocognitive and psychomotor functioning in the laboratory setting, on performance of simulated work-related tasks and of occupational tasks in actual work settings, and on mood and psychological state. The design of most of these studies involves comparisons between precall ("rested") and postcall performance in a group of residents.

Several older review articles (48–50) and a number of more recently published reviews (1,51–54) have attempted to summarize the empirical evidence that exists to date regarding the association between sleep loss and fatigue and a number of these outcome measures, including mood, neurocognitive testing, and work performance of trainees. The authors of all of these reviews largely concur that the evidence linking sleep loss to performance deficits and adverse outcomes in the medical setting, although in many studies quite compelling, may be characterized as inconsistent and inconclusive. Furthermore, they suggest that this result is not surprising, given the wide variation in the methodology, study design, and subject characteristics employed in the studies.

Thus, an important caveat to any overview of studies on sleep and fatigue in medical training, including the summary presented below, is that many of the studies that have been done in this area have substantial methodological weaknesses or design flaws. These include small sample sizes, lack of objective or reliable recording of actual sleep amounts, and use of performance outcome measures that may not be sensitive enough or may not be of adequate duration to detect more subtle levels of impairment. Even more important, most of these studies have not considered the confounding variable of chronic partial sleep deprivation in the research design, and therefore, the validity of any comparisons of performance under conditions of acute sleep restriction ("postcall") versus a "rested baseline" is likely to be compromised by the fact that most resident physicians are routinely functioning under the burden of a considerable chronic sleep debt. Moreover, the different types of outcome measures that have been used to assess the effects of sleep loss and fatigue in these studies, which have ranged from performance on psychometric tests of vigilance and reaction time, to the ability to correctly answer national-board-type questions, to performance on simulated tasks, raise concerns about the potential relevance of some of these measures to actual work performance ("ecological validity"). Alternatively, outcome measures of many potentially significant domains of impact, such as the quality of physician-patient communication and complex problem-solving skills, have not been adequately assessed in any studies.

Furthermore, because many of the outcome measures used in these studies are based on self-report, they are also vulnerable to the frequently found discrepancy between self-assessment of sleepiness/alertness level and actual physiological level of sleepiness on the one hand (10,13) and recall bias on the other; thus results may represent either an underestimation or overestimation of impairment. In addition, the role of such performance-related variables as motivation, reinforcement, feedback during the testing sessions, circadian timing of the testing sessions, and the intrinsic interest and perceived importance of the task itself have largely not been considered in these studies. Finally, very few studies to date have systematically evaluated strategies for fatigue/alertness management, such as "countermeasures" (napping, use of caffeine, etc.) or alternative work hour schedules.

### A.  Extent of Sleep Loss and Fatigue in Medical Trainees

A number of studies have attempted as either a primary or secondary focus to document the quality and quantity of sleep that medical trainees obtain, during both on-call and noncall nights. Results from a number of survey studies utilizing retrospective self-report data suggest that many trainees work more than 80 hr/week, and 100–120 hr work weeks are common (55,56), with higher average work hours in general reported in the surgical specialties (including obstetrics and gynecology) and at more junior levels of training. A number of other survey studies have included retrospective self-report data regarding typical amounts of sleep (or hours of continuous wakefulness) obtained by trainees in various specialties. Results range from 37.6 (SD 9.88) hr as the longest period of time without sleep in a random sample of over 1700 second-year residents (57) to 45.5 (SD 9.3) hr without sleep reported by surgical residents in a survey of interns from a variety of specialties (55). In the latter study, more than 20% of the residents surveyed also reported having gone without sleep for more than 48 hr on at least one occasion. Average total sleep amounts reported in the "on call condition" vary across studies, but are typically in the 2–4 hr range; most studies, however, do not include data on the length of the longest continuous (uninterrupted) sleep period on call.

Several studies (58–60) have utilized more objective measures to assess sleep amounts, including ambulatory EEG monitoring and actigraphy, a wristwatch-like device that monitors sleep-wake cycles, and have found similar levels of sleep deprivation on call. For example, one recent study of internal-medicine residents in a major teaching hospital that utilized ambulatory EEG recording to document sleep amount, found that interns spent an average of less than 5 hr/call night in bed, and obtained an average of 3.7 hr of sleep, well below the 4 hr sleep limit at which many general sleep research studies have documented significant performance impairments (58). Tov et al. (60) used actigraphy monitoring in combination with sleep diaries to compare sleep amounts during "heavy" (HWL) versus "light" (LWL) workload rotations (based on numbers of patients, admissions, and discharges) in 27 Israeli residents. In that study, residents on emergency room rotations obtained the least sleep (3.06 hr) although the average for all HWL residents was only 4.49 hr.

Furthermore, in addition to restricted sleep, many other factors potentially magnify the effects of inadequate sleep in medical trainees. These include frequent interruptions during on-call sleep periods leading to fragmented and poor-quality sleep, shift-work-related interruption of normal circadian sleep-wake rhythms, sleep inertia (characterized by confusion, poor judgment, inappropriate decision making, and impaired recall of events occurring during the immediate awakening period) (61,62), and inadequate postcall or "recovery sleep" (63). For example, in the actigraphy study cited above (60), residents in both workload groups obtained similar amounts of sleep postcall, but these recovery-sleep amounts were not significantly higher than either group's baseline sleep amounts, implying incomplete compensation for sleep loss. Furthermore, only half of the sleep-deprived residents in this study reported using naps as a strategy to compensate for insufficient sleep. In an emergency room study, night shift physicians sleeping during the day slept significantly less (496.6 min vs. 328.5 min) and had less rapid-eye-movement (REM) sleep than day shift workers, similar to what has been documented in other shift work groups (47).

Interestingly, very few studies have attempted to objectively document physiological sleepiness in medical residents as a result of inadequate sleep. One recent study (63), however, used both physiological (Multiple Sleep Latency Tests, MSLT) and subjective (Stanford Sleepiness Scale) measures to document sleepiness levels in a group of 11 anesthesia residents under three conditions: baseline "normal" work schedule, postcall, and after a period of extended sleep. Not only were the residents' postcall MSLT scores below the range typically seen with clinical sleep disorders, but physiological sleepiness levels in the "normal" condition also approached these levels and were not significantly different from those in the post-call condition. Furthermore, residents demonstrated poor ability to subjectively identify the onset of EEG-defined sleep during the MSLT, failing to report themselves as falling asleep almost half of the time that they had actually done so.

In summary, resident physicians, particularly those at more junior levels of training and those in the surgical specialties, routinely experience significant levels of sleep deprivation in the work setting, and are frequently required to function at work under conditions that are likely to lead to compromised levels of alertness.

## B. Effects on Performance

### Cognitive and Neurobehavioral Tasks

A number of studies have been conducted examining the effects of sleep deprivation in medical trainees on performance on a variety of neuropsychological and neurobehavioral tests. Many of these studies have examined the impact of short-term (on call) sleep loss on psychomotor function, sometimes in combination with simulated medical tasks. Reaction time, vigilance, and manual dexterity are among the parameters that have been shown to be negatively impacted by sleep loss in these studies, although these results are not universally found. For example, sleep deprivation in residents has also been associated with reduced performance on memory (14) and cognitive (15) tasks, as well as on tests of grammatical reasoning (16). Leonard et al. (17) found that medical residents' cognitive performance was significantly impaired postcall (average 4.5 hr sleep), while another study of anesthesiology residents (18) demonstrated impairment on a test of creative thought.

One interesting phenomenon that emerges in reviewing the literature on performance is that most of the dozen or so studies specifically examining *surgical residents* have failed to demonstrate significant performance decrements postcall. For example, Deaconson and colleagues studied the performance of 26 surgical residents under similar "rested" and unrested conditions on a 1-hr battery of validated psychomotor tests, controlling for circadian time, learning effect, and motivation (19). There were no overall differences in residents' performances after acute sleep loss. Another study of 42 surgical residents was unable to detect differences on a large battery of cognitive assays, although residents did report more subjective feelings of anger, confusion, and fatigue on the Profile of Mood States (POMS) (20). Reznick and Folse also found minimal effect of acute sleep loss in surgical residents on several neurobehavioral batteries (21), although one study did find differences on a computerized test battery after an on-call weekend (22).

However, because surgical residents may be on-call as frequently as every other night, and typically sleep less on-call than trainees in other specialties, one likely explanation for these findings is that these studies essentially failed to find any differences in performance attributable to 1 night of acute sleep deprivation superimposed on significant, ongoing chronic partial sleep loss. Furthermore, in addition to the limitation regarding the absence of a true "rested" baseline, several of the above studies had significant numbers of subject dropouts, which may have included individuals with greater impairment after sleep loss. It is also possible that some degree of self-selection results in a larger percentage of individuals who have a relatively higher tolerance for sleep loss being more likely to opt for a career in surgery, a factor that has not been well studied.

In summary, generally the speed or efficiency of neurocognitive and psychomotor task completion has been found to be more affected by restricted sleep than has the quality or accuracy of performance, although increased mental effort appears to mitigate these effects in the short term in some studies. Furthermore, studies that utilized tests that involve longer periods of sustained vigilance have been more likely to demonstrate adverse effects of sleep loss.

### Simulated Work Performance

A number of studies have included outcome variables with "real world" medical task components, either simulated or actual (see below) work performance measures. For example, one early study that examined the performance of 14 medical interns on an electrocardiogram (ECG) interpretation task in both the "rested" (mean 7.0 hr of sleep, range 5.5–8.5 hr) and the "sleep-deprived" state (mean 1.8 hr, range 0–3.8 hr) found both efficiency and accuracy of performance were impaired in the sleep-deprived condition (23). In one of the first studies to include some consideration of cumulative sleep debt (16), residents showed a deterioration in performance on a brief (3 min) task involving laboratory report interpretation, but only in association with at least 8 hr of cumulative sleep debt over several days; an increase in variability of performance was demonstrated only in those residents who slept 3 or less hr the previous night. In a more recent study that looked at the effect of training experience (first/second-year residents vs. third/fourth), Lingenfelser et al. examined the performance on a number of psychomotor tasks of residents in the "off-duty" state (at least 6 hr of sleep the previous night) and after 24 hr on-call (24). Performance on a simulated EKG task deteriorated postcall; there was no significant difference in performance between junior and senior residents, suggesting a lack of "adaptation" over time to the sleep-deprived state. However, in another study of pediatric residents that included measurement of performance on both board-type questions and several simulated tasks, including intubation, vein catheterization, and arterial catheterization (25), no significant differences were found after 24 and 36 hr of continued wakefulness on any of the tasks except efficiency of cannulation.

A number of variables, including practice effects and circadian timing of the testing, were potential confounders in many of these studies. In one study of emergency room physicians that did factor in the influence of circadian factors, Smith-Coggins et al. (26) found that accuracy of performance on a simulated intubation task deteriorated over the course of night but not day shifts, and efficiency on the intubation task was compromised on night shifts; however, performance on a case management task was not affected. In a related study that looked at the effectiveness of various countermeasures in mitigating the effects of fatigue in emergency room physicians (47), accuracy and speed of EKG interpretation did not differ between day and night shifts; although efficiency of simulated intubation was compromised on the night shift, performance actually improved over the length of the shift.

In summary, similar to what has been found with performance on neurobehavioral tasks in the laboratory setting, simulated tasks dependent on high and/or sustained levels of vigilance, those of longer duration, and those that involve newly learned procedural skills appear to be more vulnerable to the effects of short-term sleep loss in medical trainees. In addition, efficiency of performance on "real-world" tasks is often sacrificed in favor of preserving accuracy, a factor that could have significant impact in situations that require both speed and precision (intubation of a critically ill patient, for example). There is little evidence in these studies to support "adaptation" to or the development of increased tolerance for the effects of sleep loss over time in medical trainees.

### Clinical Settings

A handful of studies have examined actual work performance of residents in the fatigued state. In one of the only studies to look specifically at a clinical patient evaluation task (27), attending physicians compared the quality of the physician-patient interaction (ratings of clinical interviews and written patient evaluations) of seven medical interns in a standardized patient encounter pre- and postcall and found no significant differences in performance. In another study, the percentage of radiology residents' true-positives and false-positives in detecting pulmonary nodules on a series of radiographs was not different in the rested versus fatigued state; however, no information was included about efficiency of performance (28). Several studies have examined the performance of anesthesia residents and found less efficiency in monitoring anesthesia, especially during the night (64), and residents were also observed to actually fall asleep during anesthesia administration (65,66). Accurate ordering of medications (29) and documentation of medical histories (26) have also been shown to be impaired in both sleep-deprived medical students and physicians.

In a number of studies, surgical residents also appear vulnerable to the effects of short-term sleep loss in one key area, that of manual dexterity and surgical skills. In a very early study, videotapes of operations performed by surgical residents following greater or less than 2 hr sleep were rated on what was termed "operative inefficiency" (30); 30% more time was required because of poorly planned maneuvers in most of the residents. More recently, a large study compared the frequency of significant surgical complications (discussed at morbidity and mortality report) for three different call schedules. Although no differences were found overall among call schedules, complication rates were 45% higher when the resident had been on call the previous night (31). Finally, two recent simulated laparoscopy studies found significantly more errors and more time to perform procedures such as tissue electrocoagulation with increasing sleep loss and on mornings postcall, even in experienced surgeons (32,33).

In summary, although the data are rather sparse, clinical performance in actual medical settings, particularly in surgery and anesthesia, appears to be significantly compromised by degrees of sleep loss typically experienced by residents during training.

### C. Effects on Trainees' Health and Well-Being

*Mood, Stress, Satisfaction*

Negative effects of sleep loss on mood in medical trainees is one of the most consistent findings in the literature on this topic, paralleling what is known about the effects of sleep deprivation in humans in general. For example, a study of 40 junior and senior house staff in Germany documented a clear deterioration in "emotional condition" (increased negative mood) postcall (67). In another study, total and subscale (tension-anxiety, confusion, fatigue, and vigor) scores on the Profile of Mood States (POMS) deteriorated significantly following a 32-hr shift in a group of house officers (17). At least one study has also suggested that these negative mood effects persist for several days postcall (68). It should be noted, however, that in a large survey study of surgical residents (69), despite multiple complaints of exhaustion and sleep loss, feelings of anger, hostility, or discouragement were infrequently reported, and the surgical residents reported less substance use and fewer physical complaints than residents from other specialties. As might be expected, residents also reported that the negative psychological effects of sleep loss frequently took a toll on family life, and on their professional and personal relationships (55). For example, one study that examined the complex interaction between work- and home-related demands (termed "work-home interference") in medical residents (70) found that residents' perception of increased tension between their work and home roles strongly affected their perception of how sleep deprived they were.

Negative mood changes are particularly apparent in studies of emergency medicine residents, for many of whom shift rotations are both frequent and occur in a circadian-disruptive pattern. In one study of six emergency physicians (26) that assessed sleep amounts (sleep logs and ambulatory EEG), mood states, and performance on two simulated tasks (patient triage and intubation) as a function of day and night shift work, night shift physicians rated themselves as more sleepy, less happy, and less clear-thinking. Inadequate postcall or "recovery sleep" may further compromise mood and performance in trainees. Furthermore, the secondary effects of compromised mood may also lead to decreased motivation and initiative in the work setting. Many of these issues were highlighted in a 1998–99 national survey of PGY1 and PGY2 residents, in which these residents also perceived increased conflicts with colleagues and staff, and observed mistreatment of patients as a result of fatigue (57).

### General Health

Residents also report negative effects of sleep loss on their physical health. In one study of house officers in Scotland (71), both the number of hours worked and the number of hours slept while on call were associated with the number of somatic symptoms they reported experiencing over the previous year. In a recent resident survey study (72), sleep loss was associated with self-reported increased stress, accidents, and injuries, and alcohol and stimulant use; sleep loss was correlated with stress and illness and injury levels, and with reported significant weight change and alcohol and medication use in a dose-dependent fashion.

### Pregnancy Outcomes

A number of studies have specifically examined the effects of occupational stress and work hours on pregnancy outcomes in female residents (73–77). However, it should be kept in mind that many of these studies are based on retrospective self-reported data, and none of them have specifically examined the effects of sleep loss (separate from work load) as a risk factor. Although overall the results are somewhat mixed, an increase in a number of pregnancy-related complications [pregnancy-induced hypertension (76), abruptio placenta, and preterm labor (73), and adverse fetal outcomes (low birth weight and intrauterine growth retardation) (73)] have been reported. Even one larger study that failed to find any significant overall increase in adverse pregnancy outcomes (77) in comparison to a demographically similar control group did find an association between work week hours greater than 100 and preterm delivery.

### Drowsy Driving (See Also Chap. 14)

Several recent retrospective self-report studies have also examined the relationship between sleep loss and fatigue and traffic citations, motor vehicle crashes (MVC), and "near-miss" driving accidents. Although one study of 27 anesthesiology residents in England failed to find an increase in motor vehicle crashes compared to the general population (78), other studies that have looked at the issue in more detail have found prevalence rates for collisions as high as 8% and near-crashes up to 58% in emergency room physicians (79). In the latter study, 74% and 80% of the collisions and near-miss crashes, respectively, occurred on the drive home following the night shift. Furthermore, driving incidents were correlated with both the number of night shifts worked and residents' self-reported tolerance of shift work and adaptation to drowsiness. Marcus and Loughlin's survey comparing pediatric house officers with faculty members (80) found a significantly increased prevalence of falling asleep at the wheel either while driving or while stopped at a traffic light (49% of the residents vs. 13% of the faculty), traffic citations (25% vs. 18%), and motor vehicle accidents (20 vs. 11 MVCs), with the vast majority of these incidents occurring postcall. Finally, a recent retrospective survey of almost 700 emergency medicine residents found that they were nearly seven times more likely to have a fall-asleep MVC during, compared to prior to, residency; furthermore, these collisions were associated with rotations with more frequent call and during which less sleep was routinely obtained (81).

In summary, self-perceived negative effects on mood, motivation, and life satisfaction as a result of chronic sleep loss are almost universally reported in medical trainees. The consequences of these psychological factors on the physician-patient relationship and on interactions with other professionals in the hospital setting have been largely unexplored. The potential for significant health-related consequences in residents, particularly morbidity and mortality related to drowsy-driving accidents, is supported by a number of studies.

### D.  Effects on Learning and Medical Education

An argument that has been traditionally made in defense of the long hours of continuous duty demanded by the current system of medical training is that increased exposure to patients and disease states results in enhanced learning. Thus, the results of those few studies that have examined the impact of sleep loss on outcomes potentially related to medical education (impaired information processing, decreased retention of information, decreased motivation to learn) are important to consider. Both medical students (55) and residents (71) themselves have reported a negative correlation between long work hours and effective learning and use of skills. Decreased satisfaction with the learning environment was reported to be a consequence of sleep loss, and learning satisfaction was nega- tively correlated with reported average sleep hours in a dose-dependent fashion in one large survey study (72). In a study of 34 surgery residents that utilized sleep logs and monthly surveys of operative participation, every-other-night call was associated not only with increased levels of fatigue and stress and decreased over- all satisfaction, but also with participation in *fewer* operative cases per month, compared to every-third- and every-fourth-night call schedules (82). On the other hand, in a recent national survey of over 4500 obstetrics and gynecology resi- dents, the major reasons for opposing work hour limitations cited by those resi- dents who did oppose them (one in five) were concerns about curtailing surgical experience and limiting opportunities to see rare cases (56).

In those studies that have examined trainees' actual performance on educa- tional tasks, the results are mixed. One study (34) correlated amount of sleep obtained by a group of medical students and residents the night before the testing session with scores on a test on content recall of selected surgical journal articles. "Sleep-deprived" (defined as ≤ 4 hr of uninterrupted sleep) and "rested" trainees obtained similar scores, despite self-reported increased fatigue and decreased motivation in the sleep-deprived group. A study of pediatric residents similarly failed to find differences in factual knowledge test scores pre- and postcall (25). Several other recent studies have compared performance on standardized exami- nations, such as the American Board of Surgery In-Training Exam (ABSITE) (35,83). In contrast to a previous study that had shown a negative correlation between pretest sleep amounts and test scores for family practice residents (36), these studies failed to demonstrate any significant detrimental effect of call status or hours of sleep on test performance. However, the amount of sleep residents obtained in the 2 nights prior to ABSITE was found to contribute somewhat (approximately 7% of the variance) to ABSITE scores (35).

Finally, in one interesting study of 23 medical interns (37), there were no significant differences in medical knowledge test scores between sleep-deprived (≤ 3 hr) and "rested" residents. In addition, sleep loss did not appear to decrease the appropriateness of subjects' confidence in the accuracy of their answers. A more recent study (84) also examined the relationship between accuracy of answers and self-reported confidence in answers on a test of medical knowledge in a group of medical residents. This study found that, although length of contin- uous sleep on call was inversely correlated with the number of correct answers and confidence levels, less sleep was not associated with decreased appropriate- ness of confidence level. These study findings may suggest some subjective abil- ity to recognize impairment and, if replicated, have potential implications for the relative risk of trainees committing medical errors in the sleep-deprived state.

In summary, generally studies suggest that residents may be able to com- pensate on tests of factual knowledge for the negative effects of sleep loss and fatigue and that they are appropriately confident about their performance. However, trainees' motivation to learn appears to be significantly impacted by inadequate sleep.

### E.   Effects on Patient Safety, Medical Errors

A medical error is defined as an adverse event that results from the failure of a
health care delivery plan to be completed as intended, or the use of an incorrect
plan to reach an appropriate patient care objective (6). Medical errors may occur
at any of multiple different steps in the diagnostic and treatment process, and
often involve human factors in their genesis, such as inattention, poor communication, and fatigue,. Given the fact that most of the studies cited above show some
adverse affects of sleep loss and fatigue in medical trainees on neurocognitive
function and performance of occupational tasks, it is logical to postulate that
sleep loss in medical trainees has significant potential to compromise the margin
of safety in the delivery of patient care. In addition, fatigued residents may be less
likely to seek out additional information after an incident, thereby potentially
reducing the opportunity to avoid future similar errors. Furthermore, the almost
universal effects on affective domains such as mood and motivation and the many
negative effects on performance outcomes would be expected to have some
impact on communication and interaction with patients, and on professionalism,
and thus affect the quality of the provider-patient relationship.

   However, to date no study has conclusively demonstrated a direct causal
relationship between fatigue and medical errors in the health care setting (1).
Attempts to examine the association between sleep loss and fatigue in medical
trainees and adverse clinical outcomes have included both survey studies of
provider-identified risk factors for medical errors and studies which have examined antecedents of actual reported errors. Recent surveys of health care providers
have documented that, for example, over 60% of anesthesiologists surveyed in the
United States (85) and almost 90% of those in Australia (86) report having made
fatigue-related errors. Surveys of trainees' perceptions of risk factors for medical
errors have reported an association between prolonged work hours, fatigue, and
lack of sleep and self-reported decreased efficiency in performance of work-
related tasks (87), commission of medical errors while on call (34), and overall
compromised quality of patient care (88). In one of these studies (89), "tiredness"
in a group of 225 residents from a variety of specialties was the single most
important attribution for the lack of quality patient care, cited as a contributing
factor in almost 50% of incidents of lowered standards of care and 45.5% of incidents involving increased irritability and anger toward patients. In a recent survey
of 254 internal medicine residents, 41% of the respondents cited fatigue as a
cause of their most significant medical mistake (90).

   For a number of reasons, including the difficulties inherent in proving a
direct causal relationship between fatigue and adverse medical events and the
lack of systems for reporting various types of adverse events and errors, few studies to date have examined the specific contribution of sleep deprivation to actual
medical errors. Several recent studies, in attempting to unravel this relationship,
have employed a number of different methodologies to assess prevalence, type,
and risk factors for medical errors. For example, in one recent study of anesthetic

incidents in Australia, fatigue-related events constituted 2.7% of the 5600 reported errors occurring over a 10-year period (91), and in another Australian study, fatigue was considered a contributing factor in 10% of medication errors (92). Another study of 70 serious anesthesia incidents found that one half were related to factors potentially correlated with fatigue, such as decreased vigilance (93). More indirect evidence of an association between resident fatigue and medical errors was reported in a retrospective cohort analysis of over 19,000 patients admitted to the internal medicine service of a county teaching hospital, which found that patients admitted after midnight had a significantly higher mortality rate, which did not appear to be due to a systematically different case mix (i.e., patients admitted after midnight being more acutely ill) (94).

In summary, although results of self-report survey studies suggest that medical errors are more likely to occur in the context of sleep loss and fatigue, there is currently little empirical evidence to support or refute a direct causal link.

### F. Impact of Alertness Management Interventions

*Operational/Systems Changes*

Given the accumulation of evidence cited above, which supports the existence of a significant negative impact of sleep loss and fatigue on patient care and on trainees themselves, regulation of work hours and other operational changes such as scheduling adjustments would seem to be a necessary next step in addressing these concerns. However, there is both anecdotal and empirical evidence to suggest that operational or system changes in and of themselves do not guarantee well-rested and optimally functioning residents. There are likely to be a number of reasons for this observation. First, it is clear from recent experience that system changes may be very difficult to implement and maintain. For example, multiple violations of the Bell Commission regulations were reported in New York after their institution, as documented during unannounced inspections of teaching hospitals, revealed that about two thirds of the surgical residents were working more than 95 hr/week and for more than 24 consecutive hr (95). Second, it is unlikely that work hour regulations alone could counteract the pervasive influence of the "culture" of medical training that requires and even encourages physicians, in the interest of patient care, to survive and function on little or no sleep, nor are regulations alone likely to eliminate resistance to change in the current system on the part of the medical profession itself. Third, work hour regulations and other system changes cannot by definition govern residents' behavior outside of the workplace (e.g., "moonlighting" activities) or establish their personal priorities regarding adequate sleep, and thus cannot ensure that residents are adequately rested. Finally, it should be pointed out that many of the proposed operational changes themselves have limited or no empirical support. For example, there are no studies in any occupational settings that suggest that an 80-hr work week provides adequate opportunity for rest and recovery; furthermore, this number is well above that stipulated in federal regulations for the transportation industry where much of the research on work hours and fatigue has been conducted (96). Similarly, the proposed limit of 24 continuous hr on duty directly contradicts research data showing that the risk of human error goes up significantly at the 16–18 hr of continuous wakefulness mark.

Very few outcome-based studies have systematically assessed the positive or negative impact of regulations that limit work hours for physicians-in-training. One study that examined the quality of patient care (80-hr work week maximum) found a postregulations increase in the number of delays in ordering diagnostic tests and an increase in the number of patients suffering at least one medical complication, which persisted after controlling for a number of patient-related variables (97). Other studies (98) have demonstrated an association between preventable adverse events and interruptions in patient care continuity, and have raised concerns about the potential for inadequate communication of patient information across multiple providers resulting from work hour limitations. However, in another study that assessed the impact of instituting continuous work hour and on-call limitations in a VA hospital, not only did sleep amounts on call significantly increase, but there were: a 15% reduction in mean length of stay, a 19% reduction in median length of stay, fewer laboratory tests ordered, and fewer medication errors committed (29).

A handful of studies have examined the effects of other operational changes in medical settings. In one example of the use of operational strategies, institution of a team day/night shift on-call system resulted anecdotally in improved morale and resident learning in one obstetrics-and-gynecology residency program (99). A more recent study that examined the impact of a "night stalker" radiology resident in the emergency room on quality of care reported fewer "missed' radiological findings and less clinically significant discordant findings in the postintervention cases reviewed (100). However, in a striking illustration of the complexity and challenges involved in implementing system changes to address sleep and fatigue, one study that examined the impact of a "night float" on-call coverage system on resident performance found that, counter to expectations, the "covered" residents who had protected time for sleep actually obtained *less* sleep overall than the residents who were not relieved by the night float (38). The authors concluded that the covered residents used their protected time to catch up on work, not sleep. A number of other studies that have also addressed issues that potentially impact on the likelihood of success in implementing operational changes, such as what residents actually do when they are on call, and how individual variability in efficiency, perception of workload, etc. may impact sleep schedules and recovery sleep (101,102).

In summary, operational changes such as limitations on resident work hours, scheduling adjustments, and provision of "protected time" for sleep are necessary but unlikely to be sufficient to assure optimal levels of alertness in medical trainees, partly because of difficulties in implementation of and adherence to systems-based measures.

## Countermeasures (See Also Chaps. 20–22)

Since the most effective countermeasure for sleepiness is clearly sleep, the efficacy of napping in combating the effects of fatigue has been an active area of research in the laboratory as well as in other occupational settings. For example, "prophylactic" brief naps prior to 24 hr of sleep loss have been shown to improve alertness during 24 hr of sustained wakefulness (103), and frequent (every 2–3 hr) brief (15 min) "therapeutic" naps can significantly mitigate performance decrements during periods of prolonged sleep deprivation (104). "Maintenance" or on the job naps may also improve performance in shift workers (105). In all of these situations, however, consideration must be given to the timing and duration of naps to minimize the effects of sleep inertia on performance. Other sleep-related behavioral strategies to enhance alertness in occupational settings have included use of a variety of sleep schedules, including anchor and split-sleep periods (106).

In studies of other countermeasures, judicious use of caffeine has been shown to temporarily enhance alertness if strategically timed (107). Other alertness-enhancing pharmacological agents that have been studied in a variety of industries include the use of central nervous system stimulants such as modafinil and administration of oral melatonin. Timed manipulation of light exposure (108) and education regarding principles of sleep hygiene (109) have also been studied as potential alertness management strategies.

However, in contrast to other professions that also involve high stakes for human error (e.g., transportation, aeronautics) and have more actively developed and implemented measures to mitigate the effects of sleep and fatigue on workers' performance (110–113), only a handful of studies have addressed the issue of countermeasure strategies in medical trainees. One review article examining the impact of shift work in emergency medicine (114) proposed the use of both operational and personal strategies to optimize alertness, including rotation schedule designs based on chronobiological principles, use of regular exercise, and exposure to light on and off the job, and sleep strategies such as anchor sleep, split-sleep periods, and planned napping. Smith-Coggins et al. (47) studied the impact of a comprehensive sleep and fatigue management program on a number of sleep and performance-based outcome variables in six emergency medicine attending physicians. The program included: an educational component on sleep physiology, circadian rhythms, and sleep hygiene that was based on a fatigue countermeasure program developed by NASA; institution of a shift rotation schedule that adhered to accepted chronobiological principles (i.e., rotating shifts in a clockwise direction, limiting consecutive night shifts, etc.); and use of a variety of countermeasure strategies by the physicians (use of caffeine, napping, etc.). Outcome measures included sleep quality and quantity (measured by sleep logs and ambulatory PSG), psychomotor performance tests of vigilance/sustained attention, and simulated tasks (EKG interpretation and intubation). Despite a high rate of self-reported compliance with the countermeasure strategies and subjective reports of "quality-of-life" improvements resulting from the intervention, there was no significant improvement overall compared to the active placebo condition ("jet lag diet") on most of the outcome variables. However, the pervasiveness of the negative effects resulting from circadian disruption found in this study under all of the experimental conditions (less sleep, negative mood, impaired vigilance performance, less efficient intubation associated with night shifts) may have masked actual differences. Finally, several studies that have examined the effectiveness of oral melatonin use in emergency medicine physicians working night shifts have failed to document a significant effect (114–117).

In summary, although a potentially promising area of study, there is currently a paucity of data regarding the efficacy and utility of traditional countermeasures (napping, caffeine, etc.) and other alertness management strategies in medical residents.

## IV.  Future Directions

### A.  Research

It should be clear from the above summary of what is currently known about sleep and fatigue in medical training that an evidenced-based research approach is critical to achieving the goals of ensuring quality patient care, maintaining the health and safety of resident physicians, and optimizing graduate medical education and training. Furthermore, all changes in policy and procedures should be evidence-based and linked to results of specific studies. Therefore, a primary goal must be to continue to develop a scientifically sound and comprehensive body of evidence regarding the effects of sleep loss and fatigue on physicians in training and on the quality of health care that they deliver. To achieve this aim, the research questions need to be clearly defined and optimal research strategies identified. Expanded research methodologies and data collection techniques—such as cross-sectional and longitudinal observational studies; surveys of attending physicians, patients, and other health care personnel; examination of trainee performance on a variety of educational assessments; patient chart reviews; and qualitative studies on the working conditions and the care environment—will likely be needed for this purpose. In addition, improved information systems for reporting adverse patient outcomes will be essential to assess potential relationships between such outcomes and trainee sleep and fatigue. Key research areas must be identified and should include the following considerations:

> The scope, prevalence, and significance of the problem of inadequate sleep and fatigue in residents must be *more specifically and rigorously defined*, particularly in regard to the impact on performance in actual clinical settings, on the physician-patient relationship, on the health and safety of residents, and on the quality of their medical education.
>
> *Causal linkages* need to be established among fatigue-related variables such as resident work hours and schedules, subjective and objective

measures of fatigue, performance in the work setting, and health and safety outcomes for both patients and trainees.

Because health care delivery in teaching hospitals must operate 24 hr a day, 7 days a week, *management* rather than *elimination* of fatigue should be the driving concept, and research priorities must include studies evaluating sleep loss and fatigue management in the health care setting. Furthermore, these programs should be informed by the growing body of research and policy experience from other occupational settings, including use of a variety of specific countermeasures, education regarding sleep hygiene, and institution of technological innovations. However, because there are fundamental differences in the nature of the tasks that medical personnel are required to perform in the course of their workday, fatigue management strategies that have been successful in other occupational settings may not be applicable to medical training; therefore, strategies that are unique to the hospital setting and that incorporate the process of medical education and patient care needs must be developed and tested.

Operational metrics must be developed that will facilitate the assessment of the effects of sleep loss and fatigue on key outcomes such as patient health and safety, education effectiveness, resident health and professionalism, and health care economics. (See Table 1.)

## B. Education

The overriding goal of any recommendations or policies regarding sleep and fatigue in medical training should be to ensure that medical trainees receive adequate rest to enable them to perform and learn at their optimal level on a consistent basis. Educational interventions regarding the antecedents and consequences of sleep loss and fatigue and alertness management strategies that are targeted at faculty, medical school, and hospital administrators, and at other hospital personnel, as well as at resident physicians, are a necessary part of any comprehensive and integrated approach to this issue. Education is a necessary part of affecting any substantial and sustained behavioral change on the individual level; i.e., the individual needs to understand the rationale for the changes to "buy into" them, and also accepts personal responsibility for instituting them. Education at the systems-wide level is also a critical part of affecting change; from a social dynamic perspective, one of the most powerful identified barriers to adherence to work hour regulations is the "culture" of the workplace, and, on a pragmatic level, system-wide changes need to support and complement the changes in individuals. Furthermore, education is the only vehicle for affecting changes in lifestyle or personal behaviors that impact on fatigue and alertness, but is not likely to be amenable to external regulation.

However, medical students and house officers typically receive little or no education about normal sleep and circadian rhythms, or the essential role of sleep

**Table 1**  Important Metrics for Studying Sleep and Fatigue in Medical Education (72)

| Domain | Specific content, examples |
|---|---|
| Standard definition of trainee work hours | Actual duty hours |
| | Sleep and awake time |
| | Work intensity |
| | Moonlighting hours |
| Patient outcomes | Length of stay |
| | Medical errors |
| | Medication errors |
| | Complications |
| | Iatrogenic disease |
| | Satisfaction with care |
| Educational outcomes | Resident in training exam scores |
| | Board scores |
| | Number of medical procedures performed |
| | Educational performance in relation to on-call schedules (e.g., postcall vs. no call) |
| Trainee health outcomes | National registry of resident motor vehicle crashes and relevant covariates (e.g., work schedules, distance driven, time of day, work-related and non-work-related exposure measures) |
| | Longitudinal database of resident health outcomes relative to an appropriate control group (e.g., dentist trainees) |
| | Health outcomes from a variety of domains, including mental health and substance use disorders, pregnancy, endocrine, cardiovascular, and neurological |
| Trainee professional outcomes | Measures of doctor-patient relationships |
| | Patient satisfaction surveys |
| | Incidences of falling asleep on the job |
| Economic outcomes | Costs associated with sleep loss and fatigue (e.g., fatigue related medical errors) |
| | Cost-benefit analyses of fatigue management programs |
| | Hospital costs |
| | Patient care costs |
| | Direct and indirect costs |

in maintaining adequate health and performance. Therefore, the content of a sleep education curriculum should include basic principles of sleep and chronobiology; the impact of sleep deprivation in experimental settings, in other occupational settings, and in medical settings; common myths and misconceptions about sleep loss and fatigue; principles of sleep hygiene; use of countermeasures; and operational changes. Furthermore, because current medical education standards require application of rigorous methodological criteria for outcome measures and demonstration of efficacy of teaching methods and tools, changes in knowledge, competence, and behavior in residents, faculty (including residency and program directors), and hospital administration, as well as measures of organizational/"cultural" change at these institutions across time, must also be systematically examined.

### C. Policy

A fundamental consideration in designing and implementing policies regarding sleep and fatigue in medical training at the individual residency program, state, regional, or national level is that of the competing and often conflicting priorities of clinical service and patient care versus medical education versus quality-of-life for resident physicians. Because of the unique nature of the combined student and physician role of trainees, working conditions not only must be structured to ensure the safety of both patients and of trainees, but they should also provide an optimal learning environment that allows residents to learn in a well-rested state. In addition, it must be recognized that a number of critical stakeholders are involved in the issue of sleep and fatigue in medical education, many of whom also have competing priorities. These include student and resident organizations, graduate medical accreditation organizations (e.g., ACGME and the individual specialty residency review committees), professional organizations such as the American Medical Association (AMA), hospital staff and administrators, and patient advocacy groups. Therefore, there is clearly a need for shared responsibility among trainees, medical school faculty and administration, hospital administration, and medical education regulatory bodies for developing and incorporating effective and creative solutions. To foster this sense of collective responsibility, it is critical to include all groups with a vested interest in this issue. There is also a need to develop ongoing mechanisms to ensure *accountability* from residency program and hospital administrators in implementing and assessing the efficacy of given interventions.

It should also be pointed that a number of potentially nonexclusive pathways for regulation of resident working conditions exist, including: (a) increasing the ability of educational governing bodies such as the ACGME and the RRCs to develop and enforce regulations; (b) introducing national and state legislation regarding resident work hours; (c) encouraging government agencies and the judicial system to become involved in regulation of working conditions;, and (d) using monetary fines, sanctions from hospital accreditation groups such as Joint Commission on Accreditation of Healthcare Organizations (JCAHO), and public disclosure of any violations to increase compliance with regulations by individual hospitals.

Finally, the economics that both drive current policies and present barriers to implementing change cannot be ignored. Concerns about the fiscal and administrative aspects of the issue have been a major stumbling block in the past and are likely to continue. The parties responsible for the containment of health care costs and for funding of medical education, including third-party payers, hospitals, and federal insurance programs, usually assume that system reform necessarily involves additional professional and ancillary support staffing and, consequently, higher costs. Indeed, it was estimated in 1988 that the cost of implementing the modified New York State regulations would be upward of $226 million initially, and $15.7 billion over the subsequent 15 years. Financial and staffing considerations also need to be considered in relation to regulatory or legislative actions on work hours. Federal and state funding support for graduate medical education does not adequately cover the cost of residency training, and analyses of potential savings accrued by a more efficient resident staff must be balanced against increased costs for other health care providers.

At some fundamental level, this issue touches all deliverers and consumers of health care. Every patient who enters a teaching hospital or visits an emergency room has a reasonable chance of being treated by a professional who is competent, caring, and knowledgeable, but whose judgment and compassion may be compromised by simple lack of sleep. It is the responsibility of all physicians to embrace a leadership role in moving this issue to the forefront. To maintain credibility as educators and as advocates for the importance of good health habits for our patients, the medical profession must be willing to take a hard look at our own practices and standards in this area, and to seriously consider the implications of failing to become involved in reforming medical training practices. Not only could this effort have a lasting impact on the quality of health care delivered in the United States and abroad, but there is perhaps no more important legacy that we can leave to the next generation of physicians.

"I take the best care of people when my life is in balance and if it's totally out of balance I don't feel like I'm really giving this person the best care that I possibly can. We're a new generation of doctors and even though they're better than how they were, they shouldn't be this way. We don't want each other to die young, you know? It just shouldn't really be this way"—Medical resident, 2001.

## References

1. Gaba DM, Howard SK. Fatigue among clinicians and the safety of patients. N Engl J Med 2002; 347(16):1249–1255.
2. ACGME Approves New Proposed Common Requirements for Resident Duty Hours. Chicago: Accreditation Council for Graduate Medical Education, 2002. (Accessed September 24, 2002, at http://www.acgme.org/new/residentHours602.asp.).
3. AAMC Policy Guidance On Graduate Medical Education: Assuring Quality Patient Care and Quality Education. Washington, DC: Association of American Medical Colleges, October 2001. (Accessed September 24, 2002, at http://www.aamc.org/hlthcare/gmepolicy/gmepolicy.pdf.)
4. Asch D, Parker R. The Libby Zion case: one step forward or two steps backward? N Engl J Med 1988; 318:771–775.

5.  Petition to the Occupational Safety and Health Administration Requesting That Limits Be Placed on Hours Worked by Medical Residents (HRG publication #1570). Washington DC: Public Citizen Health Research Group, 2002. (Accessed September 24, 2002, at http://www.citizen.org/publications/release.cfm?ID=6771.).
6.  Institute of Medicine of the National Academies of Science Report. To Err Is Human: Building a Safer Health System. National Academy Press, 2000.
7.  Doran SM, Van Dongen HPA, Dinges DF. Sustained attention performance during sleep deprivation: evidence of state instability. Arch Ital Biol 2001; 139:253–267.
8.  Williams HL, Lubin A, Goodnow JJ. Impaired performance with acute sleep loss. Psychol Monogr Gen Appl 1959; 73:1–26.
9.  Pilcher JJ, Huffcutt AI. Effects of sleep deprivation on performance: a meta-analysis. Sleep 1996; 19:318–326.
10. Carskadon M, Dement WC. Cumulative effects of sleep restriction on daytime sleepiness. Psychophysiology 1981; 18:107–113.
11. Blagrove M, Alexander C, Horne JA. The effects of chronic sleep reduction on the performance of cognitive tasks sensitive to sleep deprivation. Appl Cogn Psychol.1994; 9:21–40.
12. Dinges DF, Pack F, Williams K, Gillen KA, Powell JW, Ott GE, Aptowicz C, Pack AI. Cumulative sleepiness, mood disturbance, and psychomotor vigilance performance decrements during a week of sleep restricted to 4–5 hours per night. Sleep 1997; 20:267–277.
13. Anderson CM, Maislin G, Van Dongen HP, Rogers NL, Powell JW, Carlin MM, Mullington JM, Dinges DF. Effect of chronically reduced nocturnal sleep, with and without daytime naps, on neurobehavioral performance. Sleep 2000; 23:A74.
14. Hart RP, Buchsbaum DG, Wade JB, Hamer RM, Kwentus JA. Effect of sleep deprivation on first-year residents' response times, memory, and mood. J Med Educ 1987; 52:940–942.
15. Hawkins MR, Vichick DA, Silsby HD, Kruzich DJ, Butler R. Sleep deprivation and performance of house officers. J Med Educ 1985; 60:530–535.
16. Poulton EC, Hunt GM, Carpenter A, Edwards RS. The performance of junior hospital doctors following reduced sleep and long hours of work. Ergonomics 1978; 21:279–295.
17. Leonard C, Fanning N, AttwoodJ, Buckley M. The effect of fatigue, sleep deprivation and onerous working hours on the physical and mental wellbeing of pre-registration house officers. Ir J Med Sci.1998; 167:22–25.
18. Nelson CS, Dell'Angela K, Jellish WS, Brown IE, Skaredoff M. Residents' performance before and after night call as evaluated by an indicator of creative thought. J Am Osteo Assoc 1995; 95:600–603.
19. Deaconson TF, O'Hair DP, Levy MF, Lee MB, Schueneman AL, Codon RE. Sleep deprivation and resident performance. JAMA 1988; 260:1721–1727.
20. Bartle EJ, Sun JH, Thompson L, Light AI, McCoolC, Heaton S. The effects of acute sleep deprivation during residency training. Surgery1988; 104:311–316.
21. Reznick RK, Folse JR. Effect of sleep deprivation on the performance of surgical residents. Am J Surg1987; 154: 520–525.
22. Ford CV, Wentz DK. The internship year: a study of sleep, mood states, and psychophysiologic parameters. South Med J 1984; 77:1435–1442.
23. Friedman RC, Bigger JT, Kornfeld DS. The intern and sleep loss. N Engl J Med 1971; 285:201–203.

24. Lingenfelser T, Kaschel R, Weber A, Zaiser-Kaschel H, Jakober B, Kuber J. Young hospital doctors after night duty: their task specific cognitive status and emotional condition. Med Educ 1994; 28:566–572.

25. Storer JS, Floyd HH, Gill WL, GiustiCW, Ginsberg H. Effects of sleep deprivation on cognitive ability and skills of pediatrics residents. Acad Med 1989; 64:29–32.

26. Smith-Coggins R, Rosekind MR, Hurd S, Buccino KR. Relationship of day versus night sleep to physician performance and mood. Ann Emerg Med 1994; 24:928–934.

27. Engel W, Seime R, Powell V, D'Alessandri R. Clinical performance of interns after being on call. South Med J 1987; 80:761–763.

28. Christensen EE, Dietz GW, Murry RC, Moore JG. The effect of fatigue on resident performance. Radiology 1977; 125:103–105.

29. Gottlieb DJ, Parenti CM, Peterson CA, Lofgren RP. Effect of a change in housestaff work schedule on resource utilization and patient care. Arch Intern Med 1991; 151:2065–2070.

30. Goldman LI, McDonough MT, Rosemond GP. Stresses affecting surgical performance and learning: correlation of heart rate, electrocardiogram and operation simultaneously recorded on videotapes. J Surg Res 1972; 12:83–86.

31. Haynes DF, Schwedler M, Dyslin DC, Rice JC, Kerstein MD. Are postoperative complications related to resident sleep deprivation? South Med J 1995; 88:283–289.

32. Taffinder NJ, McManus IC, Gul Y, Russell RC, Darzi A. Effect of sleep deprivation on surgeons' dexterity on laparoscopy simulator. Lancet 1998; 352:1191.

33. Grantcharov TP, Bardram L. Funch-Jensen P, Rosenberg J. Laparoscopic performance after one night on call in a surgical department: prospective study. Br Med J 2001; 323:1222–1223.

34. Browne BJ, Van Susteren T, Onsager DR, Simpson D, Salaymeh B, Condon RE. Influence of sleep deprivation on learning among surgical house staff and medical students. Surgery 1994; 115:604–610.

35. Godellas CV, Huang R. Factors affecting performance on the American Board of Surgery in-training examination. Am J Surg. 2001; 181:294–296.

36. Jacques CH, Lynch JC, Samkoff JS. The effects of sleep loss on cognitive performance of resident physicians. J Fam Pract 1990; 30:223–229.

37. Robbins J, Gottlieb F. Sleep deprivation and cognitive testing in internal medicine house staff. West J Med 1990; 12:82–86.

38. Richardson GS, Wyatt JK, Sullivan JP, Grav EJ, Ward AE, Wolf MA, Czeisler CA. Objective assessment of sleep and alertness in medical house staff and the impact of protected time for sleep. Sleep 1996; 19:718–726.

39. Light AI, Sun JH, McCool C, Thompson L, Heaton S, Bartle EJ. The effects of acute sleep deprivation on the level of resident training. Curr Surg 1989; 46:29–30.

40. Bertram DA. Characteristics of shifts and second-year resident performance in an emergency department. NY State J Med 1988; 88:10–15.

41. Klose JK, Wallace-Barnhill GL, Craythorne MWS. Performance test results for anesthesia residents over a five-day week including on-call duty. Anesthesiology 1985; 63:A485.

42. Denisco RA, Drummond JN, Gravenstein JS. The effect of fatigue on the performance of a simulated anesthetic monitoring task. J Clin Monit 1987; 3:22–24.

43. Orton DI, Gruzelier JH. Adverse changes in mood and cognitive performance of house officers after night duty. Br Med J 1989; 298:21–23.

44. Rubin R, Orris P, Lau SL, Hryhorczuk DO, Furner S, Letz R. Neurobehavioral effects of the on-call experience in housestaff physicians. J Occup Med 1991; 33:13–18.

45. Deary IJ, Tait QR. Effects of sleep disruption on cognitive performance and mood in medical house officers. Br Med J Clin Res Educ 1987; 295:1513–1516.

46. Parker JB. The effects of fatigue on physician performance—an underestimated cause of physician impairment and increased patient risk. Can J Anaesth 1987; 34:489–495.

47. Smith-Coggins R, Rosekind MR, Buccino KR, Dinges DF, Moser RP. Rotating shiftwork schedules: can we enhance physician adaptation to night shifts? Acad Emerg Med 1997; 4:951–961.

48. Asken MJ, Raham DC. Resident performance and sleep deprivation: a review. J Med Educ 1983; 58:382–388.

49. Leung L, Becker CE. Sleep deprivation and house staff performance. J Occup Med 1992; 34:1153–1160.

50. Samkoff JS, Jaques CHM. A review of studies concerning effects of sleep deprivation and fatigue on residents performance. Acad Med 1991; 66:687–693.

51. Jha AK, Duncan BW, Bates DW. Fatigue, sleepiness, and medical errors. In: Shojania KG, Duncan BW, McDonald KM, Wachter RM, eds. Making health care safer: a critical analysis of patient safety practices. Evidence report/technology assessment no. 43. Rockville, MD: Agency for Healthcare Research and Quality, 2001:519–531. (AHRQ publication no. 01–E058.) (Also availaable at http://www.ahrq.org/clinic/ptsafety/chap46a.htm.)

52. Owens JA. Sleep loss and fatigue in medical training. Curr Opin Pulm Med 2001; 7:411–418.

53. Weinger MB, Ancoli-Israel S. Sleep deprivation and clinical performance. JAMA 2002; 287:955–957.

54. Veasey S, Rosen R, Barzansky B, Rosen I, Owens J. Sleep loss and fatigue in residency training: a reappraisal. JAMA 2002; 288:1116–1124.

55. Daugherty SR, Baldwin DC. Sleep deprivation in senior medical students and first-year residents. Acad Med 1996; 71(1):S93–S95.

56. Defoe, DM, Power ML, Holzman GB, Carpentieri A, and Schulkin L. Long hours and little sleep: work schedules of residents in obstetrics and gynecology. Obstet Gynecol 2001; 97(6):1015–1018.

57. Daugherty SR, Baldwin DC, Rowley BD. Learning, satisfaction, and mistreatment during medical internship: a national survey of working conditions. JAMA 1998; 279(15):1194–1199.

58. Richardson GS, Wyatt JK, Sullivan JP, Orav EJ, Ward AE, Wolf MA, Czeisler CA: Objective assessment of sleep and alertness in medical house staff and the impact of protected time for sleep. Sleep 1996; 19:718–726.

59. Akerstedt T, Arnetz BB, Anderzen I. Physicians during the following night call duty—41 hour ambulatory recording of sleep. Electroencephalogr Clin Neurophysiol 1990; 76:193–196.

60. Tov N, Rubin A, Lavie P. Effects of workload on residents' sleep duration: objective documentation. Isr J Med Sci 1995; 31:417–423.

61.  Acherman P, Werth E, Dijk D, Borbely AA. Time course of sleep inertia after night-time and daytime sleep episodes. Arch Ital Biol 1995; 134:109–119.
62.  Bruck D, Pisani DL. The effects of sleep inertia on decision-making performance. J Sleep Res 1999; 8:95–103.
63.  Howard SK, Gaba DM, Rosekind MR, Zarcone VP. The risks and implications of excessive daytime sleepiness in resident physicians. Acad Med 2002; 77(10):1019–1025.
64.  Ou JC, Weinger MB, Mazzei WJ, et al. Further evaluation of the effects of night-time work on mood, task patterns, and workload during anesthesia care (abstr). Anesthesiology 2001; 95:A1196.
65.  Gaba DM. Physician work hours: the "sore thumb" of organizational safety in tertiary health care. In: Scheffler AL, Zipperer LA, eds. Enhancing Patient Safety and Reducing Errors in Health Care. Chicago: National Patient Safety Foundation, 1998:302–305.
66.  Weinger MB, Vora S, Herndon CN, et al. Evaluation of the effe4cts of fatigue and sleepiness on clinical performance in on-call anesthesia residents during actual nighttime cases and in simulated cases. In: Scheffler AL, Zipperer LA, eds. Enhancing Patient Safety and Reducing Errors in Health Care. Chicago: National Patient Safety Foundation, 1998:306–310.
67.  Lingenfelser T, Kaschels R, Weber A, Zaiser-Kaschels H, Jakober B, Kuper J. Young hospital doctors after night duty: their task-specific cognitive status and emotional condition. Med Educ 1994; 28:566–572.
68.  Rose MW, Ware JC, Kolm P, Risser MR. Residual effects of call on sleep and mood in medical residents. Sleep 2000; 23(abstract suppl 2).
69.  Bunch WH, Dvonch VM, Storr CL, Baldwin DC, Hughes PH. The stresses of the surgical residency. J Surg Res 1992; 53:268–271.
70.  Geurts S, Rutte C, Peeters. Antecedents and consequences of work – home inter-ference among medical residents. Soc Sci Med 1999; 48:1135–1148.
71.  Baldwin PJ, Dodd M, Wrate RW. Young doctors' health—I. How do working con-ditions affect attitudes, health and performance? Soc Sci Med 1997; 45(1):35–40.
72.  Buysse D, Barzansky B, Dinges D, Hogan E, Hunt C, Owens J, Rosekind M, Rosen R, Simon F, Veasey S, Wiest F. Sleep, fatigue, and medical training: setting an agenda for optimal learning and patient care. Sleep, Fatigue, and Medical Training: Optimizing Learning and the Patient Care Environment, Alexandria VA, Oct 28–29, 2001.
73.  Silva BM. Pregnancy during residency: a look at the issues. JAMWA 47(3):71–74.
74.  Katz VL, Miller NH, Bowes WA. Pregnancy complications of physicians. West J Med 1988; 149:704–707.
75.  Grunebaum A, Minkoff H, Blake. Pregnancy among obstetricians: a comparison of births before, during, and after residency. Am J Obstet Gynecol 1987; 157:79–83.
76.  Phelan ST. Pregnancy during residency. II. Obstetric complications. Obstet Gynecol 1988; 72:431–436.
77.  Klebanoff MA, Shiono PH, Rhoads GG. Outcomes of pregnancy in a national sam-ple of resident physicians. N Engl J Med. 1990; 323(15):1040–1045.
78.  Kua JSW, Chiu WKY. Are anesthetic trainees a high-risk group for road accidents? Anaesthesia 1999; 54:1220–1234.
79.  Steele MT, John O, Watson WA, Thomas HA, Muelleman RL. The occupational risk of motor vehicle collisions for emergency medicine residents. Acad Emerg Med 1999; 6(10):1050–1053.

80. Marcus CL, Loughlin GM. Effect of sleep deprivation on driving safety in houses-taff. Sleep 1996; 19(10):763–766.

81. Kowalenko T, Hass-Kowalenko J, Rabinovich A, Grzybowski M. Emergency medicine residency related MVC's—is sleep deprivation a risk factor? Acad Emerg Med 2000; 7(5):451.

82. Sawyer RG, Tribble CG, Newberg DS, Pruett TL, Minasi JS. Intern call schedules and their relationship to sleep, operating room participation, stress, and satisfaction. Surgery 1999; 126:337–342.

83. Stone MD, Doyle J, Bosch RJ, Bothe A, Steele G. Effect of resident call status on ABSITE performance. Surgery 2000; 128:465–471.

84. Lewis KE, Blagrove M, Ebden P. Sleep deprivation and junior doctors' performance and confidence. Postgrad Med J 2002; 78:85–87.

85. Gravenstein JS, Cooper JB, Orkin FK. Work and rest cycles in anesthesia practice. Anesthesiology 1990; 72:734–742.

86. Gander PH, Merry A, Millar MM, Wellers J. Hours of work and fatigue-related error: a survey of New Zealand anaesthetists. Anaesth Intens Care 2000; 28:178–183.

87. McKee M, Black N. Does the current use of junior doctors in the United Kingdom affect the quality of medical care? Soc Sci Med 1992; 34(5):549–558.

88. Lewittes LR, Marshall VW. Fatigue and concerns about quality of care among Ontario interns and residents. Can Med Assoc J January 1989; 140.

89. Firth-Cozens J, Greenhalgh J. Doctors' perceptions of the links between stress and lowered clinical care. Soc Sci Med 1997; 44(7):1017–1022.

90. Wu AW, Folkman S, McPhee SJ, Lo, B. Do house officers learn from their mistakes? JAMA 1991; 265(16):2089–2094.

91. Morris GP, Morris RW. Anaesthesia and fatigue: an analysis of the first 10 years of the Australian incident monitoring study 1987–1997. Anaesth Invensive Care. 2000; 28:300–304.

92. Williamson JA, Webb RK, Sellen A, Runciman WB, Van der Walt JH. Human failure: analysis of 2000 incident reports. Anesth Intens Care 1993; 21:678–683.

93. Cooper JB, Newbower RS, Kitz RJ. An analysis of major errors and equipment failures in anesthesia management: considerations for prevention and detection. Anesthesiology 1984; 60:34–42.

94. Hillson SD, Dowd B, Rich EC, Luxenberg MG. Call night and patient care: effects on inpatients at one teaching hospital. J Gen Intern Med 1992; 7:405–410.

95. Lamberg L. Long hours, little sleep: bad medicine for physicians-in-training? JAMA 2002; 287(3):303–306.

96. Code of Federal Regulations Aviation (14 CFR Part 121; 14 CFR Part 135).

97. Laine C, Goldman L, Soukup JR, Hayes JG. The impact of a regulation restricting medical house staff working hours on the quality of patient care. JAMA 1993; 269(3)374–378.

98. Petersen LA, Brennan TA, O'Neil AC, Cook EF, Lee TH Does housestaff discontinuity of care increase the risk for preventable adverse events? Ann Intern Med 1994; 121:866–872.

99. Carey JC, Fishburne JI. A method to limit working hours and reduce sleep deprivation in an obstetrics and gynecology residency program. Obstet Gynecol 1989; 74:668–672.

100. Mann FA, Danz PL. The night stalker effect: quality improvements with a dedicataed night-call rotation. Invest Radiol. 1993; 28:92–96.

101. Tanz RR, Charrow J. Black clouds: work load, sleep, and resident rotation. AJDC 1993; 147:579–584.
102. Laurie N, Rank B, Parenti C, Woolley T, Snoke W. How do house officers spend their nights? A time study of internal medicine house staff on call. N Engl J Med 1989; 320:1673–1677.
103. Gillberg M, Kecklund G, Axelsson J, Akerstedt T. The effects of a short daytime nap after restricted night sleep Sleep 1996; 19:570–575.
104. Lumley M, Roehrs T, Zorick F, Lamphere J, Roth T. The alerting effects of naps in sleep-deprived subjects. Psychophysiology 1986; 23:403–408.
105. Rosa RR, Bonnet MH, Bootzin RR, et al. Intervention factors for promoting adjustment to nightwork and shiftwork. Occup Med 1990; 5:391–415.
106. Rosekind MR, Gander PH, Gregory KB, Smith, RM, Miller DL, Oyung R, Webbon LL, Johnson JM. Managing fatigue in operational settings. 2. An integrated approach. Behav Med 1996; 21:166–170.
107. Walsh JK, Muehlbach MJ, Humm TM, Dickins QS, Sugerman JL, Schweitzer PK. Effect of caffeine on physiological sleep tendency and ability to sustain wakeful ness at night. Psychopharmacology 1990; 101:271–273.
108. Czeisler CA, Johnson MP, Duffy JF, Brown EN, Ronda JM, Kronauer RE. Exposure to bright light and darkness to treat physiologic maladaptation to night work. N Engl J Med 1990; 322:1253–1259.
109. Holbrook MI, White MH, Hutt MJ. Increasing awareness of sleep hygiene in rotating shift workers: arming law-enforcement officers against impaired performance. Percept Mot Skills 1994; 79:520–522.
110. Pilcher JJ, Lambert BJ, Huffcutt AI. Differential effects of permanent and rotating shifts on self-report sleep length: a meta-analytic review. Sleep 2000; 23:155–163.
111. Nicholson AN, Pascoe PA, Roehrs T, et al. Sustained performance with short evening and morning sleeps. Aviat Space Environ Med 1985; 56:105–114.
112. Gillberg M, Kecklund G, Akerstedt T. Sleepiness and performance of professional drivers in a truck simulator—comparisons between day and night driving. J Sleep Res 1996; 5:12–15.
113. Rosekind MR, Gander PH, Gregory KB, Smith, RM, Miller DL, Oyung R, Webbon LL, Johnson JM. Managing fatigue in operational settings 1: physiological considerations and countermeasures. Behav Med 1996; 21:157–165.
114. Whitehead DC, Thomas H, Slapper DR. A rational approach to shift work in emergency medicine. Ann Emerg Med 1992; 21:1250–58.
115. Jorgensen KM, Witting MD. Does exogenous melatonin improve day sleep or night alertness in emergency physicians working night shifts? Ann Emerg Med 1998; 31:699–704.
116. Wrenn K, Wright S. Melatonin after night shift work. Ann Emerg Med 1999; 33:479.
117. Wright SW, Lawrence LM, Wrenn KD, Haynes ML, Welch LA, Schlack HM. Randomized clinical trial of melatonin after night-shift work: efficacy and neruopsycholoigc effects. Ann Emerg Med 1998; 32:334–340.

# 19

## Legal Implications

**DANIEL W. SHUMAN**

Southern Methodist University, Dallas, Texas, U.S.A.

**ALEXANDER MCCALL SMITH**

University of Edinburgh, Edinburgh, Scotland

**CRAIG J. PRITZLAFF**

Southern Methodist University, Dallas, Texas, U.S.A.

## I. Introduction

### A. Why Sleep Deprivation Matters to the Law

In May 2002, a captain piloting a barge tow on the Arkansas River between the Oklahoma and Texas border abruptly lost consciousness as the barge approached the busy Interstate 40 Bridge (1). One of the barges drifted into the bridge causing it to collapse, resulting in over a dozen deaths. Coast Guard and National Transportation Safety Board (NTSB) investigators discovered that the captain had less than 10 hr of sleep in the previous 40 hr and also had an undiagnosed heart condition that might have contributed to his loss of consciousness. The complete NTSB investigation report has not been published as of mid-2004. Less than 6 months after the mishap a legal battle had already erupted in courts from Oklahoma to Mississippi. In early June 2002, the state of Oklahoma filed a civil lawsuit in federal court against the captain, the captain's employer, and its parent company seeking damages for the losses suffered by the state (2). In addition, relatives of an Arkansas family killed in the collapse filed suit in Mississippi, home of the tugboat's parent company (3). The parent company has made a motion under maritime law to limit its liability damages, and both Oklahoma and the survivors are attempting to move all the cases to Oklahoma so an Oklahoma judge can make a decision on the limits to damages. It is expected to take several months before any decision will be made. How far the civil as well as the criminal liability will extend remains to be seen, as more is discovered about the captain and his employer's knowledge of his heart condition and sleep deficit.

As this case illustrates, the consequences of sleep deprivation may be played out in the legal arena. The complexity of the issues the legal system faces involving sleep disorders and sleep deprivation is a function of the medical developments and technology that enhance our understanding of sleep. The law must not lag behind scientific advances, and medical professionals must work closely with their legal counterparts to ensure the law accommodates new understanding of sleep deprivation. This chapter describes the current state of the law in relation to sleep deprivation (primarily from an American perspective) and examines both criminal and civil liabilities arising out of sleep disorders and sleep deprivation.

### B.    Distinctions Between Criminal and Civil Liability

To understand the law's response to sleep deprivation, it is first important to distinguish the very different objectives of the criminal and civil law. The criminal law is primarily interested in defining the boundaries of permissible behavior and in punishing conduct that infringes the rights of others or of society in general. The criminal law does this by identifying norms that are embodied in legislation. Conduct infringing these norms is considered criminal, obvious examples being murder, rape, treason, and theft. The criminal law, for the most part, is confined to enforce what is listed in the code, and only legislative bodies may add new crimes. In a few jurisdictions the criminal law is still defined by courts (common law). The criminal law is enforced by the state and seeks to prevent the commission of socially undesirable activities through threat of punishment. Punishment for criminal acts commonly takes the form of restricting the offender's freedom, usually through imprisonment as well as fines. Punishment or the threat of punishment is intended to deter the commission of crimes.

An important feature of criminal law is that it is concerned with the punishment only of those who are considered culpable. This means that a large part of criminal law focuses on issue of what amounts to a blameworthy state of mind. A basic constituent of this state of mind—at least for most serious offenses—is what the law terms mens rea, or a guilty state of mind. *Mens rea* may be absent, for example, if a person acted unintentionally or made a relevant mistake. Juries and the courts may therefore seek to reconstruct what was happening in the accused's mind at the time of the commission of the criminal act. There are obvious difficulties in determining the subjective state of another person, and courts often have to rely on ideas of what a person was *likely* to have been thinking at the time of the commission of the offense. This may be straightforward in many cases, but in others, particularly where there is a psychopathological element in the defendant's conduct, the expert evidence of psychologists and psychiatrists may be required and may be admitted by the courts.

Tort law is a branch of the civil law that awards damages for violations of societal norms. By an award of compensatory damages, tort law seeks to compensate injured plaintiffs and to deter similar recurrences of the harm. Unlike the criminal law, where the state initiates prosecution on behalf of the state, victims may themselves choose whether to file tort claims. For the most part, courts rather than legislative bodies are the source of tort law and new torts continue to evolve. These new torts become part of what is collectively called the common law and are persuasive, though not controlling, in other jurisdictions.

### C. How Criminal and Civil Liability Is Affected by Sleep Deprivation

Human conduct does not consist of isolated acts: it occurs in the context of an unfolding sequence of events. To understand an act, then, we may need to examine what acts or other events preceded it. Decisions about criminal and civil liability may require courts to review the background to events to identify particular events that play a significant part in what happened. These events may involve choices made by individuals; this is particularly important in criminal law, where liability is often founded on the making of a choice by the defendant. For example, a person who chooses to consume excessive quantities of alcohol and later passes out while driving causing a collision that is fatal to another might not be fully conscious of his or her actions while driving. However, he or she is subject to criminal liability for the fatality because of the choice to consume the alcohol. A person who has a heart attack while driving and kills a pedestrian does not exercise a comparable choice to expose others to this risk, unless he or she has a timely warning of the heart attack. Choosing to drive in the face of high cholesterol, sedentary lifestyle, or failure to exercise is a decision too remote to the risk of a heart attack while driving to impose criminal liability. Although lifestyle or diet may be a cause of the heart attack, punishing a person for those behaviors reaches back too far. Unlike drinking and driving, poor eating habits and an unhealthy lifestyle do not carry a risk of immediate harm to others.

Civil liability generally depends on the foreseeability of the risk of harm. If, at an earlier point, it was foreseeable that a given consequence might follow from an act, and if that consequence subsequently materializes, then liability may be imposed. For instance, an employer who forces an employee to work several consecutive shifts without rest and then allows the visibly fatigued employee to drive home unaided might be civilly liable if the employee falls asleep while driving home and kills someone. Such damage may seem remote, but it is foreseeable that a tired driver will cause harm and a court may consequently decide that this harm is to be laid at the door of the employer. An award of damages might do more than merely compensate the injured party: it may deter other employers from similar risky scheduling practices and help prevent similar injuries to others. We examine this concept of causation more fully as we look in greater depth at how sleep affects the criminal and civil law.

## II.   Sleep Deprivation and Criminal Liability

### A.   Introduction

Most criminal offenses involve a deliberate decision to perform an act that is proscribed by the criminal law. The criminal law requires the state to prove that the defendant committed a guilty act (*actus reus*), while simultaneously manifesting the necessary mental state (*mens rea*, or guilty mind) that is specified for that crime. Consider a case in which a person hammers to death a family member and then claims to have been asleep at the time of the attack. Because a guilty act must be voluntary, a question of fact arises concerning the person's consciousness and the effect that impaired consciousness, or indeed unconsciousness, has on voluntariness (4). In addition, consciousness bears on the guilty state of mind and is therefore relevant to the mens rea inquiry.

The courts have grappled with how to apply the *mens rea* and *actus reus* requirements to defendants who are asleep or unconscious. The criminal law reveals two main categories of cases related to sleep deprivation. The first involves a situation where the act of falling asleep or losing consciousness causes harm, as in the case of a sleepy driver. The other concerns a person who, while asleep or unconscious, performs an act that causes harm, as in the case of a person who, while asleep, kills his roommate. Before discussing these categories in detail, we review the two essential elements of criminal liability and how they relate to sleep deprivation.

### B.   Basic Elements of Criminal Liability

To commit a crime, a person must perform some deliberate act in furtherance of the crime. A common example is a thief removing a wallet from another's pocket, or a burglar breaking the lock on a door. These acts follow upon a decision by the thief or burglar to perform the acts in question. There is deliberation and choice here—both of which are grounds for moral and legal blameworthiness. People performing actions while asleep or unconscious are normally not thought of in the law as acting voluntarily. Punishing someone for something done while unconscious would not serve the goals of the criminal law and would offend our basic moral intuition that such people are not deserving of punishment. Incarcerating an epileptic who strikes someone while in the throes of a violent seizure, for instance, would serve no deterrent or rehabilitative function.

This principle is firmly entrenched in the Model Penal Code (MPC), a model statute drafted by the American Law Institute in 1962 to help states define crimes consistently across the country (5). Many states have adopted the MPC, in whole or in part, and it has helped unify criminal law in the United States. The MPC recognized the incongruence of criminalizing actions performed by someone who is asleep or unconscious and incorporated that recognition into its definition of a voluntary act. Section 2.01 of the MPC states: "A person is not guilty of an offense unless his liability is based on conduct that includes a voluntary act or omission to perform an act of which he is physically able. . . . The following are not voluntary acts within the meaning of this section . . . a bodily movement during unconsciousness or sleep."

Every involuntary act, however, does not automatically absolve the actor from liability. Here we return to the observation above that an act that itself is not culpable may become culpable if it is shown to have been preceded by an earlier blameworthy act. For example, in *State v Olsen*, a woman became drowsy while driving and, despite opening the windows to combat her fatigue, fell asleep and killed a child playing on a sidewalk (6). She was convicted of involuntary manslaughter and the Supreme Court of Utah affirmed her conviction. The court reasoned that although an individual cannot be held accountable for actions done in an unconscious state, she may be liable for allowing herself to become unconscious. The court assumed that an individual does not fall asleep without warning, and that the decision to continue to drive in the face of extreme fatigue is sufficient to justify a conviction for involuntary manslaughter.

If the unconscious state—or the state of impaired consciousness—was self-induced through ingesting drugs or alcohol, then the voluntary act of consuming the drug is sufficient to impose criminal liability for acts performed while under their influence. For example, in *Lewis v State* the defendant consumed a pint of whisky and lapsed into unconsciousness (7). When Lewis awoke the next morning, he discovered that he had shot his roommate to death, although he had no recollection of doing this. Lewis was convicted of murder and the Supreme Court of Georgia affirmed his conviction. The court held the voluntary act of consuming the whiskey to the point that Lewis could not control his actions was sufficient to satisfy the elements of the offense. Although Lewis might have been unconscious during the commission of the crime, the court was willing to consider his earlier decision to consume alcohol as a basis for imposition of criminal responsibility.

Cases involving harm as the result of an unexpected medical condition that causes loss of consciousness present an initial set of related problems. In *People v Decina*, a motorist with a history of epileptic seizures blacked out while driving and drove into a group of six children, killing four (8). The defendant was convicted of criminal negligence in the children's deaths. Although the case was remanded on other grounds, the New York Court of Appeals affirmed the lower court's decision holding that the motorist's conduct fell within the statutory criteria for imposition of criminal liability. The court reasoned that although a sudden or unexpected loss of unconsciousness while driving normally abrogates criminal liability, in this case the motorist had prior knowledge of his propensity for epileptic seizures. Thus, the motorist should have realized the dangers in driving and took an unjustifiable risk in driving unsupervised.

In deciding whether to impose liability in respect of earlier choices made by the defendant, the courts will take into account a number of factors. The greater the risk of injury to others and the smaller the burden on the defendant to make less risky choices—the more a court will be inclined to impose criminal liability. In the case of intoxicated individuals, the risk analysis is clear. The risk of consuming intoxicants is widely recognized in society and the burden to avoid driving in an intoxicated condition small.

In cases like *Decina* involving medical conditions that cause unforeseen episodes of unconsciousness, the risk analysis is more difficult. For instance, if the motorist in *Decina* was taking medication to control his seizures, a court might find the risks of driving were sufficiently mitigated by the medication. Taking the example further, if the motorist simply forgot to take his medication, then a court might be more inclined to hold the motorist criminally liable. Reliance on a risk analysis is a necessary method of analysis; however, it may result in different decisions from court to court.

## C. Current State of Sleep and the Criminal Law

So far, our discussion has focused on those cases where the defendant's prior conduct has been such as to justify liability being imposed even if he or she was acting involuntarily (in an unconscious state) at the time of the commission of the crime. Where there is no earlier culpability, the issue becomes one of "blameless unconsciousness" and the courts are then obliged to consider their response to acts that may involve serious violence and that give rise to concerns over public safety. Such issues are not easily resolved, and there have been differing legal responses to sleep deprivation and other issues involving impaired consciousness (9). A common response, however, has been to recognize a defense known as the automatism defense. This allows for the acquittal of the person who commits a crime in a state of unconsciousness, although, as will be seen below, other approaches to automatism are possible, including treating it as a form of insanity.

### Automatism—Description and Overview

Automatism, which the law refers to as action without awareness (without regard to its cause), is generally considered a complete "defense" that negates an essential element of the prosecution's case in chief (9). Most courts treat automatism as negating the voluntary act element rather than the guilty mental state (10). Some states define automatism through case law; however, others have enacted legislation modeled after the Model Penal Code (11).

Most jurisdictions consider automatism a separate defense from that of insanity. For example, in *Fulcher v State*, an individual received a severe head injury in a drunken brawl. Subsequent to his arrest for disorderly conduct, he administered a brutal beating to a cellmate, which resulted in a conviction of aggravated assault. On appeal, the Supreme Court of Wyoming held that insanity would not be an appropriate defense in such a case. The court reasoned that this type of condition was not a disease of the mind appropriate for an insanity defense and that postacquittal civil commitment would not serve a useful purpose under these circumstances. The court affirmed the appellant's conviction, however, because there was not enough evidence to establish his unconscious state at the time of the assault. The court in *Fulcher* treated the defense of automatism as an affirmative defense. This means a defendant must not only raise the defense, but, to prevail, must prove it to the satisfaction of the fact finder by a preponderance of the evidence. Fulcher failed to meet his burden and could not overcome the presumption of consciousness the law recognizes.

It is not enough for a defendant to present uncorroborated testimony that he fell asleep or blacked out. Additional testimony, eyewitness accounts, or other forms of evidence must be presented to support a claim of unconsciousness. In *State v Jones*, Jones took a nap with his wife, and woke up to the sound of a gunshot (12). Allegedly asleep, he shot his wife in the head with a pistol she kept under her pillow. Expert testimony revealed that Jones might have had an REM sleep behavior disorder, in which he acted out his dreams. Other testimonial evidence was presented to support this diagnosis. Additional testimony was submitted, however, regarding several verbal threats he made concerning killing his wife. A jury found Jones guilty. Jones appealed his conviction for murder and argued that treating automatism as an affirmative defense required him to disprove the existence of a voluntary act. The appellate court disagreed, and held that requiring the defendant to prove his affirmative defense only shifted to him the need to overcome the presumption of consciousness. The court found no error in the instructions to the jury regarding defendant's burden of proof and upheld the conviction.

Other courts, however, hold that a defendant raising the automatism defense need only produce sufficient evidence to raise a reasonable doubt concerning the defendant's consciousness during the crime. This is less of a technical defense and more of a negation of an essential element of the state's case establishing that the defendant committed a voluntary act. California's Jury Instructions define an unconscious act as applying to "persons who are not conscious of acting but who perform acts while asleep . . . or other similar cause" (13). Evidence must be received that "tend[s] to show that the defendant was unconscious at the time and place of commission of the alleged crime" (13). If the evidence raises a reasonable doubt about the defendant's consciousness, then the jury should return a verdict of not guilty.

To defeat the prosecution's case and raise a reasonable doubt in the mind of the fact finder, it is not enough for the defendant to claim that he was unconscious at the time of the crime or that he had a sleep disorder or other malady that causes episodes of unconsciousness (14). For example, in *State v Hinkle*, Hinkle abruptly blacked out on his way home from work and collided head-on with another vehicle killing one of the passengers (15). At trial, Hinkle presented evidence of an undiagnosed brain disorder that caused the blackout. Despite this evidence, a jury convicted him of involuntary manslaughter. On appeal, Hinkle argued that he should have been entitled to an insanity defense instruction. The appellate court disagreed and held that unconsciousness (automatism) is separate from insanity and, if successful, established a reasonable doubt about the State's case. The court determined that uncorroborated testimony from the defendant would not be enough to raise a reasonable doubt. The appellate court reversed the defendant's conviction, however, because the jury was not instructed to consider whether the defendant knew of his condition and its likelihood for causing unconsciousness while driving. Without that knowledge, the appellate court reasoned, the jury would not be able to apply a classic risk analysis as described earlier in this chapter.

In one of the first cases involving sleep disorder under the automatism defense, the court in *Fain v Commonwealth* adopted the view that automatism negates an element of the prosecution's case in chief, thus exculpating the defendant (16). Fain, who had a long history of somnambulism, shot and killed a person who suddenly awakened him. He was convicted of murder, but the appellate court reversed having found error in the trial court's refusal to admit evidence of the defendant's sleep disorder. They reasoned that Fain could not be held liable for acts performed while asleep and explained that someone who is asleep would not have criminal intent, or be acting voluntarily.

### *Insanity—Description and Overview*

The insanity defense is an affirmative defense that exculpates a defendant who persuades the fact finder that, as a result of a mental disease or defect, he lacked the cognitive capacity to realize that what he was doing was wrong, or in some jurisdictions, the volitional capacity to conform his conduct to the requirements of the law (17). The modern insanity defense, with its varying iterations in different jurisdictions, is derived from the *M'Naghten Case*, an 1843 case involving a man who attempted to kill the British prime minister for various paranoid reasons (18). Instead of killing the prime minister, however, M'Naghten killed the prime minister's secretary. After the court found him insane, a panel of British judges was brought together to clarify the insanity standard. The *M'Naghten* test they developed recognizes a presumption of sanity that may be rebutted if the defendant can show that, at the time of the offense, he was "laboring under such a defect of reason, from disease of the mind as not to know the nature and quality of the act he was doing, or if he did, that he did not know what he was doing wrong" (19). Thus, the insanity defense is an affirmative defense and the burden of proving insanity at the time of the criminal act is on the defendant (20).

Some jurisdictions address sleep disorder defenses under the guise of the insanity defense. This, however, is a minority rule, and the insanity defense is usually viable only in cases involving sleep deprivation occasioned by long-term disorders such as epilepsy combined with other factors. For example, Indiana has limited the insanity defense to cases involving long-term disorders that require extended professional treatment. In *McClain v State*, McClain had only a few hours of sleep following a 25-hr flight from Japan and was allegedly in a state of dissociation caused by extreme sleep deprivation (21). After landing, McClain was pulled over for a routine traffic stop. He jumped out of his car and assaulted two police officers with a bottle, rendering one unconscious. During the trial the defendant withdrew an insanity plea and instead sought to rely on an automatism defense. McClain was found guilty of battery, among other crimes. The trial court's decision to exclude testimony related to the defendant's sleep deprivation was upheld by the intermediate appellate court because the insanity defense was withdrawn. The appellate court held that Indiana had not adopted the automatism defense because the legislature deliberately excluded such language following its adoption of the MPC. They followed the reasoning of similar jurisdictions that include automatism as a species of the insanity defense.

The defendant appealed to the Indiana Supreme Court, which reversed, holding that automatism is not a disease or defect within the meaning of the statute controlling the insanity defense (22). They found that a defense of automatism existed and hinged on the voluntariness of a defendant's actions. Citing various authorities, they defined automatism as manifesting itself in a range of conduct including sleepwalking, hypnotic states, fuges, metabolic disorders, and epilepsy or other convulsions and reflexes. The Indiana Supreme Court reasoned that by placing the requirement for a voluntary act in a separate statute from the insanity defense, the legislature implied that automatism and insanity are two defenses. They also adopted the majority rule and held that proof of automatism results in the negation of the *actus reus*.

Canadian criminal law, like U.S. criminal law, recognizes a defense of automatism in cases where the defendant has acted in a state of unconsciousness. What makes the Canadian experience in this area particularly interesting is the very full discussion of the subject to be found in a number of court decisions, including a decision of the Supreme Court of Canada in the case of *R. v Parks* (23). After the *Parks* decision the issue of somnambulism arose in a number of provincial court decisions, in which concern over the use of the automatism defense in such cases was aired.

The defendant in *Parks* was charged with the murder of his mother-in-law. On the evening of the incident, he fell asleep on a couch in his apartment and then allegedly left the building, got into his car, and drove over 14 miles to the home of his parents-in-law—all while still asleep. He entered his victims' apartment, killed the mother-in-law, and then, while assaulting the father-in-law, apparently woke up and left the apartment shouting. Psychiatric evidence was produced at the trial to establish that he was acting somnambulistically, and this evidence was accepted by the court. As a result of the conclusion that he was unconscious, the automatism defense became available to him. In Canadian law, this defense has two forms: one is intended for those cases where the unconsciousness results from a pathological condition of the brain, and the other is intended for cases where the automatism is caused by an external factor. The former results in the hospitalization of the defendant—as an insane defendant—while the latter allows for complete acquittal. A further factor in determining into which category the automatism falls is whether there is likely to be a recurrence of the automatic episode. In *Parks*, once the court accepted the expert evidence that this was unlikely to recur, it then became possible to treat the somnambulism as an instance of sane automatism, and therefore acquittal of murder would be possible, which was the eventual outcome.

The prosecution appealed unsuccessfully to the Supreme Court of Canada, which upheld the finding of the trial court. It therefore became open to a defendant in Canada to be totally exculpated, even on a charge as serious as murder, if somnambulism could be established. Not surprisingly, the *Parks* decision was controversial, not the least because the conduct in question seemed remarkably complicated for somnambulism, which is generally fairly banal and takes place over a relatively short period of time. In one view, a more likely explanation for such conduct would be dissociation, which is distinct from sleep-related activity. In the dissociative state, the defendant is not unconscious in the way in which one who is asleep is unconscious. A person in a dissociative state will be aware of his or her surroundings, even if this awareness is not normal awareness. The acts of a dissociated person are acts that he or she may take himself or herself to be doing; yet they are not acts that are referable to the "normal" or stable self, which usually constitutes the human actor. It will be important to distinguish somnambulism from dissociation because the criminal law implications may be quite different. Dissociation may form the basis of an insanity plea, although that will depend on the rules of the particular jurisdiction.

After the *Parks* case somnambulism has had a varied history in Canadian law. The defense has been invoked successfully on a number of cases, as it was, for example, in *R. v Granger* (24), where it was claimed by an adult charged with sexual interference with a young child who had climbed into his bed. In *R. v Stone* (25), however, a case involving dissociative behavior, the Supreme Court of Canada introduced a stricter standard for automatism—irrespective of the etiology of the automatism in question. Under the new test, judges will be required to start from the proposition that automatism is a concomitant of mental disease (as the law still calls it), and the more likely outcome is therefore a psychiatric disposal rather than a simple acquittal. The Supreme Court also ruled that the accused must establish automatism on the balance of probabilities and that juries must be informed of the policy issues surrounding the application of the defense. The effect of this is to suggest that it will be more difficult in the future for defendants in Canada to invoke somnambulism as a defense and, if they do, the consequences for them are more likely to be psychiatric committal rather than an uncomplicated acquittal.

### Sleep Deprivation as a Mitigating Factor in Sentencing

Courts may also consider sleep deprivation as a mitigating factor to reduce a defendant's sentence. The federal government and many states have passed laws that specify the factors a court may consider when setting its punishment (26). Sleep deprivation is an appropriate factor for a court to mitigate a sentence in many jurisdictions so long as it is not induced by voluntary consumption of drugs or alcohol (27). For example in *State v Fowler*, a man consumed alcohol and methamphetamine for 3 days during which he did not sleep. On the third day, he severely beat and robbed an acquaintance. This was Fowler's first criminal act and he claimed that the sleep deprivation caused his violent outburst. The trial court used the sleep deprivation as a mitigating factor in assessing Fowler's sentence and the state appealed. The appellate court rejected consideration of sleep deprivation as a mitigating factor because there was no evidence that the sleep deprivation was unrelated to the consumption of drugs and alcohol. The Supreme Court of Washington agreed, holding that voluntary consumption of drugs and alcohol may not be considered as a mitigating factor in sentencing.

### D. Conclusions

The criminal law embodies the general moral belief that acts performed in a state of unconsciousness are not acts deserving of punishment. The implementation of this belief is, however, difficult. In particular, it may not be easy to distinguish those cases in which there is some form of consciousness, even if impaired, and those where there is full unconsciousness. This may affect cases of somnambulism, which may in some cases share features with dissociative states. Where there is sufficient evidence that the defendant was in fact acting somnambulistically, then a defense of automatism should be available in most states. This may lead to complete acquittal, or in some circumstances it may result in hospital committal.

Where falling asleep while performing a hazardous activity has resulted in harm to others, then the enquiry as to guilt focuses on the prior conduct of the defendant. If the defendant could not have been expected to foresee a risk that this would happen, then a defense may be available. If such foresight could reasonably have been expected, or if there was culpable conduct in ingesting alcohol or drugs that might lead to unconsciousness, then there will be no defense. In such cases one might accurately say that sleep is no excuse, which sounds morally counter-intuitive, but is nonetheless legally correct.

### III.    Sleep Deprivation and Civil Liability

#### A.    Introduction

The basis of most civil liability is the negligent, rather than the intentional, harming of the legally protected interests of another. Negligence may be constituted as a failure to meet an expected standard of care, whether through a defect such as incompetence or through the taking of unreasonable risks. This standard of care is an objective one, and does not in general take into account the capacities of the individual defendant. The defendant's behavior will therefore be measured against the standard of what a reasonable person in the defendant's position could have been expected to do. If a reasonable person would have acted more prudently to avoid injury, then the court is likely to permit imposition of liability. Liability not only can be imposed on the person who was the immediate cause of the harm, but can attach to others who played a part, as an employer, for example, or even as a physician. Thus an employer who allows employees to behave in a dangerous fashion may be liable for the harm that is caused to third parties.

Cases in which civil liability claims or defenses are asserted for conduct arising out of sleep disorders or sleep deprivation generally fall into four broad categories. The first involves an action against a person for harm caused by his or her own lapse of consciousness. This category of cases includes drivers who have lost consciousness as the result of sleep deprivation, a heart attack, or other unforeseeable sudden ailment.

The second category of cases involves actions against a third person who is claimed to have breached a duty that resulted in another's loss of consciousness and consequential injury. Typical of this category of liability claims are actions against a physician by a person injured by the patient who lost consciousness while driving. The injured claimant in these cases often alleges that the physician failed to diagnose a patient's condition affecting consciousness or failed to warn a patient about the risks of unconsciousness from a prescribed medication. In addition to questions about the reasonableness of the physician's conduct, these cases present questions of whether someone who is not a party to the physician-patient relationship may sue for substandard medical care rendered the patient that caused injury to the nonpatient.

The third category of cases involves liability of employers for injuries caused by, or to, employees. The law recognizes that employers are vicariously liable for their employees' negligent acts committed within the scope of their employment, without regard to any act of negligence on the part of the employer. An employer's vicarious liability is generally limited to injuries caused by employees who are operating within the scope of their traditional work functions. Vicarious liability cases involving sleep deprivation have focused on expanding the scope of employer's liability based on job-related sleep deprivation and injury. The prototypical case involves an employer who overworks an employee who then has an accident while driving home from work, normally regarded as outside the scope of traditional work functions.

Cases involving workers who injure themselves on the job are subsumed by the workers' compensation system. The relationship between workplace-caused sleep deprivation and injury is another area in which the traditional scope of liability has been expanded.

Finally, there is a category of cases that involve contributory negligence on the part of the plaintiff. If the defendant can prove that the injured party was partly at fault, then the plaintiff's claim might be reduced by a certain percentage. For instance, if the plaintiff's own sleep deprivation helped cause his injury, then his compensation from the defendant may be reduced or denied.

## B. Current State of Sleep Deprivation and Civil Liability

*Defendant Primary Liability for Sleep Deprivation or
Disorder-Related Harm*

Motor-Vehicle-Related Accidents

Motor-vehicle accidents caused by fatigued or unconscious drivers are judged by a standard of negligence. Negligence is the breach of a duty, proximately causing injury. A driver owes a duty to other drivers to drive safely and avoid predictable accidents: a breach of that duty, whether by consuming alcohol or drugs or by driving without adequate caution, or by any other instance of defective driving, may amount to negligence and give rise to civil liability.

Tort law uses an objective standard in judging behavior; it does not seek to determine whether a person performed as well as he or she could have done but whether the performance met the standard society imposes for all of its members acting under the same circumstances (28). The objective approach looks at how an ordinary reasonable person would react in the same situation. It does not consider a person's individual unique traits, but creates a fictitious majoritarian figure and utilizes that character as a standard. The rationale for the use of this method is that it creates uniformity in the law and ensures that society as a whole can rely on a certain standard of care from their fellow citizens.

In situations involving drivers who fall asleep or become unconscious while driving, the key to assessing whether the driver met society's expectations turns on how much notice a driver has of her condition prior to the accident. Unexpected or unforeseen losses of consciousness are not usually regarded as negligent. Knowledge of the risk of unconsciousness, however, such as yawning, consumption of intoxicating substances, or previous lapses of consciousness, will generally support a finding of liability. Many courts presume that ordinary sleep does not occur without warning, and thus, a person who simply falls asleep while driving is assumed to have acted negligently without separate proof of acts that might give the driver warning of the impending loss of consciousness (29).

At one end of the spectrum are courts that hold drivers who fall asleep negligent as a matter of law (30). This means a person found to have fallen asleep while driving will be irrebuttably presumed to have acted negligently. Most courts, however, hold that a person who falls asleep at the wheel is presumed to be negligent, but may introduce proof in an effort to rebut the presumption (31).

Other courts have approached this issue more pragmatically. In *McCall v Wilder*, for example, a driver with an inoperable brain tumor had an epileptic seizure while driving and struck another vehicle (32). The defendant had prior seizures and was aware that he lost consciousness during the seizures. The Tennessee Supreme Court reversed the trial court's grant of summary judgment in favor of the defendant, finding that the seizure and accident were foreseeable. The court analyzed cases from jurisdictions around the country and articulated the general rule that the operator of a motor vehicle is not ordinarily regarded as

negligent because of a fainting spell or unforeseen loss of consciousness resulting in an inability to control the vehicle.

The court went on to describe a multifactor test to assess whether the
unconscious driver was negligent that asked whether the loss of consciousness
was reasonably foreseeable. In determining whether the loss of capacity or consciousness was foreseeable, the court suggested the following nonexclusive list of
considerations:

> the extent of the driver's awareness or knowledge of the condition that
> caused the sudden incapacity;
> whether the driver sought medical advice or was under a physician's care
> for the condition when the accident occurred;
> whether the driver had been prescribed, and had taken, medication for the
> condition;
> whether a sudden incapacity had previously occurred while driving;
> the number, frequency, extent, and duration of incapacitating episodes prior
> to the accident while driving and otherwise;
> the temporal relationship of the prior incapacitating episodes to the acci-
> dent;
> a physician's guidance or advice regarding driving to the driver, if any; and
> medical opinions regarding the nature of the driver's condition, adherence
> to treatment, foreseeability of the incapacitation, and potential advance
> warnings that the driver would have experienced immediately prior to the
> accident (32).

On a related note, automobile guest statutes bar an ordinary negligence
claim against a driver by a passenger who is riding gratuitously. Guest statutes,
however, do not bar recovery for claims of gross negligence. As contrasted with
ordinary negligence, gross negligence entails acting unreasonably in the face of a
grave risk of harm. For example, when evidence proves the driver continued operating the vehicle in the face of clear warnings of her fatigue, courts will permit a
finding that the driver was reckless or grossly negligent (33). In *Lankford v Mong*
a guest passenger in Mong's car was killed when Mong drove off a road and
struck a concrete bridge abutment (34). In the days preceding the accident, Mong
had scant amounts of sleep. The jury determined that Mong's conduct was wan-
ton, within the meaning of the guest statute that defined the term as reckless indif-
ference, and found him liable under the guest statute for the death of his
passenger. The Supreme Court of Alabama affirmed, reasoning that there was sufficient evidence for a jury to determine that Mong consciously and deliberately
disregarded a risk to his passenger by driving while severely sleep-deprived.

## Other Causes of Injury

In addition to motor vehicle accidents, sleep deprivation plays an appreciable role
in many other forms of accident, including medical ones. Scientific evidence and
general common sense reveal that sleep-deprived workers are more liable to make

mistakes that cause injuries to themselves or others while on the job (35). Courts defer to federal and state legislatures to curb maximum hours employees may work. An area of recent debate concerning resident-physicians typifies this trend (see Chap. 18). Although a case in the early 1990s helped one state change the policies of hospitals regarding resident-physician work hours, the real burden of reforming practices in this area falls upon the legislature. Legislative bodies, not courts, are the organs of government that set minimum standards for policing and controlling fatigue (36). Most often, legislative bodies or regulatory agencies such as the Occupational Safety and Health Administration (OSHA) set limits on the maximum hours that may be worked in certain professions that pose a risk to the general public such as truckers and pilots.

Efforts to regulate the hours worked by resident-physicians have gained momentum. The American Medical Student Association (AMSA) has backed a house resolution (HR 3235) that seeks to limit resident-physician work hours. Additionally, AMSA has also sponsored a petition to the Occupational Safety and Health Administration for new workplace standards for resident-physicians. In response, the American Medical Association has adopted new standards limiting resident-physician work hours to 80 hr/week (37). This policy might serve as a basis for future claims against hospitals that violate the standard.

### Health Care Provider Liability to Third Person for Patient Injury

Physicians have a duty to prevent foreseeable harm to their patients. Until the 1970s, most courts limited the liability of physicians to claims by their patients and did not recognize claims against physicians by third parties harmed by the patient. Increasingly, courts recognized that physicians have a legal duty to treat their patients properly to prevent foreseeable injuries to third persons (38). Claims against physicians involving sleep disorders arising out of harm to third persons generally fall into two categories: negligent failure to diagnose an illness affecting consciousness and negligent failure to inform a patient about the risks of unconsciousness surrounding a prescribed medication or treatment (28).

In cases involving a physician's negligent failure to diagnose a disease, courts expect the physician's diagnosis and treatment to conform to relevant professional standards and that these same standards require physicians to warn their patients about the side effects of their condition (39). Courts are becoming increasingly reluctant, however, to expose physicians to broad liabilities associated with all harms patients cause to the general public. After weighing the benefits of the warning versus the burden on the physician, many courts have retreated from imposing such broad liabilities. Some courts are now finding the utility of imposing liability—to warn patients of all side effects of their condition that might affect the general public—imposes too great a burden on physicians.

In *Praesel v Johnson*, a person with epilepsy suffered a seizure while driving and killed another motorist (40). The deceased motorist's estate brought a suit against three treating physicians for negligence in failing to warn their patient with epilepsy not to drive. The trial court granted summary judgment in favor of the physicians, holding that the physicians owed no duty to third parties. The court of appeals affirmed the judgments for all but one of the physicians. The last physician had treated the person with epilepsy for a seizure 1 year before the accident. On appeal by the third physician, the Texas Supreme Court reversed and held that physicians do not owe a duty to unknown third parties. Looking at the failure to warn, the court balanced the risk and foreseeability of the injury against the social utility and burden imposed on the physicians. The court decided that even if a physician warned a patient not to drive, the physician has no control over the patient's subsequent actions. Thus, the court reasoned that imposing liability in a vain attempt to protect the general public was too great a burden on physicians.

When considering claims of a physician's failure to warn a patient of the side effect of treatment, courts do not impose liability when the side effect is readily obvious. In *Calwell v Hassan*, a patient with long-standing problems related to daytime sleeping received various treatments and medications from her physician (41). Despite the physician's extensive treatment efforts, however, the patient's problems continued. Finally, while driving to work one morning, the patient fell asleep and struck two bicycle riders. The trial court granted summary judgment for the physician on a claim instituted by the cyclists, finding the physician owed no duty to the bicycle riders. The court of appeals reversed and found a special relationship between the physician and the general public. The Kansas Supreme Court affirmed the trial court and reversed the 1995 court of appeals decision.

The Kansas Supreme Court refused to impose liability for failure to warn of an outcome that was readily obvious to the patient. The court reasoned the patient was well aware she might fall asleep while driving, and thus it would have served no beneficial purpose for the physician to reinforce a warning not to drive as well as subjecting a physician to liability for another's acts over which he had no control. The Kansas high court also reasoned that the physician did not agree to protect third parties from a patient's actions by merely agreeing to treat her condition. The medications prescribed to the patient were meant to improve the patient's condition and did not worsen her daytime sleeping problems.

Other courts require proof that the treatment directly caused the injury to the third persons. If a patient's actions superseded the treatment's side effects, then a physician is less likely to be held liable for the harm caused by the patient. For example, in *Shortnacy v North Atlantic Internal Medicine*, a patient who received Demerol and Phenergan, medications for back pain, was warned not to drive for 12 hr (42). Despite the warning, the patient did drive, blacked out, and struck into another car head-on after driving the wrong way onto a highway. The accident occurred more than 6 hr after the injection and the patient also tested positive for marijuana in his urine. The court refused to hold the physician liable reasoning that to do so would force a physician to predict a patient's actions following treatment and balance them against the risks posed to the general public.

Here the patient's illicit drug use interfered with the treatment and could not be predicted by the physician. Absent any direct relationship between the injured family and the physician, the court declined to impose a duty.

Similarly, if too much time elapses between the treatment and the injury, courts are reluctant to impose liability on a physician for harm to third persons. In *Lester v Hall*, a patient receiving lithium treatments had a car accident 5 days after his last treatment (43). The plaintiff alleged that the treatment was negligent and left the patient in an impaired condition that caused the accident. The court found the accident was unforeseeable given the 5 days between treatment and the accident. Additionally, the court refused to hold the physician liable for the accident because he had no direct supervision over the patient's actions. In weighing public policy and social utility considerations, the court found the burden imposed on a physician would be outweighed by the incremental benefits of warning.

Another issue concerning duties of physicians involves statutes requiring physicians to report to state agencies patients who have certain sleep disorders or other conditions that might affect a patient's consciousness while driving. Physicians are normally required to maintain confidentiality regarding the care of the patient. In situations that involve high degrees of risk to the general public, however, legislative bodies have abrogated confidentiality. Many state legislatures have enacted laws requiring physicians to report sleep disorders that might affect the public to public health officials. Legislative bodies have determined that significant threats to public safety outweigh a physician's duty of confidentiality and justify disclosure.

Generally, physicians should report if an immediate and substantial risk is presented. Such risks would include those involving motor vehicle operations. State laws have not been uniform, however, with many leaving little to no guidance about which disorders to report, or when to report the disorder. Additionally, some of the laws are interpreted to be voluntary only (44). This ambiguity has led some medical associations to urge its members to err in favor of reporting (28). Others, however, recommend a more risk-based balance (28).

### Employer Liability for the Consequences of Employee Sleep Deprivation or Sleep Disorders

#### Common Law Liability for Employees' Harm to Third Parties

Employers are vicariously liable for harm caused by their employees within the employee's scope of employment under the common-law doctrine of respondeat superior, without regard to a showing of fault by the employer. Traditionally, the employer's liability is limited to the employee's work functions. The role of sleep deprivation and sleep disorders in this area of the law has been to expand the scope of vicarious liability in cases involving those harmed by fatigued employees returning home after working excessive shifts. Typically, before courts have been willing to expand the employer's vicarious liability in this manner, the employer must have some forewarning that its scheduling practices could lead to a postwork accident involving the overworked employee. An employer who has forced or allowed an employee to work excessive hours may be held liable for harm caused by the employee who fell asleep while driving home if the employer knew its employee was grossly exhausted and might pose a threat on the road (45).

In *Depew v Crocodile Enterprises*, a Crocodile Café manager fell asleep while driving home after working a double shift followed by a night shift on the day of the accident (46). After falling asleep, the manager's car struck Depew's car and killed her. Instead of pursuing a negligence claim against the manager, Depew's surviving heirs sued Crocodile Café under the doctrine of respondeat superior. The court of appeals upheld the lower courts granting of summary judgment in favor of Crocodile Café and refused to hold Crocodile vicariously liable. The court of appeals found that the manager's work schedule did not violate any statutorily imposed limitations on work hours. They also declared there was an insufficient nexus between the employer's work demands and the injury to the employee and third party. The court of appeals reasoned that the manager's 16 hr of rest between the double shift and the night shift prior to the accident were adequate buffers for an ordinary employee to secure rest. The court reasoned that any reasonable employer would feel secure that an employee with that amount of rest would not pose a threat to other motorists while driving home.

In its description of the doctrine of respondeat superior, the court noted the general rule that employers are liable for injuries caused by an employee only when the employee is acting within his/her normal job function. An employee's commute to and from work is not normally considered part of an employee's job function. There is, however, a special risk exception to this going and coming rule when the employer's actions create a risk of harm to others (46). In this case, the court concluded that Crocodile's scheduling of a double shift followed by 16 hr of rest for its manager did not meet this threshold.

The exact boundaries constituting sufficiently risky scheduling practices are imprecise. In *Hershman v New Line Productions*, a subcontractor employee who worked a continuous 19-hr shift that followed a 70-hr workweek fell asleep while driving home and was killed (47). The heirs of the deceased appealed the trial court's dismissal of their claim against the general contractor, but the California Court of Appeals upheld the dismissal. Relying on the coming-and-going rule, the court was unable to find a 70-hr workweek and a 19-hr shift sufficiently risky to meet the substantial-risk exception. The court also disregarded the fact the subcontractor's employee had no other reasonable alternative beyond driving to return home.

Similarly, in *Lesser v Nordstrom*, an employee of Nordstrom who normally worked 10-hr shifts 6 days a week worked a 12-hr shift (48). After the longer shift, she apparently fell asleep while driving home and struck another vehicle. The trial court granted the defendant's motion for summary judgment and dismissed the plaintiff's claim. The court decided the employer was not liable under the theory of respondeat superior because the employee was driving home from work and was not conducting any official business. Additionally, the employer was not negligent in scheduling the employee for a longer shift because it was not foreseeable that a shift 2 hr longer than normal would result in the employee's accident.

Some courts find an employee's voluntary decision to work extended shifts dispositive. In *Baggett v Brumfield*, a new employee worked 21 hr straight and then apparently fell asleep while driving home and killed another driver (49). On appeal, the Louisiana Court of Appeals reversed the lower court's decision holding the employer liable for not preventing the employee from working the long shift and for not providing adequate accommodations to allow the employee time to rest before driving home. The appellate court ruled that, because the employee voluntarily chose to drive home after he clocked out, the employer could not be held vicariously liable. Additionally, the employer was not negligent because the employer never forced its employee to work the extended shift, nor did it have any clear evidence the employee was grossly fatigued.

## Workers' Compensation

Workers in qualifying employment who are injured on the job must bring compensation claims against their employers through the workers' compensation system. This system is statutorily implemented and provides for an administrative remedy for workers. Thus, claims are resolved through the administrative hearing process instead of through a civil court system, which instead provides appellate review. In most workers' compensation cases, the injured worker:

> must prove that disorder/accident meets the definition of compensable injury or work-related disablement in workers' compensation laws; and
> must also show a connection between the disorder/accident and the work.

Sleep deprivation and sleep disorders question the scope of the definition of injury and work function in workers' compensation cases. Generally, unless a clear link can be shown between the sleep disorder or deprivation and the scope of employment, courts are unwilling to grant compensation to the worker. Courts have regarded sleep and work as separate and distinct.

Many cases concern workers who fall asleep while driving home after working excessive hours. Most courts refuse to extend workers' compensation benefits to workers injured while driving from home to work or work to home. In *Britt v Shelby County Health Care Authority*, an employee who regularly worked 16-hr double shifts on the weekends was injured after falling asleep while driving home after her Sunday shift (50). The court affirmed the denial of her workers' compensation claim for injury occasioned while commuting from work to home and refused to extend the special-risk exception to the facts of this case. The court ruled that although she satisfied a "but-for" causation link from her employment to the injury, she failed to show the injury was caused in the course of her job.

Similarly, in *Krushwitz v McDonald's Restaurants of Oregon*, the court refused to compensate the estate of an employee who fell asleep at the wheel and was killed in an automobile accident as he was returning home after working multiple shifts (51). Although a separate civil case held McDonald's liable for the injuries caused by Krushwitz, the Oregon Supreme Court upheld denial of Krushwitz's workers' compensation claim. Because Krushwitz had completed his work and was returning home at time of his death, he was outside of the workers' compensation realm.

Sometimes a statute governing conditions of employment may create liability when it ordinarily would not exist. In *Johnson v Stratlaw*, a 16-year-old boy was killed after falling asleep while driving home from a late shift at a local restaurant (52). State law limited the hours that minors could be scheduled to an 8-hr shift not to exceed 12:30 A.M. on nonschool nights. The minor worked past 2:00 A.M. the night of the accident. The parents filed a wrongful-death action against the employer, who successfully moved the trial court to dismiss the personal injury claim. This dismissal was on the grounds that the exclusive remedy was the workers' compensation finding that the employer's conduct met the special-risk exception to the coming-and-going rule and was thus within the scope of workers' compensation provisions.

One other area of recent debate in workers' compensation cases involves shift-work-maladaption syndrome. These cases usually involve workers who are unable to adapt to working a third shift. Workers asserting these claims usually complain of being unable to adapt their personal sleeping schedules to the late shift, and suffer from continued sleep deprivation. American courts have rejected shift-work-maladaption syndrome as a compensable injury under the workers' compensation definitions of injury, and generally hold that harm occasioned by the mere scheduling of hours is not enough to state a claim (53). A worker must show that a specific injury has been caused by a specific workplace condition or job function.

A tribunal in Nova Scotia has recently held otherwise. In *Michelin v Nova Scotia (Workers' Compensation Board)*, a worker who was in perfect health and had no outside habits that would adversely affect his sleep complained that working variable shifts adversely affected his work and private life (54). The workers' compensation tribunal found that shift-work-maladaption syndrome is a compensable injury under the workers' compensation scheme. The board found the condition disabling because the worker was too tired to work safely, and his inability to adapt to the alternating shifts was the cause of the injury. The board also found persuasive the worker's clean and healthy lifestyle that did not otherwise affect his sleep.

Despite a shrinking economy and higher-than-normal unemployment numbers, worker output in the early quarters of 2002 showed increased productivity (55). Fewer workers are being asked to do more. Whether this trend will result in increased litigation concerning sleep deprivation and workers' compensation claims is yet to be determined.

### Contributory Negligence Related to Sleep Disorder or Deprivation

If a plaintiff contributes to his or her own harm, the defendant's liability may be reduced or abrogated. In negligence claims, courts may consider the role of a plaintiff's action in a number of ways (28). The plaintiff's negligence may supersede the defendant's negligence and be regarded as the primary cause of the plaintiff's injury. If successful, this negates an element of the plaintiff's case (causation) and would abrogate the defendant's liability. Or, the plaintiff's negligence might provide the basis for an apportionment of liability based on each party's conduct and reduce the plaintiff's compensation by the percentage his or her actions contributed to the injury.

Courts generally allow defendants to submit evidence showing that a plaintiff's sleep disorder or sleep deprivation contributed to the tort in dispute. If the evidence is judged to be credible, then the plaintiff's damages will be reduced as a function of the degree to which the sleep condition contributed to the accident.

For example, in *Voohries v Cessna*, three men convinced two women to fly with them after a drinking binge at a local bar (56). In addition to evidence that the pilots were intoxicated; there was evidence that two of the three pilots were excessively fatigued. One of the men had had approximately 4 hr sleep in the past 48 hr. Once aloft, the plane plunged to the ground, killing all aboard. The mothers of the dead pilots brought a claim against Cessna, claiming the aircraft had a defective fuel tank design. Cessna countered that pilot error and negligence were the causes of the crash. A jury found for Cessna and the appellate court affirmed. The appellate court agreed with Cessna that the pilot's poor choices in flying fatigued and/or under the influence of alcohol were likely the primary causes of the accident. They reasoned that even if the aircraft had a defective design, the pilots were excessively reckless and that superseded other causes of the mishap.

In contrast, in *Bailey v Norfolk and Western Railway Company*, a railroad brakeman worked for 28 years, during which time he endured perpetual sleep deprivation owing to exhaustive work conditions (57). The sleep deprivation contributed to various health ailments that culminated in severe heart and gastrointestinal disease. The trial court found the railroad liable in a claim brought under the Federal Employer's Liability Act and the appellate court affirmed. Among many other issues, the appellate court dismissed the railroad's argument that the trial court improperly disregarded its proposed contributory negligence instruction. The railroad argued that the brakeman's failure to report his condition to the railroad helped perpetuate the poor work conditions. The appellate court disagreed based on evidence that the railroad would not have made changes to the conditions even if they were aware of the brakeman's ailments.

In *Findley v Alabama Power Company*, a utility pole installed in 1946 was the subject of several complaints owing to its proximity to a busy road (58). After working a 24-hr shift, a motorist allegedly fell asleep and struck the pole. The motorist claimed the utility company was at fault because of its failure to move the pole. The utility company countered that the motorist was contributorily negligent for the accident because she fell asleep while driving. The trial court granted a motion for summary judgment in favor of the utility company, but was reversed on appeal. The court of appeals held that a genuine issue of material fact was created concerning whether the motorist actually fell asleep and the trial judge incorrectly failed to present the issue for a jury to consider. Although a police officer at the scene of the accident took a statement from the driver indicating that she fell asleep, the defendant submitted a contradictory affidavit that claimed she was not fatigued or sleepy.

## C.  Conclusions

Tort law seeks to compensate a person who has been harmed by the wrongful conduct of another and also hopes to deter similar injuries. Tort law considers a person's decision to take a particular action and the risk involved when determining liability. As the cases above illustrate, sleep disorders and sleep deprivation can play an important role in choice and risk. Additionally, physicians who treat patients for sleep disorders have an obligation to warn their patients of the risks of the sleep condition and any treatment rendered. Failure to inform their patient of the risks could lead to injuries to others, for which the physician might be liable.

## IV.  General Conclusions

There is growing evidence of the major role that sleep disorders and sleep deprivation play in the causation of accidents. The costs of these accidents are enormous, in both economic and human terms. The barge captain who did not get enough sleep prior to piloting his barge down the Arkansas River lost his job, caused untold sums in damages, and caused the death of over a dozen people. The accident will be the focus of prolonged litigation that will cost significant sums in legal fees. Although the captain might also have suffered from a preexisting heart condition, this situation might have been avoided had he not been sleep-deprived. As medical science improves our understanding of sleep, more legal situations involving sleep deprivation are likely to arise. The incidence of sleep-related litigation will also be increased by the progress of the 24-hr society and its growing impact on normal sleep patterns. More and more people may be expected to be sleep-deprived, and more and more of these sleep-deprived people will perform below par, fall asleep at the wheel, or make decisions that pose an unreasonable risk to others. Though the resulting damage may be extensive, physicians can play an important role in minimizing the harm of sleep deprivation. This can be done through keeping abreast of developments in sleep medicine and through ensuring that their patients are aware of the risks associated with sleep deprivation and sleep disorders. For its part, the law must be open to the new insights of sleep medicine and adapt its response to take full account of these new developments. The objective should be to ensure that both the criminal and the civil law approach sleep-related issues from a position of better understanding.

## References

1. Report: Towboat Captain has Heart Blockage, Associated Press Newswires (June 1, 2002), available at WESTLAW, 06/01/02 Apwires 04:21:00.
2. Press Release, Oklahoma Attorney General, AG Files Suit in I-40 Bridge Collision, (June 5, 2002), available at http://www.oag.state.ok.us (last visited Aug. 21, 2002).
3. Walton, Rod. Family Wants I-40 Tugboat Case Moved, Tulsa World, August 2, 2002.
4. See Sallee v State, 544 P.2d 902 (Okla. Crim. App. 1976).
5. McClain C. Criminal Law Reform: Historical Development in the United States. Encyclopedia of Crime and Justice 1983; 2:510–412.
6. State v Olsen, 160 P.2d 427 (Utah 1945).
7. Lewis v State, 27 S.E.2d 659 (Ga. 1943).
8. People v Decina, 138 N.E.2d 799 (N.Y. 1956).
9. See Fulcher v State, 633 P.2d 142 (Wyo.1981).
10. LaFave WR, Scott AW. Criminal Law. 2d ed. St. Paul: West Publishing, 1986:§ 4.9.
11. See, e.g., Cal. Penal Code § 26 (West 2002) ("All persons are capable of committing crimes except those belonging to the following classes . . . Persons who committed the act charged without being conscious thereof").
12. State v Jones, 527 S.E.2d 700 (N.C. Ct. App. 2000).
13. California Jury Instructions—Criminal. 6th ed. Los Angeles: West, 1996 § 4.30.
14. See also People v Roman, No. F036067, 2002 WL 524361 (Cal. App. Dep't Super. Ct. 2002). (Defendant fondled and raped a young girl and introduced evidence that he was diagnosed with somnambulism since he was a young child. The court determined the sleep disorder was irrelevant to his sexual assault based on the defendant's actions prior and subsequent to the incident) (unpublished opinion).
15. State v Hinkle, 489 S.E.2d 257 (W. Va. 1996).
16. Fain v Commonwealth, 78 Ky. 183, 1879 WL 6704 (1879); See also Fisher v. State, 18 S.W. 90 (Tex. App. 1891) (recognizing that somnambulism is not insanity, and it is not an indication of insanity).
17. People v Grant, 377 N.E.2d 4 (Ill. 1978).
18. M'Naghten's Case, 101 Cl. & F. 200, 8 Eng. Rep. 718 (H.L. 1843).
19. Idem.; see also Rogers R, Shuman D. Conducting Insanity Evaluations, 2d ed. New York: Guilford Press, 2000.
20. State v Wilson, 514 P.2d 603 (N.M. 1973).
21. McClain v State, 670 N.E.2d 911 (Ind. Ct. App.1996).
22. McClain v State, 678 N.E.2d 104 (Ind. 1997).
23. [1992] 2 SCR 87.
24. Supreme Court of BC, 1 Feb 1996.
25. [1999] 2 SCR 290.
26. See, e.g., United States Sentencing Commission. Guidelines Manual, §5k2.0, Nov. 2001, available at http://www.ussc.gov (last visited Sept. 9, 2002).
27. State v Fowler, 38 P.3d 335 (Wash. 2002) (en banc).
28. Shuman D. Civil liability issues arising out of sleep deprivation and sleep disorders. In: Shapiro C, Smith AM, eds. Forensic Aspects of Sleep. New York: Wiley, 1997:99–114.
29. Bushnell v Bushnell, 131 A. 432 (Conn. 1925).
30. Theisen v Milwaukee Auto. Mut. Ins. Co., 118 N.W.2d 140 (Wis. 1962).
31. See, e.g., Kilburn v Bush, 223 A.D.2d 110, 646 N.Y.S.2d 429 (N.Y. App. Div. 1996); Spivak v. Heyward, 248 A.D.2d 58, 679 N.Y.S.2d 156 (N.Y. App. Div. 1998) (fol-

lowed Kilburn's rebuttable presumption of negligence for drivers who fall asleep at the wheel); Malave v Kurth, No. CV980331014S, 1999 WL 1034672 (Conn. Super. Ct.) (holding that it is a material fact for the jury whether or not an individual knows or should have reason to know he or she is about to fall asleep at the wheel).

32. McCall v Wilder, 913 S.W.2d 150 (Tenn. 1995).
33. Richards v Parks, 93 S.W.2d 639 (Tenn. Ct. App. 1935).
34. Lankford v Mong, 214 So. 2d 301 (Ala. 1968).
35. Fleming JAE. Pharmacological aspects of drowsiness. In: Shapiro C, Smith AM, eds. Forensic Aspects of Sleep. New York: Wiley, 1997:151–202.
36. Zion v New York City Hosp., 183 A.D.2d 386, 590 N.Y.S.2d 188 (N.Y. App. Div. 1992).
37. Accreditation Council for Graduate Medical Education, ACGME Highlights its Standards on Resident Duty Hours, (May 2002), at http://www.acgme.org (last visited Aug. 21, 2002).
38. See Tarasoff v Board of Regents of the University of California, 551 P.2d 334 (Cal. 1976).
39. See, e.g., Freese v Lemmon, 210 N.W.2d 576 (Iowa 1973) (doctor found liable for failing to diagnose the causes of a first-time seizure in a patient and for failing to warn the patient not to drive).
40. Praesel v Johnson, 967 S.W.2d 391 (Tex. 1998).
41. Calwell v.Hassan, 925 P.2d 422 (Kan. 1996).
42. Shortnacy v North Atl. Internal Med., 556 S.E.2d 209 (Ga. Ct. App. 2001).
43. Lester v Hall, 970 P.2d 590 (N.M. 1998).
44. See Praesel, 967 S.W.2d at 392. (Holding the reporting statute in Texas is a voluntary reporting mechanism and failure to report the condition is not negligence per se. The recording statutes control no actual conduct that leads to harm, and imposing liability for failure to report would expose physicians to an overly broad civil liability.)
45. See Faverty v McDonald Rests. of Oregon, 892 P.2d 703 (Or. Ct. App. 1995).
46. Depew v Crocodile Enters., Inc., 73 Cal. App. 4th 480, 73 Cal. Rptr. 2d 673 (1998).
47. Hershman v New Line Prods., Inc., No. B145028, 2001 WL 1470360 (Cal. Ct. App.) (unpublished opinion).
48. Lesser v Nordstrom, Inc., Nos. Civ. A.96–8121, A.97–6070, 1998 WL 480832 (E.D. Pa.).
49. Baggett v Brumfield, 758 So.2d 332 (La. Ct. App. 2000).
50. Britt v Shelby County Health Care Auth., No. 2991083, 2001 WL 367591 (Ala. Civ. App.) (unpublished opinion).
51. Krushwitz v McDonald's Rests. of Oregon, Inc., 919 P.2d 465 (Or. 1996).
52. Johnson v Stratlaw, Inc., 224 Cal. App. 3d. 1156, 274 Cal. Rptr. 363 (1990).
53. Metropolitan Edison Co. v Workmen's Comp. Appeal Bd., 718 A.2d 759 (Pen. 1998).
54. Michelin v Nova Scotia Workers Comp. Bd., Order No. 002/056/093 (2002) (decision currently on appeal to the Nova Scotia Court of Appeal).
55. U.S. Department of Labor, Bureau of Labor Statistics, at http://www.bls.gov (last visited Aug. 21, 2002) (July 2002 unemployment rate was +5.9%, preliminary second quarter 2002 worker productivity was +1.1%).
56. Voohries-Larson v Cessna Aircraft Co., 241 F.3d 707 (9th Cir. 2001).
57. Bailey v. Norfolk and Northwestern RR Co., 942 S.W.2d 404 (Mo. Ct. App. 1997).
58. Findley v Alabama Power Co., 735 So.2d 1208 (Ala. 1998).

# 20

## Stimulants

**JOHN A. CALDWELL AND J. LYNN CALDWELL**

San Antonio, Texas, U.S.A.

## I.  Introduction

A variety of automobile crashes, aviation mishaps, and industrial accidents have been at least partly attributed to sleepiness or fatigue on the job. Examples include the 30,000–90,000 car accidents each year in the United States alone; the 1993 crash of a DC-8 on approach to landing in Guantanamo Bay, Cuba; the recent crash of American Airlines flight 1420 after overrunning the end of the runway in Little Rock, Arkansas; the collision of a Korean Airlines 747 into a hillside on approach into Guam; the nuclear-power-plant mishaps at Three Mile Island and Chernobyl; and the grounding of the Exxon Valdez (1–8). The problem of on-the-job fatigue seems particularly acute in our increasingly mobile society where 24-hour-per-day operations have challenged the ability of personnel to acquire sufficient daily sleep. Prolonged work hours, shift work, lengthy periods of extended wakefulness, inadequate sleep, and pathological sleepiness are key factors responsible for compromised safety, health, and productivity (9).

To address these problems, considerable emphasis has been placed on finding operationally-useful fatigue countermeasures. However, at present, the opti-

The opinions, interpretations, conclusions, and recommendations are those of the authors and are not necessarily endorsed by the U.S. Air Force and/or the Department of Defense.

mal solution, or combination of solutions, has not been determined. A majority of the existing work has focused on "natural" or nondrug approaches to maximizing alertness on the job, but a substantial amount also has been aimed at exploring the utility of pharmacological wake-promoting strategies. After a brief overview of several of the more common nondrug interventions, a detailed overview of pharmacological strategies will be presented.

## II.  Nonpharmacological Fatigue Countermeasures

The most palatable measures for the prevention or remedy of operator sleepiness/fatigue are those of a nonpharmacological nature. These measures, described in detail in Chapters 21 and 22, are generally viewed as benign and "natural" ways of improving on-the-job alertness as they do not involve any type of "medical" intervention. Nonpharmacological strategies generally include regulatory approaches (i.e., schedules and work hour restrictions) or behavioral interventions (i.e., exercise, fitness, breaks, and/or naps), but some "environmental" countermeasures (i.e., temperature, lighting, etc.) have been attempted as well. Only the first two categories will be discussed here as the effectiveness of environmental modifications appears limited.

### A.  Limiting Time On Task

A common approach to avoiding fatigue-related operational problems is to limit the amount of duty time in an effort to ensure that the amount of time allotted for sleep is adequate. This is an approach used throughout the transportation industry (i.e., in long-haul truckers, airline pilots, etc.), but the results have been less than optimal, as evidenced by the lack of agreement regarding operator scheduling in this sector. Duty restrictions have not alleviated fatigue-related problems in part because the work requirements seem to escalate while personnel and budgetary resources remain constant or are reduced. In the Army, for instance, the mission has grown 300% while resources have declined approximately 30% over the past several years (10). Anecdotal reports from both military and civilian sectors indicate that workload factors often lead to violations of established work/rest policies. Even if such violations were not taking place, it is doubtful that duty limitations would solve the operational fatigue problem even if guidelines were rigorously followed. Time-on-task limits do not (and possibly cannot) adequately integrate all that is known about sleep and circadian physiology into an operationally-useful strategy (11). A variety of factors other than "time on task" (such as circadian phase, prior sleep quality, time since last sleep period, etc.) are directly related to performance, but are extremely difficult to account for in many real-world settings.

### B.  Physical Fitness

An alternative or additional fatigue-management strategy (which the military has traditionally used) focuses on reducing the impact of sustained work by ensuring high levels of physical fitness. Unfortunately, although it is true that fit people are able to withstand longer periods of physical labor than unfit people (thus showing a resistance to physical fatigue), there is little evidence that physical fitness offers resistance to mental fatigue. In fact, Angus, et al. (12) found that highly fit individuals were no better at sustaining intense cognitive work than those who were less fit in situations where alertness was compromised by sleep deprivation.

### C.  Exercise

Physical exercise has been considered for its potential alerting effects—the idea being that strategically placed exercise breaks can be used to significantly prolong the performance of tired workers. However, although brief periods of exercise have been shown to temporarily increase arousal in sleepy personnel (12–14), the effects are too transient to be of much benefit to people working prolonged hours day after day.

### D.  Rest Breaks

Rest breaks can provide some amelioration of the degraded performance and increased fatigue associated with sleep loss. Heslegrave and Angus (15) reported positive effects of 5–20-min breaks on performance and alertness in a 54-hr sleep deprivation protocol. Pigeau et al. (16) found immediate improvements in subjective and objective performance measures after a 15-min break during a 64-hr sleep deprivation protocol, but the effects dissipated rapidly after an hour of continuous cognitive work. Changes in physiological alertness have been observed in pilots flying a 6-hr nighttime flight (after being awake a minimum of 18 hr) in a flight simulator after receiving hourly 7-min breaks. The pilots who received the breaks showed reductions in slow eye movements, EEG theta activity, and unintended sleep episodes compared to pilots who did not receive the breaks, but the benefits did not last longer than 15–25 min (17). Thus, rest breaks are beneficial for promoting alertness; however, their effects are short-lived, making rest strategies unsuitable for maintaining long-term performance and alertness.

### E.  Napping

Napping is the most effective nonpharmacological technique for sustaining alertness in settings where some sleep is possible, but of limited duration (18). Naps have been proven extremely beneficial in several situations (19), including aviation (20). However, the efficacy of naps depends on a variety of factors such as time of day, nap length, and the availability of a sleep-conducive environment (21), which often make napping difficult to utilize in operational settings. In addition, the use of naps in close proximity to the work setting must be carefully planned to avoid problems with sleep inertia (the feeling of confusion and the reduction in performance that can occur immediately upon awakening) (22,23).

### F.   Summary of Nonpharmacological Approaches

Thus, although a variety of nonpharmacological approaches exists, they may not be sufficient or feasible in some settings. Examples might include rapid-response disaster-relief efforts, remote emergency medical care, large-scale intense fire-fighting efforts, and continuous/sustained combat military operations. In these settings, there often is little time to plan staffing ratios and schedules in advance, only narrow control (at best) over the physical work environment, and often very limited opportunities for providing adequate rest/sleep breaks owing to the high operational tempo. Under these circumstances, highly flexible, rapidly effective fatigue remedies are obviously needed to mitigate the threat that degraded cognition, mood, and performance may pose to the safety of operational personnel and those they are striving to save or defend. Here, alertness-promoting strategies are needed, not as a replacement for restorative recovery sleep, but for temporarily bridging the gap between suitable sleep periods without jeopardizing the completion of the job at hand. Stimulants (or wake-promoting) medications meet these requirements.

### III.   Pharmacological Sleep Deprivation Countermeasures

Stimulants can counter the effects of severe fatigue when adequate sleep simply is not possible. At the outset, it should be noted that stimulants are incapable of replacing sleep, and because of this, they should not be viewed as a substitute for proper staffing or adequate work/rest cycles. However, in situations where unavoidable manpower constraints, hostile environmental circumstances, or extremely high workloads prevent the effective implementation of nonpharmacological alertness management strategies, stimulants can temporarily avoid potentially serious performance decrements. Stimulants have the advantages of being effective and easy to use, and because their feasibility is not dependent on environmental manipulations or scheduling modifications, their usefulness, especially for short-term applications, is significant. This explains why pharmacological compounds such as amphetamines have been used extensively in several military conflicts. Five stimulant compounds have been studied sufficiently to warrant consideration here—methylphenidate, pemoline, caffeine, dextroamphetamine, and modafinil (24,25).* Each will be discussed in turn.

---

* Methamphetamine is not discussed in this chapter only because political factors and a lack of public and/or organizational acceptance would most likely preclude the use of this compound in operational settings. Methamphetamine is a potent CNS stimulant that, in fact, is somewhat more selective and efficacious than dextroamphetamine. However, even the military has opted to rely on dextroamphetamine rather than methamphetamine presumably to avoid associations between legitimate operational applications and the illicit sale and abuse of methamphetamine that is widely depicted almost on a daily basis in the popular media.

## A. Methylphenidate

Methylphenidate is marketed in the United States under the prescription names Concerta, Metadate, Methylin, and Ritalin (26). It is available in immediate and sustained-release formulations for the treatment of attention deficit/hyperactivity disorder (ADHD) and the symptomatic management of narcolepsy (a disorder characterized by excessive daytime sleepiness).

### *General*

A piperidine derivative, methylphenidate facilitates the release of catecholamines and blocks their reuptake and degradation (27). It is considered to be a mild central nervous system (CNS) stimulant, which appears to stimulate brain structures in a manner similar to amphetamines (26). A strongly favored treatment for ADHD, methylphenidate prescriptions account for over 90% of prescription stimulants used in the United States (28). Both children and adults who have been diagnosed with ADHD have been treated with methylphenidate with a high degree of success (29,30). A review of the studies in which stimulants were used by children with ADHD indicated significant evidence for improvement in hyperactivity, inattention, and impulsivity (28).

Clinically, methylphenidate also is used for the treatment of daytime sleepiness associated with narcolepsy. It is a mainstay treatment for this problem and has a long record of efficacy in alleviating the sleepiness symptoms (31) and maintaining alertness and performance in narcoleptic patients (32,33).

Methylphenidate also has been used to treat other medical conditions. For example, it has been used as a short-term treatment for depression in the medically ill, as an adjunct to conventional antidepressants for patients with major depressive disorder, and in combination with opiates for pain control. Methylphenidate has been prescribed to reduce apathy in patients with dementia or other brain diseases (28,34,35).

### Typical Effects

Methylphenidate is a mild CNS stimulant that affects the mental processes more than motor activities. There is no clearly established mechanism that leads to the mental and behavioral effects of methylphenidate in children (36,37). The general use of methylphenidate is for the treatment of ADHD. Doses up to 60 mg for children over 5 years of age lead to improvement in attention span, activity level, and impulsivity. The drug's alerting affects are beneficial to adults with narcolepsy, and it has been shown to have positive effects on performance, particularly reaction time and vigilance. Its physiological actions include an increase in heart rate, but not necessarily an increase in blood pressure. The alerting effects of methylphenidate have led researchers to investigate its utility for helping sleep-deprived individuals perform tasks when necessary, and it does exert some beneficial effects.

## Dosage

For the treatment of narcolepsy in adults, the usual dosage is 10 mg 2–3 times per day. Because of individual differences in responsiveness to the medication, some patients require 40–60 mg per day while others require only 10–15 mg per day (37).

## Pharmacokinetics

Methylphenidate is readily absorbed and produces peak plasma levels in approximately 2 hr (immediate-release formulation). The duration of action is 3–6 hr for the immediate-release and 8 hr for the sustained-release formulation. Approximately 90% of methylphenidate is excreted in the urine as metabolites (80% is ritalinic acid) and the remainder as unchanged drug (26,36).

## Adverse Reactions

The adverse effects associated with methylphenidate are generally mild and short-lived, with the most common effects being insomnia, decreased appetite, stomach ache, headache, and jitteriness. Although methylphenidate has been abused, the problem of abuse is generally seen in adults who use multiple substances or in adolescents experimenting with medications (28). Sweden withdrew methylphenidate from its market in 1968 because some adults dissolved tablets and injected the solution, leading to serious cases of talc granulomatosis (38). However, most cases of methylphenidate abuse apparently have led to less serious consequences (28).

## Tolerance and Toxicity

There is no evidence of sensitization or tolerance in children receiving stimulants over a long period of time (39). Data on the effects of long-term use of methylphenidate are not available, but tolerance is rare; clinically, it is not necessary to increase the dosage to maintain therapeutic benefits, at least in treating ADHD children (40). However, patients are warned about the possibility of drug dependence after chronic abuse (37). Similar to amphetamine, methylphenidate can be toxic at doses only slightly above the levels that are typically used. Benowitz (41) suggests that approximately 1 mg/kg is potentially life-threatening. In cases of overdose, he recommends (a) maintaining airways and assisting ventilation, (b) treating any symptoms of agitation, seizures, coma, and hyperthermia, (c) monitoring vital signs and electrocardiogram (ECG) for at least 6 hours, (d) treating hypertension, tachyarrhythmias, and arterial vasospasm, and (e) performing gastric lavage and administering charcoal and a cathartic.

### Effects on Physical Performance

Although some stimulants have been used in an attempt to enhance physical or athletic performance, no published studies indicate that this is the case for methylphenidate. In addition, no data were found regarding the utility of methylphenidate for the enhancement of physical performance.

### Effects on Basic Physiological Indices and Motor/Reaction Time Tasks

Almost all studies indicate that heart rate increases after administration of methylphenidate (42–44). This effect is observed in adults, ADHD children, and normal children (45). The effects on blood pressure, however, are more variable. For instance, Babkoff et al. (46) found that methylphenidate (10 mg every 6 hr) had no effect on diastolic, systolic, or mean blood pressure, while Elliot et al. (47) found that a single 20- or 40-mg dose of methylphenidate increased both systolic and diastolic blood pressure by approximately 6–7.5 mmHg (there was no difference between the two doses).

Most studies indicate that methylphenidate's effects on performance, particularly vigilance, reaction time, and memory, are beneficial, even in well-rested normal adults (48). Coons et al. (49) at first failed to detect an improvement in reaction time (RT) in healthy men who had been given 20 mg methylphenidate versus placebo. However, in a follow-up study that used a more difficult cognitive task, methylphenidate reduced rates of omission errors and produced faster reaction times in comparison to placebo. In addition, the amplitude of a late positive component of the event-related potential (ERP) (at 460 msec) was increased by methylphenidate in the more challenging task, suggesting that the drug enhanced attentional resources. These findings were confirmed in an investigation in which 0.3 mg/kg methylphenidate was compared to placebo in normal children (42). Methylphenidate reduced errors at high memory loads on the Sternberg Task, and although it did not affect pure RT, the variability in RT was decreased after drug administration. In addition, the P-300 component of the ERP tended to be larger, and the P-527 amplitude was significantly increased by methylphenidate relative to placebo during a continuous performance task. Again, these findings suggest a drug-induced enhancement in attentional resource allocation.

Naylor et al. (50) also reported beneficial effects of methylphenidate in female volunteers who received 5-, 10-, or 20-mg doses. Like Peloquin and Klorman (42), they found no significant changes in the P-300 component of the evoked response, but RT on an information-processing task was improved compared to placebo. For a task in which the target was easy to identify, the 10-mg dose significantly decreased RT (the 20-mg dose tended to have the same effect). For a task in which target selection was more difficult, both the 5- and 20-mg doses enhanced RT, but the 10-mg dose had no effect.

In summary, it appears that methylphenidate is effective in improving at least some aspects of RT in both children and adults. Generally speaking, methylphenidate shortens response times. In addition, it appears that the amplitude of the late components of the ERP is enhanced by methylphenidate, indicating that attentional resources are improved by drug administration.

### Effects on Vigilance

The effects of methylphenidate on vigilance have not been extensively studied, and the limited amount of available information is conflicting. Some studies report a positive effect (44,48), whereas others indicate a decrement in performance (43). Strauss and colleagues (44) administered 20 mg methylphenidate and placebo to 22 normal men after which a 45-min vigilance task was performed. The results indicated that methylphenidate did in fact prevent the degradation in performance normally found in lengthy tasks. This is consistent with the results of Peloquin and Klorman (42), who found a reduction in errors, RT, and RT variability on a continuous performance task with 0.3 mg/kg methylphenidate, and Camp-Bruno and Herting (48), who found improvements in RT on a 20-min vigilance task with 20 mg methylphenidate. However, this is at odds with the findings of Hink et al. (43) who administered 10 mg of methylphenidate, 100 mg of secobarbital, or placebo to 12 men prior to a 70-min target detection vigilance task. The results of this investigation indicated that performance under methylphenidate was similar to that under placebo in that methylphenidate did not prevent degradations from occurring with increased time on task. Since this latter study utilized a lower dose than the previous three, the negative results may have been due to insufficient blood levels of methylphenidate.

### Effects on Military Performance

A search of the available literature failed to produce evidence that methylphenidate has been used by the military to counteract fatigue in operational environments. However, the U.S. Navy has conducted laboratory studies in which military personnel were administered 10 mg methylphenidate or 37.5 mg pemoline during 64 hr of continuous wakefulness. The results indicated that methylphenidate did not produce improvements in objective and subjective sleepiness, or in straightforward measures of performance (27,46). However, when the performance data from a choice-reaction-time test were analyzed for trial-to-trial variance, methylphenidate was found to decrease the variance compared to placebo on the first of 2 days of sleep deprivation. The effect did not continue into the second day (51). As was the case with the vigilance studies (above), the nonsignificant or relatively small effects of methylphenidate may have resulted from the low dosage that was studied.

### Effects of Methylphenidate on Sleep-Deprived Subjects

Besides the Navy studies described above, very few investigations have been conducted to determine the efficacy of methylphenidate for counteracting the effects of sleep deprivation. However, a study conducted by Bishop et al. (25) examined the effects of 10 mg methylphenidate compared to placebo for improving attention and performance after 8 hr of sleep and again after 24 hr of continuous wakefulness. Using a within-subjects design, subjects were exposed to four conditions: placebo after 8 hr sleep, 10 mg methylphenidate (at 08:00 and 12:00) after 8 hr sleep, placebo during 24 hr of wakefulness, and 10 mg methylphenidate (at 8:00 and 12:00) during 24 hr of wakefulness. The results indicated that methylphenidate extended sleep latency to rested levels during sleep deprivation and after 8 hr of sleep (no sleep deprivation). However, methylphenidate improved divided-attention and vigilance performance only during the sleep deprivation period.

A later study supported the findings that methylphenidate's benefits are most apparent in sleep-deprived/sleep-restricted volunteers. Roehrs et al. (52) compared the effects of 09:00 doses of 10 mg methylphenidate to placebo on sleepiness (Multiple Sleep Latency Test, MSLT), Profile of Mood States (POMS) ratings, and divided-attention performance after either 4 or 8 hr of sleep. After these test days, the 4- and 8-hr sleep conditions were repeated, but this time subjects were given their choice of drug or placebo. Results indicated that performance was improved by methylphenidate, most notably after the 4-hr condition. Methylphenidate also improved sleep latency and mood, but only after restricted sleep. During the "choice" phase of the study, subjects showed a preference for methylphenidate after 4 hr sleep (in 88% of opportunities), but not after 8 hr sleep (in only 29% of opportunities), suggesting that the preference for methylphenidate depended on the perceived sleepiness level of the individual.

These results were later replicated in a follow-up study in which 5, 10, and 20 mg of methylphenidate were used. The results indicated that 5- and 10-mg doses of methylphenidate were chosen over placebo after restricted sleep (4 hr time in bed), but not after a full 8 hr in bed. No clear indication of preference was found for the 20-mg dose (53).

### Effects on Mood and Motivation

A series of three experiments explored the relative effects of *d*-amphetamine (10 mg), methylphenidate (10 mg), chlordiazepoxide hydrochloride (10 mg), and placebo on memory and mood (54). After drug administration, subjects were tested on the Paced Sequential Memory Task (PSMT) and the Nowlis Mood Adjective Check List over a 4-hr test period. The results indicated that *d*-amphetamine significantly reduced subjective ratings of fatigue and increased subjective ratings of vigor compared to the other drugs. In addition, performance on the PSMT was enhanced by *d*-amphetamine compared to placebo and methylphenidate. Methylphenidate was not found to enhance either mood or performance in this experiment.

In other studies, methylphenidate has been shown to improve subjective mood evaluations in both adults (44) and children (42). A comparison between *d*-amphetamine, *l*-amphetamine, and methylphenidate (administered in dosages equimolar to 10 mg or 20 mg) indicated that methylphenidate's euphoric effects were between those found with *d*-amphetamine and *l*-amphetamine (55). In the earlier-mentioned study by Coons et al. (49), methylphenidate increased subjective ratings of concentration and aggression compared to placebo. In the study by Peloquin and Klorman (42), 0.3 mg/kg methylphenidate prevented the increased ratings of dysphoria over time, and produced an overall lower dysphoria rating than placebo. In Roehrs et al. (53), methylphenidate (10 mg) remedied the adverse mood effects of 4 hr of sleep restriction. Thus, it appears that methylphenidate exerts beneficial mood effects, but the magnitude of these effects is lower than those observed with more potent stimulants.

### Summary

In summary, methylphenidate has not been well studied in sleep-deprived subjects, but the data that do exist indicate mild stimulant effects on mood and some aspects of performance, particularly RT. The effects are more consistent in fatigued versus nonfatigued individuals, but there is evidence that methylphenidate's alerting characteristics may not persist beyond 1 day of sleep deprivation (although a dose escalation strategy or an overall higher dose could be the answer to this problem). Methylphenidate is particularly beneficial during the early-morning hours when the circadian trough in performance and alertness is most pronounced. Although methylphenidate is not the most potent wake-promoting agent available, it has the advantage of relatively low abuse potential as evidenced by the fact that subjects given a choice frequently will not take the drug unless they are sleep-deprived.

## B. Pemoline

Pemoline is marketed in the United States under the prescription names Cylert and PemADD (56). It is available in immediate and sustained release formulas for the treatment of ADHD, but should not be considered as the first-choice therapy owing to its association with hepatic failure (57). Like methylphenidate, pemoline has not been well studied in sleep-deprived humans.

### General

Pemoline, an oxizolidine compound, acts similarly to methylphenidate—through catecholamine uptake inhibition in the CNS (27) with minimal sympathomimetic effects (57). Although pemoline is not the first-line stimulant for the treatment of ADHD, it has been successfully used for the treatment of this disorder in both children and adults (28,30). Pemoline has also been used for the treatment of daytime sleepiness associated with narcolepsy (31), and although it is somewhat effective for this purpose (33), it is not a first-line choice owing to its potentially lethal liver toxicity.

### Typical Effects

Pemoline is a mild psychostimulant with CNS effects that are not clearly understood; the exact mechanism and site of action of the drug are not known. While it is structurally different from amphetamine and methylphenidate, its actions are similar to those of the other stimulants (56). The typical use of pemoline is for the treatment of the symptoms of distractibility, hyperactivity, and impulsivity in ADHD. It has not been approved for the treatment of narcolepsy, but it does have alerting effects in adults (31,33). Researchers have examined the use of pemoline as an aid to fatigued individuals. Although it has been shown to improve some aspects of performance and alertness, it does not appear to affect mood. Its physiological effects are mild, and it does not exert pronounced effects on blood pressure or heart rate. However, it is not recommended as a first line treatment for ADHD or as an alerting drug owing to potentially lethal liver toxicity (57).

## Dosage

The usual starting dose for the treatment of ADHD in children over 5 years of age is 37.5 mg/ day, increased gradually by 18.75 mg/week until the desired response is reached. The usual therapeutic dose range is from 56.25 to 75 mg/day, with a maximum dose of 112 mg/day (57). Since pemoline is not approved for the treatment of narcolepsy, dosage recommendations for this indication are not readily available; however, in the subsequent section, dosage information can be extrapolated from a small number of sleep deprivation studies.

## Pharmacokinetics

Pemoline has a peak effect of 4 hr with an 8-hr duration of action and a half-life of 12 hr in adults. It is metabolized by the liver, with approximately 50% excreted unchanged in the urine (57). Although drug levels peak fairly quickly, clinical improvement may not be seen until after 3–4 weeks of treatment (36).

## Adverse Reactions

As with methylphenidate, the adverse effects associated with pemoline are generally mild. The most common effects are insomnia, decreased appetite, stomachache, headache, and jitteriness (28). Periodic monitoring of liver enzymes is necessary because of the potential for hepatic toxic effects.

## Tolerance and Toxicity

Information on pemoline's tolerance and toxicity is not available. However, as with almost any drug, there is a chance of psychological and/or physical dependence with excessive doses and/or long-term misuse (57). In comparison to methylphenidate and amphetamine, pemoline has the least potential for abuse (39). Benowitz (41) suggests that approximately 3 mg/kg pemoline should be considered life-threatening. Treatment for overdose is similar to what has been recommended for methylphenidate and amphetamine. In cases of overdose, the administration of chlorpromazine has been found useful for decreasing the amount of CNS overstimulation (57).

### *Effects on Physical Performance*

There have been no published studies in which pemoline was administered and physical performance was tested. Thus, there are no known ergogenic properties of this medication.

### *Effects on Basic Physiological Indices and Motor/Reaction-Time Tasks*

Pemoline has not been shown to exert pronounced effects on blood pressure or heart rate (46,58). Although Babkoff and associates (46) found an increase in diastolic blood pressure after administration of pemoline, systolic blood pressure, mean blood pressure, and the rate-pressure product were not affected by the drug.

Evaluations of pemoline in normal adults are rare. However, tests in fatigued adults indicate that in general, pemoline promotes a faster RT when compared to placebo (46,59). This effect was clear when 37.5 mg pemoline was administered every 12 hr starting on the first night of a 64-hr sleep deprivation period. However, when only a single 37.5 mg dose was given on the second night of a 64-hr period of continuous wakefulness, Kelly et al. (58) found RT improvements on only a single task, whereas accuracy benefited in a more general way (i.e., on three tests).

### Effects on Vigilance

Since pemoline is intended primarily as a treatment for ADHD, its effects on vigilance have not been well established. However, Orzack et al. (60) compared 25 mg and 50 mg pemoline to 100 mg and 200 mg caffeine, 15 mg methylphenidate, and placebo on the performance of a 2-hr psychomotor task (pressing keys corresponding to visual stimuli). They found that performance deteriorated as a function of time on task under the influence of placebo, but that 50 mg pemoline, 200 mg caffeine, and 15 mg methylphenidate maintained consistent performance throughout the 2 hr.

### Effects on Military Performance

There is no evidence that pemoline has been used by military personnel in operational settings despite the fact that the Royal Air Force at one time felt pemoline may be the optimal choice of stimulants in specific circumstances (24). However, despite the absence of data from the field, militarily-relevant research has been conducted both in the United States and in the United Kingdom. The U.S. Naval Health Research Center examined the efficacy of pemoline for the mitigation of performance and mood decrements associated with 3 days and 2 nights of sleep deprivation (27,46,51,58,59). Because some of the results from these studies have already been presented and others will be highlighted in the next section, they will not be explained here. However, the general conclusions from the U.S. military investigations indicate that pemoline could be a viable fatigue countermeasure, but it appears that dose timing would be a critical issue for ensuring benefits during the circadian trough.

### Effects of Pemoline on Sleep-deprived Subjects

An early study by Gelfand and colleagues (61) investigated the effects of pemoline on the performance of subjects who had been awake for a minimum of 20 hr before testing. Subjects received either placebo, 20 mg methylphenidate, 15 mg *d*-amphetamine, 25 mg pemoline, 50 mg pemoline, or 100 mg pemoline at 07:15 and were tested on an arithmetic task until 11:15. Generally, the results indicated that 100 mg pemoline maintained performance, but 25 mg and 50 mg pemoline did not. These findings agree with those of Mitler et al. (32), who found that only the highest dose of pemoline (112.5 mg/day vs. either 18.75 or 56.25 mg/day) improved the performance of narcoleptics (not subjected to experimental sleep deprivation) on a Wilkinson addition test or a digit-symbol substitution task, while lower doses failed to produce beneficial effects.

As mentioned earlier, the U.S. Naval Health Research Center has investigated the efficacy of pemoline over long periods without sleep. Naitoh et al. (59) compared four groups of subjects exposed to 64 hr of continuous wakefulness who received either a 20-min nap every 6 hr, no nap for the duration of the study, 37.5 mg pemoline every 12 hr, or placebo. Performance effects were measured using a four-choice reaction time task administered every 3 hr. While both pemoline and a nap were successful at attenuating fatigue-related degradations in accuracy, response speed, and number of stimuli attempted, the effects on these latter two variables were more robust under pemoline (compared to naps).

Supportive results were found by Matteson et al. (27) in a study that compared 37.5 mg pemoline to 10 mg methylphenidate. Once again, a 64-hr period of continuous wakefulness was used, but this time the napping intervention was absent, and subjects received either 10 mg methylphenidate every 6 hr, 37.5 mg pemoline every 12 hr, or placebo. Results indicated that pemoline significantly reduced both subjective and objective sleepiness (determined via visual analog scales and lapses on a tapping task), but did not affect mood (as measured with the POMS). Pemoline's effects on sleepiness were particularly pronounced in the early morning hours during the circadian trough. Based on these findings, the authors made a positive appraisal of the potential utility of pemoline in sustaining performance; however, this was tempered by indications that pemoline might interact with prolonged sleep deprivation in a negative way. This is because Kelly et al. (62) found that pemoline administration, while for the most part beneficial, adversely affected the accuracy of performance on some tests toward the end of a 64-hr period of sleep loss.

This concern was to some extent alleviated by a follow-up study in which placebo was administered on the first night of continuous wakefulness followed by a single dose of pemoline on the second night of continuous wakefulness (58). After subjects received pemoline, they self-reported less sleepiness, and their performance on simple tasks (such as mental rotation, addition, and tapping), was improved relative to placebo despite significant sleep loss. The authors concluded that this dosing schedule (one dose rather than repeated doses) was effective in decreasing sleepiness and increasing performance accuracy without the negative effects that occurred toward the end of the wakefulness period in the earlier multiple-dosing study. However, it should be noted that such a single-dose strategy should not be expected to sustain performance for much longer than 1 night.

Nicholson et al. (63) summarized the research performed by the Royal Air Force (RAF) Institute of Aviation Medicine that showed that pemoline (30 and 40 mg) was beneficial for a 12-hr period of high-workload, overnight performance, and that the positive effects of the drug extended somewhat beyond the work shift. In fact, the long duration of effect ultimately reduced the quality of recovery sleep. A lower dose (20 mg) was efficacious for 8–12 hr, and did not produce the sleep disturbances. This generally agrees with another RAF study in which the effects of 10, 20, 30, and 40 mg pemoline on subjective alertness and performance were evaluated during a 12-hr night shift (the doses were administered at 20:00). The 30- and 40-mg doses began to produce positive effects on alertness 4.5 hr postdose, and the benefits again persisted beyond the end of the work shift, even into the subsequent recovery sleep period. The 20-mg dose also was effective, and it once again had the advantage of not disrupting recovery sleep. The 10-mg dose apparently was insufficient for attenuating the impact of sleep loss to a significant degree.

Thus, it is clear that pemoline can sustain some aspects of performance and alertness in sleep-deprived personnel, especially for relatively short periods (approximately 24 hr). However, questions remain about whether the multiple administrations necessary for longer-term maintenance of functioning may ultimately create problems in the accuracy of some types of cognitive performance.

### Effects on Mood and Motivation

Generally, pemoline has not been shown to affect mood, either positively or negatively. In a study in which 37.5 mg pemoline was administered to adult male volunteers, the drug did not affect mood as measured by the POMS (27). These results were confirmed in other studies in which pemoline did not alter mood when administered during 64 hr of continuous wakefulness (46,58).

### Summary

In summary, the literature suggests pemoline could be useful for sustaining alertness and performance over short periods of sleep deprivation (24 hr). In fact, there are some indications that pemoline is more efficacious for this purpose than methylphenidate, although the drug may have a slower onset of action. Pemoline seems to affect reaction time more so than accuracy in various performance tasks, and it exerts no substantial effect on mood. One study raised the possibility that multiple doses may actually produce performance decrements in some tasks after the second day of continuous wakefulness, and this issue remains unresolved. In light of this fact and the fact that pemoline has been associated with hepatic failure, pemoline should not be considered for the maintenance of wakefulness in sleep-deprived people.

### C.   Caffeine

Caffeine is a psychostimulant that is available in a number of forms, including 100- and 200-mg tablets (i.e., Vivarin and NoDoz), 50- and 100-mg chewing-gum preparations (i.e., Stay Alert), and even 15- and 20-mg candies (i.e., Penguin peppermints and Moovitz candies). Caffeine also is a component in a wide variety of beverages. A 5-oz cup of drip-brewed coffee contains an average of 120 mg of caffeine, a 5-oz cup of brewed tea contains approximately 33 mg of caffeine, and a 12-oz cola drink contains an average of 42 mg of caffeine (64). It is important to note that these are *averages* and that different preparations of the same type of beverage may contain greater or lesser amounts of caffeine. For instance, based on the information presented above, it might be assumed that an 8-oz cup of coffee from the local coffee shop contains approximately 192 mg caffeine, but the Center for Science in the Public Interest (65) reports that an 8-oz cup of Starbucks (Starbucks short) contains 250 mg. In addition to the caffeine present in foods and beverages, caffeine is present in medications, including over-the-counter analgesic compounds, such as Excedrin Migraine (which has 65 mg caffeine per tablet). Caffeine is one of the three methylxanthines (caffeine, theophylline, and theobromine) that occur naturally in foods and drugs (66).

### General

The effects of methylxanthine compounds generally include relaxation of smooth muscles, CNS stimulation, diuresis, and stimulation of the heart. The actions of methylxanthines are thought to be mediated by the inhibition of phosphodiesterases, the mobilization of intracellular calcium, and the antagonism of adenosine receptors, but the latter effect appears to account for the most important pharmacological actions of these substances (67). In animals, it has been found that adenosine levels covary with sleep and wakefulness, that extracellular adenosine levels in the basal forebrain increase with sleep deprivation, that activation of adenosine receptors in the basal forebrain enhances slow-wave sleep, and that antagonism of A1 adenosine receptors decreases sleep and increases wakefulness (68). A variety of animal studies have shown that heightened adenosine levels reduce vigilance, promote sleep, and decrease locomotor activity, whereas adenosine antagonism, via methylxanthine administration (such as would be the case with caffeine), improves wakefulness and increases activity (69). Adenosine antagonists, such as methylxanthines, reverse the inhibition of CNS neurotransmitter release associated with the presence of adenosine. Theophylline is a more potent form of methylxanthine than caffeine, but as caffeine is more widely available and better studied, it will receive the greatest attention here.

Caffeine is the most widely used behaviorally active pharmacological compound in the world (70). Caffeine has been self-administered in the form of caffeine-containing foods possibly for as long as 4700 years (71), it is regularly ingested by more than 80% of the adults in North America (72), and its use exceeds that of alcohol and nicotine—the second and third most widely ingested mind-altering drugs in the world (73). In North America and Europe, the majority of dietary caffeine is consumed in the form of coffee (74,75).

Throughout the past 100 years, numerous investigations have examined the pharmacological effects of caffeine on metabolism, cardiovascular, respiratory, gastrointestinal, renal, and CNS functioning in humans. These studies have contributed greatly to our understanding of the general effects of caffeine, but it should be noted that conflicting results are common. For instance, Curatolo and Robertson (76) cite differing reports of whether caffeine increases or decreases lower esophageal sphincter pressure, raises or lowers blood pressure, increases or decreases heart rate, or raises or fails to affect epinephrine and norepinephrine levels. Kuznicki and Turner (77) cite discrepant information on whether caffeine relieves or causes headaches, produces or relieves anxiety, and improves or disturbs reaction time. Such inconsistencies may in part be due to a failure to differentiate between the testing of habitual versus nonhabitual consumers of caffeine, as tolerance has been shown to occur in hemodynamic and other parameters (66,76). Furthermore, Lieberman et al. (78) point out that methodological differences across studies (presence or absence of a caffeine washout period, choice of tests, etc.) may account for the lack of consensus regarding many of caffeine's effects. All of this notwithstanding, there is general agreement that caffeine's actions on human subjects are consistent with what would be expected from a stimulant medication.

## Typical Effects

Caffeine exerts stimulatory effects both on the CNS and in the periphery. Serafin (67) indicates that ingestion of caffeine or theophylline can affect the circulatory system by increasing peripheral vascular resistance, elevating blood pressure, stimulating the heart, increasing blood flow to the organs, and inducing a diuretic effect. Cardiovascular effects of 250–350 mg caffeine are more noticeable in caffeine-naive individuals (slight increase in heart rate and blood pressure) whereas regular caffeine users experience little change. Caffeine increases physical work capacity, possibly by improving neuromuscular transmission or muscular contractility. Methylxanthines (caffeine and theophylline) enhance the production of urine, although the exact mechanisms underlying this effect remain unclear. Caffeine, ingested either in beverages or in other forms, can produce decreased sensations of drowsiness and fatigue accompanied by improvements in the clarity of thought. Dose-dependent elevations in CNS stimulation can include nervousness, anxiety, restlessness, and insomnia. Doses ranging from 85 to 200 mg have been shown to enhance cognitive vigilance and improve reaction time, but fine motor control, accurate timing, and the ability to perform mathematical tests may be impaired. Zarcone (79) and Landolt et al. (80) report caffeine can impair sleep quality by increasing the time to sleep onset, reducing slow-wave sleep, and increasing the amount of wake time after sleep onset.

## Dosage

Establishing dosing recommendations for caffeine is somewhat difficult because of individual variability in response to the drug. Factors influencing dosing include the level of habitual caffeine usage, the time of caffeine administration, whether or not the individual is a smoker, and whether or not fatigue is present (81). With regard to habitual usage, it should be noted that the average daily per capita consumption of 211 mg caffeine by adults in the United States (82) must be considered when choosing an effective dose of caffeine. In the United Kingdom, per capita consumption is even higher, at 444 mg daily (70). Given that tolerance to the subjective, sleep-disrupting, and physiological effects of caffeine develops rapidly—within 1–14 days depending on the variable of interest and the dosage (71)—the individualized dose required for alleviation of fatigue-induced decrements should exceed the amount of average daily consumption to ensure effectiveness. Generally speaking, it appears that between 70 mg and 210 mg is the minimum dose required to produce observable behavioral effects (83), while anywhere from 100 to 600 mg will be necessary to improve or sustain the vigilance, mood, and performance of sleep-deprived personnel (81).

## Pharmacokinetics

After oral ingestion of caffeine, peak plasma concentrations are reached within 1 hr, sometimes as early as 15 min (84). The half-life falls within the range of 3–7 hr, with an average half-life of 4.9 hr (67,85). The rate of caffeine metabolism is significantly higher in smokers than in nonsmokers, producing a shorter half-life (86). Caffeine's pharmacokinetics are generally thought to be linear and dose-independent, but Kamimori et al. (87) recently reported that higher doses of caffeine (150 vs. 300 vs. 600 mg) are metabolized and cleared more slowly than lower doses in sleep-deprived individuals.

## Adverse Reactions

The ingestion of excessive caffeine has been associated with several adverse reactions constituting a syndrome termed "caffeine intoxication" (88). The symptoms include restlessness, nervousness, excitement, insomnia, flushed face, diuresis, gastrointestinal disturbance, muscle twitching, rambling flow of thought and speech, rapid heartbeats, feelings of inexhaustibility, and/or psychomotor agitation.

## Tolerance and Toxicity

As noted earlier, tolerance to many of caffeine's effects develop rather quickly (i.e., often within 14 days). Therapeutic doses of caffeine cover a wide range, and caffeine is rarely associated with serious toxicity (89). However, an acute dose of 10 g is considered lethal, and the effects of such a dose may include vomiting, confusion, delirium, seizures, and tachyarrhythmias. In the event of acute caffeine intoxication, Brown (89) recommends: (a) maintaining the airway and assisting with ventilation, (b) treating seizures and hypotension, (c) monitoring the ECG and vital signs for 6 hr or until serum levels begin to decline, (d) administering beta blockers to reverse cardiotoxic effects, (e) inducing vomiting or performing gastric lavage, and (f) administering activated charcoal and a cathartic.

### Effects on Physical Performance

Caffeine is widely used as an ergogenic aid by competitive athletes and "weekend warriors" alike (90), but its effects appear to be variable depending on the type of physical activity undertaken. Evidence for caffeine-related improvements in muscle strength, work capacity, and performance on short-duration, intense physical activities is not convincing (69), but there is little doubt that caffeine is beneficial for athletes engaged in long-term endurance exercises in which fatigue occurs within 30–60 minutes (91). On the one hand, caffeine's failure to improve performance during short, intense bursts of physical activity is typified in a recent report by Paton et al. (92) in which approximately 420 mg caffeine (6 mg/kg) or placebo was administered to 16 athletes prior to measuring the amount of time it took to complete 20-m sprints. Caffeine led to negligible effects on both the speed of running and the rate of fatigue over the 10 trials, leading the authors to conclude that caffeine does not enhance team sprinting performance. On the other hand, caffeine's benefits in longer-duration activities are exemplified by MacIntosh and Wright (93) who found that 6 mg/kg of caffeine enhanced the speed of a 1500-m swim by 23 sec. Although the mechanisms responsible for caffeine's effects on prolonged exercise remain unclear, some reports indicate that glycogen sparing and elevated plasma epinephrine levels are involved (94), others suggest that caffeine's benefits are related to reductions in beta-endorphin and cortisol release thresholds (95), and still others point to improved motor-unit force production related to caffeine-induced muscle tissue alterations in calcium and potassium levels (91). This latter explanation is consistent with evidence that at least some of caffeine's ergogenic effects occur at the skeletal muscle level (96).

### *Effects on Basic Physiological Indices and Motor/Reaction-Time Tasks*

Curatolo and Robertson (76) summarized the basic physiological effects of caffeine in a report designed to address whether caffeine poses a health risk. Their review of the literature reported that oral caffeine is rapidly absorbed, yielding peak plasma levels within 15–45 min, and the half-life ranges from 3 to 7.5 hr. Although caffeine was observed to increase blood pressure, plasma catecholamine levels, plasma renin activity, and urine production (primarily in non-habitual users), there appeared to be no association with myocardial infarction, cancers of the urinary/renal tract or pancreas, teratogenic effects, or fibrocystic disease. With regard to blood pressure effects, Robertson et al. (97) found that a single 250-mg dose of caffeine administered to non-coffee-drinkers produced an average 11 mmHg increase in systolic blood pressure within 60 min of ingestion, which tended to persist for approximately 2 hr. In habitual caffeine users, a similar increase occurred on the first caffeine dose of the day after abstinence, but over the course of 4 days (with repeated dosing 3 times/day), the effect dissipated. Diastolic blood pressures in both groups of subjects showed similar patterns, but the increase was only about 60% of what was seen in systolic pressures. Caffeine did not affect heart rate. Kenemans and Lorist (98) found that administration of approximately 200 mg caffeine (3 mg/kg) to moderate caffeine users following a

12-hr period of abstinence reduced electroencephalographic (EEG) power in the delta, alpha, and beta bands (with the smallest effect in the higher EEG frequencies), suggesting conflicting stimulatory and sedative effects. This is inconsistent with the finding that a 6-mg/kg dose of caffeine (but not lower doses) increased the dominant alpha frequency (suggesting a slight stimulatory effect) in female subjects who were regular coffee drinkers, while both a 3-mg/kg and a 6-mg/kg dose increased the dominant beta frequency, indicating a clear increase in cortical arousal (99). Nehlig et al. (69) point out that discrepancies in the caffeine literature with regard to EEG effects may stem from the differing methodologies employed across studies.

With regard to basic motor skills, Weiss and Laties (100) indicate that caffeine's effects on reaction time are equivocal—an assessment that was later echoed by Lieberman (66). A quick overview of the published literature reveals several examples of why this is the case. On the positive side, Rapoport et al. (101) found that high-dose versus low-dose caffeine (10 mg/kg vs. 3 mg/kg) decreased the reaction time of children (but not adults) during the performance of a continuous performance task, and Horst and Jenkins (102) reported improved reaction time after administration of 3 or 4 mg/kg of caffeine to adult men. Clubley et al. (103) found that simple reaction time was improved following administration of either 75- or 150-mg doses of caffeine; and Lorist et al. (104,105) reported similar effects with 200 mg followed by a 50-mg maintenance dose in both fatigued and well-rested subjects. However, Kuznicki and Turner (77) failed to detect changes in choice reaction time following either a 20- or a 160-mg dose of caffeine. Ruijter et al. (106) determined that 250 mg of caffeine did not affect reaction time in a 10-min sustained-attention task. Lane (107) likewise failed to find differences in choice reaction times after ad lib consumption of caffeinated beverages (vs. abstinence) in habitual coffee drinkers during caffeine withdrawal, and Phillips-Bute and Lane (108) later supported these results in a comparable group of subjects given a 250 mg dose of caffeine in a similarly designed study. Discrepancies in the literature may be due to the testing of habitual versus nonhabitual caffeine users, the evaluation of caffeine-deprived versus non-caffeine-deprived subjects, and/or the divergent test methods and/or dosing levels. With regard to the effects of caffeine dose, Jacobsen and Edgley (109) found that an acute 300-mg dose significantly improved the reaction time of non-sleep-deprived volunteers whereas a 600-mg dose did not.

### Effects on Vigilance

Although the effects of caffeine on some aspects of performance may be difficult to establish, the impact of this compound on tasks requiring vigilance or sustained attention is clearer. Lieberman et al. (110) evaluated the impact of 32-, 64-, 128-, and 256-mg doses of caffeine on a four-choice visual reaction time test (10 min), a continuous-performance task (variable duration), and the Wilkinson auditory vigilance test (1 hr). Results indicated that every dose of caffeine improved four-choice reaction time without increasing the number of errors. Every dose also increased the number of signal tones detected on the Wilkinson test without changing the number of false alarms. Similar results were observed with a shorter (30-min) version of the Wilkinson task when the effects of 64 mg of caffeine were evaluated (78). Lieberman (66) reports that caffeine reliably enhances vigilance in male, female, and elderly individuals, and the impact of caffeine is not dependent upon baseline intake levels (at least within the 0–400-mg range). Lane and Phillips-Bute (111) found caffeine-related vigilance improvements in moderate to heavy caffeine users as well. In a caffeine deprivation study, they found that while withdrawal and subsequent caffeine administration did not affect performance of psychomotor tests such as tapping, serial memory, digit-symbol substitution, or a 2-min reaction time test (107,108), ad lib caffeine consumption did alleviate deprivation-related accuracy losses and response slowing on a 30-min vigilance task. Rosenthal et al. (112) found that twice-daily administrations of both 75- and 150-mg doses of caffeine improved reaction time in an auditory vigilance task, and they further reported that there were no differences in the efficacy of caffeine based on whether subjects had slept 5 hr versus 8 hr prior to testing. There were, however, no effects on a shorter (15-min) divided attention task. Reyner and Horne (113) found that a 200-mg dose of caffeine administered to sleep-restricted subjects significantly improved lane-tracking behavior in an automobile simulator during a monotonous, 2-hr, afternoon drive. In this study, the caffeine condition reduced the number of driving errors by 66% in comparison to placebo. Similar results were later obtained with sleep-restricted and sleep-deprived volunteers during an early-morning 2-hr drive (114). Following 200 mg of caffeine, lane tracking was improved throughout the entire experimental session for the sleep-restricted subjects and for the first 30 min in sleep-deprived volunteers. In general, caffeine's effects on vigilance are quite consistent from one study to another (69), and it appears that even relatively small doses (32 mg) can have beneficial effects in well-rested subjects.

### Effects on Military Performance

Military operations often include the requirement for continuous work schedules in which personnel may not be able to gain sufficient sleep for extended periods of time (115,116). Since these requirements ultimately will produce decrements that could jeopardize the well-being and effectiveness of soldiers (117), the stimulant properties of caffeine have long been of interest in this context. Since caffeine has been shown to improve alertness without producing significant side effects, and since this compound appears to have a low abuse potential, some investigators have suggested that it may be the stimulant of choice for use in military air operations (63).

Unlike methylphenidate and pemoline, caffeine has been used as a fatigue countermeasure in operational environments. A survey of 125 aircrew members involved in flight operations over Iraq in 1992 indicated that sleep restriction and circadian disruptions were common during the 18 days of intensive carrier operations in Operation Southern Watch (118). Aviation personnel reported using several strategies to maintain performance, but some form of caffeine use (coffee, tablets, or sodas) was indicated in numerous (49%) responses. Only one negative effect of caffeine was reported, and this was by a non-caffeine-user who ingested a tablet on an empty stomach and experienced subsequent problems with agitation and in-flight refueling. Generally, aircrew members felt that the availability of caffeine tablets was important from the standpoint of knowing that a fatigue countermeasure was available if needed. This is consistent with a recent survey of Israeli Air Force commanders that indicated a favorable view toward using alertness-enhancing drugs such as caffeine or amphetamine as secondary fatigue countermeasures, (i.e., 88% of survey respondents supported the use of stimulants after other types of nondrug strategies were found to be insufficient) (119).

The acceptance of caffeine as a fatigue remedy in air operations extends beyond the military community to civilian aviation as well. Gander et al. (120) found that short-haul, fixed-wing pilots working 10.6-hr duty days experienced significant fatigue due to a variety of operational factors, including sleep restriction. In an attempt to counter the effects of tiredness on performance and alertness, crew members reported consuming 1.5 times more caffeine on flight days than on pretrip days. This is similar to what has been observed in long-haul transport pilots, who have reported consuming a daily average of 3.1 cups of coffee during trips as opposed to only 1.9 cups prior to trips (121), and in helicopter pilots servicing North Sea oil rigs who have been found to increase their duty-day caffeine consumption by 42% (122).

A recent report by the Committee on Military Nutrition Research (81) recommended using caffeine doses of 100–600 mg to sustain the cognitive performance and physical endurance of military personnel, especially during periods of sleep deprivation. The Committee noted the fact that caffeine's effects appear particularly consistent in fatigued individuals.

### Effects of Caffeine on Sleep-deprived Subjects

Caffeine's effects on sleep-deprived volunteers have been explored more thoroughly than those of methylphenidate and pemoline. Although reviews of the literature by Weiss and Laties (100) and Dews (83) indicate that caffeine's efficacy is modest compared to amphetamine, studies show that caffeine is beneficial with regard to enhancing alertness and sustaining aspects of performance in fatigued people. Approximately 300 mg caffeine taken between 22:00 and 01:30 has been found effective for reducing sleepiness during nighttime shift work (123,124), and doses ranging from 250 to 400 mg have proven beneficial for sustaining both alertness and psychomotor performance until approximately 05:30 (125).

Penetar et al. (126,127) examined the efficacy of 150, 300, and 600 mg/70 kg on subjects kept awake for a total of 63.5 hr (caffeine or placebo was administered after 48 hr). After the dose, data were collected on sleep latencies, psychomotor performance, subjective sleepiness ratings, mood, and alertness. The 600-mg dose restored sleep latency to approximately 50% of well-rested levels (up from approximately 20%) and continued to exert a positive effect for 3 hr. Throughput on the choice reaction time test was significantly improved for 8 hr by 600 mg of caffeine and for 4 hr by 300 mg of caffeine. Serial addition/subtraction benefited for 3 hr from all three doses. Performance on the logical reasoning task was better after 600 mg and 300 mg than after placebo, and the effect lasted for 12 hr. All three doses returned subjective sleepiness ratings to near baseline levels, but only for 2 hr. Ratings of vigor were improved and ratings of fatigue were attenuated similarly by all three doses and these improvements persisted for 2 hr postdose. Self-ratings of confusion were affected only by the 150-mg dose at the 2-hr postdose point. Kelly et al. (58) failed to support the sleep latency results (collected with standard multiple-sleep-latency-test procedures) or the performance results in a later study that used a 300-mg dose of caffeine across a 64-hr sleep deprivation period (300 mg every 6 hr from 23:20 on the first day through 17:20 on the third day). However, when sleep latencies were collected using a maintenance-of-wakefulness protocol, subjects receiving the caffeine were able to sustain near-baseline levels of alertness whereas placebo subjects were not. Some of the differences between the Penetar et al. (126) and Kelly et al. (58) studies no doubt stem from the fact that one study was designed to restore performance that had already deteriorated, whereas the other study attempted to prevent decrements from ever occurring.

In an investigation having some basic similarities to the strategy taken by Penetar et al. (126), Tharion et al. (128) evaluated the efficacy of 100-, 200-, and 300-mg doses of caffeine on Navy Seal trainees after 72 hr of sleep deprivation. Two test sessions followed caffeine administration (either 1–1.5 hr postdose or 8–10 hr postdose) and included auditory and visual vigilance tasks, four-choice reaction time, matching to sample, repeated acquisition (learning a sequence of key presses), rifle marksmanship, mood, and subjective sleepiness assessments. The two higher doses of caffeine were found to attenuate deprivation-induced performance decrements in all of the tasks except for auditory vigilance, matching to sample, and marksmanship. Although target detection in visual vigilance was significantly impaired by sleep deprivation, it was improved by 11% after 300 mg of caffeine. Caffeine produced a dose-dependent attenuation of fatigue-related reaction time decrements (significance was found between the 300-mg-vs. the 100-mg-caffeine and placebo groups). Fatigue ratings increased significantly less in the high-dose group than in all of the other groups, and this effect persisted for 8–10 hr. Sleepiness ratings increased the least, relative to baseline, in the 300-mg group, and a similar pattern was observed in the 200-mg group.

Kamimori et al. (129) tested the effects of approximately 150, 300, and 600 mg caffeine on noradrenaline and adrenaline levels, sleep latency, Stanford Sleepiness Scale ratings, and choice reaction time in volunteers who were dosed after 49 hr of continuous wakefulness (and kept awake for an additional 12 hr).

Although statistical comparisons were not performed on data other than the catecholamine levels, it was found that adrenaline levels were consistently higher 60–240 min after the 600-mg dose relative to placebo, and higher 60–150 min after the 600-mg dose relative to the 150-mg dose. Sleep latencies, sleepiness scores, and reaction times correlated with serum caffeine levels in the predicted direction, showing that caffeine improved alertness in a dose-dependent fashion.

A recent study by Dinges (130) explored the possibility of using frequent low doses of caffeine to sustain the performance of sleep-deprived subjects during 88 hr of continuous wakefulness. The equivalent of approximately 578 mg of caffeine per 80 kg of body weight was given every 24 hr—but instead of being administered as a single large dose, it was divided into 0.3 mg/kg every hour (for the last 66 hr). Caffeine attenuated attention lapses throughout the second of 4 days of deprivation, and it tended to improve the fastest reaction times. However, low-dose caffeine had no effect on digit-symbol substitution, short-term memory, or, surprisingly, self-reports of sleepiness/alertness.

Recently, a new galenic, slow-release form of caffeine has been investigated as a countermeasure for sleep loss. The primary emphasis behind this work centers on the fact that larger doses of caffeine (i.e., 600 mg) appear more efficacious than lower doses for attenuating the effects of sleep loss, but high-dose caffeine also tends to produce deleterious cardiovascular and/or CNS side effects. Slow-release caffeine may offer a solution to this dilemma because it peaks more slowly (within 4 hr) and at lower levels, and it maintains relatively level plasma concentrations longer (4–6 hr) than the typically available form (131). Sicard et al. (132) found that a 600-mg dose of slow-release caffeine was well tolerated in a large group of young, healthy, male subjects, despite the fact that they were well rested at the time of testing. The only adverse effect was a decrease in self-ratings of calmness at 2, 5, and 10 hr postdose. Patat et al. (133) supported the usefulness of 600 mg slow-release caffeine in subjects who were sleep deprived for 36 hr while being tested on EEG status, critical flicker fusion (CFF), choice reaction time, tracking, sustained attention, body sway, subjective sleepiness, and Stroop test performance. Caffeine, administered at 21:00, attenuated deprivation-related increases in delta and theta EEG, improved choice and Stroop reaction time, decreased body sway, increased accuracy on the sustained-attention test, and reduced self-rated sleepiness. The majority of these effects occurred within 4 hr postdose and persisted for 19–21 hr.

Lagarde et al. (131) found consistent beneficial effects of slow-release caffeine in a later study of sleep-deprived subjects. This investigation of the effects of 150, 300, and 600 mg slow-release caffeine on volunteers who remained awake from 06:00 on the morning of one day through 17:00 the next day (32 hr of continuous wakefulness) revealed at least some positive impact on objective and subjective wakefulness from all three doses; however, the 300- and 600-mg doses were most effective. The 300-mg dose was considered "optimal." With 300 mg, there were positive effects on self-ratings of "awake," "peppy," "attentive," "capable," "quick-witted," "happy," and "interested," and all of these occurred within 2 hr postdose (but only the effect on "happy" was sustained). This dose also produced better performance (relative to placebo) on spatial processing, memory search, and tracking at 9 hr postdose, an effect that was sustained to 13 hr on the search and tracking tasks. Although results with 600 mg were similar, it was associated with "shivering" and tachycardia in female volunteers. Lagarde et al. (131) concluded that slow-release caffeine works well as a vigilance and mood regulator in sleep-deprived volunteers, and suggested that it may be a useful adjunct to prophylactic napping in sustained operations.

### Effects on Mood and Motivation

The literature is replete with evidence for the mood-enhancing effects of caffeine, especially in habitual consumers; however, it is difficult to determine the degree to which caffeine's positive effects on mood are straightforward and which effects simply are the result of alleviating withdrawal symptoms (134). Nevertheless, Lieberman (66) has summarized a large body of evidence suggesting that caffeine in doses ranging from 64 to 400 mg enhances feelings of alertness in a dose-dependent fashion, although doses of 300 mg or more increase reports of anxiety. In well-rested adolescents, caffeine administered via ad lib consumption of caffeinated soft drinks was found to decrease ratings of depression, drowsiness, and fatigue compared to levels seen during caffeine abstinence (135). In a group of 18–35-year-old men, 64 mg of caffeine was found to improve self-ratings of clear-headedness, efficiency, vigor, sleepiness, and alertness (110). A study of college students revealed that a morning cup of coffee decreased fatigue prior to a midday test session, although effects were negligible earlier in the day (136). In both fatigued and well-rested university students, a 200-mg dose of caffeine followed by a 50-mg maintenance dose was found to increase ratings of energy (relative to placebo) and reduce feelings of fatigue, especially in the fatigued subjects. Overall, caffeine reduced anger ratings as well (104).

### Summary

In summary, caffeine is a known psychostimulant that exerts positive effects on physical endurance, alertness, and vigilance. The effects on reaction time and EEG activity are debatable. Caffeine may cause small, but inconsequential, increases in blood pressure, particularly in people who do not habitually use this compound. Although the effects on mood are generally positive, increased anxiety may result from doses of 300 mg or more. Caffeine's most reliable effects appear to occur in sleep-deprived personnel in whom doses ranging from 250 to 600 mg (including sustained-release caffeine doses of 300–600 mg) have been shown to improve wakefulness, mood, and various aspects of performance.

Caffeine's efficacy relative to pemoline and methylphenidate is unknown since side-by-side comparisons have not been performed. However, caffeine's effects are purported to be modest compared to those of amphetamine (100,126,131), and there is evidence that caffeine may be most useful for shorter (i.e., 36-hr) rather than longer periods of sleep deprivation (116). In part, this may be due to the fact that tolerance to at least some of caffeine's effects occurs rapidly (71), suggesting that it may be necessary to significantly elevate the dose to sustain level performance despite increasing amounts of fatigue (although evidence on this last point is currently unavailable). It may be that escalating the dose sufficiently to maintain alertness would be contraindicated by the introduction of unwanted side effects, but again, this issue has not been studied. Akerstedt and Ficca (24) recently indicated the need for further research, but in the meantime, suggested that caffeine is appropriate for occasional use in attenuating the negative effects of fatigue from irregular work hours in the performance of short- or medium-duration tasks. Caffeine almost certainly is a better choice than pemoline since caffeine is safer and more readily available.

### D. Dextroamphetamine

Dextroamphetamine is available in 5-mg tablets as Dexedrine (GlaxoSmithKline) and in 5- and 10-mg tablets as DextroStat (Shire US). Both products consist of the dextro isomer of *d,l*-amphetamine sulfate (137). Dexedrine also comes in *Spansule* sustained-release capsules (both 5 and 10 mg). The U.S. Food and Drug Administration (FDA) has classified amphetamines as Schedule II controlled substances, meaning that they are available only by physician prescription because, although these compounds have recognized therapeutic value, there is a high potential for abuse coupled with a high liability for psychological or physical dependence. Although amphetamine compounds are well known for their psychostimulant properties and their usefulness for promoting wakefulness in a variety of situations, the FDA-approved indications for these medications include only the treatment of narcolepsy and attention deficit disorder, and not the promotion of wakefulness in sleep-deprived personnel. Common forms of amphetamine are dextroamphetamine and methamphetamine.

### General

Amphetamine (and dextroamphetamine) are among several drugs that belong to the general category of compounds referred to as sympathomimetic agents. Although the various sympathomimetic amines differ in their effects based on differing amounts and types of central and peripheral stimulation (41), they have broad actions, which Hoffman and Lefkowitz (36) enumerate as: (a) peripheral excitatory (stimulates certain smooth muscles like those in blood vessels of the skin, mucous membranes, and glands like salivary and sweat glands); (b) peripheral inhibitory on other smooth muscles (like those in the gut, blood vessels supplying skeletal muscles, and the bronchial tree); (c) cardiac excitatory (increased heart rate and/or force of contraction); (d) metabolic actions (increased glycogen conversion in liver and muscle and liberation of fatty acids from fat stores); (e) endocrine actions (modulation of insulin, renin, and pituitary hormones); (f) CNS effects (increased wakefulness and motor activity with reduced appetite); and (g) presynaptic inhibition or enhancement of the release of neurotransmitters such as norepenephrine and acetylcholine. Amphetamines have many, but not all, of these effects.

Amphetamine's primary effects (increased wakefulness, appetite suppression, and increased locomotor activity) are thought to be mediated by the release of norepinephrine from noradrenergic neurons in the CNS (36). However, research points to the role of plasma transport inhibition of dopamine, norepinephrine, and serotonin as well as inhibition of the vesicular monoamine transporter (138). Wisor et al. (139) summarize evidence that dopamine reuptake inhibition produces a greater alerting effect than norepinephrine transport blockade.

Amphetamines became available as early as 1887, but the medical utility of these compounds was not discovered until the 1930s. Early on, amphetamines were considered risk-free medications, and as a result, they were available without prescription for use in the treatment of a variety of conditions until 1951 (140). During World War II, amphetamines were used by the predominant military forces as a way to sustain alertness despite sleep loss. Unfortunately, widespread abuse became a problem in the general U.S. population between the mid 1950s and late 1960s (141) before public awareness campaigns, law enforcement activities, and other factors resulted in a substantial decline in the 1970s (140). Since that time, amphetamines have been used more for their medically recognized purposes, although evidence of abuse, particularly of methamphetamine, appears daily in the popular media. Despite this drawback, properly controlled administration of amphetamine compounds remains a viable strategy for the sustainment of combat performance in select military operations where sleep is difficult or impossible to obtain, and in these settings, amphetamines are generally considered more effective than caffeine. The U.S. Navy's guide for flight surgeon's and the Army's guide for leaders both mention the use of dextroamphetamine for the sustainment of aviator performance in continuous-flight operations (142,143), the U.S. Air Force has authorized the use of dextroamphetamine in certain types of lengthy single-seat and dual-seat aviation missions, and a recent NATO Research and Technology Organization publication discusses amphetamine's value as an antifatigue measure for aviation personnel (63).

## Typical Effects

Amphetamine is a potent psychostimulant, having both CNS and peripheral effects. As summarized by Hoffman and Lefkowitz (36), these include: (a) increased systolic and diastolic blood pressure with an initial slowing of the heart rate; (b) some smooth muscle stimulation (contraction of the sphincter in the urinary bladder, increased uterine tone) with unpredictable gastrointestinal effects; (c) potent CNS stimulation thought to be related to cortical and reticular-activating-system activation (particularly with the *d* isomer); (d) an increase in psychological arousal (decreased fatigue, increased wakefulness/alertness, improved mood and self confidence, increased initiative and ability to concentrate, and often feelings of elation and euphoria accompanied by increased activity and talkativeness); (e) the attenuation of fatigue, sustainment of performance, reduction of attentional lapses, and postponement of sleep; and (f) the temporary suppression of appetite. Some individuals report side effects of headache, palpitation, dizziness, agitation, dysphoria, anxiety, or fatigue when administered amphetamine.

## Dosage

The usual chronic oral dose of dextroamphetamine is 5 mg, 2–3 times daily; however, studies employing the drug to prolong wakefulness and performance typically employ larger doses in the range of 10–20 mg (100). Prior to administering normal therapeutic doses to humans, a test dose of 2.5 mg is recommended since toxic manifestations have been seen (as an idiosyncrasy) after even a 2-mg dose, although reactions are rare with doses under 15 mg.

## Pharmacokinetics

A single dose of two 5-mg tablets has been shown to produce an average peak blood level of 29.2 ng/mL at approximately 2 hr. The average half-life is 10.25 hr (144).

## Adverse Reactions

The most common cardiovascular adverse effects are palpitations, tachycardia, and elevated blood pressure. The most common adverse CNS reactions are overstimulation, restlessness, dizziness, insomnia, euphoria, dyskinesia, tremor, and headache. The most common adverse gastrointestinal reactions are dryness of mouth, unpleasant taste, diarrhea, and constipation. Other adverse reactions can include urticaria, impotence, and/or changes in libido (137).

## Tolerance and Toxicity

Although the amphetamines can be toxic at doses only slightly higher than the recommended dose, tolerance develops quickly with repeated use. Ingestion of an acute dose of 1 mg/kg is considered life-threatening in the case of a nonhabitual user (41), although doses of 400–500 mg are not necessarily fatal (137). In the event of acute intoxication, chlorpromazine and an alpha-receptor blocking agent should reduce both the CNS and the pressor effects of amphetamine (145); however, Benowitz (41) reports that there is no specific antidote. He recommends: (a) maintaining airways and assisting ventilation, (b) treating any symptoms of agitation, seizures, coma, or hyperthermia, (c) monitoring vital signs and ECG for at least 6 hr, (d) treating hypertension, tachyarrhythmias, and arterial vasospasm, and (e) performing gastric lavage and administering charcoal and a cathartic.

### Effects on Physical Performance

It has long been accepted that amphetamines produce beneficial effects in athletic endeavors (146), and amphetamines also have been shown to be particularly beneficial in the performance of activities that are physically exhausting (100).

Although one early study raised doubts concerning the benefits of 10- and 20-mg doses of amphetamine for improving running time, endurance, and recovery, and the speed with which athletes swam 100-yd and 440-yd courses (147), an examination of the methodology revealed that the dose-administration times may have been too close to the experimental sessions (30 min–1 hr). In another study, during which amphetamine was administered 2–3 hr prior to the experimental sessions, 14 mg/70 kg was observed to generally improve swimming speed in 100- and 200-yd races (although there were exceptions); decrease the time it took to run courses of 600 yd, 1000 yd, and 1 mile; decrease the time it took for marathon runners to run 4.5–12.7 miles; improve shot-putting and weight-throwing distances; and increase the speed with which swimmers completed 100- and 200-yd swims (148). These data are consistent with the finding that 15 mg/70 kg amphetamine produced improvements in the strength, acceleration, anaerobic capacity, and endurance of athletes (149). In athletic competition, stimulants have been used at least as early as the latter part of the nineteenth century, when cyclists took caffeine to improve endurance (150). By the early 1950s, amphetamines were being used by athletes, and over the next several years, the problem of amphetamine abuse was severe enough to prompt special investigations by the medical community. It is estimated that about 3% of athletes continue to use amphetamines for their ergogenic effects. This is understandable given the positive effects of these drugs (150), especially when it comes to the enhancement of physical strength and endurance (149).

### Effects on Physiology and Simple Task Performance

Martin et al. (151) assessed the physiological effects of 15 and 30 mg/70 kg amphetamine on 12 men and found increases in blood pressure, respiration rate, body temperature, pupillary dilation, and heart rate. In addition, dextroamphetamine increased the excretion of epinephrine, but did not affect overall urinary output or the excretion of norepinephrine, dopamine, or creatinine. Caldwell (152) studied the effects of three successive 10-mg doses of dextroamphetamine (administered at midnight, 04:00, and 08:00) on healthy male and female aviators. In men, a noticeable increase in systolic pressure was observed within 1 hr postdose, with a peak increase 12 hr later or 5 hr after the last 10-mg dose (21 mmHg higher than what was observed under placebo). In women, there was only a transient elevation in systolic pressure 20 min after their second 10-mg dose. A persistent increase was not observed until 50 min after the third 10-mg dose, and the peak effect (a 20 mmHg increase over placebo) was not seen until 6 hr after the last dose. Diastolic blood pressures in both groups increased approximately 10 mmHg over placebo levels after the second 10-mg dose of dextroamphetamine, and this persisted for 8 hr. Peak heart rates averaged 85 beats/min under dextroamphetamine versus 67 beats/min under placebo. Heart rates were not elevated until 2 hr after the second 10-mg dose, but once the increases occurred, they tended to last the remainder of the testing day (until 22:20).

Morselli et al. (153) studied the effects of two different 20-mg preparations of amphetamine (salt-based and resinate) on physiological parameters. Blood work indicated that average peak plasma levels with these compounds occurred 4 hr postadministration while the peak blood levels occurred at 4 hr for the resinate and 6 hr for the salt-based form. Increases in blood pressure (34 mmHg systolic and 25 mmHg diastolic after the salt, and 15 mmHg systolic and 7 mmHg diastolic after the resinate) were observed but subsided completely within 4 hr. There was a slight decrease in heart rate during the first 45 min (in four of six subjects) with a subsequent slight (10–15 bpm) increase lasting 60–90 min. Additionally, there were EEG amplitude reductions in the alpha range and increased fast activity 45–60 min post drug. Some side effects (nausea, cramps, dry mouth, headache, etc.) were seen with both preparations, although those with the salt base were more pronounced. As far as the effects on performance were concerned, it was found that skill on a letter-matching test, a number comparison test, a memory test, and a test in which subjects placed metal pins into holes was improved under both forms of amphetamine. No conclusive relationship was seen between blood levels and performance, but there was an apparent relationship between the rate at which amphetamine entered the blood stream and the occurrence of side effects.

Earlier investigations reviewed by Cole (154) found similar results with regard to the pressor effects and task performance. It was reported that amphetamine increased both blood pressure and metabolic activity as well as improved performance on a diversity of tasks. Additionally, there was evidence that amphetamine enhanced motor task performance, but it was postulated that the drug-induced facilitation was not simply a function of enhanced motor activity. This is consistent with findings that 10–15 mg dextroamphetamine improves other types of performance as well, such as paced sequential-memory tasks and arithmetic tasks (155), as well as performance on noncompetitive paired associate learning tasks and simple (but not difficult) coding tests (156). Cole (154) suggested that amphetamine improves some task performance by facilitating the monitoring of task-relevant cues, rather than by enhancing motor responses to task-relevant stimuli. Data summarized by Weiss and Laties (100) indicate more consistent improvements in simple reaction time with amphetamine than with caffeine, and they indicate that tracking accuracy is rather reliably improved, while the effects of amphetamine on "steadiness" appear to be equivocal. Kennedy et al. (157) found that 10 mg dextroamphetamine given to well-rested subjects enhanced two-handed tapping speed (but not non-preferred-hand or preferred-hand tapping) and the percentage of correct responses on a speed-related short-term memory task, but degraded grammatical reasoning and exerted no clear effects on a mental-rotation task. There is evidence that amphetamine generally improves speed, but does not exert a substantial influence on high-level intellectual functioning (100,156,158).

### Effects on Vigilance

The vigilance-enhancing effects of amphetamine during extended work periods are well documented. Payne (159) and Payne and Hauty (160) studied the ability of 5 mg dextroamphetamine and 20 mg of a caffeine derivative, as well as instructional manipulations, to prolong performance in a task where subjects were required to monitor four dials and minimize pointer deviations throughout a 4-hr session. The results clearly indicated that both dextroamphetamine and caffeine prevented the performance decrements that occurred across time under the placebo and control conditions. Dextroamphetamine maintained performance longer than the caffeine (4 vs. 2 hr). A follow-up study (161) examined the impact of enhanced task cues, different instructional manipulations, and the effects of *d*-amphetamine (5 mg), time-released *d*-amphetamine, a caffeine derivative, and two compounds of diphenhydramine (50 mg) combined with other drugs on several parameters. Results showed that providing additional cues and intermediate work breaks improved overall task performance, and both preparations of *d*-amphetamine (and to some extent the caffeine) significantly reduced declines in vigilance during the 7 hr. The amphetamines were clearly the most effective performance sustainers.

A later investigation of various doses of *d*-amphetamine (162) confirmed the performance-sustaining effects noted earlier, and it was found that with normal (presumably non-sleep-deprived) subjects, a 5–7.5-mg dose was optimal. However, a 10-mg dose was also effective. In Speigel's (163) summary of the literature, it was concluded that "mostly positive effects of amphetamine were reported in various tasks requiring sustained attention (letter canceling, card sorting, tracking, pursuit rotor, signal detection, arithmetic)" (p. 192). Speigel (163) suggests that amphetamine's positive effects may stem from the drug's ability to maintain consistent levels of arousal and vigilance, thus minimizing the transient troughs that typically occur in these parameters. In support of this assertion, Speigel (163) states that evaluations of relatively long (30–60 min) EEG recordings have shown that 10 mg dextroamphetamine does not produce hypervigilance, but rather suppresses the naturally occurring fluctuations in various EEG activity bands.

### Effects on Military Performance

The positive effects of amphetamine are of particular relevance to the military, where it is often necessary for personnel to remain "on task" for extended duty periods without prolonged breaks. Babkoff and Krueger (164) point out that stimulants have been used by the military since World War II to reduce fatigue and increase performance of soldiers assigned to special duties such as long-range reconnaissance and extended transport flights. Although such stimulant use has not been well studied in a field setting, reports tend to substantiate their operational utility. Winfield (165) reported that 5-mg Benzedrine (amphetamine) tablets given to aircrews involved in Royal Air Force antisubmarine patrols and offensive coastal patrols significantly delayed the onset of fatigue and reduced boredom-related decrements in one third of personnel. Based on these findings, Winfield (165) suggested that amphetamine (10–15 mg) would be effective for warding off fatigue in particularly demanding flights. Tyler (166) reported consistent results with volunteers from the Army, Marines, and civilian work camps, who were better at marksmanship, steadiness, and reaction time, and were more able to stay alert after 48 hr of sleep deprivation under the influence of 10 mg benzedrine sulfate given every 8–12 hr. McKenzie and Elliot (167) examined the use of secobarbital (to promote premission sleep) and dextroamphetamine (to alleviate in-flight fatigue) in fighter pilots performing 5–12 hr flight missions. Prior to detailing the results of their study, they reported on a survey that indicated that 64% of 200 pilots said they had taken the dextroamphetamine with them on the flight, and 24% had used at least one 5-mg dextroamphetamine in flight (about the same number also took a second in-flight dose). Ninety-six percent of the pilots who took dextroamphetamine reported satisfactory effects. In terms of experimental results, McKenzie and Elliot (167) found that performance during a 12-hr flight-simulation task was adversely affected in those who had received secobarbital the previous evening, and that dextroamphetamine only partly attenuated this effect. When dextroamphetamine was administered to subjects who had not previously received secobarbital, 7 hr into the simulation, there was a marked improvement in performance, which lasted for approximately 4 hr. These findings tended to support the results of the survey conducted earlier.

According to Cornum et al. (168), amphetamines were used during the Vietnam conflict to sustain aircrew performance during 8–12 hr overseas deployments which often required multiple aerial refuelings. Such use appears justified based on the experimental data of McKenzie and Elliot (167) and the field observations made by Senechal (169). Senechal (169) indicated that jet crews who were administered 5 mg dextroamphetamine approximately 13 hr into an Air Force strike on Libya in April of 1986 (EF-111 Ravens performing electronic jamming) experienced positive effects in terms of overcoming the fatigue of the mission itself and the sleep deprivation that occurred during earlier preparation for the mission. There were no in-flight or landing problems and all aircraft returned safely to base.

Cornum (170) reported that dextroamphetamine was also used with 35 F15-C pilots who were flying combat air patrol missions during Operation Desert Shield/Storm. These pilots were not only flying long missions (6–11 hr), but they were sleep-deprived and suffering from circadian desynchronization as well. To counteract potentially lethal performance decrements, the pilots were issued five to six, 5-mg dextroamphetamine tablets at the beginning of flights and were told to self-administer one tablet every 2–4 hr as needed to maintain alertness until landing (K. Cornum, personal communication, 1993). The aviators reported clear benefit from the drug and the unit's commander ultimately concluded that dextroamphetamine administration contributed significantly to the safety of operations. There were no reported adverse effects, even in personnel who took 10 mg at a time, and no aviators reported a need to continue the drug once proper work/sleep schedules were reinstated. Cornum et al. (168) later investigated the experiences of two F-15C squadrons who had deployed in support of Operation

Desert Shield, and reported that 58% of respondents stated they had used amphet-amines during combat air patrol missions protecting Airborne Warning and Control Systems (AWACS) and other valuable assets. The overwhelming majority stated they used the medication at night during low-task missions, when alertness was most adversely affected. Cornum et al. concluded that dextroamphetamine was preferable to caffeine for the sustainment of fighter-pilot performance because it has more pronounced alertness-enhancing properties, it has no diuretic side effects, and it reduces vestibular disturbances. Emonson and Vanderbeek (171) likewise reported benefits from dextroamphetamine administration in Air Force aircrews during Operation Desert Shield/Storm. A survey of all Tactical Air Command squadrons (including pilots of F-16s, F-15s, A-10s, and F-4s) indicated that 65% had occasionally used amphetamines as a fatigue countermeasure during the deployment, and of these, 58–61% felt they were beneficial or essential. No major side effects were reported with 5-mg doses administered at 4-hr intervals.

Studies summarized by Weiss and Laties (100) provide further evidence of the facilitative effects of amphetamine in a nonaviation military performance con-text. In one study by Seashore and Ivy (172), two doses of either amphetamine (10 mg) or methamphetamine (5 mg) were shown to improve subjective reports of alertness and motor tests after subjects performed an 18–20-mile march and a night of guard duty. In another investigation, by Somerville (173), it was shown that 30 or 35 mg amphetamine (given in divided doses) enhanced rifle-firing speed and accuracy during the final 22 hr of a 56-hr training exercise. However, it appeared from an earlier study that enhancements in marksmanship and obsta-cle course performance did not occur under amphetamine (15 mg) after only the road march alone (without guard duty). Thus, the effects of amphetamine may be more pronounced in the presence of higher levels of fatigue, such as those asso-ciated with sleep loss, rather than the fatigue associated with only increased phys-ical activity.

### Effects on Performance Sustainment After Sleep Deprivation

As is the case with caffeine, the effects of dextroamphetamine are particularly noticeable during periods of sleep deprivation. Although some investigators have reported only minimal performance benefits from amphetamine administration even in subjects who have been deprived of sleep for 44–68 hr (174), many other studies suggest that properly timed drug administration, at sufficient dose levels, can restore performance that has already declined, or prevent decrements that stem from significant sleep loss. Newhouse et al. (175) conducted an experiment in which three groups of subjects were sleep-deprived for over 48 hr and given either oral *d*-amphetamine (5, 10, or 20 mg), intravenous nicotine (0.39, 0.53, 0.79, or 1.05 mg), or oral *l*-deprenyl (20 or 30 mg). Alertness, performance, and physiological changes were measured. Results indicated nicotine produced only minor changes in performance and physiology without affecting alertness. *l*-Deprenyl (30 mg) was better than nicotine in terms of accuracy improvement on logical reasoning, but again, alertness was unaffected. In contrast, the 20-mg dose of d-amphetamine produced marked improvements in addition/subtraction (lasting more than 10 hr), a gradual improvement in logical reasoning (significant between 5.5 and 7.5 hr postdose), and a long-lasting improvement in the speed of responding during the choice reaction-time task (10 hr). Also, there was an increase in alertness for 7 hr, blood pressure for 5 hr, heart rate (only after 8–10 hr), and temperature. The 10-mg dose exerted fewer effects, and those that were seen (addition/subtraction performance and alertness) were shorter in duration than was the case with the 20-mg dose. No physiological effects were observed. The 5-mg dose did not affect any of the measures. Interestingly, the observed performance enhancements with 20 mg continued even after the subjects' subjective feelings of increased vigor had subsided. Overall, amphetamine improved performance without impairing judgment.

These results are consistent with those of Hartmann et al. (176), who studied the effects of *l*-amphetamine (10 mg) and *d*-amphetamine (10 mg) on the mood, EEG, and performance of subjects exposed to a much shorter period of sleep deprivation (1 night). The authors found that subjective reports of decreased vigor and increased fatigue associated with sleep deprivation were not alleviated by either drug; however, cumulative omission errors in the vigilance task were reduced by *d*-amphetamine, and *d*-amphetamine was also effective in restoring EEG alpha activity to predeprivation levels in comparison to either placebo or *l*-amphetamine. The fact that *d*-amphetamine was the most potent of the two preparations supports the contention by others (177) that *d*-amphetamine is approximately twice as effective as *l*-amphetamine.

Caldwell et al. (178,179) investigated the prophylactic administration of repeated 10-mg doses of dextroamphetamine (given at midnight, 04:00, and 08:00) for the mitigation of fatigue-related decrements in aviators kept awake for 40 continuous hr. In male aviators, performance on four of nine fight maneuvers, EEG indicators of arousal, and subjective impressions of the ability to think clearly and feel alert were significantly better under dextroamphetamine than under placebo. In female pilots, similar effects were found in that simulator flight performance on six of the nine maneuvers, EEG activation (less slow-wave activity), and self-ratings of alertness were better after dextroamphetamine than placebo. These effects were especially noticeable between 03:00 and 11:00, when fatigue-related problems were most severe. Performance on a 10-min task of short-term memory, arithmetic ability, and monitoring was unaffected by the drug, probably because the task was too short. However, despite the lack of basic cognitive effects, it appeared that the prophylactic administration of dextroamphetamine maintained performance and alertness close to well-rested levels even though significant fatigue from sleep loss was present.

These results were later confirmed in an actual in-flight study in which 10 pilots completed a series of 1-hr flights in a specially-instrumented UH-60 helicopter throughout 40 hr of continuous wakefulness (180). When 10-mg doses of dextroamphetamine were given at midnight, 04:00, and 08:00, the performance of straight-and-level maneuvers as well as climbs, descents, right standard-rate turns, and a left-descending turn was significantly better than the performance of these same maneuvers under placebo. In addition, dextroamphetamine markedly attenuated fatigue-related elevations in EEG theta activity and decreased subjective feelings of fatigue, confusion, and depression, while improving self-ratings of vigor. With regard to cognitive effects, dextroamphetamine sustained the ability to monitor warning lights and dials, monitor radio communication calls, and track an unstable target during a divided-attention, computerized performance battery (181). As was the case with the earlier simulator studies, the most noticeable drawbacks of dextroamphetamine were (a) its pressor effects (not clinically significant in healthy pilots), and (b) its moderate disturbance of the recovery sleep period. However, despite the observed increases in stages 1 and 2 of this recovery sleep and the delay in onset of rapid eye movement (REM) sleep, a comparison of next-day mood and performance revealed no differences as a function of whether dextroamphetamine versus placebo had been administered during the preceding sleep deprivation period (182).

In a follow-up investigation, it was determined that dextroamphetamine also was useful for sustaining pilot performance and alertness for periods longer than 40 hr. Caldwell et al. (183) exposed aviators to 64 hr of continuous wakefulness while providing either 10-mg doses of dextroamphetamine at midnight, 04:00, and 08:00 (on 2 successive nights), or matching placebos. Evaluations of simulator flight performance, EEG activity, mood, and cognitive performance revealed several positive amphetamine effects. Flight performance was maintained close to well-rested levels until the last flight of the study (after 58 hr of continuous wakefulness), and this sustainment of performance was accompanied by a suppression of slow-wave EEG activity and reduced self-perceptions of fatigue and confusion. Again, the negative effects included increased cardiovascular stimulation and a reduction in recovery sleep quality. However, it was concluded that while dextroamphetamine is no replacement for adequate work/rest scheduling or restful sleep, it can attenuate the performance, alertness, and mood degradations associated with significant sleep loss. This conclusion is consistent with the findings of Pigeau et al. (16), who indicated that strategically placed 20-mg doses of dextroamphetamine (as well as 300-mg doses of modafinil) produced superior reaction time, logical reasoning, and short-term memory performance, in addition to improved ratings of mood and sleepiness in comparison to placebo.

### Effects on Mood and Motivation

Typically, the effects of dextroamphetamine on mood and motivation are positive and can be summarized as increased euphoria, exhilaration, energy, talkativeness, mental capacity, and desire for work, while the negative effects are increased restlessness and anxiety (100). Smith and Davis (177), confirm these effects, but go on to suggest there might also be a tendency toward increased end-of-day depression with amphetamine, although this has not been confirmed statistically. Nash (184) reported that 10 mg of sustained-release dextroamphetamine improved subjects' evaluations of their abstract-reasoning performance and their subjective ratings of feeling "fresh and alive." Cameron et al. (185) combined data across several studies and found that Benzedrine (usually 10 mg) and Dexedrine (5 mg) made subjects feel "more optimistic, friendly, energetic, talkative, decisive, egotistic, keyed-up, and light-headed" while simultaneously feeling "less drowsy, languid, bored, dissatisfied, depressed, and grouchy" (p. 118). Smith and Davis (177) found that 10- and 20-mg doses of dextroamphetamine increased ratings of vigor, talkativeness, friendliness, and anxiousness, while only the 20-mg dose increased ratings of confidence, euphoria, and speeding. Studies of sleep-deprived volunteers are consistent with many of the above findings in that dextroamphetamine has been observed to improve ratings on dimensions such as vigor, alertness, energy, and talkativeness, while reducing feelings of fatigue, confusion, and sleepiness (183,186).

While the positive effects of amphetamine on psychological mood are generally considered to be beneficial, concerns have been raised over the tendency of amphetamine-treated subjects to experience overconfidence and, by implication, poor judgment. Early on, Davis (187) reported that amphetamine improves the speed of performance at the expense of accuracy, and that research subjects often judge the effects of amphetamine more favorably than the experimenter. Marshall and Beech (188) later found that subjects who were given 14 mg/70 kg amphetamine significantly overestimated the number of correctly solved calculus problems in comparison to the estimates made under the influence of placebo, and Hurst (189) reported that 10 mg $d$-amphetamine increased the amount of risk subjects were willing to take when gambling with cigarettes. These reports introduced the persistent worry that amphetamine impairs judgment or that amphetamine impairs accuracy for the sake of speed. However, experimental evidence of overconfidence, response bias, poor judgment, or unfavorable speed/accuracy tradeoffs related to amphetamine is difficult to find in more recent studies. Newhouse et al. (186) reported that amphetamine restored a sleep-loss-induced liberal response bias to predeprivation levels, and Hurst and Weitzner (155) determined that neither 10- nor 15-mg doses of dextroamphetamine caused inaccurate assessments of performance on a sequential memory test or an arithmetic test. Baranski and Pigeau (190) found that subjects who were administered either placebo or 20-mg doses of dextroamphetamine were consistently able to monitor their own performance status throughout a period of sleep deprivation whereas subjects given 300-mg modafinil were not. Finally, Shappell et al. (191) reported that a group of Marine flight students chose an increasingly risky response strategy (higher speed with lower accuracy) under placebo during a simulated sustained-operations mission, but that administration of 10 mg/70 kg of dextromethamphetamine prevented this problem. It is likely that amphetamine tends to promote risky behavior only in normally alert people who inappropriately use the drug, whereas those who take amphetamine to prevent fatigue or to recover from the effects of sleep loss actually experience an improvement relative to their untreated sleep deprivation state.

### Summary

Amphetamine is a potent psychostimulant that is capable of counteracting many of the problems associated with fatigue and sleep deprivation. Amphetamines enhance physical strength and endurance, simple motor and tracking performance, and the monitoring of task-relevant cues, although the impact on basic reaction time is debatable. Amphetamine administration significantly increases blood pressure and heart rate, so it is not recommended for people with compromised cardiovascular function. The effects on mood are generally positive (more optimistic, friendly, energetic, talkative, and decisive) but anxiety has been reported, and higher doses produce euphoric effects that may be associated with increased risk-taking behavior, particularly in nonfatigued individuals. Amphetamine's effects are most clearly observed in fatigued or sleep-deprived personnel suffering from degraded alertness and performance. Single or divided multiple doses ranging from 10 to 20 mg appear most effective for restoring degraded alertness or maintaining level performance throughout periods of sleep loss.

In comparison to caffeine, pemoline, and methylphenidate, amphetamine appears to offer a more consistent and prolonged alerting effect (100,192), and both the benefits and drawbacks are fairly well known because amphetamines have a long history of use in real-world settings, particularly in military aviation. It has been concluded that "to date, the most promising stimulants to counteract performance decrements attributed to aircrew sustained operations are the amphetamines" (191, p. 269). Furthermore, Cornum et al. (193) have stated that the proper administration of amphetamines to severely fatigued personnel can make the difference between a mission that ends safely and one that ends in disaster.

Despite the significant advantages of amphetamines for sustaining alertness while postponing sleep, it must be kept in mind that these compounds have a high abuse potential, and they may produce physical dependence and other problems if not administered in a controlled fashion. While it is estimated that less than 10% of those who use amphetamine compounds will risk addiction (192), this risk must be weighed against the benefits of using amphetamines to mitigate the known decrements associated with sleep deprivation. In some military or emergency operations, the cost/benefit ratio is clear as there often is no choice but to complete the mission despite severe fatigue, either with or without pharmacological support. In the general civilian sector, the cost/benefit ratio is less certain because people are rarely required to work beyond the normal limits of human endurance. These factors must be considered before employing amphetamines or any other countermeasure but sleep to remedy fatigue-related decrements. However, if sleep is not possible and a high level of performance is required, amphetamines are likely the best option.

### E. Modafinil

In comparison to the scientific data that are available on both caffeine and dextroamphetamine, relatively little information is published on modafinil. Primarily, this is due to the fact that modafinil was not available by prescription in France (under the trade name Modiodal) until 1994, and it was not available in the United States (under the trade name Provigil) until December 1998 (194,195). Since the development of modafinil was targeted for the treatment of narcolepsy, research on healthy, normal volunteers is rare. Modafinil is available for oral administration in 100- and 200-mg tablets (196). The U.S. Food and Drug Administration (FDA) has classified modafinil as a Schedule IV controlled substance, meaning that it is available only by physician prescription because, although it has little abuse potential with only a small possibility of producing dependence, modafinil nonetheless should be used with the same level of care as drugs such as the benzodiazepines. The existing research indicates that modafinil has significant alertness-enhancing properties useful for alleviating the fatigue associated with sleep loss. It is FDA-approved for the treatment of excessive daytime sleepiness in patients with narcolepsy and obstructive apnea/hypopnea, and it is approved for bolstering wakefulness in patients with excessive sleepiness associated with shift work sleep disorders.

#### General

Modafinil ([diphenylmethyl]sulfinyl-2 acetamide) is a novel antinarcoleptic compound that promotes wakefulness and vigilance in animals and in humans without producing many of the side effects that occur with amphetamine administration (197). Modafinil was once thought to be an alpha-1 adrenergic agonist (198), but more recent evidence suggests that although an intact central alpha-adrenergic system is essential to modafinil's wake-promoting effects, the drug does not act directly on this system (199). Instead, research performed by Ferraro et al. (200) found that modafinil uniquely inhibited GABA release in the nucleus accumbens of rats while having little impact on the dopaminergic system relative to *d*-amphetamine. Other evidence exists concerning the role of GABA-mediated neurotransmission in modafinil's effects. McClellan and Spencer (199) summarized studies showing reduced GABA release in the cerebral cortex of both guinea pigs and rats in addition to GABA inhibition in the nucleus accumbens of rats. They also cite evidence pointing toward serotonergic involvement in modafinil's effects while reiterating that unlike amphetamines, modafinil's wake-promoting properties are not dependent on the dopaminergic system. However, it seems that the role of the dopaminergic system remains debatable because large doses of modafinil have been shown to produce an increase in dopamine levels in the nucleus accumbens of rats, although this effect is probably secondary to the inhibition of GABA (194). Further evidence for distinct differences between the mechanisms responsible for amphetamine's and modafinil's actions come from Engber et al. (201). Using 2-deoxyglucose autoradiography, Engber et al. found that both amphetamine and modafinil increased glucose utilization in the hippocampus and the centrolateral nucleus of the thalamus, but only modafinil increased activity in the amygdala. Amphetamine increased glucose utilization in the basal ganglia, other parts of the thalamus, the frontal cortex, the nucleus accumbens, the ventral tegmental area, and the pontine reticular fields, but modafinil had no effect on these areas. These data show that modafinil is more selective than amphetamine in targeting systems that affect sleep/wakefulness regulation, and this may explain why modafinil appears to have fewer side effects than other psychostimulants.

Modafinil was developed by Lafon Ltd. in France in the early 1980s, and it was tested for the treatment of narcolepsy and idiopathic hypersomnia using twice-daily divided doses of 200–400 mg (202). After clinical trials revealed that modafinil significantly reduced sleepiness, the first double-blind, placebo-controlled study was conducted in 1987. The results of this first investigation were similar to those of Bastuji and Jouvet (197), who found that morning and noon doses ranging from 200 to 500 mg decreased sleep attacks and drowsiness in 83% of the hypersomniacs and 71% of the narcoleptics. Furthermore, it was concluded that patients using modafinil generally did not suffer from peripheral side effects or nighttime sleep disturbances. Broughton et al. (203) recently supported the efficacy of 200- or 400-mg divided doses in the treatment of excessive daytime sleepiness in narcoleptics. At the end of a 2-week treatment period, patients on both doses suffered from less sleepiness (as measured by a Maintenance-of-Wakefulness test), fewer daytime sleep episodes, and a reduced probability of inadvertently falling asleep compared to placebo. As was the case in the earlier Bastuji and Jouvet (197) study, there were no nocturnal sleep disturbances and no elevations in blood pressure or heart rate. The only adverse events were increased nausea and nervousness with the 400-mg dose. Interestingly, modafinil administration did not interfere with the ability of patients to take voluntary naps during the day. Data from these types of studies, as well as the few investigations conducted on sleep-deprived normals (to be discussed shortly), have led to a great deal of interest in the possibility of using modafinil to temporarily remedy the effects of sleep loss in operational settings.

## Typical Effects

Modafinil exerts significant CNS effects with virtually no peripheral effects (204). Modafinil increases wakefulness, decreases EEG indications of fatigue, improves concentration, enhances mood, and facilitates cognitive performance without elevating psychomotor activity (198). In monkeys, Largarde and Milhaud (205) found modafinil is able to produce prolonged wakefulness across 4 days and nights with no behavioral side effects and no residual effects on sleep architecture. Hermant et al. (206) confirmed the finding regarding side effects after administration of the drug to monkeys over 5 consecutive days. Although modafinil was approved for use in the United States in 1998, at that time the drug already had been used to treat narcolepsy on well over 1000 patients in Europe (207). As noted above, in narcoleptics, modafinil has been shown to reduce the frequency of daytime sleep attacks while improving performance on cognitive tests (208,209). In addition to the more objective findings that modafinil attenuates drowsiness in patients, Besset et al. (210) indicated that 64% of narcoleptic/cataplectic patients rated modafinil either "good" or "excellent" for effectively reduced excessive daytime sleepiness. These results have been supported by Phase III and IV clinical studies conducted in the United States in which modafinil significantly improved wakefulness and reduced disease severity among narcoleptic patients (211).

### Dosage

The recommended dose of modafinil is 200 mg/day for the treatment of excessive daytime sleepiness associated with narcolepsy; however, doses of 400 mg/day are FDA-approved. While there is evidence that the higher dose is well tolerated, it has not been established that it confers additional therapeutic benefit (196). In sleep-deprived subjects, doses of 600 mg/day have been administered, but the preponderance of evidence suggests that 300–400 mg/day is probably sufficient and less likely to produce unwanted side effects.

### Pharmacokinetics

Modafinil is rapidly absorbed and produces peak plasma levels in 2–4 hr (196,211). The overall half-life after multiple doses is approximately 15 hr.

### Adverse Reactions

The most common adverse reactions to this medication are headache, nausea, nervousness, anxiety, and insomnia (211). Generally, these reactions are mild or moderate. The frequencies with which the most common treatment-emergent whole-body, digestive, respiratory, and nervous-system adverse experiences have occurred with daily 200- and 400-mg doses in patient populations were: headache 50%, nausea 13%, rhinitis 11%, and nervousness 8%. Unlike amphetamine, modafinil is not associated with significant cardiovascular stimulation.

### Tolerance and Toxicity

Modafinil has relatively low toxicity (compared to amphetamine) as evidenced by the fact that, in one study, doses of up to 1400 mg/day did not produce significant peripheral effects in patients with decreased motivation, and although blood pressure was found to be elevated in elderly patients receiving 1000 mg/day, these effects were not clinically significant. Furthermore, Bastuji and Jouvet (197) reported that a female hypersomniac who attempted suicide via the acute ingestion of 4500 mg modafinil suffered only tachycardia and 24 hr of nervousness, nausea, and insomnia prior to a full recovery. Cephalon (211) reported that a total of 151 doses of 1000 mg/day or more have been recorded in 32 patients, and that these produced only limited adverse experiences (i.e., excitation, agitation, insomnia, etc.), which resolved completely by the following day. In the event of overdose, the *Physicians' Desk Reference* (196) recommends supportive care to include cardiac monitoring and consideration of induced vomiting or gastric lavage. There is no specific antidote to the toxic effects of modafinil.

### Effects on Physical Performance

Unlike caffeine and amphetamine, which have long been used for ergogenic purposes, the effects of modafinil on physical performance have not been well researched. However, a review of the literature revealed one investigation in which the effects of 4 mg/kg of modafinil on time to exhaustion were evaluated. In 15 healthy subjects exercising on a cycle ergometer at 50% $\dot{V}O_{2max}$ and then at 85% $\dot{V}O_{2max}$, modafinil prolonged the time to exhaustion from 15.6 min to 18.3 min, and lowered subjective ratings of perceived exertion (212). Oxygen uptake, minute ventilation, and respiratory exchange were unaffected.

### Effects on Physiology and Simple Task Performance

The effects of acute oral doses of modafinil (200, 400, and 600 mg) were examined in a group of 10 elderly subjects (mean age 66 years) (213). Measurements taken at 0, 1, 2, 4, 6, and 8 hr postdose indicated modafinil generally increased EEG alpha activity and decreased delta, theta, and beta activity consistent with improved vigilance. Blood pressure, pulse rate, and skin conductance level were unaffected. Pupil diameter was increased under 400 mg modafinil at the sixth and eighth hr postdose, and concentration, complex reaction time, mood, and affect were improved especially by 200 mg modafinil in comparison to placebo. The 600-mg dose was sometimes deleterious. Generally speaking, effects were seen as early as 1 hr postdose and as late as 6 hr postdose, and the EEG effects occurred earlier than the performance effects. Ellis et al. (214) corroborated the alertness-promoting effect of modafinil (400 mg) in narcoleptics and normals, and concurred with the absence of pressor effects; however, the expected changes in cortical activation were not observed with functional magnetic resonance imaging. In contrast, Laffont (215) reported that administering 200 mg modafinil to young subjects caused increased CNS activation as evidenced by a reduction in slow-wave EEG activity (delta and theta) concurrent with an increase in alpha. These effects occurred within 1 hr postdose and persisted for 22 hr.

Brun et al. (216) evaluated the mental performance, hormone levels, and temperatures of eight sleep-deprived volunteers given 300-mg of modafinil at 22:00 and 08:00. Modafinil did not affect melatonin, cortisol, or growth hormone levels, but it did attenuate performance decrements, attenuate the nocturnal decrease in body temperature, and increase daytime body temperature. These temperature effects are different from what has been observed in non-sleep-deprived subjects. Bourdon et al. (217) found no effects of 200 mg of modafinil on thermal balance in neutral conditions and no effect on thermoregulation in cold conditions (despite a tendency toward greater reductions in core temperature when modafinil was applied in a cold environment). However, these authors did not examine temperature effects beyond 3 hr in the morning. The differences with regard to modafinil's effects on body temperature in sleep-deprived versus non-sleep-deprived subjects partly result from the fact that modafinil attenuates the amplitude of the daily temperature rhythm. This results in nighttime and postdeprivation temperatures that are higher under modafinil than under placebo (218). Effects on normal daytime temperatures are minimal.

With regard to modafinil's effects on task performance, the drug appears to have minimal impact on simple psychomotor tests (at least in untreated narcoleptics), whereas there are tendencies toward improvement in more complex tasks requiring concentration, dexterity, and the coordination of cognitive and motor resources (215). In non-sleep-deprived normals, it has been determined that 200 mg had no effect on the performance of a digit symbol substitution test despite improved EEG activation (measured by theta/alpha ratios) for up to 6 hr postdose (219).

### Vigilance Effects

Because modafinil has only recently become available, performance studies with normal subjects are scarce. In addition, the majority of performance studies have been conducted on sleep-deprived rather than well-rested volunteers, making the effects of modafinil on vigilance in nonfatigued individuals relatively uncertain. However, the earlier-cited findings of Saletu et al. (213) suggest that modafinil has a beneficial effect on vigilance even in non-sleep-deprived subjects since it attenuated the progressive deteriorations in attention and concentration that were seen throughout 8 hr of testing under placebo (the dose effects were somewhat variable in terms of magnitude and time).

### Effects on Military Performance

To date, no published studies could be found in which modafinil has been used to sustain alertness or performance in real-world military or other environments. Although laboratory studies of modafinil conducted on military volunteers have produced promising results (see the next section), actual field data apparently do not exist (24), although there is anecdotal evidence that the French armed forces may have employed modafinil during Operation Desert Storm.

### Effects on Performance After Sleep Deprivation

In terms of the effects of modafinil in sleep-deprived individuals, several beneficial effects have been reported. Lagarde et al. (220) studied the efficacy of 200-mg doses of modafinil, given at 8-hr intervals (for a total of 600 mg/day), for maintaining the alertness of eight normal volunteers throughout a 60-hr sleep deprivation period and found that modafinil reduced episodes of microsleeps and permitted subjects to maintain more normal (i.e., rested) mental states than placebo without inducing the anxiety that is sometimes associated with psychostimulant administration. Lagarde and Batejat (221) further reported that modafinil, given to these same subjects, significantly attenuated the precipitous drop in cognitive performance that became especially noticeable starting at 03:00 on the second day (after 20 hr of continuous wakefulness). In fact, modafinil maintained performance at well-rested levels for approximately 44 hr. Modafinil attenuated decrements in reaction times on a reaction time task, and on mathematics, memory search, spatial-processing, grammatical-reasoning, and letter memory tasks. Modafinil likewise reduced fatigue-related exacerbations of tracking errors. The benefits of the medication were most apparent during the circadian trough (on both deprivation days), although on the psychomotor tracking task, the differences between modafinil and placebo diverged at a fairly consistent rate from hour 34 to hour 59 of continuous wakefulness.

Bensimon et al. (222) examined the efficacy of a single 200-mg dose of modafinil for sustaining the performance of normal sleep-deprived subjects. On the sleep deprivation nights, the participants were given drug or placebo at 22:00 hours and then tested at 04:00 and 16:00 on critical flicker fusion (an indicator of CNS activation), choice reaction time, and memory. The results showed that in comparison to placebo, modafinil significantly sustained alertness, reaction time, and short-term (but not long-term) memory at 04:00, but that a majority of these effects dissipated by 16:00. These findings partly confirm an earlier study by Benoit et al. (223) in which a single 200-mg dose of modafinil was found to improve subjective ratings of alertness and, to some extent, performance on a search-and-memory task in normal subjects during 24 hr of sleep deprivation. Although this dose of modafinil did not sustain postdeprivation alertness at predeprivation levels, the perceived effects on activation persisted throughout the testing period. When Stivalet et al. (224) used a slightly higher dose (100 mg modafinil given 3 times/day), they found a more persistent performance effect. In fact, modafinil maintained the speed of high-level attentional processing (scanning) at well-rested levels throughout 60 hr of continuous wakefulness. In addition, target identification errors associated with fatigue under the placebo condition were reduced by half during modafinil administration.

Baranski et al. (225) investigated the ability of modafinil (100 mg every 6 hr) to sustain the performance of subjects throughout 40 hr of sleep deprivation in a warm (30°C) environment. Modafinil significantly lessened the impact of fatigue on the cognitive performance tests that were degraded by sleep deprivation (serial reaction time, addition, vigilance, logical reasoning, and multitasking) under placebo, but it did not maintain performance at baseline levels. Although subjective estimates of fatigue increased and ratings of motivation decreased as a function of sleep loss, modafinil significantly attenuated this effect.

Pigeau et al. (226) assessed the usefulness of modafinil for preventing fatigue-related declines in alertness and performance and for recovering from decrements that had already occurred. Forty-one soldiers were subjected to 64 hr of continuous wakefulness during which 300-mg doses of modafinil, 20 mg doses of dextroamphetamine, or placebo were administered at 17.5, 47.5, and 57.5 hr. Compared to placebo, both modafinil and amphetamine suppressed the amplitude of the core temperature rhythm. The initial doses of both drugs attenuated the performance and mood decrements relative to placebo (from 17.5 to 27.5 hr), while the second doses improved performance and mood relative to placebo (from 47.5 to 57.5 hr). The third doses did not appear to confer added benefit beyond what was observed after the second dose. Pigeau et al. (226) summarized the study by pointing out that unmedicated subjects suffered a 30–40% performance decline after 24 hr without sleep and a 55–65% decline after 48 hr without sleep. Both modafinil and dextroamphetamine reduced these decrements to 5–10%, and 20–30% at the two testing times, respectively. Recovery sleep after modafinil was shortened, suggesting a reduced requirement for sleep compared to placebo or dextroamphetamine. In addition, the sleep appeared to be less disturbed than the recovery sleep after amphetamine (227). The only drawback to modafinil was that subjects appeared to suffer from an impaired ability to monitor their own performance status, particularly during the first few hours after taking the drug. Modafinil was associated with 12.6% overestimation of accuracy on an addition task and a 9.5% overestimation of accuracy on a perceptual-comparison task. A similar effect was not observed with amphetamine or placebo (190). If this finding is validated, concerns about modafinil producing an "overconfidence effect" may limit the application of this compound in situations where risk-taking behavior may pose a serious threat to safety. However, at present, the only study that has explicitly sought to further explore this issue failed to replicate the judgment impairment (225).

Caldwell et al. (228) conducted a flight simulation study with modafinil in which six U.S. Army pilots were exposed to two 40-hr periods of continuous wakefulness. In one of the periods, three 200-mg doses of modafinil were given and in the other, matching placebos were administered. Results indicated that modafinil attenuated sleep deprivation effects (improved control accuracy) on four of six flight maneuvers, reduced the deprivation-related increase in slow-wave EEG activity, and lessened self-reported problems with mood and alertness in comparison to placebo. Similar to what was observed by Lagarde and Batejat (221), the most noticeable benefits occurred at times when the combined impact of sleep loss and the circadian trough was most severe. In many cases, modafinil maintained performance at well-rested levels similar to what has been observed with dextroamphetamine (183); however, there were some side effects that must be further examined. Under modafinil four of six pilots offered spontaneous reports of vertigo, nausea, and dizziness. This suggests that modafinil may not be an optimal fatigue countermeasure for aviators. However, like the "overconfidence effect" discussed earlier, these findings have not been confirmed, which leaves open the possibility that they were idiosyncratic to this group of volunteers. It is noteworthy that Eddy and colleagues (229) were unable to find vestibular disturbances in sleep-deprived volunteers treated with 200- and 400-mg doses of modafinil. Thus, it may be that lowering the dosage of modafinil from the 600 mg used by Caldwell et al. (228) to the 200 or 400 mg used by the majority of other investigators may offer a solution. A dose-response relationship in the incidence of adverse events has been reported with doses ranging from 200 to 800 mg (230). While most of the problems were headache, insomnia, anxiety, and palpitations rather than the nausea and dizziness symptoms found by Caldwell et al. (228), the 800-mg dose was associated with significant elevations in both blood pressure and pulse rate.

### Effects on Mood and Motivation

In non-sleep-deprived normals, modafinil tended to improve self-rated mood during the 8 hr after 200 mg of modafinil, and affectivity (as measured with a semantic differential polarity profile) was significantly better under 200 and 400 mg of modafinil at 6 and 8 hr postdose, respectively (213). Modafinil does not have the noticeable euphoric or stimulatory effect produced by amphetamine (231). This is consistent with the results of animal studies that indicate that modafinil's reinforcing effects are weak compared to those of amphetamine (232). In fatigued subjects, modafinil increases self-reported vigor and positive mood and decreases fatigue, confusion, and negative mood (226,228).

### Summary

In summary, modafinil is an effective wake-promoting substance that exerts its effects through different mechanisms than the classic psychostimulants. Although the potential benefits of modafinil on physical performance have not been well studied, there is limited evidence that it may prolong the time to exhaustion. There also are indications that modafinil improves cortical activation, reaction time, and mood in nonfatigued subjects and fatigued subjects, although the effects are certainly more robust under conditions of fatigue. In many cases modafinil has been shown to substantially attenuate the decrements in mood and performance that occur as a result of sleep deprivation. Positive assessments of modafinil are bolstered by findings that, unlike amphetamine and to some extent caffeine (at typical doses), this compound usually does not increase either blood pressure or heart rate, and it has relatively few effects on sleep parameters even when given close to bedtime. The negative side of modafinil is that it may produce overconfidence that could increase risk-taking behavior and it has been found to cause nausea and dizziness in sleep-deprived aviators and in some other individuals. In addition, it has not been well tested in real-world settings (such as industrial or military environments).

In comparison with caffeine, modafinil at 200 and 400 mg was found to have similar effects to 600 mg of caffeine in a sleep deprivation study conducted by Wesensten et al. (233). In this study, it was found that both compounds enhanced alertness and performance (especially during the circadian trough) without inducing noteworthy side effects. Wesensten et al. (233) concluded that since modafinil apparently offered no distinct benefit over and above what was seen with caffeine, the latter drug would be a better alternative because of its ready availability without prescription. However, this assessment is contrary to the one made by Lagarde and Batejat (221), who concluded that caffeine is a less powerful wake-promoting compound than modafinil, and that its effects are more dose-dependent, more variable across subjects, and more easily affected by the preexisting level of caffeine use (i.e., tolerance).

In comparison to amphetamine, Pigeau et al. (226) concluded that modafinil may be a better alternative, based on the fact that both compounds are efficacious for attenuating the impact of sleep loss, but modafinil produced 10% fewer side effects than dextroamphetamine and lacked the euphoriant effects that make amphetamine a more probable drug of abuse. Other reports likewise indicate that modafinil may be preferable to amphetamine as it exerts only a minimal impact on sleep quality whereas amphetamine has more disruptive effects (227,234,235). In addition, it is well established that modafinil produces far less cardiovascular stimulation than dextroamphetamine. However, these positive assessments notwithstanding, it should be kept in mind that modafinil may be slightly less effective than amphetamine (192); some side effects (nausea, dizziness) have been reported, which would limit the usefulness of modafinil in aviation (228); there may be judgment impairments with modafinil (190); and, as noted earlier, real-world experience with this compound is quite limited (24).

## IV. Conclusions

Each of the stimulants (or wake-promoting agents) discussed in this chapter is to some extent capable of mitigating the effects of sleep deprivation. While they cannot significantly enhance the alertness and performance of well-rested individuals, they are in most cases effective either for *preventing* (or attenuating) the decrements associated with sleep loss or for *restoring* alertness and performance that have already suffered from fatigue-related declines. This is particularly the case for amphetamines, which have been widely evaluated in the laboratory and in the field for over 50 years, but also true, in varying degrees, for methylphenidate, pemoline, caffeine, and modafinil. Because of this, it seems logical that stimulants should be considered a viable short-term remedy to the sweeping deleterious effects of fatigue in settings where administrative or behavioral countermeasures simply are not feasible. The choice of which stimulant is appropriate for a specific circumstance will depend on a variety of factors, including the availability, pharmacokinetics, and potential side effects (some of which are briefly mentioned in Table 1).

Although potential drawbacks are associated with pharmacological interventions, the problems attributable to untreated fatigue seem more immediate and severe, especially when there are few alternatives other than to accomplish the task at hand with a high degree of skill regardless of the extent of sleep debt. A case in point is the fact that several military mishaps have been attributed to fatigue, but none have thus far been attributed to stimulants (i.e., amphetamines)

**Table 1**  Stimulant Medications

| Name | Usual dose | Half life | Pros | Cons | Comments |
|---|---|---|---|---|---|
| Caffeine | 200–400 mg every 4 hr (1 6-ounce cup of coffee contains about 75–100 mg) | 4–5 hr | Plentiful<br>Legal<br>High user acceptance | Mildly effective<br>Tolerance exists in moderate to heavy users (possibly reducing effectiveness)<br>Side effects (tremor, diarrhea, diuretic) | May not be effective in those who normally consume caffeine from other sources<br>Avoid in people with heart problems and/or high blood pressure |
| Methylphenidate | 10 mg every 4–6 hr | 1–2 hr | Short half-life<br>Low abuse potential<br>Few cardiovascular effects | Prescription<br>Only mildly effective compared to amphetamine | Brand name Ritalin™<br>Has not been approved or extensively tested in aviators or other sleep-deprived normals |
| Pemoline | 37.5 mg once per day to start (effective daily dose is 56.25–75 mg) | 12 hr | Low abuse potential<br>Few cardiovascular effects | Prescription<br>Mildly effective compared to amphetamine<br>Delayed onset of action | Brand name Cylert™<br>Has not been approved or extensively tested in aviators or other sleep-deprived normals |
| Dextro-Amphetamine | 5–10 mg every 4–6 hr (not to exceed 60 mg per day) | 10 hr | Very effective<br>Extensively studied in the laboratory and under realworld conditions | Prescription<br>Moderate abuse potential<br>Cardiovascular side effects (elevated heart rate and blood pressure)<br>Low user acceptance because of '60s/70s abuse | Brand name Dexedrine™<br>Has been approved for military aviators<br>Has been well-tested in a variety of sleep-deprived normals<br>Avoid in people with heart problems and/or high blood pressure |
| Modafinil | 100–200 mg every 8 hr (manufacturer recommends a single 200-mg or 400-mg dose at start of day for narcoleptics) | 14 hr | Effective<br>Low abuse potential<br>Few cardiovascular effects<br>FDA approved for sleepiness associated with shift work | Prescription<br>Moderately effective compared to amphetamine<br>May have some nausea as side effect | Brand name Provigil™<br>Has not been as extensively studied as amphetamine in sleep-deprived normals |

despite the fact that these compounds have been used by military aviators during several conflicts (193).

The choice of which stimulant is most appropriate depends on the situation at hand. At present, amphetamines would seem best suited for short-term, specialized applications in which a powerful alerting effect is absolutely essential. Years of laboratory studies and field experience have substantiated the utility of using dextroamphetamine to safely counter the effects of sleep loss in operational contexts. However, to avoid/minimize dependency and/or abuse, amphetamines must not be used unless their administration can be controlled under the supervision of a physician. In addition, the use of amphetamine compounds is dependent on direct knowledge of the health status of each individual as these drugs are known to stress the cardiovascular system. When there is little possibility of medical oversight and when fatigued individuals will be responsible for self-administering their own medication, caffeine is a better choice than amphetamine from a risk reduction standpoint. Caffeine ingestion is beneficial for the maintenance of performance in sleep-deprived personnel, and it has the advantages of being widely available and posing little risk of abuse. However, the efficacy of caffeine may be compromised in habitual heavy users (of which there are many in our society), and it is at present unclear how to counteract this difficulty or the extent to which this is a serious concern. In addition, the diuretic properties of caffeine may make its use impractical in some settings. Pemoline was at one time an alternative worthy of serious consideration in light of its efficacy for alertness enhancement, but it is no longer an option because its use has been associated with hepatic injury. Methylphenidate also does not appear to be a promising choice because, despite its demonstrated utility for combating the effects of sleepiness, the magnitude of methylphenidate's effects, compared to those of caffeine, do not appear large enough to warrant the additional administrative and medical oversight that would be required. Modafinil appears to hold promise for use in the near future. Laboratory studies have shown modafinil to be an effective tool for alleviating many of the decrements associated with insufficient sleep, ranging from basic cognitive/psychomotor degradations to accuracy losses in the performance of skilled tasks (such as flying an aircraft simulator). However, the optimal dosing scheme has not yet been determined and additional data with regard to efficaciousness in real-world settings are needed. It is expected that these issues will soon be resolved.

In conclusion, stimulants should be viewed as one of many tools for preventing or overcoming the problems associated with sleep deprivation in operational environments. Although not a substitute for proper staffing levels, well-designed work schedules, or adequate daily sleep, stimulants can enhance safety and effectiveness in sleep-deprived people who are nonetheless required to be vigilant and productive. As Lagarde and Batejat (221) point out, the choice of whether or not pharmacological strategies should be considered depends on risk assessment. *Is it better and safer to perform a job under conditions of sleep deprivation without the aid of a stimulant, or should a pharmacological aid be used to temporarily overcome the known effects of fatigue until adequate sleep is once again possible?* As is often true in life, it is necessary to carefully consider and then balance the risks and benefits of each alternative.

### References

1.  Akerstedt T. Work hours, sleepiness and the underlying mechanisms. J Sleep Res 1995; 4(suppl 2):15–22.
2.  Dinges DF. An overview of sleepiness and accidents. J Sleep Res 1995; 4(suppl 2):4–14.
3.  Mitler MM, Carskadon MA, Czeisler CA, Dement WC, Dinges DF, Graeber RC. Catastrophes, sleep, and public policy: Consensus report. Sleep 1988; 11(1):100–109.
4.  NTSB. Marine accident report-grounding of the US. tankship Exxon Valdez on Bligh Reef, Prince William Sound, near Valdez, Alaska, 24 Mar 1989. Report No. NTSB/Mar-90/04. Washington, DC: National Transportation Safety Board, 1990.
5.  NTSB. Uncontrolled collision with terrain American International Airways flight 808, Douglas DC-8-61, N814CK, U.S. Naval Air Station Guantanamo Bay, Cuba, August 18, 1993. Report No. NTSB/AAR-94-04. Washington, DC: National Transportation Safety Board, 1994.
6.  NTSB. A review of flightcrew-involved, major accidents of U.S. air carriers, 1978 through 1990. NTSB Safety Study No. SS-94-01. Washington DC: National Transportation Safety Board, 1994.
7.  NTSB. Aircraft accident report: Controlled flight into terrain, Korean Air flight 801, Boeing 747-300, HL7468, Nimitz Hill, Guan, August 6, 1997. Report No. NTSB/AAR-99-02. Washington, DC: National Transportation Safety Board, 1999.
8.  NTSB. Aviation accident report: Runway overrun during landing, American Airlines Flight 1420, McDonnell Douglas MD-82, N215AA, Little Rock, Arkansas, June 1, 1999. Report No. NTSB/AAR-01-02. Washington, DC: National Transportation Safety Board, 2002.
9.  Akerstedt, T. Consensus statement: Fatigue and accidents in transport operations. J Sleep Res 2000; 9:395.
10. Department of the Army. Force of Decision: Capabilities for the 21st century. White paper. Washington, DC: Department of the Army, 1996.
11. Dinges DF, Graeber RC, Rosekind MR, Samel A., Wegmann HM. Principles and guidelines for duty and rest scheduling in commercial aviation. NASA Technical Memorandum No. 110404. Moffett Field, CA: NASA Ames Research Center, 1996.
12. Angus RG, Pigeau RA, Heslegrave RJ. Sustained operation studies: From the field to the laboratory. In: Stampi C, ed. Why We Nap: Evolution, Chronobiology, and Functions of Polyphasic and Ultrashort Sleep. Boston: Birkhäuser, 1992:217–244.
13. LeDuc PA, Caldwell JA, Ruyak PS. The effects of exercise as a countermeasure for fatigue in sleep-deprived aviators. Milit Psychol 2000; 12(4):249-266.
14. Horne JA, Reyner LA. Driver sleepiness. J Sleep Res 1995; 4(suppl 2):23-29.
15. Heslegrave RJ, Angus RG. The effects of task duration and work-session location on performance degradation induced by sleep loss and sustained cognitive work. Behav Res Methods Inst Comput 1985; 17:592-603.
16. Pigeau R, Naitoh P, Buguet A, McCann C, Baranski J, Taylor M, Thompson M, Mack I. Modafinil, *d*-amphetamine, and placebo during 64 hours of sustained men-

tal work. I. Effects on mood, fatigue, cognitive performance and body temperature. J Sleep Res 1995; 4:212-228.

17. Neri DF, Oyung RO, Colletti LM, Mallis MM, Tam PY Dinges DF. Controlled breaks as a fatigue countermeasure on the flight deck. Aviat Space Environ Med 2002; 73:654-664.

18. Dinges DF, Broughton RJ. Sleep and Alertness: Chronobiological, Behavioral, and Medical Aspects of Napping. New York: Raven Press, 1989.

19. Stampi C. Why We Nap: Evolution, Chronobiology, and Functions of Polyphasic and Ultrashort Sleep. Boston: Birkhäuser, 1992.

20. Rosekind MR, Graeber RC, Dinges DF, Connell LJ, Rountree MS, Spinweber CL, Gillen KA. Crew factors in flight operations. IX. Effects of planned cockpit rest on crew performance and alertness in long-haul operations. NASA Technical Memorandum No. 108839 Moffett Field, CA: NASA Ames Research Center, 1994.

21. Caldwell, JL. Efficacy of napping strategies to counter the effects of sleep deprivation. NATO-RTO Report No. RTO-EN-016. Neuilly-sur-Seine Cedex, France: North Atlantic Treaty Organization, 2001.

22. Muzet A, Nicolas A, Tassi P, DeWasmes G, Bonneau A. Implementation of napping in industry and the problem of sleep inertia. J Sleep Res 1995; 4(suppl 2):67–69.

23. Ferrara M, DeGennaro F, Bertini M. Time-course of sleep inertia upon awakening from sleep with different sleep homeostasis conditions. Aviat Space Environ Med 2000; 71(3):225–229.

24. Akerstedt T, Ficca G. Alertness-enhancing drugs as a countermeasure to fatigue in irregular work hours. Chronobiol Int 1997; 14(2):145-158.

25. Bishop C, Roehrs T, Rosenthal L, Roth T. Alerting effects of methylphenidate under basal and sleep-deprived conditions. Exp Clin Psychopharmacol 1997; 5(4):344-352.

26. UpToDate Online 10.2. Methylphenidate: Drug information. 2002.

27. Matteson L.T, Kelly TL, Babkoff H, Hauser S, Naitoh P. Methylphenidate and pemoline: effects on sleepiness and mood during sleep deprivation. Naval Health Research Center Technical Report No. 90–41, 1990.

28. Goldman LS, Genel M, Bezman RJ, Slanetz PJ. Diagnosis and treatment of attention-deficit/hyperactivity disorder in children and adolescents. JAMA 1998; 279(14):1100–1107.

29. Kinsbourne M, DeQuiros, GB, Rufo DT. Adult ADHD: Controlled medication assessment. Ann NY Acad Sci 2001; 931:287–296.

30. Wender PH, Wolf LE, and Wasserstein J. Adults with ADHD: an overview. Ann NY Acad Sci 2001; 931:1–16.

31. Littner M, Johnson SF, McCall WV, Anderson, WM, Davila D, Hartse K, Kushida CA, Wise MS, Hirshkowitz M, Woodson BT. Practice parameters for the treatment of narcolepsy: an update for 2000. Sleep 2001; 24(4):451–466.

32. Mitler MM, Shafor R, Hajdukovich R, Timms RM, Browman CP. Treatment of narcolepsy: objective studies on methylphenidate, pemoline, and protriptyline. Sleep 1986; 9(1):260–264.

33. Mitler MM. Evaluation of treatment with stimulants in narcolepsy. Sleep 1994; 17:S103–S106.

34. Chiarello RJ, Cole JO. The use of psychostimulants in general psychiatry. Arch Gen Psychiatry 1987; 44:286–295.

35. Satel SL, Nelson JC. Stimulants in the treatment of depression: a critical overview. J Clin Psychiatry 1989; 50:241–249.

36.  Hoffman BB, Lefkowitz RJ. Catecholamines, sympathomimetic drugs, and adrenergic receptor antagonists. In: Hardman JG, Limbird LE, Molinoff PB, Ruddon RW, Gilman AG, eds. Goodman and Gilman's The Pharmacological Basis of Therapeutics, 9th ed. New York: McGraw-Hill, 1996:199-248.

37.  Physician's Desk Reference. Ritalin Hydrochloride Tablets, Ritalin-SR Tablets (Novartis). Montvale, NJ: Medical Economics, 2001.

38.  Perman ES. Speed in Sweden. N Engl J Med 1970; 283:760-761.

39.  Santosh PJ, Taylor E. Stimulant drugs. Eur Child Adolesc Psychiatry 2000; 9:I27-I43.

40.  Safer DJ, Allen, R.P. Absence of tolerance to the behavioural effects of methylphenidate and inattentive children. Pediatrics 1989; 115:1003-1008.

41.  Benowitz NL. Amphetamines. In: Olson KR, ed. Poisoning and Drug Overdose, 1st ed. CA: Appleton & Lange, 1990:62-63.

42.  Peloquin LJ, Klorman R. Effects of methylphenidate on normal children's mood, event-related potentials, and performance in memory scanning and vigilance. J Abnorm Psychol 1986; 95(1):88-98.

43.  Hink RF, Fenton WH, Tinklenberg JR, Pfefferbaum A, Kopell BS. Vigilance and human attention under conditions of methylphenidate and secobarbital intoxication: an assessment using brain potentials. Psychophysiology 1978; 15(2):116-125.

44.  Strauss J, Lewis JL, Klorman R, Peloquin L, Perlmutter RA, Salzman LF. Effects of methylphenidate on young adults' performance and event-related potentials in a vigilance and a paired-associates learning test. Psychophysiology 1984; 21(6):609-621.

45.  Brumaghim JT, Klorman R, Strauss J, Lewine JD, Goldstein MG. Does methylphenidate affect information processing? Findings from two studies on performance and P3b latency. Psychophysiology 1987; 24(3):361-373.

46.  Babkoff H, Kelly, TL, Matteson, LT, Gomez SA, Lopez A, Hauser S, Naitoh P, Assmus J. Pemoline and methylphenidate: interaction with mood, sleepiness, and cognitive performance during 64 hours of sleep deprivation. Milit Psychol 1992; 4(4):235-265.

47.  Elliot R, Sahakian BJ, Matthews K, Bannerjea A, Rimmer J, Robbins TW. Effects of methylphenidate on spatial working memory and planning in healthy young adults. Psychopharmacology 1997; 131:196-206.

48.  Camp-Bruno JA, Herting RL. Cognitive effects of milacemide and methylphenidate in healthy young adults. Psychopharmacology 1994; 115:46-52.

49.  Coons HW, Peloquin L, Klorman R, Bauer LO, Hyan RM, Perlmutter RA, Salzman LF. Effect of methylphenidate on young adults' vigilance and event-related potentials. Electroencephalogr Clin Neurophysiol 1981; 51:373-387.

50.  Naylor H, Halliday R, Callaway E. The effect of methylphenidate on information processing. Psychopharmacology 1985; 86:90-95.

51.  Babkoff, H., Kelly, TL, Naitoh, P. Trial-to-trial variance in choice reaction time as a measure of the effect of stimulants during sleep deprivation. Milit Psychol 2001; 13(1):1-16.

52.  Roehrs T, Papineau K, Rosenthal L, Roth T. Sleepiness and the reinforcing and subjective effects of methylphenidate. Exp Clin Psychopharmacol 1999; 7(2):145-150.

53.  Roehrs T, Johanson CE, Meixner R, Asti T, Fortier J, Roth T. Methylphenidate preference and subjective effects: time-in-bed and dose. Sleep 2002 ; 25:A44-A45.

54.  Hurst PM, Weidner MF. Drug effects upon cognitive performance under stress. Report No. ONR-H-66-3 1966.

55.  Smith RC, Davis JM. Comparative effects of *d*-amphetamine, *l*-amphetamine, and methylphenidate on mood in man. Psychopharmacology 1977; 53:1-12.

56. UpToDate Online 10.2 Pemoline: Drug information. 2002.
57. Physician's Desk Reference. Cylert Chewable Tablets, Cylert Tablets (Abbott). Montvale, NJ: Medical Economic, 2001.
58. Kelly TL, Ryman DH, Schlangen K, Gomez SA, Elsmore, TF. The effects of a single dose of pemoline on performance and mood during sleep deprivation. Milit Psychol 1997; 9(3):213-225.
59. Naitoh P, Kelly TL, Babkoff H. Napping, stimulant, and four choice performance. Naval Health Research Center Report No. 90-17. San Diego, CA: Naval Health Research Center, 1990.
60. Orzack MH, Taylor CL, Kornetsky C. A research report on the anti-fatigue effects of magnesium pemoline. Psychopharmacology 1968; 13:413-417.
61. Gelfand S, Clark LD, Herbert EW, Gelfand DM, Holmes ED. Magnesium pemoline: Stimulant effects on performance of fatigued subjects. Clin Pharmacol Ther 1968; 9(1):56-60.
62. Kelly TL, Babkoff H, Matteson L, Gomez S, Naitoh P. The effect of moderate doses of methylphenidate and pemoline on the maintenance of performance speed during 64 hours of sleep deviation (abstr). Sleep Res 1990; 19:67.
63. Nicholson AN, Stone BM, Turner C. Drug and air operations. In: Medication for Military Aircrew: Current Use, Issues, and Strategies for Expanded Options, NATO Research and Technology Organization Technical Report 14. Neuilly-sur-Seine, France: NATO Research and Technology Organization, 2001:57-65.
64. Food and Drug Administration. Caffeine content of various products. Talk paper T80-45, October 9. Rockville, MD: FDA. 1980.
65. Center for Science in the Public Interest. Caffeine: the inside scoop. Nutrition Action Health Letter, Dec. 1996. Washington, DC: Center for Science in the Public Interest.
66. Lieberman HR. Caffeine. In: Jones D, Smith A, eds. Factors Affecting Human Performance. Vol II. The Physical Environment. London: Academic Press, 1992.
67. Serafin WE. Drugs used in the treatment of asthma. In: Hardman JG, Limbird LE, Molinoff PB, Ruddon RW, Gilman AG, eds. Goodman and Gilman's The Pharmacological Basis of Therapeutics, 9th ed. New York: McGraw-Hill, 1996:659-682.
68. Basheer R, Porkka-Heiskanen T, Strecker RE, Thakkar MM, McCarley RW. Adenosine as a biological signal mediating sleepiness following prolonged wakefulness. Biol Signals Recept 2000; 9:319-327.
69. Nehlig A, Daval JL, Debry G. Caffeine and the central nervous system: mechanisms of action, biochemical, metabolic and psychostimulant effects. Brain Res Rev 1992; 17:139-170.
70. Gilbert RM. Caffeine consumption. In: Spiller GA, ed. The Methylxanthine Beverages and Foods: Chemistry, Consumption, and Health Effects. New York: Liss, 1984:185–213.
71. Griffiths RR, Mumford GK. Caffeine—a drug of abuse? In: Bloom FE, Kupfer DJ, eds. Psychopharmacology: The Fourth Generation of Progress. New York: Raven Press, 1995:1699-1713.
72. Gilbert RM. Caffeine as a drug of abuse. In: Gibbins RJ, Israel IY, Kalant H, Popham RE, Schmidt W, Smart RG, eds. Research Advances in Alcohol and Drug Problems, vol 3. New York: Wiley, 1976:49-176.
73. Gilbert RM. Betel-nut chewing in Toronto. In: The Journal, 5. Toronto: Addiction Research Foundation of Ontario, April 1, 1986.

74. Barone JJ, Roberts H. Human consumption of caffeine, In: Dews, ed. Caffeine. New York: Springer, 1984:59-73.
75. Hirsh K. Central nervous system pharmacology of the dietary methylxanthines. In: Spiller GA, ed. The Methylxanthine Beverages and Foods: Chemistry, Consumption, and Health Effects. New York: Liss, 1984:235-301.
76. Curatolo PW, Robertson D. The health consequences of caffeine. Ann Intern Med 1983; 98(part 1):641-653.
77. Kuznicki JT, Turner LS. The effects of caffeine on caffeine users and non-users. Physiol Behav 1986; 37:397-408.
78. Lieberman HR, Wurtman RJ, Emde GG, Coviella ILG. The effects of caffeine and aspirin on mood and performance. J Clin Psychopharmacol 1987; 7(5):315-320.
79. Zarcone VP. Sleep hygiene. In: Kryger MH, Roth T, Dement WC, eds. Principles and Practice of Sleep Medicine, 3rd ed. Philadelphia: Saunders, 2000:657-651.
80. Landolt HP, Werth E, Borbely AA, Dijk JJ. Caffeine reduces low-frequency delta activity in the human sleep EEG. Neuropsychopharmacology 1995; 12:229-238.
81. Committee on Military Nutrition Research. Caffeine for the Sustainment of Mental Task Performance: Formulations for Military Operations. Washington, DC: National Academy Press, 2002.
82. Griffiths RR, Woodson PP. Caffeine physical dependence: a review of human and laboratory animal studies. Psychopharmacology 1988; 94:437-451.
83. Dews PB. Behavioral effects of caffeine. In: Dews PB, ed. Caffeine. Berlin: Springer-Verlag, 1984:87-103.
84. Arnaud MJ. The pharmacology of caffeine. Prog Drug Res 1987; 31:273-313.
85. Benet LZ, Oie S, Schwartz JB. Design and optimization of dosage regimens; pharmacokinetic data. In: Hardman JG, Limbird LE, Molinoff PB, Ruddon RW, Gilman AG, eds. Goodman and Gilman's The Pharmacological Basis of Therapeutics, 9th ed. New York: McGraw-Hill, 1996:1707-1792.
86. Parsons WD, Neims AH. Effect of smoking on caffeine clearance. Clin Pharmacol Ther 1978; 24:40-45.
87. Kamimori GH, Lugo SJ, Penetar DM, Chamberlain AC, Brunhart GE, Brunhart AE, Eddington ND. Dose-dependent caffeine pharmacokinetics during severe sleep deprivation in humans. Int J Clin Pharmacol Ther 1995; 32(3):182-186.
88. Strain EC, Griffiths RR. Caffeine use disorders. In: Tasman A, Kay J, Lieberman JA, eds. Psychiatry. Philadelphia: Saunders, 1997:779-794.
89. Brown CR. Caffeine. In: Olson KR, Becker CE, Benowitz NL, Buchanan JF, Mycroft FJ, Osterloh J, Woo OF, eds. Poisoning and Drug Overdose. Norwalk, CT: Appleton & Lange, 1990:100-102.
90. Applegate E. Effective nutritional ergogenic aids. Int J Sport Nutr 1999; 9:229-239.
91. Graham TE. Caffeine and exercise: metabolism, endurance, and performance. Sports Med 2001; 31(11):785-807.
92. Paton CD, Hopkins WG, Vollebregt L. Little effect of caffeine ingestion on repeated sprints in team-sport athletes. Med Sci Sports Exerc 2001; 33(5):822-825.
93. MacIntosh BR, Wright BM. Caffeine ingestion and performance of a 1500 meter swim. Can J Appl Physiol 1995; 20:168-177.
94. Graham TE, Rush JWE, Van Soren MH. Caffeine and exercise: metabolism and performance. Can J Appl Physiol 1994; 19(1):111-138.
95. Laurent D, Schneider KE, Prusaczyk WK, Franklin C, Vogel SM, Krssak M, Petersen KF, Goforth HW, Shulman GI. Effects of caffeine on muscle glycogen uti-

lization and the neuroendocrine axis during exercise. J Clin Endocrinol Metab 2000; 85(6):2170-2175.

96. Tarnopolsky M, Cupido C. Caffeine potentiates low frequency skeletal muscle force in habitual and nonhabitual caffeine consumers. J Appl Physiol 2000; 89:1719-1724.

97. Robertson D, Wade D, Workman R, Woosley RL, Oates JA. Tolerance to the humoral and hemodynamic effects of caffeine in man. J Clin Invest 1981; 67:1111-1117.

98. Kenemans JL, Lorist MM. Caffeine and selective visual processing. Pharmacol Biochem Behav 1995; 52(3):461-471.

99. Hasenfratz M, Battig K. Acute dose-effect relationships of caffeine and mental performance, EEG, cardiovascular, and subjective parameters. Psychopharmacology 1994; 114(2):281-287.

100. Weiss B, Laties VG. Enhancement of human performance by caffeine and the amphetamines. Pharmacol Rev 1962; 14:1-36.

101. Rapoport JL, Jensvold M, Elkins R, Buchsbaum MS, Weingartner H, Ludlow C, Zahn T, Berg CJ, Neims AH. Behavioral and cognitive effects of caffeine in boys and adults. J Nerv Ment Dis 1981; 169:726-732.

102. Horst K, Jenkins WL. The effect of caffeine, coffee and decaffeinated coffee upon blood pressure, pulse rate and simple reaction time of men of various ages. J Pharmacol 1935; 53:384-400.

103. Clubley M, Bye CE, Henson TA, Peck AW, Riddington CJ. Effects of caffeine and cyclizine alone and in combination on human performance, subjective effects and EEG activity. Br J Clin Pharmacol 1979; 7:157-163.

104. Lorist MM, Snel J, Kok A. Influence of caffeine on information processing stages in well rested and fatigued subjects. Psychopharmacology 1994; 113:411-421.

105. Lorist MM, Snel J, Kok A, Mulder G. Influence of caffeine on selective attention in well-rested and fatigued subjects. Psychophysiology 1994; 31:525-534.

106. Ruijter J, Lorist MM, Snel J, DeRuiter MB. The influence of caffeine on sustained attention: an ERP study. Pharmacol Biochem Behav 2000; 66(1):29-37.

107. Lane JD. Effects of brief caffeinated-beverage deprivation on mood, symptoms, and psychomotor performance. Pharmacol Biochem Behav 1997; 58(1):203-208.

108. Phillips-Bute BG, Lane JD. Caffeine withdrawal symptoms following brief caffeine deprivation. Physiol Behav 1998; 63(1):35-39.

109. Jacobson BH, Edgley BM. Effects of caffeine on simple reaction time and movement time. Aviat Space Environ Med 1987; 58:1153-1156.

110. Lieberman HR, Wurtman RJ, Emde GG, Roberts C, Coviella ILG. The effects of low doses of caffeine on human performance and mood. Psychopharmacology 1987, 92:308-312.

111. Lane JD, Phillips-Bute BG. Caffeine deprivation affects vigilance performance and mood. Physiol Behav 1998; 65(1):171-175.

112. Rosenthal L, Roehrs T, Zwyghuizen-Doorenbos A, Plath D, Roth T. Alerting effects of caffeine after normal and restricted sleep. Neuropsychopharmacology 1991; 4(2):103-108.

113. Reyner LA, Horne JA. Suppression of sleepiness in drivers: combination of caffeine with a short nap. Psychophysiology 1997; 34:721-725.

114. Reyner LA, Horne JA. Early morning driver sleepiness: effectiveness of 200 mg caffeine. Psychophysiology 2000; 37:251-256.

115. Haslam R. The military performance of soldiers in continuous operations: exercises "Early Call" I and II. In: Burch N, Altshuler HL, eds. Advances in Sleep Research, vol 7. New York: Plenum, 1981:435-458.

116. Lagarde D, Batejat D. Some measures to reduce effects of prolonged sleep deprivation. Neurophysiol Clin 1995; 25:376-385.

117. Opstead P, Ekanger R, Nummestad M, Raabe N. Performance, mood and clincial symptoms in men exposed to prolonged, severe physical work and sleep deprivation. Aviat Space Environ Med 1978; 49:1065-1073.

118. Belland KM, Bissell C. A subjective study of fatigue during Navy flight operations over southern Iraq: Operation Southern Watch. Aviat Space Environ Med 1994; 65:57-561.

119. Rosenberg E, Caine Y. Survey of Israeli Air Force line commander support for fatigue prevention initiatives. Aviat Space Environ Med 2001; 72:352-356.

120. Gander PH, Gregory KB, Miller DL, Graeber RC, Connell LJ, Rosekind MR. Flight crew fatigue. V. Long-haul air transport operations. Aviat Space Environ Med 1998; 69(9 suppl):B37-B48.

121. Gander PH, Gregory KB, Graeber RC, Connell LJ, Miller DL, Rosekind MR. Flight crew fatigue. II. Short-haul fixed-wing air transport operations. Aviat Space Environ Med 1998; 69(9 Suppl.):B8-B15.

122. Gander PH, Barnes RM, Gregory KB, Graeber RC, Connell LJ, Rosekind MR. Flight crew fatigue. III. North Sea helicopter air transport operations. Aviat Space Environ Med 1998; 69(9 suppl):B16-B25.

123. Muehlbach MJ, Walsh JK. The effects of caffeine on simulated night-shift work and subsequent daytime sleep. Sleep 1995; 18(1):22-29.

124. Walsh JK, Muehlbach MJ, Humm TM, Dickins QS, Sugerman JL, Schweitzer PK. Effect of caffeine on physiological sleep tendency and ability to sustain wakefulness at night. Psychopharmacology 1990; 101:271-273.

125. Walsh JK, Muehlbach MJ, Schweitzer PK. Hypnotics and caffeine as countermeasures for shiftwork-related sleepiness and sleep disturbance. J Sleep Res 1995; 4(suppl 2):80-83.

126. Penetar D, McCann U, Thorne D, Kamimori G, Galinski C, Sing HC, Thomas M, Belenky G. Caffeine reversal of sleep deprivation effects on alertness and mood. Psychopharmacology 1993; 112(2-3):359-65.

127. Penetar DM, McCann U, Thorne D, Schelling A, Galinski C, Sing H, Thomas M, Belenky G. Effects of caffeine on cognitive performance, mood, and alertness in sleep-deprived humans. In: Marriott BM, ed. Food Components to Enhance Performance. Washington, DC: National Academy Press, 1994:407-431.

128. Tharion MS, Shukitt-Hale B, Coffey B, Desai M, Strowman SR, Tulley R, Lieberman HR. The use of caffeine to enhance cognitive performance, reaction time, vigilance, rifle marksmanship, and mood states in sleep-deprived Navy SEAL (BUD/S) Trainees. USARIEM Technical Report No. ADA331982. Natick, MA: U.S. Army Research Institute of Environmental Medicine 1997.

129. Kamimori GH, Penetar DM, Headley DB, Thorne DR, Otterstetter R, Belenky G. Effect of three caffeine doses on plasma catecholamines and alertness during prolonged wakefulness, Eur J Clin Pharmacol 2000; 56:537-544.

130. Dinges DF. Homeostatic and circadian regulation of wakefulness during jet lag and sleep deprivation: effect of wake-promoting countermeasures. AFOSR Technical Report No. 31-08-2000. Arlington, VA: Air Force Office of Scientific Research. 2000.

131. Lagarde D, Batejat D, Sicard B, Trocherie S, Chassard D, Enslen M, Chauffard F. Slow-release caffeine: a new response to the effects of a limited sleep deprivation. Sleep 2000; 23(5):651-661.

132. Sicard BA, Perault MC, Enslen M, Chauffard F, Vandel B, Tachon P. The effects of 600 mg of slow release caffeine on mood and alertness. Aviat Space Environ Med 1996; 67:859–862.

133. Patat A, Rosenzweig P, Enslen M, Trocherie S, Miget N, Bozon M, Allain H, Gandon J. Effects of a new slow release formulation of caffeine on EEG, psychomotor, and cognitive functions in sleep-deprived subjects. Hum Psychopharmacol 2000; 15:153-170.

134. Rogers PJ, Richardson NJ, Dernoncourt C. Caffeine Use: Is there a net benefit for mood and psychomotor performance? Neuropsychobiology 1995; 31:195-199.

135. Hale KL, Hughes JR, Oliveto AH, Higgins ST. Caffeine self-administration and subjective effects in adolescents. Exp Clin Psychopharmacol 1995; 3(4):364-370.

136. Smith AP, Clark R, Gallagher J. Breakfast cereal and caffeinated coffee: effects on working memory, attention, mood, and cardiovascular function. Physiol Behav 1999; 67(1):9–17.

137. Physicians' Desk Reference. Dexedrine (brand of dextro-amphetamine sulfate) and DextroStat (brand of dextro-amphetamine sulfate), PDR Electronic Library. Montvale, NJ: Medical Economics, 2001.

138. Sciden JS, Sabol KT, Ricaurte GA. Amphetamine: effects on catecholamine systems and behavior. Annu Rev Pharmacol Toxicol 1993; 32:639-677.

139. Wisor JP, Nishino S, Sora I, Uhl GH, Mignot E, Edgar DM. Dopaminergic role of stimulant-induced wakefulness. J Neurosci 2001; 21(5):1787-1794.

140. Miller MA. History and epidemiology of amphetamine abuse in the United States. In: Klee H, ed. Amphetamine Misuse: International Perspectives on Current Trends. Amsterdam: Harwood Acad Pub, 1997:113-134.

141. Grinspoon L, Hedblom P. The Speed Culture, Amphetamine Use and Abuse in America. Cambridge: Harvard University Press, 1975.

142. U.S. Navy Aerospace Medical Research Laboratory. Performance maintenance during continuous flight operations. Pensacola, FL: U.S. Navy Aerospace Medical Research Laboratory. 2001.

143. U.S. Army Aeromedical Research Laboratory (in conjunction with the Army Safety Center). Leader's guide to crew endurance. Fort Rucker, AL: U.S. Army Safety Center.1996.

144. Physicians' Desk Reference. Dexedrine (brand of dextroamphetamine sulfate). PDR, 3043, 3044. Montvale, New Jersey: Medical Economics, 1999.

145. Weiner N. Norepinephrine, epinephrine, and the sympathomimetic amines. In: Gilman AG, Goodman LS, Gilman A, eds. The Pharmacological Basis of Therapeutics, 6th ed. New York: Macmillan, 1980:138-173.

146. Friedl KE. Performance-enhancing substance: Effects, risks, and appropriate alternatives. In: Baechle TR, ed. Essentials of Strength Training and Conditioning. Champaign, IL: Human Kinetics, 1994:188-209.

147. Karpovich PV. Effect of amphetamine sulfate on athletic performance. JAMA 1959; 170(5):558-561.

148. Smith GM, Beecher HK. Amphetamine sulfate and athletic performance. J Am Med Assoc 1959; 170(5):542-557.

149. Wagner JC. Abuse of drugs used to enhance athletic performance. Am J Hosp Pharm 1989; 46:2059-2067.
150. Wagner JC. Enhancement of athletic performance with drugs: an overview. Sports Med 1991; 12(4):250-265.
151. Martin WR, Sloan JW, Sapira JD, Jasinski DR. Physiologic, subjective, and behavioral effects of amphetamine, methamphetamine, ephedrine, phenmetrazine, and methylphenidate in man. Clin Pharmacol Ther 1971; 12(2):245-258.
152. Caldwell JA. Effects of operationally effective doses of dextroamphetamine on heart rates and blood pressures of Army aviators. Milit Med 1996; 161(11):673-678.
153. Morselli PL, Placidi GF, Maggini C, Gomeni R, Guazelli M, DeLisio G, Standen S, Tognoni G. An integrated approach for the evaluation of psychotropic drug in man. Psychopharmacology 1976; 46:211-217.
154. Cole SO. Experimental effects of amphetamine: a review. Psychol Bull 1967; 68(2):81–90.
155. Hurst PM, Weitzner MF. Drug effects upon cognitive performance under stress. Office of Naval Research Report No. ONR-H-66-3. Washington, DC: Office of Naval Research. 1966.
156. Weitzner M. Manifest anxiety, amphetamine and performance. The anesthesia laboratory of the Harvard Medical School, DTIC report no. AD601455. Fort Belvoir, VA: Defense Technical Information Center. 1963.
157. Kennedy RS, Odenheimer RC, Baltzley DR, Dunlap WP, Wood CD. Differential effects of scopolamine and amphetamine on microcomputer-based performance tests. Aviat Space Environ Med 1990; 61:615-621.
158. Smith GM, Weitzner M, Levenson SR, Beecher HK. Effects of amphetamine and secobarbital on coding and mathematicl performance. J Pharmacol Exp Ther 1963; 141:100–104.
159. Payne RB. The effects of drugs upon psychological efficiency. J Aviat Med 1953; 24:523-529.
160. Payne RB, Hauty GT. The effects of experimentally induced attitudes upon task proficiency. J Exp Psychol 1954; 47(4):267-273.
161. Payne, RB and Hauty GT. Mitigation of work decrement. J Exp Psychol 1955; 49:60-67.
162. Payne RB, Hauty GT, Moore EW. Restoration of tracking proficiency as a function of amount and delay of analeptic medication. J Comp Physiol Psychol 1957; 50:146-149.
163. Spiegel R. Effects of amphetamines on performance and on polygraphic sleep parameters in man. Adv Biosci 1978; 21:189-201.
164. Babkoff H, Krueger GP. Use of stimulants to ameliorate the effects of sleep loss during sustained performance. Milit Psychol 1992; 4(4):191-205.
165. Winfield RH. The use of benzedrine to overcome fatigue on operational flights in coastal command. Flight. Personnel Research Committee Report No. FPRC-361. London: Flying Personnel Research Committee. 1941.
166. Tyler DB. The effect of amphetamine sulfate and some barbiturates on the fatigue produced by prolonged wakefulness. Am J Physiol 1947; 150:253-262.
167. McKenzie RE, Elliot LL. Effects of secobarbital and d-amphetamine on performance during a simulated air mission. Aerospace Med 1965; 36:774-779.
168. Cornum K, Cornum R, Storm W. Use of psychostimulants in extended flight operations: a Desert Shield experience. In Advisory Group for Aerospace Research and Development conference Proceedings No. 579, Neurological Limitations of

Aircraft Operations: Human Performance Implications, 371-374. Nuilley sur Seine, France: NATO Advisory Group for Aerospace Research and Development. 1995.

169. Senechal PK. Flight surgeon support of combat operations at RAF Upper Heyford. Aviat Space Environ Med 1988; 59:776-777.

170. Cornum K. Sustained operations: an F-15 squadron in the Gulf War. Minutes of the Human Factors Engineering Technical Group, 29th meeting, Huntsville, AL, November, 1992.

171. Emonson DL, Vanderbeek RD. The use of amphetamines in U.S. Air Force tactical operations during Desert Shield and Storm. Aviat Space Environ Med 1995; 66:260-263.

172. Seashore RH, Ivy AC. Effects of analeptic drugs in relieving fatigue. Psychol Monogr 1953; 67(15):1-16.

173. Somerville W. The effect of benzedrine on mental or physical fatigue in soldiers. Can Med Assoc J 1946; 55:470–476.

174. Kornetsky C, Mirsky AF, Kessler EK, and Dorff JE. The effects of dextro-amphetamine on behavioral deficits produced by sleep loss in humans. J Pharmacol Exp Ther 1959; 127:46-50.

175. Newhouse PA, Penetar DM, Fertig JB, Thorne DR, Sing HC, Thomas ML, Cochran JC, Belenky GL. Stimulant drug effects on performance and behavior after prolonged sleep deprivation. Milit Psychol 1992; 4(4):207-233.

176. Hartmann E, Orzack MH, and Branconnier R. Sleep deprivation deficits and their reversal by *d*- and *l*-amphetamine. Psychopharmacology 1977; 53:185-189.

177. Smith RC, Davis JM. Comparative effects of *d*-amphetamine, *l*-amphetamine, and methylphenidate on mood in man. Psychopharmacology 1977; 53:1-12.

178. Caldwell JA, Caldwell JL, Crowley JS, Jones HD. Sustaining helicopter pilot performance with Dexedrine during periods of sleep deprivation. Aviat Space Environ Med 1995; 66:930-937.

179. Caldwell JA, Caldwell JL, Crowley JS. Sustaining female helicopter pilot performance with Dexedrine during sleep deprivation. Int J Aviat Psychol 1997; 7(1):15-36.

180. Caldwell JA, Caldwell JL. An in-flight investigation of the efficacy of dextroamphetamine for sustaining helicopter pilot performance. Aviat Space Environ Med 1997; 68(12):1073-1080.

181. Caldwell JA, Caldwell JL, Lewis JA, Jones HD, Reardon MJ, Jones R, Colon J, Pegues A, Dillard R, Johnson P, Woodrum L, Higdon A. An in-flight investigation of the efficacy of dextroamphetamine for the sustainment of helicopter pilot performance, USAARL Technical Report No. 97-05. Fort Rucker, AL: US Army Aeromedical Research Laboratory. 1996.

182. Caldwell JL, Caldwell JA. Recovery sleep and performance following sleep deprivation with dextroamphetamine. J Sleep Res 1997; 6:92-101.

183. Caldwell JA, Smythe NK, LeDuc PA, Caldwell JL. Efficacy of Dexedrine for maintaining aviator performance during 64 hours of sustained wakefulness: a simulator study. Aviat Space Environ Med 2000; 71:7-18.

184. Nash, H. Psychologic effects of amphetamines and barbituates. J Nerv Ment Dis 1962; 134:203-217.

185. Cameron JS, Specht PG, Wendt GR. Effects of amphetamins on moods, emotions, and motivations. J Psychol 1965; 61:93-121.

186. Newhouse PA, Belenky G, Thomas M, Thorne D, Sing HC, Fertig J. The effects of *d*-amphetamine on arousal, cognition, and mood after prolonged total sleep deprivation. Neuropsychopharmacology 1989; 2(2):153-164.

187.  Davis DR. Psychomotor effects of analeptics and their relation to "fatigue" phenomena in aircrew. Br Med Bull 1947; 5:43-45.
188.  Marshall G, Beech HK. Drugs and judgement: effects of amphetamine and secobarbital on self-evaluation. J Psych 1964; 52(2):397-405.
189.  Hurst, PM. The effects of *d*-amphetamine on risk taking. Psychopharmacology 1962; 3:283-290.
190.  Baranski JV, Pigeau RA. Self-monitoring cognitive performance during sleep deprivation: effects of modafinil, *d*-amphetamine, and placebo. J Sleep Res 1997; 6:84-91.
191.  Shappell SA, Neri DF, DeJohn CA. Simulated sustained flight operations and performance. Part 2. Effects of dextro-methamphetamine. Milit Psychol 1992; 4(4):267-287.
192.  Mitler MM, Aldrich MS. Stimulants: efficacy and adverse effects. In: Kryger MH, Roth T, Dement WC, eds. Principles and Practice of Sleep Medicine. Philadelphia: Saunders, 2000:429-440.
193.  Cornum R, Caldwell J, Cornum K. Stimulant use in extended flight operations. Airpower J 1997; 11(1):53-58.
194.  Pierard C, Lallement G, Peres M, Lagarde, D. Modafinil: a molecule of military interest. In: Medication for Military Aircrew: Current Use, Issues, and Strategies for Expanded Options, NATO Research and Technology Organization Technical Report 14. Neuilly-sur-Seine, France: NATO Research and Technology Organization, 2001.
195.  U.S. Food and Drug Administration. Drug approvals for December, 1998. Center for Drug Evalulation and Research, *http://www.fda.gov/cder/da/da1298.htm*.
196.  Physicians' Desk Reference. Provigil tablets (Cephalon), PDR Electronic Library. Montvale, NJ: Medical Economics, 2001.
197.  Bastuji H, Jouvet M. Successful treatment of idiopathic hypersomnia and narcolepsy with modafinil. Prog Neuro-psychopharmacol Biol Psychiatry 1988; 12:695-700.
198.  Lyons TJ. French J. Modafinil: The unique properties of a new stimulant. Aviat Space Environ Med 1991; 62(5):432-435.
199.  McClellan KJ, Spencer CM. Modafinil: a review of its pharmacology and clinical efficacy in the management of narcolepsy. CNS Drugs 1998; 9(4):311-324.
200.  Ferraro L, Antonelli T, O'Connor WT, Tenganelli S, Rambert FA, Fuxe K, Modafinil: an antinarcoleptic drug with a different neurochemical profile to *d*-amphetamine and dopamine uptake blockers. Biol Psychiatry 1997; 42:1181-1183.
201.  Engber, T.M., Dennis, S.A., Jones, B.E., Miller, MS, Contreras, PC. Brain regional substrates for the actions of the novel wake-promoting agent modafinil in the rat: comparison with amphetamine. Neuroscience 1998; 87(4):905-911.
202.  Billiard M. Introduction: Modafinil, a new treatment of narcolepsy and idiopathic hypersomnia. Drugs Today 1996; 32(suppl I):1-5.
203.  Broughton RJ, Fleming JA, George CF, Hill JD, Kryger MH, Moldofsky H, Montplaisir JY, Morehouse RL, Moscovitch A, Murphy WF. Randomized, double-blind, placebo-controlled crossover trial of modafinil in the treatment of excessive daytime sleepiness in narcolepsy. Neurology 1997; 49(2):444-451.
204.  Drugs of the future. 1990; 15(2):130.
205.  Largarde D, Milhaud C. Electroencephalographic effects of modafinil, an alpha-1-adrenergic psychostimulant, on the sleep of rhesus monkeys. Sleep 1990; 13(5):441-448.

206. Hermant J, Rambert FA, Duteil J. Awakening properties of modafinil: effect on nocturnal activity in monkeys after acute and repeated administration. Psychopharmacology 1991;103:28-32.

207. Drug news and perspective. Cephalon licenses modafinil from Laboratoire L. Lafon. R and D briefs. Drug News Perspect, 1993; 6(2):113.

208. Boivin DB, Montplaisir J, Petit D, Lambert C, Lubin S. Effects of modafinil on symptomatology of human narcolepsy. Clin Neuropharmacol 1993; 16(1):46-53.

209. Besset A, Tafti M, Villemin E, Billiard M. Effets du modafinil (300 mg) sur le sommeil, la somnolence et la vigilance du narcoleptique. Neurophysiol Clin 1993; 23:47-60.

210. Besset A, Chetrit M, Carlander B, Billiard M. Use of modafinil in the treatment of narcolepsy: a long term follow-up study. Clin Neurophysiol 1996; 26:60-66.

211. Cephalon. Provigil (Modafinil) tablets. FDA approved package insert. West Chester, PA: Cephalon, 1998.

212. Jacobs I, Bell D. Modafinil prolongs time to exhaustion during high intensity submaximal exercise (abstr). Med Sci Sports Exerc 1997; 29(suppl 5):S39.

213. Saletu B, Grunberger J, Linzmayer L, Stohr H. Pharmaco-EEG, psychometric and plasma level studies with two novel alpha-adrenergic stimulants CRL 40476 and 40028 (adrafinil) in elderlies. New Trends Exp Clin Psychiatry 1986; 2(1):5-31.

214. Ellis CM, Monk C, Simmons A, Lemmens G, Williams SCR, Brammer M, Bullmore E, Parkes JD. Functional magnetic resonance imaging neuroactivation studies in normal subjects and subjects with the narcoleptic syndrome: actions of modafinil. J Sleep Res 1999; 8:85-93.

215. Laffont F. Clinical assessment of modafinil. Drugs Today 1996; 32(suppl I):35-44.

216. Brun J, Chamba G, Khalfallah Y, Girard P, Boissy I, Bastuji H, Sassolas G, Claustrat B. Effect of modafinil on plasma melatonin, corisol and growth hormone rhythms, rectal temperature and performance in healthy subjects during a 36 hour sleep deprivation. J Sleep Res 1998; 7:105-114.

217. Bourdon L, Jacobs I, Bateman WA, Vallerand AL. Effect of modafinil on heat production and regulation of body temperatures in cold-exposed humans. Aviat Space Environ Med 1994; 65:999-1004.

218. Pigeau, R, Naitoh, P. The effect of modafinil and amphetamine on core temperature and cognitive performance using complex demodulation during 64 hours of sustained work. In: Neurological Limitations of Aircraft Operations: Human Performance Implications, AGARD Conference Proceedings No. 579, 39-1 - 39-11. Neuilly-sur-Seine, France: NATO Advisory Group for Aerospace Research and Development, 1996.

219. Goldenberg F, Weil JS. Effects of a central alpha stimulant (CRL-40476) on quantified vigilance in young adults. Proceedings of the 8th European Congress on Sleep Research. New York: Gustav Fischer Verlag, 1986:343-345.

220. Lagarde D, Batejat D, Van Beers P, Sarafian D, Pradella S. Interest of modafinil, a new psychostimulant, during a sixty-hour sleep deprivation experiment. Fundam Clin Pharmacol 1995; 9:271-279.

221. Lagarde D, Batejat D. Disrupted sleep-wake rhythm and performance: advantages of modafinil. Milit Psychol 1995; 7(3):165-191.

222. Bensimon G, Benoit D, Lacomblez L, Weiller E, Warot D, Weil JS, Puech AJ. Antagonism by modafinil of the psychomotor and cognitive impairment induced by sleep-deprivation in 12 healthy volunteers. Eur Psychiatry 1991; 6:93-97.

223. Benoit O, Clodore M, Touron N, Pailhous E. Effects of modafinil on sleepiness in normal sleep deprived and symptomatic subjects (abstr). Sleep Res 1987; 16:74.

224. Stivalet P, Esqivie, D, Barraud P, Leifflen D, Raphel C. Effects of modafinil on attentional processes during 60 hours of sleep deprivation. Hum Psychopharmacol Clin Exp 1998; 13:501-507.

225. Baranski JV, Gil V, McLellan TM, Moroz D, Buguet A, Radomski M. Effects of modafinil on cognitive performance during 40 hours of sleep deprivation in a warm environment. Milit Psychol 2002; 14(1):23-47.

226. Pigeau R, Naitoh P, Buguet A, McCann C, Baranski J, Taylor M, Thompson M, Mack I. Modafinil, d-amphetamine and placebo during 64 hours of sustained mental work. I. Effects on mood, fatigue, cognitive performance and body temperature. J Sleep Res 1995; 4:212-228.

227. Buguet A, Montmayeur A, Pigeau R, Naitoh P. Modafinil, d-amphetamine, and placebo during 64 hours of sustained mental work. II. Effects on two nights of recovery sleep. J Sleep Res 1995; 4:229-241.

228. Caldwell JA, Caldwell JL, Smythe NK, Hall KK. A double-blind, placebo-controlled investigation of the efficacy of modafinil for sustaining the alertness and performance of aviators: a helicopter simulator study. Psychopharmacology 2000; 150:272-282.

229. Eddy D, Gibbons J, Storm W, Miller J, Cardenas R, Stevens K, Hickey P, Barton E, Beckinger R, Fischer J, Whitmore J. The effect of modafinil upon cognitive and vestibular performance under a single night of sleep loss. Proceedings of the 15th international symposium on night and shiftwork, 10–13 Sep, Hayama, Japan, 2001.

230. Wong YN, Simcoe D, Hartman LN, Laughton WB, King SP, McCormick GC, Grebow PE. A double-blind, placebo-controlled, ascending-dose evaluation of the pharmacokinetics and tolerability of modafinil tablets in healthy male volunteers. J Clin Pharmacol 1999; 39:30–40.

231. Warot D, Corruble E, Payan C, Weil JS, Puech AJ. Subjective effects of modafinil, a new central adrenergic stimulant in healthy volunteers: a comparison with amphetamine, caffeine, and placebo. Eur Psychiatry 1993; 8:201-208.

232. Gold L.H, Balster RL. Evaluation of the cocaine-like discriminative stimulus effects and reinforcing effects of modafinil. Psychopharmacology 1996; 126:286-292.

233. Wesensten NJ, Belenky G, Kautz MA, Thorne DR, Reichardt RM, Balkin TJ. Maintaining alertness and performance during sleep deprivation: modafinil versus caffeine. Psychopharmacology 2002; 159(3):238-247.

234. Saletu B, Frey R, Krupka M, Anderer P, Grunberger J, Barbanoj MJ. Differential effects of a new central adrenergic agonist—modafinil—and d-amphetamine on sleep and early morning behaviour in young healthy volunteers. Int J Clin Pharmacol Res 1989; 9(3):183–195.

235. Saletu B, Frey R, Krupka M, Anderer P, Grunberger J, Barbanoj MJ. Differential effects of a new central adrenergic agonist—modafinil—and d-amphetamine on sleep and early morning behaviour in elderlies. Arzneim-Forsch/Drug Res 1989; 39(2):1268-1273.

# 21

# Behavioral and Environmental Countermeasures

**TIMOTHY ROEHRS AND THOMAS ROTH**

**Henry Ford Hospital, Sleep Disorders and Research Center,
and Wayne State University, School of Medicine, Detroit, Michigan, U.S.A.**

## I.  Introduction

Population-based surveys typically have found that a substantial percentage of people report that they do not get sufficient sleep (1). While the exact prevalence may be disputed, it is an accepted fact that many people get insufficient sleep. In addition to those recognizing their insufficient sleep are other individuals who show objective evidence of excessive sleepiness, deny difficulty with sleepiness, and yet show normalization of their alertness with extended time in bed (TIB) (2). Consciously or subconsciously, people employ various stratagems to counteract the disruptive effects of their sleep loss. While the functionally disruptive effects and health risks associated with sleep loss and its consequent daytime sleepiness are generally recognized, questions remain regarding what behavioral and environment factors act as countermeasures to sleep loss and daytime sleepiness, as well as to their effectiveness and duration of effect.

This chapter will review all of the behavioral and environmental interventions that may act as countermeasures to the disruptive effects of sleep loss on waking function. The literature addressing this question is very limited, not well organized, and quite diverse. Many questions remain unanswered. Before reviewing the evidence regarding countermeasures, we will provide a conceptual analysis of the issues surrounding them.

## II. Countermeasures: A Conceptual Analysis

### A. Sleep Loss Activates a Biological Drive State

Sleep loss can be conceptualized as activating a basic biological drive state much like hunger or thirst. Deprivation of sleep increases this drive state, sleepiness. As hunger and thirst are reversed by food and fluid, so sleep reverses sleepiness. Again, as with hunger and thirst, the presence and intensity of this drive state can be inferred by observing the characteristics of the consumption of sleep: its speed of onset, ease of disruption, and duration. Sleep scientists' understanding of how sleep loss occurs and how the consequent biological drive state of sleepiness develops has changed.

Over the last two decades with the development of the field of sleep disorders medicine, there has been a paradigm shift in our understanding of sleep loss. First, the disruptive effects on performance and alertness of small reductions of TIB and its capacity to accumulate over nights is now generally accepted. Prior to the 80s the cumulative effects of a reduced TIB had not been addressed. Furthermore, the impact of small reductions of sleep time was not appreciated. In fact, two pre-80s studies were conducted with the intent of finding the shortest tolerable TIB (3,4). In each study the participants' TIB was gradually reduced from 8 hr to a point at which they were not able to tolerate the sleep restriction. A TIB of between 4.5 and 5 hr was the break point for the participants. The participants in those studies felt a 6-hr TIB was tolerable and some adopted that sleep schedule after the study was over. But more recent studies have shown the cumulative performance-disruptive and alertness-impairing effects of a 6-hr TIB (5,6). While not the purpose of those earlier studies, whether there were countermeasures, either consciously or unconsciously employed by those subjects that facilitated adaptation to the 6-hr TIB, would be interesting to know. The recent Drake et al. study did show that some adaptation to sleep loss occurs when it is accumulated at a slow rate (6). A question emerges as to whether the adaptation is due to a natural change in the sensitivity of sleepiness-alertness system or a result of countermeasures.

A second advance in our understanding of sleep loss relates to the construct of sleep fragmentation, a disruption of sleep by brief arousals without complete awakening, which was introduced to explain the excessive daytime sleepiness of patients with sleep apnea or periodic leg movements during sleep (7). Studies clearly showed the number of brief arousals during sleep relate systematically to the level of daytime sleepiness, and treatments that reduce arousal frequency are associated with improvements in daytime sleepiness (8). Thus, it is now accepted that small cumulative reductions of TIB or the fragmentation of sleep produces sleep loss and its consequent sleepiness and impaired memory and performance. Again, many individuals in the population function with routinely reduced TIB or with sleep-fragmenting disorders and the question is whether and which countermeasures allow this adaptation.

## B. Countermeasures as Opponent Processes

Any countermeasure might be viewed as the activation of an opponent process that diminishes the impact of sleep loss. However, our understanding of these processes and how they operate is limited, in part because the substrates of sleepiness have yet to be determined. It is assumed that sleepiness is a central nervous system phenomenon with identifiable neural mechanisms and neurochemical correlates. Various electrophysiological events have been identified that are suggestive of incipient sleep processes as they appear in behaviorally awake organisms undergoing sleep deprivation. Some neuroimaging studies have implicated the involvement of specific brain regions in sleepiness, and pharmacological studies provide several hypotheses regarding the neurochemistry of sleepiness. Discussing all the evidence in detail is beyond the scope of this chapter; it is reviewed in other sources (8).

The neurobiology underlying any given countermeasure is somewhat less elusive. To the extent that any countermeasure stimulates the reticular activation system, either primarily or secondarily, one would predict a counteractive effect to sleepiness. But the important issue is how quickly adaptation to the stimulatory effects occurs. Reticular stimulation most likely occurs with sensory stimuli, but an adaptation to their effects is also likely. Other countermeasures may operate through different and possibly specific mechanisms (i.e., motivation, posture, movement, etc.) and then secondarily have reticular-activating effects.

It may also have heuristic value to conceptualize countermeasures in terms of intensity of effect, or "dose," and duration of effect, or "half-life," much as a pharmacologist does for a drug and its potential for effects. For example, parametric analyses of the different intensities of a physical stimulus relative to different levels of sleepiness would be important to advancing our understanding of the effectiveness of that countermeasure. Very few studies have done that. With some limitations, quantification of the level of sleepiness is possible using the Multiple Sleep Latency Test (MSLT). Thus, for example, a study compared the alerting capacity of 75 and 150 mg of caffeine after a 4-hr TIB and an 8-hr TIB the previous night using the MSLT (9). Average daily sleep latency on the MSLT was increased by 4 min with 150 mg and 2 min with 75 mg after both the 4- and 8-hr TIB, although the absolute level of alertness still differed in the 4- and 8-hr TIB. Such an approach could then also facilitate a comparison among different classes of countermeasures. Thus, in the above-cited study, substitution of two different physical stimuli for the two caffeine doses can be made. Finally, this approach can also be used to evaluate the cumulative effects of two or more countermeasures, as multiple interventions are the rule rather than the exception.

The analysis above and the literature reviewed below approach the definition of a countermeasure as the external application of stimuli or conditions that counteract the impact of sleep loss. However, in the "real world" people often either consciously or unconsciously make behavioral choices when experiencing sleep loss. Those behavioral choices might also be considered as countermeasures, albeit personally imposed. That is, under sleep loss conditions people may choose stimulus-rich (i.e., bright, noisy) environments and tasks and/or tasks that are less physically or intellectually demanding. The behavioral choices made may also depend on one's current level of sleepiness. Furthermore, there may be individual differences in one's preferred behavioral choice to counteract sleep loss. Such an approach to understanding countermeasures and sleep loss has not been attempted or studied.

## III.  Countermeasures: The Evidence

### A.   Motivation

Motivation is probably the most studied countermeasure. Some of the earliest studies showed that participants could be motivated to overcome the performance-disruptive effects of sleep loss, at least for brief periods (10). The classic motivational variable is incentive or reward and a sleep deprivation study was conducted in which monetary rewards were given for "hits" and fines for "false alarms" on a vigilance task (11). The high-reward condition maintained performance at baseline levels over the first 36 hr of the 72 hr deprivation and produced better performance than the low reward condition throughout the deprivation. Clearly, tolerance to the effectiveness of reward developed over time. Another motivator is competition. The publication of daily performance results for all participants to view was sufficient to maintain performance at baseline levels during 1 night of sleep loss (12). Another classic motivational variable, knowledge of results, without public disclosure as in the previous study, was found to improve performance during sleep deprivation (13). On the other hand, feedback on one's level of electroencephalogram alpha-frequency power during a sleep deprivation, as opposed to performance level feedback, had no impact on the ability to maintain basal performance (14). And finally, knowledge about the time to conclusion of the deprivation provides a boost to performance (15).

The impact of sleep loss on performance, however, is more than a motivational deficit. First, the impact of motivation during sleep loss is time-limited. As the deprivation continues, motivation has a lessened effect; in the majority of studies its effects are limited to a single night of sleep loss. Second, its effectiveness is limited. In a clever study of sleep deprivation, one task was targeted for incentives, while other tasks were presented as filler tasks (16). On the targeted task, performance was maintained, while on the nontargeted tasks performance declined with the deprivation. The same has been observed informally on divided-attention tasks in which individuals, during conditions of sleep loss or sedative drug administration, will adopt the strategy of concentrating their attention to only one component of the task.

Task interest is another relevant, but difficult-to-study, motivational variable. There are wide divergences among individuals in interest, interest is difficult to quantify as a variable, and interest is not independent of task complexity, a variable known to impact the effects of sleep loss. One study did show that individuals could maintain basal performance for the first 50 hr of a 60-hr sleep deprivation on a task rated by each participant as being "interesting" (17). The fact that some people stay awake for long periods of time engaged in tasks (i.e., artists and writers) or in games (i.e., all-night poker and gambling) that have intense interest to them attests to the effectiveness of this variable. Nearly every review of the sleep deprivation literature includes the statement that "long and boring tasks are necessary to reveal the impact of sleep deprivation on performance."

## B.  Physical Stimulation

Probably the most frequently used "real-world" countermeasure to sleep loss and its consequent sleepiness is physical stimulation. But sensory adaptation to physical stimuli is a characteristic of all organisms, which raises questions regarding its utility as a countermeasure. There are stimuli that have survival value and for which adaptation does not occur. The hypoxia stimulus in patients with sleep apnea syndrome remains quite potent regardless of the number of apnea events and sleepiness level. However, even in apnea the degree of sleepiness, as manipulated by sleep loss or sleep extension, modulates the level of hypoxemia needed to cause an arousal. In attempts to model the sleep fragmentation of apnea patients in healthy normals using tones delivered via earphones, the intertone interval, tone frequency, and tone complexity were all varied, and yet on the second night of fragmentation some adaptation to the arousing effect of the stimuli occurred (18). The informational value of the stimulus is a critical factor, as well. The mother of a newborn child will awaken to the slightest whimper of her child, but not to loud traffic noises. Yet, for most stimuli, adaptation does occur and thus, the speed of the adaptation becomes the issue in considering physical stimulation as a countermeasure.

Auditory stimulation in the form of noise in a work environment or of a radio or tape player in automobile driving has been studied for its beneficial effect in maintaining performance during sleep deprivation. But studies show that the beneficial effects are minimal and short-lived (12,19–21). For example, Reyner and Horne studied the use of a radio set to the subject's station choice during a 2.5-hr simulated automobile drive after a night of restricted sleep (22). The radio only had a trend in reducing the number of driving incidents observed in the no-stimulation condition. Compared to caffeine or a brief nap that the authors had assessed in previous studies using the same methods, the radio was a very temporary and impotent countermeasure.

Another physical stimulus studied as a countermeasure is bright light, which has been primarily studied in the context of shift- or night work. However, a distinction has to be made between an alerting and performance-enhancing effect of bright light due to its circadian-phase-shifting capacity versus its direct alerting effects. For example, Dawson et al. showed that a 4-hr exposure of 7000 lux bright light from 24:00–04:00 hr on each of 3 nights improved cognitive and psychomotor performance compared to a dim-red-light control (23). While the bright light indeed produced a shift in the circadian rhythm over the 3 nights, performance was improved on the first night before the benefit of a circadian shift could be realized. So bright light would appear to have an "alerting" effect beyond its phase-shifting capacity, but this needs further study as to the degree of brightness, duration of exposure, and duration of effectiveness.

A typical countermeasure used by sleepy drivers is to turn on the air conditioner or open a window. Two aspects of this stimulus can be considered in analyzing it as a countermeasure. The first is the cold temperature of the stimulus, or in the least a change in temperature. There has been very little study of the effectiveness of cold temperature as a countermeasure. The simulated automobile drive study cited above also included a cold-air condition produced by the automobile air conditioner (22). As with the radio, cold air had a minimal and transitory alerting effect. The fact that temperature change may be the critical factor is seen in a study that showed heat (92°F) improved performance from basal levels during sleep deprivation, although the impact was very time-limited (24).

The second critical aspect is the cutaneous stimulation produced by the rushing air from the air conditioner or the moving car. We are not aware of any studies of this stimulus as a countermeasure. But, in the "real world" cutaneous stimulation is a frequently used countermeasure, washing one's face with cold water or slapping one's face. These stimuli probably have some effects that could be quantified and documented, but again the effects are probably quite short-lived.

The use of "rumble strips" on highways to prevent sleepiness-related accidents represents the clearest example of society adapting a countermeasure. "Rumble strips" combine multiple stimuli (i.e., noise, cutaneous stimulation) in an attempt to arouse the driver and prevent accidents. Like the other countermeasures discussed, there is no question about its acute effectiveness. There is a decrease in accidents proximal to the "rumble strip." However, a question remains about its overall efficacy. Some research has described a phenomenon called "migration," the movement of accidents from the location of the "rumble strips" to other locations on the highway. The question yet to be resolved is whether "rumble strips" prevent accidents or merely postpone them.

## C.  Posture

The potential of posture to act as a countermeasure to sleep loss has not been studied in a systematic manner. It is known that there are species-specific postures for sleep, and in humans recumbency is sleep-conducive and an erect posture is not. Although studies of the impact of posture on the ability to maintain alertness and performance efficiency during sleep loss have not been done, one study of the impact of posture on the continuity of sleep may be germane. A polysomnographic study of the sleep of healthy normals in chairs with back angles of 40, 53, and 72 degrees from the horizontal found progressive increases in wakefulness and decreases in duration of sleep compared to sleep in the horizontal position in a bed (25). Given that the factors important to maintaining sleep may differ in some respects from those for maintaining alertness, these results still would suggest that as posture moves to the horizontal the disruptive effects of sleep loss become more likely. On the other hand, a 90-degree seated posture or even an erect standing posture is not an absolute countermeasure. During sustained sleep loss when sitting at 90 degrees to the horizontal and standing erect, EEG signs of sleep have been observed (26).

### D. Physical Activity

Maintaining continuous physical activity is one of the most commonly used methods in sleep-depriving animals, and often physical activity is encouraged to maintain alertness in human sleep deprivation studies. However, a distinction between rhythmic and arrhythmic activity is important because the two have very different effects on maintaining alertness and reducing the likelihood of sleep. While arrhythmic activity facilitates alertness, rhythmic physical activity, at least a gentle rocking motion, in fact induces sleep.

The degree to which physical activity is effective as a countermeasure appears to be dependent on the extent of the sleep loss. A study in which nocturnal sleep time was reduced by about 50% for 1 night found that a brief 5-min walk prior to testing reversed the reduction in sleep latency on the Multiple Sleep Latency Test (MSLT) the following day associated with the sleep restriction (27). On the other hand, in studies of extensive total sleep deprivation (40–64 hr) physical activity showed no benefit in lessening the sleepiness and performance impairment of the deprivation (28—30). The same question remains as to the degree of effectiveness of physical activity. It attenuated the effects of a 50% reduction in sleep time for 1 night, but not 40–64 hr of sleep deprivation. And second, *what is the duration of its efficacy?* Although activity was able to postpone sleep onset on the MSLT for a few minutes, it was not able to maintain performance over the entire testing session.

### IV. Remaining Questions and Research Needs

As the above brief review indicates, very little systematic study has been done to address any of the many countermeasures reported to be beneficial to individuals experiencing sleep loss. Studies comparing the effectiveness and duration of the various countermeasures are critical to defining their use. It is only after these two questions are answered that any particular countermeasure can be appropriately used. *Will the countermeasure help the sleepy driver get to the next exit or all the way home?*

It seems apparent that people adapt to shortened sleep times and fragmented sleep and the question is: *what countermeasures are being employed, how effective are they, and what risks remain?* To thoroughly understand these issues, parametric analyses of the various countermeasures would be quite helpful and important. Beyond the behavioral analyses are the questions regarding the neuro-biological mechanisms that underlie sleepiness and the counteractive effects of any countermeasure. The critical questions for all the countermeasures is how enduring their effects are and if they have to be continuously reapplied, how rapidly adaptation to their effect occurs.

## V. Conclusions

The literature on countermeasures, while incomplete and limited, suggests that most of the countermeasures studied have small and time-limited capacities to counteract the impact of sleep loss. The most difficult problem for any of the various countermeasures is the inevitable adaptation that occurs to their alerting effects. Ultimately the most effective countermeasure to sleep loss is sleep.

Second to sleep as a countermeasure is knowledge. People tend to underestimate the impairment and risks associated with sleep loss and to overestimate the effectiveness of any given countermeasure. Risks increase when individuals are sleepy, working and driving in isolation, in a quiet darkened environment, and on long, boring tasks and roads. When one is sleepy, the potential of any countermeasure is limited in effectiveness and duration but knowledge about these facts can be a countermeasure.

## Acknowledgments

This study was supported by National Institutes of Health grants # R01 AA07147, #R01-DA05086 awarded to Dr. T. Roehrs and #R01-MH59338 awarded to Dr. T. Roth.

## References

1.  Gallup Organization. Sleep in America 1995. Princeton, NJ: The Gallup Organization, 1995.
2.  Levine B, Roehrs T, Zorick F, Roth T. Daytime sleepiness in young adults. Sleep 1988; 11:39–46.
3.  Johnson L, MacLeod WL. Sleep and awake behavior during gradual sleep reduction. Percept Motor Skills1973; 36:87–97.
4.  Friedman J. Globus G. Huntley A. Mullaney D, Naito P. Johnson L. Performance and mood during and after gradual sleep reduction. Psychophysiology 1978; 14:245–250.
5.  Dinges DF, Pack F, Williams K, Gillen KA, Powell JW, Ott GE, Aptowicz C, Pack AI. Cumulative sleepiness, mood disturbance, and psychomotor vigilance performance decrements during a week of sleep restricted to 4–5 hours per night. Sleep 1997; 20:267–277.

6.  Drake CL, Roehrs TA, Burduvali E, Bonahoom A, Rosekind M, Roth T. Effects of rapid versus slow accumulation of eight hours of sleep loss. Psychophysiology. 2001; 38:979–987.

7.  Roth T, Hartse KM, Zorick F, Conway W. Multiple naps and the evaluation of daytime sleepiness in patients with upper airway sleep apnea. Sleep 1980; 3:425–439.

8.  Roehrs T, Carskadon MA, Dement WC, Roth T. Daytime sleepiness and alertness. In: Kryger MH, Roth T, Dement WC, eds. Principles and Practice of Sleep Medicine, 3rd ed. Philadelphia: Saunders, 2000:43–52.

9.  Rosenthal L, Roehrs TA, Zwyghuizen-Doorenbos A, Plath D, Roth T. Alerting effects of caffeine after normal and restricted sleep. Neuropsychopharmacology 1991; 4:103–108.

10. Williams HL, Lubin A, Goodnow JJ. Impaired performance with acute sleep loss. Psychol Monogr: Gen Appl. 1959; 73:1–26.

11. Horne JA, Pettitt AN. High incentive effects on vigilance performance during 72 hours of total sleep deprivation. Acta Psychol 1985; 58:123–139.

12. Wilkinson RT. Interaction of lack of sleep with knowledge of results, repeated testing, and individual differences. J Exp Psychol 1961; 62:263–271.

13. Wilkinson RT. Muscle tension during mental work under sleep deprivation. J Exp Psychol 1962; 64:;565–571.

14. Hord DJ, Lubin A, Tracy ML, Jensma BW, Johnson LC. Feedback for high EEG alpha does not maintain performance or mood during sleep loss. Psychophysiology 1976; 13:58–61.

15. Haslam DR. The incentive effect and sleep deprivation. Sleep 1983; 6:362–368.

16. Bonnet MH, Webb WB. The effect of repetition of relevant and irrelevant tasks over day and night work periods. Ergonomics 1978; 21:999–1005.

17. Wilkinson RT. Effects of up to 60 hours' sleep deprivation on different types of work. Ergonomics 1964; 7:175–186.

18. Roehrs T, Merlotti L, Petrucelli N, Stepanski E, Roth T. Experimental sleep fragmentation. Sleep 1994; 17:438–443.

19. Gunter TC, van der Zande RD, Wiethoff M, Mulder G, Mulder LJ. Visual selective attention during meaningful noise and after sleep deprivation. Electroencephalogr Clin Neurophysiol Suppl 1987;4099–107.

20. Hartley L, Shirley E. Sleep-loss, noise and decisions. Ergonomics 1977; 20:481–489.

21. Tassi P, Nicolas A, Seegmuller C. Interaction of the alerting effect of noise with partial sleep deprivation and circadian rhythmicity of vigilance. Percept Mot Skills 1993; 77:1236–1248.

22. Reyner LA, Horne JA. Evaluation of "in-car" countermeasures to sleepiness: cold air and radio. Sleep 1998; 21:46–50.

23. Dawson D, Encel N, Lushington K. Improving adaptation to simulated night shift: timed exposure to bright light versus daytime melatonin administration. Sleep 1995; 18:11–21.

24. Poulton EC, Edwards RS, Colquhoun WP. The interaction of the loss of a night's sleep with mild heat: task variables. Ergonomics 1974; 17:59–73.

25. Nicholson AN, Stone BM. Influence of back angle on the quality of sleep in seats. Ergonomics 1987; 30:1033–1041.

26. Torsvall L, Akerstedt T, Gillander K, Knutsson A. Sleep on the night shift: 24–hour EEG monitoring spontaneous sleep/wake behavior. Psychophysiology 1989; 26:352–358.

27. Bonnet MH, Arand DA. Sleepiness as measured by modified multiple sleep latency testing varies as a function of preceding activity. Sleep 1998; 21:477–483.

28. Webb WB, Agnew HWJ. Effects on performance of high and low energy-expenditure during sleep deprivation. Percept Mot Skills 1973; 37:511–514.

29. Lubin A, Hord DJ, Tracy ML, Johnson LC. Effects of exercise, bedrest and napping on performance decrement during 40 hours. Psychophysiology 1976; 13:334–514.

30. Angus RG, Heslegrave RJ, Myles WS. Effects of prolonged sleep deprivation, with and without chronic physical exercise, on mood and performance. Psychophysiology 1985; 22:276–282.

# 22

## Naps

**AMBER (TIETZEL) BROOKS AND LEON LACK**

**Flinders University, Adelaide, South Australia, Australia**

### I. Introduction

Given the social and economic burden of impaired performance, productivity. and safety arising from sleep deprivation, it is not surprising that there has been considerable industrial and scientific interest in napping as a solution for maximizing alertness. Napping offers an effective solution for increasing alertness after sleep deprivation, thereby enhancing performance, productivity and safety. This chapter reviews the current literature pertaining to the recuperative value of naps.

A nap has been defined as "any sleep period with a duration of less than 50 per cent of the average major sleep period of an individual" (1, pp. 313–314). The recuperative effects of a nap are "those beneficial effects that restore human behavioural efficiency and subjective feelings of vigor and arousal" (2, p. 555).

Indeed the sheer prevalence of napping in the population is good reason to suggest that napping may be beneficial. Dinges (3) conducted an extensive literature review of napping patterns among adults, and reported that on average, 61% of adults napped at least once a week, with an average duration of 73 min. A more recent survey of napping behavior conducted by Pilcher et al. (4) revealed that approximately 74% of young and middle-aged adults napped at least once within a 7-day sleep log period, with almost half napping for less than 20 min, for a total mean duration for the sample of less than 18 min. The difference in mean nap durations reported in the Dinges and Pilcher et al. studies may reflect changing social trends in napping behavior, with a shift toward brief napping.

*Why do people nap?* Typically, people nap to restore their alertness and performance after a sustained period of wakefulness. Indeed, a nap taken after reduced nighttime sleep has been shown to improve performance to levels comparable to a normal night of sleep (5). This type of napping strategy, referred to as recuperative napping, has been differentiated from prophylactic napping in the napping literature. Prophylactic napping, which occurs in anticipation of nighttime sleep loss (6), is often utilized by shift workers with a view to improving their alertness and performance on the subsequent work shift. Prophylactic naps have been shown to be effective in enhancing alertness (7) and minimizing performance decrements (8) overnight.

The recuperative effects of napping have been established through a variety of measurement techniques, including subjective self-report assessments, performance measures, and objective psychophysiological indices. Subjective self-report measures serve as a simple and ready means of assessing self-perceived sleepiness, alertness, fatigue, and vigor. A variety of performance assessments have also been shown to be sensitive to the effects of napping and are more relevant to productivity issues. Objective psychophysiological measures, which are relevant to safety issues and less susceptible to motivational and demand characteristics, have also evidenced improvement following napping. A commonly used and reliable objective measure of sleepiness is the Multiple Sleep Latency Test (MSLT) (9), which requires participants to attempt sleep over a number of trials. The underlying assumption of the MSLT is that the time taken to initiate sleep (i.e., sleep latency) indicates sleepiness, with short sleep latencies reflecting "sleepiness" and long sleep latencies reflecting "alertness."

## II.  Factors Affecting the Recuperative Value of Naps

The extent to which naps will be beneficial, in terms of improved self-perceived alertness, performance, and objective alertness, is likely to depend on a number of factors. The factors of particular significance that will be addressed in this chapter include: (a) sleep inertia, (b) nap duration, (c) nap sleep infrastructure, (d) circadian timing, (e) prior wake time, (f) napping strategies for periods of extended wakefulness, (g) individual differences, and (h) the setting (laboratory vs. applied settings). The discussion will now turn to the first of these factors, sleep inertia.

### A. Sleep Inertia

Sleep inertia, the experience of "inferior task performance and/or disorientation occurring immediately after awakening from sleep" (10, p. 226), is a well-documented consequence of napping (11). Although sleep inertia is said to dissipate in an exponential manner (11–13), effects may endure for up to 4 hr after awakening (14), although most negative effects appear to dissipate within 35 min (15).

The reduced performance capacity that characterizes sleep inertia has been documented for an extensive array of behavioral tasks, including reaction time, grip strength, short-term memory, complex cognitive and visual tasks (2), and a decision-making task (16). Although sleep inertia also suppresses subjective experiences of alertness, self-reported alertness does not generally reflect the magnitude of the performance decrements (11,17). Sleep inertia is also characterized by a stage 1 sleep electroencephalographic (EEG) pattern (10) rather than a fully wakeful EEG pattern (18).

Sleep inertia generally occurs after sleep durations greater than 30 min but has been shown to occur after naps as short as 20 min of sleep (19,20). It has been suggested that sleep inertia is more likely to follow longer naps because longer naps comprise more slow-wave sleep of stages 3 and 4 (15,21,22). Accordingly, brief naps generate minimal sleep inertia because they consist mainly of stage 1 sleep and are generally not long enough to allow time for slow-wave sleep to develop. Of note, sleep inertia may be enhanced by prior sleep deprivation (14) and napping coinciding with the circadian trough (e.g., Refs. 2, 21), conditions during which slow-wave sleep duration is enhanced.

Sleep inertia also appears to be related, in part, to the sleep stage at arousal, with poorest performance incurred from awakening from slow-wave sleep of stages 3 and 4 (14,15,23,24) and lesser deficits resulting from awakening from sleep stages 1, 2 or REM sleep (14,15). Thus, one possible strategy for minimizing the effects of sleep inertia after longer naps is to curtail the period of the nap to less than 20 min, or otherwise after a complete sleep cycle (i.e., 80–100 min), thereby reducing the likelihood of waking from the slow-wave sleep portion of the sleep cycle (25).

To summarize, sleep inertia is a factor to consider when implementing a napping strategy. As sleep inertia appears to be affected by the duration of slow-wave sleep within the sleep period and slow-wave sleep occurring at arousal, sleep inertia tends to accompany naps in excess of 20–30 min. For this reason, as well as the fact that naps greater than 20 min appear to produce characteristically different postnap effects compared to naps of shorter duration, naps in excess of 20 min duration will henceforth be referred to as long naps and those 20 min and shorter will be termed brief naps.

### B. Nap Duration

*Long Naps*

Notwithstanding the initial effects of sleep inertia that may accompany long naps, they have been shown to produce beneficial effects after normal nocturnal sleep (26–29), sleep restriction (30), total sleep deprivation (31), as well as during experimental night shifts (32,33) and periods of sustained wakefulness (1). Reported benefits include increased post-nap sleep latency (30,31,33), improved

subjective alertness (26–29), reduced fatigue (26,28,29), and improved performance accuracy (29,32), performance productivity (32), response speed (i.e., reaction time) (1,27–29,33), and short-term memory (28,29).

However, as an additional factor to consider, the benefits of long naps may
be tempered by the fact that they may disrupt the duration and architecture of the
subsequent sleep period (3,34). In this capacity, long naps may lead to further
sleep loss (15). Brief naps, on the other hand, do not appear to affect subsequent
sleep duration and quality (35).

### Brief Naps

Research has shown that deficits resulting from nocturnal sleep restriction can be
ameliorated by brief naps of mean durations as short as 19.8 (5), 10.8 (36), 10.2
(37), and 10 min (20,38,39). Brief naps of mean durations of 7.3 min (40) and 20
min (41,42) after normal nocturnal sleep, and brief workplace naps during the
night shift (35,43) have also been shown to be beneficial. Reported benefits of
brief naps include increased sleep latency (20,38,39), EEG indicators of increased
alertness (5,36,37,41,42,44), improved subjective alertness (5,20,39–41,44),
reduced fatigue (20,39), and improved performance accuracy (5,40,41,44,45), performance productivity (20,38,39,45), response speed (20,35,43,45) and simulated
driving performance (36).

### Ultrabrief Naps

In a review of the minimal amount of sleep required for maintaining performance,
Naitoh (46), concluded that 4 min was the minimum amount of sleep required for
producing recuperative effects. In a study investigating the recuperative effects of
30-sec, 90-sec, and 10-min nap conditions with respect to a no-nap condition,
Tietzel and Lack (39) sought to determine the minimum duration of nap sleep
required for improving alertness and performance after nocturnal sleep restriction. The ultrabrief naps of 30 sec and 90 sec produced no measurable benefits,
while the 10-minute nap significantly improved subjective and objective alertness, fatigue, and cognitive performance.

In their most recent study, Tietzel and Lack (20) found that a 5-min nap provided only limited postnap benefits (evidencing improvements relative to no-nap on
one of eight measures examined), but was clearly not as effective as a 10-min nap.
Takahashi et al. (40) found that a 15-min nap opportunity (resulting in a mean sleep
duration of 7.3 min) improved subjective alertness and performance; however, the
precise duration of nap sleep that produced these benefits was not elucidated.

Taken together, these findings suggest that while a nap on the order of 5
min may produce some benefit, consistent benefits are achieved by a nap of 10
min duration. This conclusion is supported by Bonnet (47), who investigated the
effects of sleep continuity and the recuperative benefits of different-length sleep
periods and concluded that continuous sleep periods longer than 10 min are
required for sleep to have recuperative value.

### Brief Naps Versus Long Naps

Although there is ample evidence to suggest that both long and brief naps can be effective in improving or even restoring daytime alertness and performance, there has been only limited research comparing brief naps with naps of longer duration.

The existing evidence suggests that longer naps (i.e., 1–2 hr) appear to be more alerting than brief naps after total sleep deprivation (31,48). Lumley et al. (31) compared nap opportunities of 0, 15, 30, 60, and 120 min duration and found that the 30-, 60-, and 120-min naps increased sleep latency compared to the no-nap condition, with such improvements emerging 4 hr after napping. The 15-min nap did not significantly improve alertness, which may be attributed to the scheduling of the naps in the morning, the fact that subjects were totally sleep-deprived, and/or that the first assessment of objective alertness was 2 hr after the nap. Of note, the 120-min nap did not produce improvements superior to the 60-min nap. Helmus et al. (48) compared a 2-hr nap with a 15-min nap and revealed greater improvements in sleep latency from the 2-hr nap, relative to the 15-min nap, but only after a 3-hr postnap delay.

However, under conditions of mildly restricted nocturnal sleep, brief afternoon naps appear to be at least as effective as naps of longer duration. For example, Tietzel and Lack (38) found that a brief afternoon nap of precisely 10 min was at least as recuperative as a 30-min nap in terms of improved alertness and performance in the hour following napping. In a more comprehensive study examining the recuperative effects of brief naps of varying duration, Tietzel and Lack (20) found that a 10-min nap generally produced greater benefits than 20- and 30-min naps over the three-hour period following the naps. The 10-min nap produced consistent alertness and performance benefits for more than 2.5 hr, whereas 20- and 30-min naps appeared to produce a period of sleep inertia immediately after waking before improving to levels comparable to the 10-min condition.

After normal nocturnal sleep, brief naps also appear to be at least as effective as longer naps in improving alertness and performance. Specifically, Taub et al. (27) observed significant improvements in subjective arousal and auditory reaction time for both 30-min and 2-hr napping opportunities, with no significant differences between the two nap conditions. Takahashi et al. (40) compared a 15-min nap opportunity (mean duration 7.3 min) with a 45-min nap opportunity (mean duration 30.1 min) and observed significantly improved alertness 30 min after the 15-min nap opportunity and comparable improvements for the 15-min and 45-min nap conditions 3 hr after napping. Furthermore, Helmus et al. (48) compared a 2-hr nap with a 15-min nap after a normal night of sleep and revealed comparable sleep latencies for the 3 hr after both nap opportunities.

On balance, while long naps appear to be more beneficial following total sleep deprivation, any benefit must be weighed against their limitations of sleep inertia and possible disruptions to the subsequent nocturnal sleep period. After normal nocturnal sleep or mildly restricted nocturnal sleep, brief naps would be the preferred strategy. Brief naps on the order of 10 min provide immediate and consistent benefits, seemingly avoid the negative effects of sleep inertia, appear to be at least as effective as longer naps, and require only a minimal investment of time. However, any informed judgment regarding the optimal napping strategy for improving alertness and performance would need to take account of how long the benefits of brief and long naps endure.

### Time Course of Napping Effects

Findings obtained by Takahashi and Arito (37) provide some insight into the length of time one can expect the benefits of brief naps to last. Takahashi and Arito explored the effects of a brief afternoon nap (mean duration 10.2 min) on alertness and performance after nocturnal sleep restriction (4 hr) and observed significantly improved logical reasoning performance 30 min after napping. However, when performance was assessed at 2, 3.5 and 5 hr after napping, post-nap effects were not significantly different from the no-nap condition. Such findings would indicate that the effects of a brief nap last for less than 2 hr. However, Takahashi et al. (40) observed that a brief nap produced beneficial effects that lasted for as long as 3 hr.

A recent study by Tietzel and Lack (20) is informative when considering the time course of effects after naps of different durations. They comprehensively plotted the 3-hr time course of effects after 5-, 10-, 20- and 30-min naps with respect to a no-nap condition. The ultrabrief 5-min nap exhibited a trend of improved alertness and performance lasting approximately 1 hr, while the 10-min nap produced immediate and consistent benefits in alertness and performance lasting approximately 2.5 hr. Although the 20-min nap evidenced a suppression of alertness and performance immediate after napping, significant improvements were observed 35 min after napping and appeared to last for at least 2 hr. Finally, the 30-min nap produced an immediate period of reduced alertness and performance, even more pronounced than after the 20-min nap (indicative of greater sleep inertia), followed by alertness and performance improvements comparable to the 10- and 20-min naps, lasting at least 2.5 hr.

In terms of the time course of effects after longer naps, Lumley et al. (31) showed that increased alertness after 1- and 2-hr-long naps emerged 4 hours after napping and was maintained for at least 4 hr. Two-hour-long naps taken 6 or 18 hr into a 56-hr period of otherwise sustained wakefulness have been shown to produce performance improvements lasting at least 24 hr, while a 2-hr nap taken after 30 hrs awake improved performance for 8 hr (1).

To summarize the findings presented thus far, one would conclude that naps are differentially beneficial over time according to the duration of the nap. The available evidence suggests that brief naps (of approximately 10 min) produce immediate improvements in alertness and performance lasting for at least 3 hr. On the other hand, longer naps typically produce an initial period of sleep inertia upon awakening, the duration of which may vary according to the amount of

slow-wave sleep accumulated during the nap, followed by alertness and performance improvements lasting for several hours up to 24 hr.

### C.  Nap Sleep Infrastructure

The issue of comparing the effects of different-duration naps (brief vs. long) is
complicated by the fact that sleep is not one homogeneous state but varies in
depth (stages 1, 2, 3, and 4) and state (non-REM and REM) over the duration of
the nap.

One of the primary neurophysiological forces that regulates sleepiness and
performance is the homeostatic drive for sleep (Process S). Process S proposes
increased sleepiness with increasing time spent awake, as well as increased alertness potential with increasing sleep (49). Theoretical proponents of Process S
maintain that the increase in alertness potential produced by sleep is determined
almost exclusively by slow-wave sleep (49,50). Process S would therefore predict
greater benefits associated with longer naps as longer naps comprise a greater
proportion of slow-wave sleep.

Some researchers have documented significant positive correlations
between slow-wave sleep during naps and reaction time performance improvements after normal nocturnal sleep (51) and sleep deprivation (52). Moreover,
Lavie (53) documented preliminary laboratory findings that naps containing more
of stages 3 and 4 sleep were associated with improved postnap sleepiness levels.
Examining naps of 0, 15, 30, 60, and 120 min duration, Lumley et al. (31) also
demonstrated that alertness increased as a function of duration of slow-wave
sleep. Consistent with sleep homeostasis, Helmus et al. (48) also observed that a
2-hr nap opportunity was more recuperative than a 15-min nap opportunity, 2 hr
after napping.

However, given that a brief nap comprises mainly stage 1 sleep with limited slow-wave sleep, the significant improvements in alertness and performance
produced by brief naps are disproportionate to the recuperative effect that would
be predicted by Process S. Furthermore, Process S is not consistent with findings
that brief naps may be at least as recuperative as longer naps (e.g., Ref. 20, 38,
40). Evans et al. (26) also reported that nonnappers, who had significantly more
slow-wave sleep in their naps than habitual nappers, actually obtained less subjective benefit.

It is not surprising that the homeostatic theory does not completely account
for the beneficial effects of brief naps, as the theory was derived from experimental studies of long nocturnal sleep episodes rather than comparably shorter-
duration napping studies. Hence the homeostatic theory may simply not be an
appropriate theory of the recuperative effects of napping. The incongruence
between existing scientific evidence from napping studies and Process S warrants
the consideration of an alternative explanation.

Several alternative explanations regarding the mechanism of nap benefits
have been proposed. For example, in a study of napping during the night shift,

Signal and Gander (43) concluded that stage 1 sleep significantly contributed to nap benefits. In a review of polyphasic sleep schedules, Stampi (54) proposed that "every time the organism falls asleep some process related to the recuperation might be activated, which may be independent from sleep episode duration, and therefore, that overall beneficial effects are related to the number of times the sleep system is activated (within reasonable limits)" (p. 172)

Tietzel and Lack (39) sought to determine whether the benefits of naps arose from the initiation of stage 1 sleep. Examining ultrabrief (30-sec and 90-sec) and brief (10-min) naps, they concluded that the operative mechanism determining nap benefits did not appear to be the onset of stage 1 sleep, but rather nap benefits might arise from the onset of stage 2 sleep, the accumulation of stage 2 sleep, or a fixed period of nap sleep between 90 sec and 10 min. Subsequent findings by Tietzel and Lack (20) were not consistent with the notion that the beneficial effects of brief naps may be due to the onset of stage 2 sleep or the total accumulation of stage 2 sleep. In view of nap sleep infrastructure data obtained from 5-, 10-, 20-, and 30-min naps and a no-nap control condition, they concluded that the beneficial effects of napping may be due to the onset of slow-wave activity during the nap or the attainment of a fixed duration of stage 2 sleep (in the order of 8–9 min), which is directly opposed by the accumulation of slow-wave sleep occurring during the naps (i.e., sleep inertia). This would assume that, after the dissipation of sleep inertia, all naps during which slow-wave activity is initiated or 8–9 min of stage 2 sleep obtained would produce comparable benefits.

In summary, while the theory of sleep homeostasis appears to adequately account for the effects associated with longer sleep episodes, particularly in reversing the effects of total and thus slow-wave sleep deprivation, its application to brief naps after mild sleep loss appears to be inadequate. Hence, further research is necessary to determine the mechanism by which brief naps exert their effects. Indeed, an understanding of the mechanism that improves behavioral efficiency after a brief nap is clearly an integral component of any comprehensive theory of sleep regulation.

### D.   Circadian Timing

Naps may also be differentially beneficial to alertness and performance, depending on the timing of the nap with respect to the 24-hr circadian rhythm of core body temperature. In accordance with the biphasic circadian rhythm of core body temperature, periods of greatest sleepiness occur during the morning between 02:00 and 06:00 hours (55) and the afternoon between 13:00 and 16:00 hours (56).

Research has shown that naps taken near the circadian nadir (circa 05:00) may lack recuperative value. Indeed, Naitoh (1981) reported that naps taken between 04:00 and 06:00 hours were of little recuperative value compared to naps taken in the afternoon between 12:00 and 14:00 hours. Other researchers have also shown that a 3-hr nap taken in the circadian nadir (Naitoh et al., 1982, as cited in Ref. 1), a 30-min nap opportunity scheduled at either 01:00 or 03:30 hours (57), and a nap at 03:00 hours (58) produce little to no benefit. Contrary to these findings, 20-min naps scheduled between 01:00 and 03:00 hours (35), 30- or 50-min naps taken at 01:00 or 04:00 hr (33), 1-hr naps taken at 02:00 hours (32), and 2-hr naps taken between 04:00 and 06:00 hours (59) have been shown to improve cognitive performance and/or alertness. Nevertheless, the findings generally support the notion that naps taken near the circadian nadir have less recuperative value than naps taken in the afternoon.

Studies comparing evening naps with early-morning naps (60,61) and naps taken at late morning (28) have shown no differential effects due to circadian placement. When evening naps (19:00–21:00 hours) were compared with naps scheduled in the midafternoon (15:00–17:00 hours), greater postnap sleepiness and mood decrements were associated with the evening naps (Lavie and Veler, in press, as cited in Ref. 10). On balance, these findings suggest that although evening naps are no more or less effective than morning naps, evening naps are less effective than naps scheduled in the afternoon.

In terms of the optimal timing of napping in the afternoon, Hayashi and his colleagues showed that a 20-min nap scheduled in the midafternoon (14:00 hours) provided greater recuperative value than a nap scheduled in the early afternoon (12:20 hours) (41,42). Data indicating that regular nappers tend to nap in the midafternoon period also evidences the superior recuperative power of midafternoon naps. For example, Webb and Dinges (62) analyzed the Human Relations Area Files, a cross-cultural survey that compiles and classifies information on more than 1700 cultures worldwide, and reported that "virtually all of the siesta cultures described in the file have preferred times for napping between 1200 and 1600 hr" (p. 255). In college student populations, the "nap zone" has been shown to occur between 14:00 and 18:00 hours (3) with the peak number of nap sleep onsets occurring at 16:00 hours (63).

MSLT data for young adults have also identified the period near 15:30 as a time of increased sleepiness (64). Furthermore, the endogenous circadian rhythm of sleep propensity as derived from a laboratory-controlled, constant-routine procedure confirmed the timing of the afternoon sleepy period to be 13:40 in a midtwenties, full-time-employed sample (56) and about 15:30 in a young-adult student sample (65).

The above findings indicate that sleepiness, and therefore the tendency for napping, is increased in the early to midafternoon. One may argue that napping occurring at this time represents time of greater opportunity to nap, rather than an underlying circadian predisposition. Opportunity may indeed be the reason for some people to nap in the midafternoon. Nevertheless, evidence obtained by Dinges et al. (1983, as cited in Ref. 3) suggests midafternoon napping is temporally bound to the circadian cycle. Sleep log data of 58 regular nappers in a college student population revealed that subjects averaged longer nocturnal sleep durations on weekends relative to weekdays and a significant phase shift in nocturnal sleep time on weekends (mean delay of 47 min in midnocturnal sleep times). Midnap sleep time was also delayed on weekends, by an average of 36 min. In addition, Lack and Lushington (56) found the afternoon sleepy period to be significantly correlated ($r = .81$) with the endogenous core temperature minimum. Thus, napping in the afternoon does appear to be regulated by the circadian system and is not simply the function of opportunity.

In accordance with research pertaining to the timing of naps during the 24-hr day, it appears that circadian constraints determine not only when a nap is most likely to occur, but also when a nap is most likely to have recuperative value. The time at which naps appear to have the greatest recuperative power is the early- to midafternoon period, which coincides with the endogenous afternoon peak in sleepiness. In terms of designing sleep management schedules for operational settings, it would make sense to schedule napping during the afternoon sleepy period because this is a time when individuals are looking for countermeasures to their sleepiness, when sleep latency will be relatively short and therefore when sleep efficiency will be maximized.

### E.  Prior Wake Time

In addition to the circadian timing of naps, the effectiveness of napping may also depend on the length of wakefulness preceding the nap, such that napping occurring after prolonged wakefulness will be less effective or produce shorter-lasting effects than napping occurring after a shorter period of sleep loss (i.e., prophylactic napping) (66). Indeed, Dinges et al. (1) found that the benefits associated with prophylactic naps exceeded the benefits derived from napping after prolonged wakefulness. Specifically, 2-hr naps taken 6 and 18 hr into a 56-hr period of otherwise sustained wakefulness produced more robust and longer-lasting reaction time performance improvements relative to a control group than 2-hr naps taken after 30–42 hr of sustained wakefulness.

Nevertheless, prophylactic napping is not always feasible; hence it is worthwhile considering the duration of nap sleep required for restoring cognitive functioning to baseline levels after different-length periods of prolonged wakefulness. This issue has been addressed in studies conducted by Morgan and Coates (1974, as cited in Ref. 10) and Rosa (67). After 36 hr of continuous work, 2 or 3 hr of "rest" (i.e., sleep, eating and other activities) appears to be necessary to restore performance to 60% of baseline, 4 hr to restore to 70% and 12 hr to restore to 100%, while after 44 hr of work, 4 hr of "rest" appears to be required to restore performance to 40% of baseline levels (Morgan & Coates, 1974, as cited in Ref. 10). In a study incorporating sleep periods (as opposed to rest periods) it was found that after 48 hr of continuous work, 4 hr of sleep restored reaction time performance to baseline levels, whereas after 64 hr of continuous work, 8 hr of sleep was required to return performance to baseline levels (67).

Taken together, these findings suggest that naps will be differentially beneficial according to the duration of prior wakefulness. Naps taken earlier into the period of prolonged wakefulness will be more effective than naps taken later into the sleep loss period. Furthermore, the longer the period of sleep loss preceding the nap, the longer the length of the nap required to compensate for sleep loss.

### F. Napping Strategies for Periods of Extended Wakefulness

In considering a napping strategy under periods of prolonged wakefulness, it is important to recognize that many occupations that require employees to be engaged in prolonged periods of activity cannot accommodate a long monophasic sleep period. Frequently occurring shorter naps may offer a flexible approach to maintaining an acceptable level of functioning over such an extended period, without significantly interfering with operational demands. For example, yachtsmen involved in long-distance solo races are able to avert long episodes of continuous sleep by repeatedly taking brief naps (68). Several experimental studies have been undertaken to investigate whether multiple shorter sleeps can be used to maintain alertness and performance during long continuous periods of work that do not allow less frequent, longer sleeps.

Naitoh et al. (45) employed a sleep/wake schedule of 20-min naps every 6 hr during a 64-hr period of continuous work, comparing this experimental condition against a second condition comprising total sleep deprivation for the entire 64-hr period. Compared to the sleep deprivation condition, the 20-min naps significantly reduced the cumulative effects of sleep loss on a four-choice reaction time task.

In a study employing a 42-hr period of otherwise continuous work, Mullaney et al. (69) tracked the effects of six evenly spaced 1-hr naps (polyphasic sleep group) and a single 6-hr nap taken after 18 hr of wakefulness (monophasic sleep group), with respect to a no-nap condition (sleep deprivation group). In the first 18 hr of the experiment, the polyphasic sleep group showed superior cognitive performance relative to the other two conditions. Although performance was superior for the monophasic sleep group over the entire 42-hr period, this finding is confounded by the fact that participants obtained more sleep in the monophasic sleep condition than the polyphasic sleep condition. In addition, performance measures derived immediately after the naps were included in the overall analyses; hence six incidences of sleep inertia were included in analyses for the polyphasic sleep group compared to once for the monophasic sleep group.

Other research suggests that under extreme sleep deprivation conditions, multiple shorter naps may be more effective than single longer periods of sleep (54). For example, over a period of 4 consecutive days, three 80-min naps per day have been shown to be more effective than one 4-hr nap per day, in offsetting vigilance performance decrements (Hartley, 1974, as cited in Ref. 10). However, in interpreting these results, it should be noted that the interval between waking and performance testing was considerably longer after the longer nap compared to the shorter naps (10).

Haslam (70) observed, during 4 days of quasi-continuous work after a 23-hr period of wakefulness, that four 1-hr naps per day were comparable to a single

4-hr nap, in terms of effects on cognitive performance and mood. The utility of both nap schedules was evidenced on the final experimental day, during which cognitive performance and mood were comparable to baseline values.

Taken together, these findings suggest that multiple naps may be effective in offsetting performance impairments during prolonged periods of wakefulness. Furthermore, while monophasic sleep may be superior to polyphasic sleep under conditions of prolonged wakefulness (69), polyphasic sleep schedules may be more effective under conditions of extreme sleep deprivation (54). For a comprehensive review of polyphasic sleep schedules, refer to Ref. 54.

### G.  Individual Differences

The duration of a nap, level of sleep deprivation, circadian timing of a nap, and nap sleep infrastructure are considered among the most important factors that determine the effectiveness of daytime napping. However, the effectiveness of daytime napping may also vary according to whether the individual is a habitual napper or nonnapper. Taub and Berger (71) asserted that optimal levels of behavioral functioning are contingent upon the maintenance of an established sleep schedule, suggesting that napping will be more beneficial to individuals who habitually nap. In their studies of habitual nappers, Taub et al. (27,28) found that an afternoon nap improved mood and performance in these subjects. They did not, however, compare habitual nappers with unaccustomed nappers.

Consistent with Taub and Berger's assertion, Evans et al. (26) found that individuals who habitually napped obtained greater subjective benefit from an afternoon nap than individuals who were not accustomed to napping. Habitual nappers felt less tired and sleepy after the afternoon nap and were more satisfied with the nap, compared to nonnappers.

Contrary to Taub and Berger (71) and Evans et al. (26), Daiss et al. (72) reported that an afternoon nap improved mood from prenap to postnap irrespective of whether the individual was a habitual napper or not. Further, several research groups have studied the effects of napping with subjects who were not habitual nappers and documented improved performance and subjective alertness after napping (e.g., Refs. 20,36,38,39,41). However, these researchers did not compare the improvement of these nonnappers with a group of regular nappers.

In summary, relevant research pertaining to napper type is limited and findings are mixed. Some research suggests differential improvements following napping, between nappers and nonnappers, whereas other research has demonstrated improvements irrespective of napper type. One could conclude, however, that demonstrating beneficial effects of napping for nonnappers would imply that napping would be beneficial to habitual nappers also.

### H.  Workplace Napping

The discussion thus far has revealed the complex interaction of factors that contribute to the effectiveness of naps in well-controlled, laboratory-based research.

The real-life situation presents another dimension to this complexity. For example, naps that occur in the workplace may be shorter and more fragmented compared to naps examined under laboratory conditions (43), there may be more noise in the workplace (35), and suitable bedding may not be available in workplace settings. Of the limited research investigating the recuperative value of napping in the workplace, the aviation industry has been at the forefront of research.

A study conducted by the National Aeronautics and Space Administration and the Federal Aviation Administration investigated the benefits of a planned nap opportunity for pilots in long-haul flight operations (Rosekind et al., 1994, as cited in Ref. 15). Pilots in the rest group were permitted a 40-min nap opportunity (mean sleep duration of 25.8 min) in the cockpit seat, followed by a 20-min recovery period to allow for the dissipation of sleep inertia. The rest group showed a 34% improvement in vigilance performance and 54% improvement in physiological alertness [as indicated by EEG electro-oculographic (EOG) activity] after napping, relative to a no-rest group, who were not permitted an in-flight nap opportunity. In addition, the rest group totaled 34 "microsleeps" of 5 sec or more (and none during the descent and landing phases), compared to 120 microsleeps in the no-rest group, of which 22 occurred during the descent and landing phases. Controlled rest strategies have since been successfully implemented by some airlines, with a view to maintaining alertness and performance during long-haul flights (15).

A recent study of Air Traffic Controllers in New Zealand (43) examined whether a 40-min workplace nap opportunity, scheduled during a break on the night shift, improved psychomotor vigilance performance. The 40-min nap opportunity, resulting in a mean sleep duration of 17.7 min of fragmented sleep, significantly improved psychomotor performance, with stage 1 sleep significantly contributing to this improvement. In a study examining the impact of a 20-min nap opportunity during the night shift of aircraft maintenance engineers, Purnell et al. (35) found that a 20-min nap improved response speed on a vigilance task on the first night shift but not on the second. There were no significant effects of the nap on subjective sleepiness and fatigue or subsequent sleep duration and quality.

On balance, the applied research investigating napping provides evidence for the utility of workplace napping. To the extent that naps are beneficial in the workplace, they have important practical implications for many individuals and industry alike. With particular regard to industry, management may avoid the adverse effects of impaired performance, productivity, and workplace safety that accompanies sleepiness (15) by allowing employees to interject a nap into their work routines.

On a practical level, however, it would not be feasible for some organizations to implement a napping strategy incorporating a long nap, as substantial company time would need to be invested to allow sufficient opportunity for napping and subsequent recovery from sleep inertia. Thus, long naps are simply not practical in many operational settings, particularly those that require effective employee performance promptly after awakening. On the other hand, management may be more likely to implement a 10-min napping strategy as only slightly more than 10 min of company time would need to be invested, with immediate and identifiable benefits.

Nevertheless, although napping may provide a useful strategy for promoting alertness and performance after sleep deprivation, the implementation of a napping strategy in industry may raise issues of concern for management. To make the most effective use of company time, that is, to maximize sleep efficiency, managers would need to ensure that the environment for napping was conducive to sleep (22). Providing adequate ventilation, minimal noise, ambient temperature, pillows, and so forth may be a significant financial burden for many organizations. However, the cost of modifying the workplace environment to supplement the napping strategy needs to be balanced against the potential benefits of improved alertness, productivity, and safety in the workplace.

Another hurdle for the napping strategy is the attitude of many managers and employees who believe that napping represents substandard motivation and questionable work ethic (22). The first steps toward convincing management and employees to implement napping during hours of operation are to increase industry awareness of: (a) the detrimental and sometimes devastating consequences of daytime sleepiness (22), and (b) the opportunity provided by the napping strategy for improving employee alertness and performance during work hours.

## III.  Conclusions

In summary, as people continue to compromise their physiological sleep requirement in accordance with increased work, domestic, and social demands, there is an enormous opportunity afforded by napping for improving alertness, performance, and productivity. Indeed, even people who obtain adequate nocturnal sleep may derive some benefit from napping. However, as outlined in this chapter, napping is a complex issue. When devising a napping strategy, one would need to take into account the dissipation of sleep inertia, the time available for napping, the period of improvement sought by individuals, the circadian timing of the nap, the degree of sleep deprivation, individual differences, and the napping environment.

The following summary of the aforementioned research in this chapter may serve as a useful guide when devising a napping strategy:

Long naps have been shown to improve subjective and objective measures of alertness and performance.

Long naps may produce an immediate period of impaired alertness and performance (i.e., sleep inertia).

Long naps may disrupt the duration and architecture of subsequent sleep.

Brief naps on the order of 10 min appear to effectively ameliorate the adverse effects of sleep restriction.

Brief naps appear to be at least as effective as longer naps under conditions of restricted sleep and normal nocturnal sleep, and longer naps may be more effective under conditions of total sleep deprivation.

The benefits of brief naps may last up to 3 hr, whereas longer naps may have more long-lasting benefits.

The early- to midafternoon period is the time during which naps appear to be most recuperative.

Naps taken earlier into a period of prolonged wakefulness may be more effective than naps taken later into the period.

The longer the period of wakefulness preceding the nap, the longer the nap duration required to compensate for the sleep loss.

The mechanism by which naps produce benefits is poorly understood and further research is required.

There is some suggestion that nappers may obtain greater benefit from napping than nonnappers.

Multiple naps may be effective in offsetting performance impairments during prolonged periods of wakefulness.

Research (albeit limited) indicates that napping produces alertness and performance benefits in operational settings.

From a practical viewpoint, brief naps are more amenable to incorporation into an existing work schedule compared to naps of longer duration.

## References

1. Dinges DF, Orne MT, Whitehouse WG, Orne EC. Temporal placement of a nap for alertness: contributions of circadian phase and prior wakefulness. Sleep 1987; 10:313–329.
2. Naitoh P. Circadian Cycles and Restorative Power of Naps. 1981:553–580.
3. Dinges DF. Napping patterns and effects in human adults. In: Dinges DF, Broughton RJ, eds. Sleep and Alertness: Chronobiological, Behavioral, and Medical Aspects of Napping. New York: Raven Press, 1989:171–204.
4. Pilcher JJ, Michalowski KR, Carrigan RD. The prevalence of daytime napping and its relationship to nighttime sleep. Behav Med 2001; 27:71–76.
5. Gillberg M, Kecklund G, Axelsson J, Åkerstedt T. The effects of a short daytime nap after restricted night sleep. Sleep 1996; 19:570–575.
6. Broughton R, Dinges DF. Napping: A ubiquitous enigma. In: Dinges DF, Broughton RJ, eds. Sleep and Alertness: Chronobiological, Behavioral, and Medical Aspects of Napping. New York: Raven Press, 1989:1–7.
7. Sugerman JL, Walsh JK. Physiological sleep tendency and ability to maintain alertness at night. Sleep 1989; 12:106–112.
8. Dinges DF. Adult napping and its effects on ability to function. In: Stampi C, ed. W W N: Evolution, Chronobiology, and Functions of Polyphasic and Ultrashort Sleep. Boston: Birkhauser, 1992:118–134.
9. Carskadon MA, Dement WC, Mitler MM, Roth T, Westbrook PR, Keenan S. Guidelines for the Multiple Sleep Latency Test (MSLT): A standard measure of sleepiness. Sleep 1986; 9:519–524.

10. Naitoh P, Angus RG. Napping and human functioning during prolonged work. In: Dinges DF, Broughton RJ, eds. Sleep and Alertness: Chronobiological, Behavioral, and Medical Aspects of Napping. New York: Raven Press, 1989:221–246.

11. Jewett ME, Wyatt JK, Ritz-De Cecco A, Khalsa SB, Dijk D-J, Czeisler CA. Time course of sleep inertia dissipation in human performance and alertness. J Sleep Res 1999; 8:1–8.

12. Achermann P, Werth E, Dijk D-J, Borbély AA. Time course of sleep inertia after nighttime and daytime sleep episodes. Arch Ital Biol 1995; 134:109–119.

13. Folkard S, Åkerstedt T. A three-process model of the regulation of alertness-sleepiness. In: Broughton RJ, Ogilvie RD, eds. Sleep, Arousal, and Performance. Boston: Birkhauser, 1992:11–26.

14. Tassi P, Muzet A. Sleep inertia. Sleep Med Rev 2000; 4:341–353.

15. Rosekind MR, Smith RM, Miller DL, et al. Alertness management: strategic naps in operational settings. J Sleep Res 1995; 4:62–66.

16. Bruck D, Pisani DL. The effects of sleep inertia on decision-making performance. J Sleep Res 1999; 8:95–103.

17. Dinges DF. Are you awake? Cognitive performance and reverie during the hypnopompic state. 1990; 159–175.

18. Naitoh P, Kelly T, Babkoff H. Sleep inertia: best time not to wake up? Chronobiol Int 1993; 10:109–118.

19. Guido P, Rosenthal L, Nykamp K, et al. Sleep inertia following one and twenty minute nap opportunities. Sleep 1998; 21:165.

20. Tietzel AJ, Lack LC. A brief afternoon nap following nocturnal sleep restriction: what is the optimal nap duration? Sleep. Under review.

21. Dinges DF, Orne MT, Orne EC. Sleep depth and other factors associated with performance upon abrupt awakening. Sleep Res 1985; 14:92.

22. Muzet A, Nicolas A, Tassi P, Dewasmes G, Bonneau A. Implementation of napping in industry and the problem of sleep inertia. J Sleep Res 1995; 4:67–69.

23. Fort A, Mills JN. Influence of sleep, lack of sleep and circadian rhythm on short psychometrics tests. In: Colquhoun WP, ed. Aspects of Human Efficiency: Diurnal Rhythm and Loss of Sleep. London: English University Press, 1972:115–127.

24. Stampi C, Mullington J, Rivers M, Campos JP, Broughton R. Ultrashort sleep schedules: sleep architecture and recuperative value of 80–, 50– and 20–min naps. In: Horne J, ed. Sleep '90. Bochum: Pontenagel Press, 1990:71–74.

25. Ferrara M, De Gennaro L. The sleep inertia phenomenon during the sleep-wake transition: theoretical and operational issues. Aviat Space Environ Med 2000; 71:843–848.

26. Evans FJ, Cook MR, Cohen HD, Orne EC, Orne MT. Appetitive and replacement naps: EEG and behavior. Science 1977; 197:687–688.

27. Taub JM, Tanguay PE, Clarkson D. Effects of daytime naps on performance and mood in a college student population. J Abnorm Psychol 1976; 85:210–217.

28. Taub JM, Hawkins DR, Van de Castle RL. Temporal Relationships of napping behavior to performance, mood states and sleep physiology. Sleep Res 1978; 7:164.

29. Taub JM. Effects of scheduled afternoon naps and bedrest on daytime alertness. Int J Neurosci 1982; 16:107–127.

30. Carskadon MA, Dement WC. Effects of a daytime nap on sleepiness during sleep restriction. Sleep Res 1986; 15:69.

31. Lumley M, Roehrs T, Zorick F, Lamphere J, Roth T. The alerting effects of naps in sleep-deprived subjects. Psychophysiology 1986; 23:403–408.

32. Rogers AS, Spencer MB, Stone BM, Nicholson AN. The influence of a 1 h nap on performance overnight. Ergonomics 1989; 32:1193–1205.

33. Sallinen M, Härmä M, Åkerstedt T, Rosa R, Lillqvist O. Promoting alertness with a short nap during a night shift. J Sleep Res 1998; 7:240–247.

34. Åkerstedt T, Torsvall L, Gillberg M. Shift work and napping. In: Dinges DF, Broughton R, eds. Sleep and Alertness: Chronobiological, Behavioral and Medical Aspects of Napping. New York: Raven Press, 1989:205–220.

35. Purnell MT, Feyer A-M, Herbison GP. The impact of a nap opportunity during the night shift on the performance and alertness of 12–h shift workers. J Sleep Res 2002; 11:219–227.

36. Horne JA, Reyner LA. Counteracting driver sleepiness: effects of napping, caffeine, and placebo. Psychophysiology 1996; 33:306–309.

37. Takahashi M, Arito H. Maintenance of alertness and performance by a brief nap after lunch under prior sleep deficit. Sleep 2000; 23:813–819.

38. Tietzel AJ, Lack LC. The short-term benefits of brief and long naps following nocturnal sleep restriction. Sleep 2001; 24:293–300.

39. Tietzel AJ, Lack LC. The recuperative value of brief and ultra-brief daytime naps. J Sleep Res 2002; 11:213–218.

40. Takahashi M, Fukuda H, Arito H. Brief naps during post-lunch rest: effects on alertness, performance, and autonomic balance. Eur J Appl Physiol Occup Physiol 1998; 78:93–98.

41. Hayashi M, Watanabe M, Hori T. The effects of a 20 min nap in the mid-afternoon on mood, performance and EEG activity. Clin Neurophysiol 1999; 110:272–279.

42. Hayashi M, Ito S, Hori T. The effects of a 20–min nap at noon on sleepiness, performance and EEG activity. Int J Psychophysiol 1999; 32:173–180.

43. Signal L, Gander PH. Psychomotor performance improvements with a short workplace nap on the night shift: the benefits of stage 1 sleep. Sleep 2002; 25:A116.

44. Tamaki M, Shirota A, Hayashi M, Hori T. Restorative effects of a short afternoon nap (<30 min) in the elderly on subjective mood, performance and EEG activity. Sleep Res Online 2000; 3:131–139.

45. Naitoh P, Kelly TL, Babkoff H. Napping, Stimulant, and Four-Choice Performance. In: Broughton RJ, Ogilvie RD, eds. Sleep, Arousal, and Performance: A Tribute to Bob Wilkinson. Boston: Birkhauser, 1992:198–219.

46. Naitoh P. Minimal sleep to maintain performance: the search for sleep quantum in sustained operations. In: Stampi C, ed. WHY WE NAP: Evolution, Chronobiology, and Functions of Polyphasic and Ultrashort Sleep. Boston: Birkhauser, 1992:199–216.

47. Bonnet MH. Performance and sleepiness as a function of frequency and placement of sleep disruption. Psychophysiology 1986; 23:263–271.

48. Helmus T, Rosenthal L, Bishop C, Roehrs T, Syron ML, Roth T. The alerting effects of short and long naps in narcoleptic, sleep deprived, and alert individuals. Sleep 1997; 20:251–257.

49. Borbély AA. A Two process model of sleep regulation. Hum Neurobiol 1982; 1:195–204.

50. Borbély AA, Achermann P. Concepts and models of sleep regulation: an overview. J Sleep Res 1992; 1:63–79.

51. Taub JM. Effects of habitual variations in napping on psychomotor performance, memory and subjective states. Int J Neurosci 1979; 9:97–112.

52. Davidson JR, Radomski MWM, Heslegrave RJ, Angus RG, Montelpare WJ. Sleep structure of a nap following 40 hours of sleep deprivation and its relation to performance upon awakening. Sleep Res 1986; 15:213.

53. Lavie P. To nap, perchance to sleep—ultradian aspects of napping. In: Dinges DF, Broughton RJ, eds. Sleep and Alertness: Chronobiological, Behavioral, and Medical Aspects of Napping. New York: Raven Press, 1989:99–120.

54. Stampi C. The effects of polyphasic and ultrashort sleep schedules. In: Stampi C, ed. W W N: Evolution, Chronobiology, and Functions of Polyphasic and Ultrashort Sleep. Boston: Birkhauser, 1992:137–179.

55. Dijk D-J, Czeisler CA. Paradoxical timing of the circadian rhythm of sleep propensity serves to consolidate sleep and wakefulness in humans. Neurosci Lett 1994; 166:63–68.

56. Lack LC, Lushington K. The rhythms of human sleep propensity and core body temperature. J Sleep Res 1996; 5:1–11.

57. Gillberg M, Kecklund G, Åkerstedt T. Sleepiness and performance of professional drivers in a truck simulator—comparisons between day and night driving. J Sleep Res 1996; 5:12–15.

58. Saitoh Y, Sasaki T. Sleepiness and fatigue during early morning hours after a 30 minute nocturnal nap. Shiftwork Int Newslett 1995; 12:53.

59. Angus RG, Pigeau RA, Heslegrave RJ. Sustained-operations studies: from the field to the laboratory. In: Stampi C, ed. W W N: Evolution, Chronobiology, and Functions of Polyphasic and Ultrashort Sleep. Boston: Birkhauser, 1992:217–241.

60. Gillberg M. Effects of naps on performance. In: Folkard S, Monk T, eds. Hours of Work. New York: Wiley, 1985:77–86.

61. Gillberg M, Åkerstedt T. Effect of a 1–hour nap on performance following restricted sleep. In: Koella WP, ed. Sleep 1982. Basel: Karger, 1983:392–394.

62. Webb WB, Dinges DF. Cultural perspectives on napping and the siesta. In: Dinges DF, Broughton RJ, eds. Sleep and Alertness: Chronobiological, Behavioral, and Medical Aspects of Napping. New York: Raven Press, 1989:247–265.

63. Dinges DF, Orne MT, Orne EC, Evans FJ. Behavioral patterns in habitual nappers. Sleep Res 1981; 10:136.

64. Carskadon MA. Ontogeny of human sleepiness as measured by sleep latency. In: Dinges DF, Broughton RJ, eds. Sleep and Alertness: Chronobiological, Behavioral, and Medical Aspects of Napping. New York: Raven Press, 1989:53–69.

65. Lack LC, Patrick S. Evidence that the "post-lunch dip" is endogenous to the circadian system. Sleep 2000; 23:A46–A47.

66. Dinges DF. An overview of sleepiness and accidents. J Sleep Res 1995; 4:4–14.

67. Rosa RR. Recovery of performance during sleep following sleep deprivation. Soc Psychophysiolog Res 1983; 20:152–159.

68. Stampi C. Ultrashort sleep/wake patterns and sustained performance. In: Dinges DF, Broughton RJ, eds. Sleep and Alertness: Chronobiological, Behavioral, and Medical Aspects of Napping. New York: Raven Press, 1989:139–169.

69. Mullaney DJ, Kripke DF, Fleck PA, Johnson LC. Sleep loss and nap effects on sustained continuous performance. Psychophysiology 1983; 20:643–651.

70. Haslam DR. Sleep deprivation and naps. Behav Res Meth, Instrum Comput 1985; 17:46–54.

71. Taub JM, Berger RJ. Performance and mood following variations in the length and timing of sleep. Psychophysiology 1973; 10:559–570.

72. Daiss SR, Bertelson AD, Benjamin LT Jr. Napping versus resting: effects on performance and mood. Psychophysiology 1986; 23:82–88.

# 23

## Sleep Restriction as Therapy for Insomnia

**CHARLES M. MORIN, MÉLANIE LEBLANC, AND
MEAGAN DALEY**

Université Laval, Québec, Canada

### I.  Introduction

Insomnia is a prevalent health complaint affecting between 9% and 12% of the
adult population on a chronic basis and up to one third occasionally (1). Several
therapeutic options, including behavioral and pharmacological approaches, are
available for the management of insomnia. Pharmacotherapy is by far the most
frequently used approach in clinical practice. While it is effective for the short-
term treatment of insomnia, a number of drawbacks are associated with the use
of hypnotics, including their daytime residual effects and the risks of tolerance
and dependence associated with long-term use. Several behavioral interventions
have also been developed and validated for this condition (2–4). These methods
include stimulus control, relaxation training, cognitive therapy, sleep hygiene,
and sleep restriction therapy. Their use is predicated on the assumption that mal-
adaptive sleep habits and dysfunctional sleep cognitions perpetuate insomnia.
This chapter addresses the nature and use of sleep restriction as a therapeutic
approach for insomnia. After describing the rationale and specific methods of this
clinical procedure, we review the evidence regarding its efficacy, mechanisms of
action, and limitations, as well as some practical issues concerning its implementation in clinical practice.

## II.  Sleep Restriction Therapy: Background and Rationale

Sleep restriction therapy (SRT), as a therapeutic intervention for insomnia, was first described by Spielman and his colleagues (5). It involves a systematic curtailing of *time allowed in bed* at night. This restriction is intended to counteract an important factor involved in the perpetuation of insomnia—that of spending too much time in bed (6). Indeed, individuals with chronic insomnia often spend excessive amounts of time awake in bed in a misguided effort to compensate for poor sleep or lack of sleep. This may involve going to bed early in the evening, staying in bed later in the morning, or napping during the day. The main objective of SRT is to consolidate the sleep episode(s) into a more restricted period of time allowed in bed (i.e., sleep window). Such a countermeasure to insomnia appears somewhat paradoxical, at least upon first presentation, because insomnia is often equated with sleep loss/deprivation. Although there is some sleep loss in insomnia, the main features of this condition involve difficulties initiating and maintaining sleep, with reduced sleep efficiency. The extent of sleep loss per se is often not excessive (7). Furthermore, SRT involves a curtailment of time spent in bed, not necessarily sleep time, as most of this curtailment involves time that is usually spent awake. As such, SRT should not be equated with sleep deprivation per se; perhaps SRT is a misnomer because the time that is taken away from the insomnia patient is usually time that is spent awake.

The theoretical rationale behind SRT is derived from our current understanding of the mechanisms regulating the sleep-wake cycles (8). At least two factors regulate the propensity and the timing of sleep, namely homeostatic and circadian processes. Homeostasis involves the natural drive to seek sleep after extended periods of wakefulness. This drive increases with the duration of the current episode of wakefulness. Indeed, Webb and Agnew (9,10) showed that good sleepers who were sleep-deprived subsequently fell asleep faster and experienced more slow-wave sleep during recovery nights. As such, SRT is a procedure that capitalizes on these effects, while controlling the duration and intensity of the sleep deprivation and sleepiness that follows. Circadian rhythms, which are controlled predominantly by the suprachiasmatic nucleus located in the hypothalamus, regulate the timing of sleep-wake cycles over the 24-hr period. Homeostasis and circadian processes work in tandem to influence sleep/wake cycles. There may be a disruption of one or both of these mechanisms among insomnia sufferers. Interventions such as bright-light therapy and melatonin target the circadian processes, whereas sleep restriction addresses directly the homeostatic drive to sleep.

The postulated mechanisms of action of SRT are twofold, physiological and psychological. First, SRT produces a mild sleep deprivation, which increases the homeostatic drive to sleep. In addition, sleep anticipatory anxiety is a common feature among insomnia sufferers. Indeed, there is often a great deal of apprehension about bedtime, about the fear of not being able to fall asleep, and about the potential consequences of insomnia the next day. As SRT involves a postponement of bedtime, it also produces a paradoxical effect, i.e., whereas the patient fears insomnia, he/she is now required to deliberately postpone bedtime to a later hour than usual. The patient's focus of attention often changes from worrying about one's inability to sleep to wondering what he/she will do until the prescribed bedtime. Consequently, SRT produces a paradoxical effect that decreases sleep anticipatory anxiety and the conditioned arousal that often perpetuates insomnia (7,11).

## III. Treatment Implementation

Keeping a daily sleep diary is essential to implement SRT effectively. Although the sleep diary is subject to distortions (12), it is a standard assessment procedure for collecting the daily estimates of sleep-wake parameters necessary for SRT. The diary serves several functions, including that of determining baseline values of total sleep time and time spent in bed to set an appropriate sleep window during the intervention. Ideally, those baseline values are based on at least 1 week and, preferably, 2 weeks of self-monitoring.

Several sleep-wake parameters are derived from the diary. Time in bed (TIB) is based on the total time elapsed from initial bedtime to final rising time. Total sleep time (TST) is then derived by subtracting from TIB the amount of time required to fall asleep, the total amount of time spent awake during nighttime awakenings, and the amount of time spent awake in the morning before rising. A sleep efficiency (SE) percentage for each night is then derived (TST/TIB x 100) and a weekly average calculated. For example, an individual, who reports sleeping during baseline an average of 6 hr while spending 8 hr in bed has a sleep ratio of 3:4, or a sleep efficiency of 75%. The objective of SRT is to come as close as possible to a perfect match between TST and TIB, or a 1:1 ratio.

The average time asleep per night becomes the basis upon which a sleep window (bedtime and rising time) is derived. For the present example, TIB would be restricted to 6 hr/night, with the individual selecting his bedtime and rising times. Although there is some flexibility in changing bedtime and rising times, as treatment unfolds it is preferable to keep the rising times as stable as possible to establish a consistent sleep-wake rhythm. To control the degree of daytime sleepiness and to enhance treatment compliance, it is not advisable to restrict time in bed (the sleep window) below 4.5 or 5 hr/night, regardless of the reported sleep time during baseline. These parameters can also be adjusted as a function of the patient's acceptance of and adherence to these prescriptions. The prescribed sleep window does not represent a mandatory period to be spent in bed; rather, it specifies the maximal duration an individual is allowed to spend in bed. Sleeping, napping, or lying down is usually not permitted between rising and retiring times, although some exception to this rule are discussed below for the treatment of insomnia in older adults.

Periodic adjustments to the sleep window are made contingent upon the SE ratio for the previous week. In Spielman et al.'s original study (5), patients had to call in their sleep data on a daily basis and adjustments to the sleep window were made based on a moving average for the preceding 5 days. The original criteria for changing the prescribed TIB were as follows: if the average SE was >90%, TIB was increased by 15 min, usually by going to bed earlier. If the average SE was <85%, TIB was decreased by 15 min. No TIB changes were made when SE fell between 85% and 90%.

Different investigators have used several variations of Spielman's original protocol. For example, adjustments to the sleep window are typically done on a weekly basis to coincide with follow-up consultation visits. In addition, some investigators have used different cutoff SE values (e.g., 80% rather than 85%) to adjust the sleep window (13,14). Others have introduced the restriction of TIB gradually over time, rather than abruptly at the beginning of treatment (15,16). Indeed, while SRT reduces TIB on the very first session to a value equal to subjectively reported TST, with subsequent adjustments made based on SE variations, sleep compression, in contrast, allows the patient to gradually *reduce* TIB to more closely match TST (16). Although napping is forbidden in most insomnia treatment studies, some investigators (17,18) have made napping optional with older adults, especially in the early phase of treatment to promote adherence with SRT. Finally, TIB is usually increased until an optimal sleep duration/sleep efficiency balance is achieved.

## IV.  Empirical Support

In their original clinical case series (5), Spielman and his colleagues evaluated SRT with 35 middle-aged patients presenting to a sleep clinic with various subtypes of chronic insomnia (i.e., primary and secondary). The results indicated that SE was increased by 20% from baseline to posttreatment (67% to 87%), with a correspondingly increased TST (average of 33 min), and decreased total wake time by an average of 108 min. TIB was reduced from an average of 8 hr to 6.5 hr. In addition, follow-up data showed that sleep improvements were well maintained over time, with TST remaining stable, and SE decreasing slightly. There was a significant reduction of the variability of several sleep parameters with treatment, a positive outcome given the extensive night-to-night variability in the sleep patterns of insomnia patients. The outcomes were similar for medicated and unmedicated patients and for patients with primary insomnia and those with insomnia associated with psychiatric disorders.

Subsequently, several authors have tested SRT, either alone or as one component in multifactorial interventions. The majority of the studies evaluating SRT alone have focused on elderly populations. As sleep becomes fragmented, daytime alertness is reduced, and insomnia vulnerability increases with aging. Older adults often spend more time in bed to cope with these changes. Although this response is adaptive in the short term, it may also perpetuate/exacerbate sleep difficulties. The use of SRT is, therefore, very relevant for this segment of the population (11,19,20). Studies employing SRT with elderly individuals suffering from insomnia have generally shown a significant improvement in sleep continuity (i.e., reduced sleep onset latencies and wake after sleep onset), sleep efficiency, subjective sleep quality, and a reduction of stage 1 sleep (14,16,18,21–23). The outcomes on TST and daytime sleepiness have been more variable across studies (see Table 1). For subjective TST measures, some studies have reported an increment (5,14,23–27) and another study reported no change (22). For polysomnographic measures, no study reported a significant change of TST. One study reported no change at all (25), one reported a trend to increment (24), and one a trend to decrement (18). Finally, one study using actigraphy reported a decrement of TST after SRT (18). For daytime sleepiness, two studies found no significant changes on the Epworth Sleepiness Scale (ESS) (22) and on the Stanford Sleepiness Scale (SSS) (18), whereas one reported a slight decrease of daytime sleepiness on the SSS (16) and those using the Multiple Sleep Latency Test (MSLT) reported an increment of daytime sleepiness with SRT (18,24).

The preventive value of SRT has also been tested for slowing down the decline of sleep quality often experienced with aging (19). Hoch and colleagues examined the potential benefits of a simple variation of SRT (i.e., delaying bedtime by 30 min) in self-defined good sleepers without sleep disorders. The results showed that this minimal intervention increased sleep efficiency, slow-wave sleep, and the EEG delta power, and reduced sleep onset latency. These results suggest that a modest curtailment of time spent in bed is effective in preventing age-related declines in the sleep quality of otherwise healthy elderly good sleepers.

Two meta-analyses on the efficacy of nonpharmacological interventions for insomnia have shown that SRT produces, along with stimulus control therapy, among the largest effect sizes on sleep onset latency and wake after sleep onset variables (3,4). However, SRT alone has been evaluated in significantly fewer studies than other interventions. Furthermore, results from meta-analyses have also shown that SRT produces a reduction of TST, particularly at posttreatment, with a rebound/gain at short-term follow-ups. Three treatment studies of late-life insomnia have directly compared the relative efficacy of SRT to other nonphar-

**Table 1**  Effects of Sleep Restriction Therapy

| Parameters | Effects | References |
|---|---|---|
| Sleep continuity | ↓ Sleep onset latency | 5,14,19,21,22,25,26 |
| | ↓ Time awake after sleep onset | 14,16,22,25,26 |
| | ↑ Sleep efficiency | 5,16,19,22,25 |
| | ↔ or ↓ or ↑ Total sleep time | ↔22; ↓18; ↑5,14,25–27 |
| Sleep architecture | ↓ % stage 1 | 21 |
| | ↓ Stage shifts | |
| | ↑ Stages 3–4 and delta power | 19 |
| Daytime sleepiness | ↔ or ↑ or ↓ | ↔ 22; ↑24; ↓16 |
| Mood | ↓ Depressive symptoms | 27 |

macological interventions. In one unpublished study (24), SRT yielded comparable benefits to stimulus control therapy, and in two other studies it increased TST and SE significantly more than relaxation therapy (14,25).

In clinical practice, SRT is typically combined with other nonpharmacological interventions like stimulus control, relaxation, or cognitive therapy. Several studies employing a multicomponent treatment have reported significant improvements in sleep continuity and quality, but the specific contribution of SRT is unknown because of the multicomponent nature of those interventions (2). In one study (26), patients who had completed cognitive-behavioral therapy for insomnia were asked about their use of the program's 10 treatment components. The reported use of the stimulus control/sleep restriction component was the best predictor of improvements in sleep latency and nighttime wakefulness. Although relaxation was the most commonly endorsed strategy, it was not related to clinical outcomes. Finally, several case studies have also documented the benefits of SRT for other populations (27–29), including for the inpatient management of insomnia secondary to depression and chronic pain (28).

## V. Clinical and Practical Issues

SRT is indicated for the management of chronic insomnia (primary or secondary) involving difficulties initiating and/or maintaining sleep (30). Individuals with fragmented sleep or even with sleep state misperception may also be responsive to this approach by gaining a more consolidated and deeper sleep and, perhaps, improving the perception of having slept. On the other hand, sleep restriction is not indicated for individuals with sleep apnea or other conditions producing excessive daytime sleepiness or for patients with a bipolar disorder, and special caution is needed with patients for whom daytime alertness cannot be compromised (e.g., transport drivers, emergency staff). Sleep restriction is also contraindicated for patients with insomnia complaints when there is additional evidence of night terrors or sleepwalking; the possible increase in slow-wave sleep produced by sleep restriction might increase the propensity of the parasomnia.

As for most behavioral therapies, the success of SRT is entirely dependent on the patient's compliance with the prescribed sleep window (7,22). Despite the apparent simplicity of this clinical procedure, therapist guidance is often essential to optimize compliance with the clinical recommendations (16). The first hurdle is making it clear to the patient *what* is expected and *why*. Indeed, the idea of curtailing even further the sleep of someone who presents with insomnia is somewhat paradoxical. For many patients, it is counterintuitive when sleep quality is unsatisfactory—from their vantage point, time in bed should be *increased* to obtain more satisfactory sleep. Thus, it is essential to explain the basic principles of sleep homeostasis and the rationale behind SRT, which should help patients better understand why time in bed should be restricted (27). The addition of sleep education is also useful for elderly individuals to explain the nature and extent of sleep changes associated with aging (16,18,22,25).

Another factor that may hinder compliance is the sleep loss experienced early in treatment. SRT initially produces a mild sleep deprivation, with associated daytime fatigue and drowsiness experienced in midafternoon and evening hours. Sometimes, patients worry that they will not be able to tolerate these effects (5,30). Education, reassurance, and support are important to alleviate fears, increase treatment compliance, and help reduce dropouts. Warning patients about this potential short-term effect is important, especially when full alertness at work or for other tasks is a concern (30).

Treatment compliance can also be thwarted for logistical reasons. Patients may complain of boredom or uncertainty as to what activities to perform during the time freed up by the new sleep schedule. In addition, they may be resistant to the idea that they should get out of bed and begin their day's activities as soon as they awaken in the morning, or leave the comfort of their bed if they waken during the night and cannot fall back asleep. These challenges are amplified for the elderly population, whose retirement schedule allows more flexibility for activities, including napping, bedtime, and rising time. Accordingly, some minor adjustments may be needed when using SRT with older adults. First, the 90% SE cutoff criterion should be decreased to 85% or even 80% to reflect age-related changes in sleep continuity (30). Some authors also allow a short afternoon nap to alleviate daytime sleepiness caused by restriction of time in bed (17,18). The impact of such modifications, however, is not entirely clear.

Attrition is a potential problem with SRT, as for most therapies. It is more likely to occur in the first 2 weeks of treatment, and particularly in the absence of therapist guidance. Thus, special attention, support, and compromise are needed to enhance compliance and minimize attrition. Dropout rates are a reflection, to some extent, of special challenges or dissatisfaction with an intervention. Vincent and Lionberg (31) examined treatment preference for and satisfaction with group treatment in 43 individuals with chronic insomnia. In general, cognitive-behavioral treatment was preferred over pharmacological treatment. Moreover, it seems that a more favorable attitude toward the therapy at pretreatment was associated with better adherence. Of the interventions studied, participants showed a higher preference for sleep hygiene and a lower preference for sleep restriction (also seen as the least useful). Interestingly, however, results showed that sleep restriction was associated with the largest improvements in sleep efficiency, sleep-related impairment, and quality of life. Furthermore, the more favorable the treatment was perceived, the more substantial were the improvements.

## VI. Conclusions

SRT has become a standard therapeutic approach, either alone or in combination with other methods, for the management of insomnia. Although it was formally described only 15 years ago, sleep restriction has probably been used as a naturalistic countermeasure to insomnia for much longer. The evidence available, although not very extensive, indicates that SRT is an effective intervention for treating insomnia. Its main effects are to consolidate sleep by reducing the time needed to initiate sleep and the amount of time spent awake at night. As such, it consolidates sleep over a shorter period of time and increases sleep efficiency. Aside from some daytime sleepiness during the initial part of the intervention, there are no side effects to this treatment. One of the limitations to existing research on SRT is that it has relied almost exclusively on subjective sleep data gathered from sleep diaries and questionnaires. Only a few studies have employed objective sleep measures such as polysomnography and wrist actigraphy to document the effects of SRT on sleep (18,21). More objective data of this nature are needed to develop a more thorough understanding of SRT effects on sleep, daytime functioning, and subjective well-being.

## Acknowledgments

Preparation of this chapter was supported in part by grants from the National Institute of Mental Health (Grant #60413) and the Canadian Institutes of Health Research (Grant #MT42504).

## References

1.  Ohayon MM. Epidemiology of insomnia: what we know and what we still need to learn. Sleep Med Rev 2002; 6:97–111.
2.  Morin CM, Hauri PJ, Espie CA, Spielman AJ, Buysse DJ, Bootzin RR. Nonpharmacological treatment of chronic insomnia. Sleep 1999; 22:1134–1156.
3.  Morin CM, Culbert JP, Schwartz SM. Nonpharmacological interventions for insomnia: a meta-analysis of treatment efficacy. Am J Psychiatry 1994; 151:1172–1180.
4.  Murtagh DR, & Greenwood KM. Identifying effective psychological treatments for insomnia: a meta-analysis. J Consul Clin Psychol 1995; 63:79–89.
5.  Spielman AJ, Saskin P, Thorpy MJ. Treatment of chronic insomnia by restriction of time in bed. Sleep 1987; 10:45–56.
6.  Spielman AJ, & Glovinsky P. The varied nature of insomnia. In: Hauri PJ, ed. Case Studies in Insomnia. New York: Plenum Press, 1991:1–15.
7.  Morin CM. Insomnia: Psychological Assessment and Management. New York: Guilford Press, 1993.
8.  Borbély AA, Achermann P. Sleep homeostasis and models of sleep regulation. In: Kryger MH, Roth T, Dement WC, eds. Principles and Practice of Sleep Medicine, 3rd ed. Philadelphia: Saunders, 2000: 377–390.
9.  Webb W, Agnew H. Sleep: effects of a restricted regime. Science 1965; 150:1745–1747.
10. Webb W, Agnew H. The effects of a chronic limitation of sleep length. Psychophysiology 1974; 11:265–274.
11. Wohlgemuth WK, Edinger JD. Sleep restriction therapy. In: Lichstein KL, Morin CM, eds. Treatment of Late-Life Insomnia. Sage: London, 2000:147–165.
12. Edinger JD, Fins AI. The distribution and clinical significance of sleep time misperceptions among insomniacs. Sleep 1995; 18:232–239.

13. Edinger JD, Hoelscher TJ, Marsh GR, Lipper S, Ionescu-Pioggia M. A cognitive-behavioral therapy for sleep-maintenance insomnia in older adults. Psychol Aging 1992; 7: 282–289.

14. Friedman L, Bliwise DL, Yesavage JA, Salom SR. A preliminary study comparing sleep restriction and relaxation treatments for insomnia in older adults. J Gerontol 1991; 46: P1–8.

15. McCurry SM, Logsdon RG, Vitiello MV, Teri L. Successful behavioral treatment for reported sleep problems in elderly caregivers of dementia patients: a controlled study. J Gerontol 1998; 53B:122–129.

16. Riedel BW, Lichstein KL, Dwyer WO. Sleep compression and sleep education for older insomniacs: self-help versus therapist guidance. Psychol Aging 1995; 10: 54–63.

17. Morin CM, Colecchi C, Stone J, Sood, R, Brink, D. Behavioral and pharmacological therapies for late-life insomnia. JAMA 1999; 28:991–999.

18. Friedman L, Benson, K, Noda A, Zarcone V, Wicks DA, O'Connell K, Brooks JO III, Bliwise DL, Yesavage, JA. An actigraphic comparison of sleep restriction and sleep hygiene treatments for insomnia in older adults. J Geriatr Psychiatry Neurol 2000; 13:17–27.

19. Hoch CC, Reynolds III CF, Buysse DJ, Monk TH, Nowell P, Begley AE, Hall F, Dew MA. Protecting sleep quality in later life: a pilot study of bed restriction and sleep hygiene. J Gerontol 2001; 56B:P52–P59.

20. Lichstein KL, Morin CM, eds. Treatment of Late-life Insomnia. California: Sage Publications, 2000.

21. Anderson MW, Zendell SM, Rubinstein ML, Spielman AJ. Daytime alertness in chronic insomnia: diagnostic differences and response to behavioral treatment. Sleep Res 1994; 23: 217.

22. Riedel BW, Lichstein KL. Strategies for evaluating adherence to sleep restriction treatment for insomnia. Behav Res Ther 2001; 39:201–212.

23. Bliwise DL, Friedman L, Nekich JC, Yesavage JA. Prediction of outcome in behaviorally based insomnia treatments. J Behav Ther Exp Psychiatry 1995; 26:17–23.

24. Anderson MW, Zendell SM, Rosa DP, Rubinstein ML, Herrera CO, Simons O, Caruso L, Spielman AJ. Comparison of sleep restriction therapy and stimulus control in older insomniacs: an update. Sleep Res 1988; 17:141.

25. Lichstein KL, Riedel BW, Wilson NM, Lester KW, Aguillard, RN. Relaxation and sleep compression for late-life insomnia: a placebo-controlled trial. J Consult Clin Psychol 2001; 69:227–239.

26. Harvey L, Inglis SJ, Espie C. Insomniacs' reported use of CBT components and relationship to long-term clinical outcome. Behav Res Ther 2002; 40:75–83.

27. Lichstein KL. Sleep compression treatment of an insomnoid. Behav Ther 1988; 19:625–632.

28. Morin CM, Kowatch RA, O'Shanick G. Sleep restriction for the inpatient treatment of insomnia. Sleep 1990; 13:183–186.

29. Hoelscher TJ, Edinger JD. Treatment of sleep-maintenance insomnia in older adults: Sleep period reduction, sleep education, and modified stimulus control. Psychol Aging 1988; 3:258–263.

30. Glovinsky PB, Spielman AJ. Sleep restriction therapy. In: Hauri PJ, ed. Case Studies in Insomnia. New York: Plenum Press, 1988.

31. Vincent N, Lionberg C. Treatment preference and patient satisfaction in chronic insomnia. Sleep 2001; 24:411–417.

# 24

## Recovery from Sleep Deprivation

**THOMAS S. KILDUFF**

SRI International, Menlo Park, California, U.S.A.

**CLETE A. KUSHIDA**

Stanford University, Stanford, California, U.S.A.

**AKIRA TERAO**

SRI International, Menlo Park, California, U.S.A.

## I.  Introduction

Sleep is commonly thought to be restorative in some way from prior wakeful activities. Although the function of sleep remains elusive, intracellular energy stores, membrane ionic gradients, and macromolecules have all been proposed to be restored during sleep. An assumption that underlies many experimental paradigms is that the restorative process(es) can be amplified or exacerbated by sleep deprivation (SD). Thus, by focusing on the sleep that occurs after a period of SD sometimes called "recovery sleep" (RS), it may be possible to identify restorative processes related to the function of sleep. In this chapter, we will discuss various aspects of RS and new observations regarding the genetic bases and molecular processes that occur during RS.

## II.  Sleep Deprivation and Recovery Sleep

### A.  Characteristics of Recovery Sleep

In humans, RS is typically studied by depriving subjects of sleep and then either allowing them to sleep ad libitum or scheduling them an extended time in bed. Loss of 1 night of sleep usually results in an extension of the subsequent night's sleep by approximately 10–20% (1,2). However, when subjects spend the subsequent 24 hr in bed, they recover 72% and 42% of the total amount of sleep lost during 24- and 48-hr SD periods, respectively (3). This study also showed that, although the majority of the RS occurred during the first 8 hr, significant recovery continued through a fourth 4-hr block after SD. Fragmentation of sleep during the recovery period diminishes its recuperative value; the mean sleep latencies of recovery naps after 1 night of SD increased linearly as the rate of arousal during the recovery naps decreased (4).

The role of circadian factors in RS has been investigated in both human and animal studies since the 1970s. In humans, a "90-min day" study placed subjects on a schedule of 60 min of wakefulness and 30 min of sleep for 5 1/3 24-hr periods, followed by two 24-hr recovery periods (5,6). Circadian patterns of sleep-wake behavior persisted despite increasing sleep debt, thus providing evidence for a circadian process associated with sleep and alertness independent of the homeostatic sleep drive. Sleep studies of humans maintained in temporal isolation indicated that sleep onset was coupled to the body temperature rhythm and that sleep duration was linked to the phase of temperature rhythm at sleep onset (7). Rapid-eye-movement (REM) sleep, in particular, was found to be tightly coupled to the circadian pacemaker (8). More recently, forced desynchrony studies have demonstrated dramatic alerting effects of the circadian system across the circadian day even after prolonged wakefulness (9,10). Other investigators have found that the composition of RS, especially the level of REM sleep, was relatively unaffected by circadian factors; instead, the response of the sleep system appeared to be primarily determined by non-REM (NREM) stage 4 debt (11). However, during the subjective day when melatonin was not produced, recovery after 24-hr SD did not occur in delayed-sleep-phase- syndrome patients, while RS occurred during the subjective day in controls (12).

Elimination of the circadian pacemaker in the suprachiasmatic nuclei (SCN) of the hypothalamus was first shown to result in arrhythmicity of the sleep/wake cycle in the mid-1970s (13). This observation led to the question of the role of the SCN in regulating the homeostatic response to sleep. Mistlberger et al. (14) assessed recovery sleep for 3–5 days after 24 hr of total sleep deprivation (TSD) in normal rats and in rats in which the SCN was surgically ablated. All groups showed immediate rebounds of high-amplitude NREM sleep and paradoxical (or REM) sleep, confined mostly to the first 12–18 hr of recovery, and decreases in moderate and low-amplitude NREM sleep during the first 6–12 hr of recovery. Sleep rebound was distributed over a longer period in SCN-lesioned rats but total accumulated rebound sleep was similar in all groups. Thus, the SCN were proposed to modulate the timing, but not the amount, of accumulated total sleep rebound. Tobler et al. (15) also assessed the effect of 24-hr TSD on sleep in SCN-lesioned rats. As found in the above study, SD caused an increase in total sleep, REM sleep, and the slow-wave sleep (SWS) portion of NREM sleep. On the basis of these results, the authors concluded that "the homeostatic component of sleep regulation is 'morphologically and functionally distinct' from the circadian component." In a study designed to assess the necessity of the SCN for the soporific effects of the benzodiazepine triazolam, state-specific electroencephalographic (EEG) power spectra profiles in SCN-lesioned rats were similar to those of intact animals although EEG slow-wave activity (SWA) in NREM sleep was markedly lower in SCN-lesioned rats (16). As recovery from 6-hr SD was characterized by a short-lasting reduction of REM sleep and a long-lasting increase of NREM sleep time at the cost of wakefulness and because EEG SWA rebounded during the first 8 hr in recovery, the authors concluded that major features of homeostatic sleep EEG regulation are present in SCN-lesioned rats. Thus, studies by three different laboratories support the concept that, although the circadian system is clearly involved in sleep expression, sleep homeostasis itself is not dependent upon an intact circadian system.

## B. Age-dependent Changes in Recovery Sleep

In SD studies on adolescents, Carskadon (17) found: (a) evidence of RS in subjects who were not only not sleep-deprived, but were on a sleep-"optimizing" schedule and had been awake only 10 hrs; (b) extended sleep starting 4 hr in advance of entrained sleep onset phase was not associated with a return of SWS; and (c) the homeostatic sleep/wake process becomes less robust or "sleep responsive" during adolescent development. After 25 hr of SD, middle-aged subjects (40–60 yrs) showed a steeper increase in the duration of wakefulness during daytime RS than younger subjects (18). In addition, middle-aged subjects showed a reduced rebound of SWS and SWA than that of the younger subjects.

In RS studies on a geriatric population, Bonnet (19,20) showed that subjective sleepiness did not return to baseline levels until early in the second recovery night after 64 hr of SD and that some of the subjects had a shortened REM latency, which was interpreted as evidence of decreased pressure for SWS in aging. Although subjects 80 years and older have lower sleep efficiencies and less delta sleep compared to younger subjects, sleep continuity and delta sleep are similarly enhanced in both age groups (21). Surprisingly, the young subjects had shorter daytime sleep latencies than the old, and mood and performance were disturbed by sleep loss to a greater extent among the young, leading the investigators to conclude that acute total sleep loss is a more disruptive procedure for the young than the old. Gender effects are evident in healthy elderly subjects sleep deprived for 36 hr; elderly women had better RS than elderly men, as evidenced by higher sleep maintenance/efficiency and more SWS (22).

Age-dependent changes in RS are not only restricted to humans; significant changes also occur in rats after 48 hr of SD (23). Young (3 months) and middle-aged (12 months) rats had large (21–24%) increases in total sleep time during RS whereas old (24 months) rats had a quantitatively small (8%) increase in total sleep. The young and middle-aged rats had increases in REM sleep, respectively, of 96% and 93% during RS compared to their baseline, which was significantly greater than the 65% increase observed in the old rats. These increases in total and REM sleep during recovery were largely confined to the first 6 hr in young and middle-aged rats, but the maxima for the old rats occurred in the second 6 hr. Finally, NREM sleep significantly increased during the recovery period in the young and middle-aged rats, and high-voltage NREM sleep declined by 30% during recovery compared to baseline in the young rats.

### C. Performance and Behavioral Changes During Recovery Sleep

The majority of studies indicate complete recovery of performance and behavioral indices in humans with RS after SD. Reaction time in a visual vigilance task returned to baseline values with RS after 40 hr of SD (24). Similarly, after 2 nights of SD, young adults showed recovery to baseline levels in performance on the Wilkinson Addition Test after 1 or 2 full nights of sleep (25). In the same study, self-reported mood and sleepiness recovered to baseline levels after 1 full night of sleep, although sleep latency scores measured at 2-hr intervals during all waking periods did not return to baseline until after the second recovery night. Subjects who were sleep restricted to an average of 4.98 hr, or 33% below their habitual sleep duration for a week, showed similar findings, with cumulative sleepiness, mood disturbance, and psychomotor vigilance performance decrements recovering after 2 full nights of RS (26). However, some elements of performance vigilance tasks did not return to baseline levels with 3 days of RS after one week of 3, 5, or 7 hr of sleep restriction (27). The authors in this latter study theorized that the brain adapts to chronic sleep restriction, that this adaptation is sufficient to stabilize performance, albeit at a reduced level, and that the adaptation may persist for several days after normal sleep duration is restored.

### D. Physiological Changes During Recovery Sleep

Rechtschaffen's group in the University of Chicago conducted detailed studies of the physiological changes of RS in rats. Everson and colleagues (28) found that the effects of total and partial SD were reversible and baseline or near-baseline levels were restored within 15 days of RS. These effects consisted of a debilitated appearance, lesions on the paws and tails, increased energy expenditure, increased plasma epinephrine (in totally sleep deprived rats) and norepinephrine, and decreased plasma thyroxine. In the rats that underwent TSD, there was a high priority in sequence and amount for a REM sleep rebound and an absence of an early high-voltage NREM (HS2) sleep rebound in the TSD rats.

The reversal of increased energy expenditure with RS has also been observed in humans with measurements of metabolism ($O_2$ uptake and $CO_2$ output) after 1 night of brief frequent experimental arousals (29). Given the debilitated appearance, lesions of the paws and tail, and progressive elevations in white cell counts of the TSD rats, immune function was studied in these animals.

Surprisingly, no difference in immune function as measured by spleen cell counts, in vitro lymphocyte proliferation responses to mitogens, and in vitro and in vivo plaque-forming cell responses to antigens was observed (30). However, human studies have shown changes in natural killer cell activity after TSD and during RS (31,32).

Feng and colleagues (33) studied peritoneal temperature in wake and sleep during recovery from short-term (5 days) and long-term (14–21 days) TSD. On the first recovery day, both short- and long-term TSD rats showed mean temperature values during NREM and REM sleep that were slightly above mean temperature during wakefulness. Interestingly, this phenomenon has also been reported in humans in the first NREM sleep episode of RS after 40 hr of SD (34). In short-term TSD rats, wake-NREM sleep and wake-REM sleep differences were significantly reduced from baseline on the first recovery day and nonsignificantly on the remaining 3 recovery days. In long-term TSD rats, wake-NREM sleep and wake-REM sleep differences were significantly reduced from baseline on the first 4-recovery-day block. The authors concluded that the reduction of the wake-sleep temperature differences in recovery did not support either energy reduction or cooling functions for sleep. However, the temperature decline suggested that vasoconstrictor defenses against heat loss in the regions of major heat dissipation in the rat (hindpaws and tail) were impaired during SD. Zenko and colleagues (35) tested this hypothesis by examining peripheral vascular resistance (PVR) in rats deprived of sleep for 10–22 days. Although PVR was near baseline levels during the latter half of the TSD period, there was a small decline in PVR early in the deprivation and these rats showed significantly lower PVR than the yoked control rats. A rapid PVR rebound was found during the recovery period, suggesting a release from a TSD-related blockade of vasomotor compensation for heat loss. In summary, the physiological changes associated with SD appear to be reversible during RS.

### III. Homeostatic Regulation of Sleep

Numerous studies of SD in both humans and animals support the idea that sleep is homeostatically regulated. As illustrated in Figure 1, sleep loss produces proportional increases in the "drive" to sleep, in subsequent sleep expression, and in SWA recorded in the EEG during NREM sleep. This property of homeostatic regulation, along with a circadian input, has been incorporated into the "two-process model" of sleep regulation (Fig. 2) which addresses the timing of sleep (36,37). In this model, the homeostatic sleep-related "Process S" is proposed to interact with input from the circadian system ("Process C") to gate the occurrence of sleep and wakefulness. Process S is proposed to be a neurochemical process(es) that begins to build up at the onset of wakefulness. Once a threshold value is reached, sleep will ensue only if Process C is in the appropriate circadian phase. This model, although seemingly simplistic, accounts remarkably well for the timing of sleep in humans and several other species (38–44).

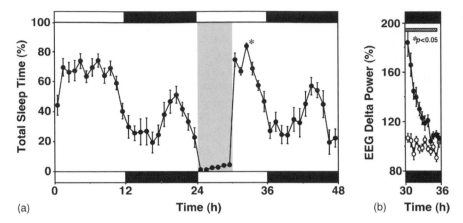

(a)    Time (h)    (b)    Time (h)

**Figure 1** (a) Distribution of sleep across a 24-hr baseline, a 6-hr sleep deprivation (SD) period, and the subsequent 18 hr of recovery in C57BL/6 male mice (*n* = 10). SD was induced by disturbing cage bedding around the mouse using an artist's brush, stroking the vibrissae or, toward the end of the SD period, stroking the fur. (b) *Closed circles*: EEG delta power values (mean ± SEM) in male C57BL/6 mice during hours 30–36, the first 6 hr of the recovery period subsequent to the SD period illustrated in (a) *Open circles*: Baseline EEG delta power values (mean ± SEM) during the same period on the prior baseline day (ZT 6–12). Note that sleep intensity, as measured by EEG delta power during NREM sleep, is significantly increased for the first 5.5 hr of the recovery period. (From Ref. 73.)

Electrical activity measured in the EEG is widely accepted to reflect underlying thalamocortical activity. A number of studies have suggested that EEG slow waves, i.e., activity in the 0.5–4.0-Hz (delta) range of the EEG during NREM sleep, are a characteristic of sleep that is related to the underlying Process S. When slow waves recorded in the delta range during sleep are subjected to Fourier analysis, the spectral power measured increases in proportion to prior wake duration in humans and many other species (38–44). The level of "EEG delta power" is almost entirely determined by the prior history of sleep and wakefulness: delta power after prolonged wakefulness increases in a dose-dependent manner, decreases after daytime naps, and decreases over the course of the nighttime sleep period, reflecting a diminution of Process S during sleep. Thus, EEG delta power has been interpreted to represent the cortical manifestation of the recovery from prior waking activities that occurs during sleep (36,45).

Mathematical analyses of EEG SWA have yielded quantitative information about the time course of accumulation and discharge of sleep need. The dynamics of the sleep/wake-dependent changes in delta power have been quantified with the use of computer simulations, and delta power can now be predicted in detail. The increase of "sleep need" during waking can be described by an exponentially saturating curve with a time constant ($\tau_i$) of 18.2 hr in humans (37) and 8.6 hr in

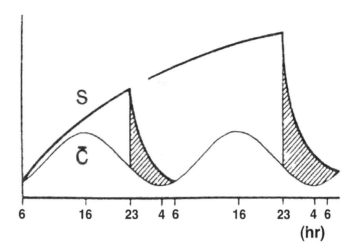

**Figure 2** Several models have been proposed to conceptualize the interaction of circadian and homeostatic processes in sleep regulation. In the "two-process model," a sleep homeostatic process increases during waking and decreases during sleep ("Process S") and interacts with input from the circadian system that is independent of sleep and waking ("Process C") to gate the occurrence of sleep and wakefulness. (Adapted from Ref. 1.)

rats (46). Conversely, the decrease in EEG SWA during sleep is an exponentially decaying function with a time constant ($\tau_d$) of 4.2 hr in humans (37), 3.2 hr in rats (46), and 1.7 hr in mice (44). These calculated values presumably reflect not only the buildup and discharge of sleep need during wake and NREM sleep, respectively, but also the neurochemical substrates that correlate with EEG SWA. These and other observations lead to the conclusion that EEG delta power reflects a homeostatically regulated recovery process that drives sleep need (47). As described in the next section, $\tau_d$ is highly conserved among mouse strains whereas the buildup of sleep need ($\tau_i$) is a characteristic that varies by genotype (44). Since $\tau_d$ is highly conserved, we can infer that the neurochemical or molecular processes that occur either during spontaneous sleep or during RS after SD must be crucial for organismal function.

## IV. Genetic Regulation of Sleep Homeostasis

In the last several years, an increasing number of studies have been published on sleep in mice owing to the advent of various transgenic and knockout strains. The use of inbred strains to identify the genetic basis of sleep characteristics has also been of great interest. For example, C57BL/6 and C57BR strains of mice are characterized by long REM sleep episodes, short SWS episodes, and significant circadian variation under light:dark conditions (48,49). At the opposite end of the spectrum, BALB/c mice have very short REM sleep episodes and weak diurnal rhythms, while D2 mice are intermediate for these characteristics (48). Qualitative differences in EEG signals are also observed: CBA/Ca and BALB/c but not C57BR mice display high-amplitude spindles, and REM-associated theta frequency varies significantly between strains. Early investigations (50) concluded that many genes are likely to be involved in the expression of each trait, as the interactions observed are complex. However, more recent studies (51) have identified provisional quantitative trait loci (QTL) associated with paradoxical (or REM) sleep (PS), which suggests that a complex behavior like PS may be controlled by only a few genes. In BALB/c x C57BL (CXB) recombinant inbred mice, PS during the light period was associated with markers on chromosome 7 between 7 and 20 centimorgans from the centromere, whereas PS during the dark period was associated with a single QTL on chromosome 5 near the *clock* gene. Markers on chromosomes 2, 17, and 19 influenced the daily amount of REM sleep.

The physiological response to SD also appears to be under genetic control (44). A comparison of six inbred mouse strains revealed that homeostatic sleep regulation follows the same basic rules that govern sleep regulation in humans and rats. As indicated in the prior section, the rate at which sleep need decreases during sleep ($\tau_d$) seems to be species-specific, being slowest for humans and fastest for mice. The sleep-dependent $\tau_d$ was highly conserved across mouse strains whereas the buildup of sleep need ($\tau_i$) was strain-specific and thus is likely to be subject to genetic influence (44). Figure 3 shows that the rebound in delta power after 6-hr SD was greatest in AK mice and least in the D2 mice during the first 3 hr of RS after SD (52). Simulations indicated that the time constant for the buildup of Process S during wakefulness ($\tau_i$) is more than twice as fast in AK mice ($\tau_i = 5.3 \pm 0.3$ hr) as in D2 mice ($\tau_i = 12.6 \pm 1.6$ hr). Thus, in the mouse, relatively short periods of SD will yield a large increase in sleep need.

A 6-hr SD period appears to be optimal for studying homeostatic sleep regulation in mice (44,52). As indicated in Figure 3, 6-hr SD achieved by gentle handling elicits a robust increase in EEG delta power and REM sleep. Curiously, SD protocols longer than 6 hr are not followed by larger increases in SWA; lower values for delta power were obtained after 9-hr SD than after 6-hr SD (44). Such diminished responses with longer SD durations are likely due to two factors. First, wake-dependent increases in EEG delta power follow an exponential function that saturates around 6 hr. Second, with SD durations greater than 6 hr, sleep drive becomes so high that mice constantly try to enter sleep, resulting in brief (~10 sec) but frequent sleep episodes that cannot be avoided and that are sufficient to counter a further increase in EEG delta power. Nonetheless, the interstrain variability in the EEG spectral profiles for SWS and for the time course of EEG delta power during RS after SD (Fig. 3) suggest that interstrain comparisons are likely to be a useful tool to help identify the cellular and molecular bases of Process S.

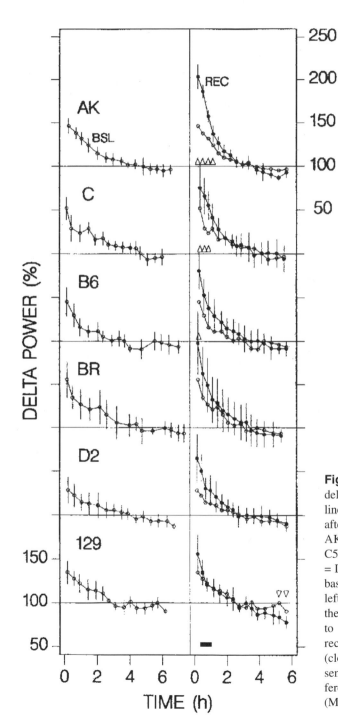

**Figure 3** Time course of EEG delta power in SWS during baseline (BSL) and recovery (REC) after a 6 h SD regimen. AK = AKR/J; C = BALB/c; B6 = C57BL/6; BR = C57BR/cdJ; D2 = DBA/2J; 129 = 129/OLA. The baseline data presented on the left (open circles) are repeated on the right to facilitate comparison to delta power recorded during recovery after the 6-hr SD (closed circles). Triangles represent bins in which significant differences in delta power occur. (Modified from Ref. 52.)

## V.  Gene Expression During Sleep Deprivation and Recovery Sleep: Candidate Gene Studies

At least four experimental approaches have been used to study the role of gene expression in association with arousal states: (a) gene expression in association with spontaneous variation in arousal state; (b) gene expression associated with SD; (c) gene expression associated with RS after SD; and (d) gene expression associated with drug-induced sleep. In this section, we will primarily focus on approaches in which specific "candidate" genes have been studied in association with SD and RS.

The expression of the immediate early gene (IEG) c-*fos* has been extensively used as a functional marker of brain activity in neuroscience including sleep research (53–55). In most cell types, the basal level of c-*fos* expression is relatively low; however, c-*fos* messenger ribonucleic acid (mRNA) and Fos protein can be rapidly and transiently induced by a diverse range of extracellular stimuli. Several laboratories have found that both c-Fos protein and mRNA levels decrease in the cerebral cortex during sleep relative to wakefulness (56–59). This decline has been linked to a reduction in the firing rate of the locus ceruleus during sleep and the consequent reduction of norepinephrine release in the cortex (60).

When studied in relation to SD, Fos expression was not directly proportional to time kept awake; the largest increases in many brain areas were found after 3-hr SD (58). SD for 24 hr increased Fos protein in some specific brain areas (61). Our early studies of SD (56) found that c-*fos* mRNA was increased after both 45 min and 6 hr of SD in every brain region examined. The induction of c-*fos* mRNA at 45 min was attributed to the initial sensory stimulation of deprivation, whereas the induction at 6 hr was thought to more likely reflect an increase due to sleep homeostasis. Others have found a greater increase in c-*fos* mRNA after 8 hr than after 4-hr SD (57). In rat cortex, Fos protein remained high during 6 or 12 hr of enforced wakefulness but declined rapidly (within 1 hr) with increasing time of RS (59). Similarly, in transgenic mice in which lacZ expression is driven from the c-*fos* promoter, β-galactosidase activity was higher after enforced wakefulness and declined with increasing amounts of sleep (59). These results suggest that the decrease in Fos protein in cortical neurons during sleep may be attributable to cessation of c-*fos* expression, activation of a process that degrades the wake-induced c-*fos*, or both. In contrast to these results, experiments utilizing long-term (10-day) TSD did not reveal significant changes in the expression of the IEG *egr-1* (*NGFI-A*) mRNA or immunoreactivity in most of the 25 brain regions examined (62).

Although the homeostatic drive to sleep accrues primarily during wakefulness, its physiological manifestation, Process S, is measured only during the ensuing sleep period. Since SWA can be directly measured during RS, determination of gene expression during RS is an attractive paradigm because mRNA or protein levels can be directly correlated with SWA levels. Although this approach is yet to be extensively used in molecular studies of sleep, it has led to the identification of the ventrolateral preoptic area (VLPO) as a sleep-active region through correlation of Fos expression with increased SWA during NREM sleep (63). Fos expression in the VLPO has been positively correlated with the preceding amount of both naturally occurring (63) and pharmacologically induced sleep (64). A positive correlation with sleep induced by warming has also been found in the median preoptic nucleus (65). These and other studies indicate that gene expression varies with behavioral state in a brain region-specific manner.

The results of the studies summarized here suggest that there is not a simple relationship between the expression of *c-fos* and other IEGs in brain and the amount of prior wakefulness; this may be due, at least in part, to the transient nature of *c-fos* induction and the refractory period subsequent to induction (53). Expression of *c-fos* is of interest because this gene encodes the transcription factor Fos, which dimerizes with other DNA-binding proteins such as Jun family proteins to form the activator protein-1 (AP-1). The resultant heterodimers bind at AP-1 sites in the promoter region of numerous genes, regulating the expression of "target" genes bearing this element and thereby the long-term response of a cell to stimulation (53,54). Therefore, to systematically examine the expression of major IEGs in response to SD and RS, we measured seven *fos/jun* family members (*c-fos, fosB, fra-1, fra-2, junB, c-jun,* and *junD*), two members of the *egr* family (*egr-1* and *egr-3*), and *nur77* by real-time quantitative polymerase chain reaction (RT-PCR) (Taqman) in seven regions of mouse brain after 6-hr SD and a subsequent period of RS (66). During SD, there was widespread increase of IEG mRNAs in cortex, basal forebrain, thalamus, and cerebellum but no significant change in brainstem areas (Fig. 4a,b). In these four brain regions, *c-fos* and *fosB* mRNA levels were elevated during SD whereas *junB* mRNA was elevated only in the cerebral cortex and *fra-1* and *fra-2* mRNA increased in the basal forebrain in this condition, suggesting the possibility of region-specific dimerization. In contrast to SD, only two genes exhibited increased mRNA levels during RS: *fra-2* and *egr-3*. Thus, among the 10 IEGs examined, only two genes showed elevated expression during RS and these changes were restricted to the cerebral cortex. Interestingly, the expression of *fosB* and *nur77* expression was very similar to that of *c-fos* across the experimental conditions, indicating that these IEGs might also be useful markers of functional activity.

## VI. Gene Expression During Sleep Deprivation and Recovery Sleep: "Unbiased" Approaches

Rather than describing changes in expression of a known class of genes, several studies have utilized "unbiased" approaches to determine changes in expression of a large number of genes in association with arousal state using cDNA arrays, DNA chips, or other molecular techniques. Subtractive hybridization was used to isolate two mRNAs whose expression was altered in forebrain after 24-hr SD

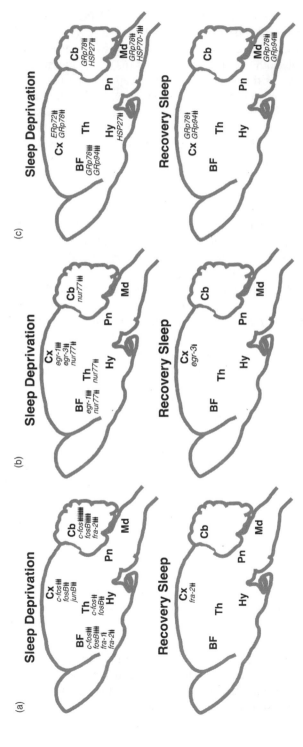

**Figure 4**  Summary of the gene expression changes observed during sleep deprivation and recovery sleep across seven brain areas. (a) Fos and Jun family genes. (b) Other IEGs. (c) HSP family genes. Number of arrows indicates x-fold change as determined by Taqman analysis. ↑ indicates gene is significantly upregulated but the magnitude is 1.5-fold or less; ↑↑ indicates gene is significantly upregulated and the magnitude is 1.5–2.5-fold; ↑↑↑ indicates gene is significantly upregulated and the magnitude is 2.5–3.5-fold, etc. BF, basal forebrain; Cx, cortex; Th, thalamus; Hy, hypothalamus; Pn, pons; Cb, cerebellum; Md, medulla. (Modified from Ref. 66 and 73.)

induced by forced locomotion (67). Subsequent studies revealed that one of the clones was the 17-kDa rat protein neurogranin, a phosphoprotein that contains a consensus sequence for protein kinase C phosphorylation (68), and the other was dendrin, which exists in both 81-kD and 89-kD variants (69). Subtractive hybridization has also led to the identification of cortistatin, a molecule proposed to have sleep-inducing properties (70). A differential-display-PCR (DD-PCR) study of the cerebral cortex of rats that had been spontaneously asleep, spontaneously awake, or sleep-deprived for 3 hr (71) identified several mRNAs that were expressed at higher levels during waking, including the transcription factors *c-fos, NGFI-A,* and *rlf* as well as three transcripts encoded by the mitochondrial genome (*subunit 1 of cytochrome c oxidase, subunit 2 of NADH dehydrogenase, and 12S rRNA*). A survey using both DD-PCR and cDNA arrays identified 44 genes that had higher mRNA levels in the rat cortex after waking and/or SD than during sleep (72). These genes clustered into the following functional categories: IEGs/transcription factors, energy metabolism, growth factors/adhesion molecules, chaperones/heat shock proteins, vesicle- and synapse-related genes, neurotransmitter/hormone receptors, neurotransmitter transporters, enzymes, and a miscellaneous group.

Our DNA array studies in the mouse also find increased mRNA levels of chaperone/heat shock protein and IEG/transcription factor family members in the cortex after SD (66,73). To thoroughly evaluate the expression of the heat-shock protein (HSP) family members in response to SD and RS, we examined the expression of six HSP family members (*erp72, grp78, grp94, hsp27, hsp-70-1, hsp84*) by Taqman in seven brain regions. Our studies revealed increased mRNA levels for several HSPs in cortex, basal forebrain, hypothalamus, cerebellum, and medulla during SD, whereas increased mRNA levels during RS were limited to *grp78* and *grp94* and were anatomically restricted to the cortex and medulla (Fig. 4c). Immunohistochemical studies confirmed these results by identifying increased numbers of GRp78-, GRp94-, and ERp72-immunoreactive cells in the dorsal and lateral cortex during SD. During RS, however, the number of these cells increased only in the lateral cortex. In the medulla, increased numbers of GRp94-immunoreactive cells were observed in the nucleus tractus solitarius, the dorsal motor nucleus of the vagus, and the rostroventrolateral medulla during RS. The widespread increase of HSP family mRNAs in brain during SD may be a neuroprotective response to prolonged wakefulness. In contrast, the relatively limited HSP family mRNA expression during RS may be related to the role of HSPs in protein biogenesis and thus to the restorative function of sleep. Although this and other studies indicate that changes in the expression of genes other than the IEGs can occur in association with arousal state changes, the results summarized in the lower half of Figure 4 indicate that increased mRNA expression during sleep is rare and may be anatomically restricted.

Although the focus of the foregoing discussion has been on total SD and the subsequent RS, gene expression has also been studied in relation to selective SD. Selective REM sleep deprivation has been reported to increase the expression of tyrosine hydroxylase mRNA in the locus ceruleus (74) and galanin mRNA in the preoptic area and periventricular nucleus (75) and to have differential effects on the expression of m1, m2, and m3 muscarinic receptor mRNAs in the pontine nuclei (76). Fos immunochemistry has also been used to determine functional activation within neurochemically identified cell groups after REM sleep deprivation and recovery (77-79).

## VII. Summary

The studies summarized in this chapter indicate that there is a profound homeostatic response to SD that can be readily quantified. Genetic studies in mice indicate that this response is highly conserved among mouse strains, indicating that some important neurochemical process is occurring during RS. The nature of the restorative process is yet to be identified but restoration of intracellular energy stores, membrane ionic gradients, and macromolecules have all been proposed to occur during sleep. To pursue the latter possibility, molecular biological studies using both candidate gene and unbiased approaches have been undertaken. The results to date indicate that increased mRNA expression during sleep is rare and may be anatomically restricted. With the recent completion of the DNA sequence of the mouse genome, it will soon be possible to assay the expression of the entire mouse genome in response to SD and RS as well as during spontaneously occurring sleep and wakefulness. Such studies are likely to provide unique insights into the nature of the restorative process that occurs during sleep.

## References

1. Webb WB, Agnew HW Jr. The effects on subsequent sleep of an acute restriction of sleep length. Psychophysiology 1975; 12:367–370.
2. Benoit O, Foret J, Bouard G, Merle B, Landau J, Marc ME. Habitual sleep length and patterns of recovery sleep after 24 hour and 36 hour sleep deprivation. Electroencephalogr Clin Neurophysiol 1980; 50:477–485.
3. Rosenthal L, Merlotti L, Roehrs TA, Roth T. Enforced 24-hour recovery following sleep deprivation. Sleep 1991; 14:448–453.
4. Levine B, Roehrs T, Stepanski E, Zorick F, Roth T. Fragmenting sleep diminishes its recuperative value. Sleep 1987; 10:590-599.
5. Carskadon MA, Dement WC. Sleep studies on a 90-minute day. Electroencephalogr Clin Neurophysiol 1975; 39:145-155.
6. Carskadon MA, Dement WC. Sleepiness and sleep state on a 90-min schedule. Psychophysiology 1977; 14:127-133.
7. Czeisler C, Weitzman E, Moore-Ede M, Zimmerman J, Knauer R. Human sleep: its duration and organization depend on its circadian phase. Science 1980; 210:1264-1267.
8. Czeisler C, Zimmerman J, Ronda J, Moore-Ede M, Weitzman E. Timing of REM sleep is coupled to the circadian rhythm of body temperature in man. Sleep 1980; 2:329-346.

9. Dijk DJ, Czeisler CA. Paradoxical timing of the circadian rhythm of sleep propensity serves to consolidate sleep and wakefulness in humans. Neurosci Lett 1994; 166:63-68.

10. Dijk DJ, Czeisler CA. Contribution of the circadian pacemaker and the sleep homeostat to sleep propensity, sleep structure, electroencephalographic slow waves, and sleep spindle activity in humans. J Neurosci 1995; 15:3526-3538.

11. Tilley AJ. Recovery sleep at different times of the night following loss of the last four hours of sleep. Sleep 1985; 8:129-136.

12. Uchiyama M, Okawa M, Shibui K, et al. Poor recovery sleep after sleep deprivation in delayed sleep phase syndrome. Psychiatry Clin Neurosci 1999; 53:195-197.

13. Ibuka N, Kawamura H. Loss of circadian rhythm in sleep-wakefulness cycle in the rat by suprachiasmatic nucleus lesions. Brain Res 1975; 96:76-81.

14. Mistlberger RE, Bergmann BM, Waldenar W, Rechtschaffen A. Recovery sleep following sleep deprivation in intact and suprachiasmatic nuclei-lesioned rats. Sleep 1983; 6:217-233.

15. Tobler I, Borbely AA, Groos G. The effect of sleep deprivation on sleep in rats with suprachiasmatic lesions. Neurosci Lett 1983; 42:49-54.

16. Trachsel L, Edgar DM, Seidel WF, Heller HC, Dement WC. Sleep homeostasis in suprachiasmatic nuclei-lesioned rats: effects of sleep deprivation and triazolam administration. Brain Res 1992; 589:253-261.

17. Carskadon MA, Acebo C, Seifer R. Extended nights, sleep loss, and recovery sleep in adolescents. Arch Ital Biol 2001; 139:301-12.

18. Gaudreau H, Morettini J, Lavoie HB, Carrier J. Effects of a 25-h sleep deprivation on daytime sleep in the middle-aged. Neurobiol Aging 2001; 22:461-468.

19. Bonnet MH. Recovery of performance during sleep following sleep deprivation in older normal and insomniac adult males. Percept Mot Skills 1985; 60:323-334.

20. Bonnet MH. Effect of 64 hours of sleep deprivation upon sleep in geriatric normals and insomniacs. Neurobiol Aging 1986; 7:89-96.

21. Brendel DH, Reynolds CF, 3rd, Jennings JR, et al. Sleep stage physiology, mood, and vigilance responses to total sleep deprivation in healthy 80-year-olds and 20-year-olds. Psychophysiology 1990; 27:677-685.

22. Reynolds CF, 3rd, Kupfer DJ, Hoch CC, Stack JA, Houck PR, Berman SR. Sleep deprivation in healthy elderly men and women: effects on mood and on sleep during recovery. Sleep 1986; 9:492-501.

23. Mendelson WB, Bergmann BM. Age-dependent changes in recovery sleep after 48 hours of sleep deprivation in rats. Neurobiol Aging 2000; 21:689-693.

24. Corsi-Cabrera M, Arce C, Ramos J, Lorenzo I, Guevara MA. Time course of reaction time and EEG while performing a vigilance task during total sleep deprivation. Sleep 1996; 19:563-569.

25. Carskadon MA, Dement WC. Effects of total sleep loss on sleep tendency. Percept Mot Skills 1979; 48:495-506.

26. Dinges DF, Pack F, Williams K, et al. Cumulative sleepiness, mood disturbance, and psychomotor vigilance performance decrements during a week of sleep restricted to 4–5 hours per night. Sleep 1997; 20:267-277.

27. Belenky G, Wesensten NJ, Thorne DR, et al. Patterns of performance degradation and restoration during sleep restriction and subsequent recovery: a sleep dose-response study. J Sleep Res 2003; 12:1-12.

28. Everson CA, Gilliland MA, Kushida CA, et al. Sleep deprivation in the rat. IX. Recovery. Sleep 1989; 12:60-67.

29.  Bonnet MH, Berry RB, Arand DL. Metabolism during normal, fragmented, and recovery sleep. J Appl Physiol 1991; 71:1112-1118.

30.  Benca RM, Kushida CA, Everson CA, Kalski R, Bergmann BM, Rechtschaffen A. Sleep deprivation in the rat. VII. Immune function. Sleep 1989; 12:47-52.

31.  Dinges DF, Douglas SD, Zaugg L, et al. Leukocytosis and natural killer cell function parallel neurobehavioral fatigue induced by 64 hours of sleep deprivation. J Clin Invest 1994; 93:1930-1939.

32.  Heiser P, Dickhaus B, Schreiber W, et al. White blood cells and cortisol after sleep deprivation and recovery sleep in humans. Eur Arch Psychiatry Clin Neurosci 2000; 250:16-23.

33.  Feng PF, Shaw P, Bergmann BM, et al. Sleep deprivation in the rat. XX. Differences in wake and sleep temperatures during recovery. Sleep 1995; 18:797-804.

34.  Dijk DJ, Czeisler CA. Body temperature is elevated during the rebound of slow-wave sleep following 40-h of sleep deprivation on a constant routine. J Sleep Res 1993; 2:117–120.

35.  Zenko CE, Bergmann BM, Rechtschaffen A. Vascular resistance in the rat during baseline, chronic total sleep deprivation, and recovery from total sleep deprivation. Sleep 2000; 23:341-346.

36.  Borbely AA. A two process model of sleep regulation. Hum Neurobiol 1982; 1:195-204.

37.  Daan S, Beersma DG, Borbely AA. Timing of human sleep: recovery process gated by a circadian pacemaker. Am J Physiol 1984; 246:R161-183.

38.  Borbely AA, Baumann F, Brandeis D, Strauch I, Lehmann D. Sleep deprivation: effect on sleep stages and EEG power density in man. Electroencephalogr Clin Neurophysiol 1981; 51:483-495.

39.  Borbely AA, Tobler I, Hanagasioglu M. Effect of sleep deprivation on sleep and EEG power spectra in the rat. Behav Brain Res 1984; 14:171-182.

40.  Tobler I, Jaggi K. Sleep and EEG spectra in the Syrian hamster (*Mesocricetus auratus*) under baseline conditions and following sleep deprivation. J Comp Physiol [A] 1987; 161:449-459.

41.  Dijk DJ, Daan S. Sleep EEG spectral analysis in a diurnal rodent: *Eutamias sibiricus*. J Comp Physiol [A] 1989; 165:205-215.

42.  Deboer T, Franken P, Tobler I. Sleep and cortical temperature in the Djungarian hamster under baseline conditions and after sleep deprivation. J Comp Physiol [A] 1994; 174:145–155.

43.  Huber R, Deboer T, Tobler I. Effects of sleep deprivation on sleep and sleep EEG in three mouse strains: empirical data and simulations. Brain Res 2000; 857:8-19.

44.  Franken P, Chollet D, Tafti M. The homeostatic regulation of sleep need is under genetic control. J Neurosci 2001; 21:2610-2621.

45.  Borbely AA, Tobler I. Endogenous sleep-promoting substances and sleep regulation. Physiol Rev 1989; 69:605-670.

46.  Franken P, Tobler I, Borbely AA. Sleep homeostasis in the rat: simulation of the time course of EEG slow-wave activity [published erratum appears in Neurosci Lett 1991 Nov 11;132(2):279]. Neurosci Lett 1991; 130:141-144.

47.  Borbely AA. From slow waves to sleep homeostasis: new perspectives. Arch Ital Biol 2001; 139:53-61.

48.  Valatx JL, Bugat R. [Genetic factors as determinants of the waking-sleep cycle in the mouse (author's transl)]. Brain Res 1974; 69:315-330.

49. Valatx JL, Cespuglio R, Paut L, Bailey DW. [Genetic study of paradoxical sleep in mice: connection with coloration genes]. Waking Sleeping 1980; 4:175-183.
50. Friedmann JK. A diallel analysis of the genetic underpinnings of mouse sleep. Physiol Behav 1974; 12:169-175.
51. Tafti M, Franken P, Kitahama K, Malafosse A, Jouvet M, Valatx JL. Localization of candidate genomic regions influencing paradoxical sleep in mice. Neuroreport 1997; 8:3755-3758.
52. Franken P, Malafosse A, Tafti M. Genetic determinants of sleep regulation in inbred mice. Sleep 1999; 22:155-169.
53. Morgan JI, Curran T. Stimulus-transcription coupling in the nervous system: involvement of the inducible proto-oncogenes fos and jun. Annu Rev Neurosci 1991; 14:421-451.
54. Karin M, Liu Z, Zandi E. AP-1 function and regulation. Curr Opin Cell Biol 1997; 9:240–246.
55. Cirelli C. How sleep deprivation affects gene expression in the brain: a review of recent findings. J Appl Physiol 2002; 92:394-400.
56. O'Hara BF, Young KA, Watson FL, Heller HC, Kilduff TS. Immediate early gene expression in brain during sleep deprivation: preliminary observations. Sleep 1993; 16:1–7.
57. Grassi-Zucconi G, Menegazzi M, De Prati AC, et al. c-fos mRNA is spontaneously induced in the rat brain during the activity period of the circadian cycle. Eur J Neurosci 1993; 5:1071-1078.
58. Cirelli C, Pompeiano M, Tononi G. Sleep deprivation and c-*fos* expression in the rat brain. J. Sleep Res 1995; 4:92-106.
59. Basheer R, Sherin JE, Saper CB, Morgan JI, McCarley RW, Shiromani PJ. Effects of sleep on wake-induced c-*fos* expression. J Neurosci 1997; 17:9746-9750.
60. Cirelli C, Pompeiano M, Tononi G. Neuronal gene expression in the waking state: a role for the locus coeruleus. Science 1996; 274:1211-1215.
61. Pompeiano M, Cirelli C, Tononi G. Effects of sleep deprivation on fos-like immunoreactivity in the rat brain. Arch Ital Biol 1992; 130:325-335.
62. Landis CA, Collins BJ, Cribbs LL, et al. Expression of Egr-1 in the brain of sleep deprived rats. Brain Res Mol Brain Res 1993; 17:300-306.
63. Sherin JE, Shiromani PJ, McCarley RW, Saper CB. Activation of ventrolateral preoptic neurons during sleep. Science 1996; 271:216-219.
64. Scammell T, Gerashchenko D, Urade Y, Onoe H, Saper C, Hayaishi O. Activation of ventrolateral preoptic neurons by the somnogen prostaglandin D2. Proc Natl Acad Sci USA 1998; 95:7754-7759.
65. Gong H, Szymusiak R, King J, Steininger T, McGinty D. Sleep-related c-Fos protein expression in the preoptic hypothalamus: effects of ambient warming. Am J Physiol Regul Integr Comp Physiol 2000; 279:R2079-2088.
66. Terao A, Greco MA, Davis RW, Heller HC, Kilduff TS. Region-specific changes in immediate early gene expression in response to sleep deprivation and recovery sleep in the mouse brain. Neuroscience 2003; 120:1115-1124.
67. Rhyner TA, Borbely AA, Mallet J. Molecular cloning of forebrain mRNAs which are modulated by sleep deprivation. Eur J Neurosci 1990; 2:1063-1073.
68. Neuner-Jehle M, Rhyner TA, Borbely AA. Sleep deprivation differentially alters the mRNA and protein levels of neurogranin in rat brain. Brain Res 1995; 685:143-153.

69. Neuner-Jehle M, Denizot JP, Borbely AA, Mallet J. Characterization and sleep deprivation-induced expression modulation of dendrin, a novel dendritic protein in rat brain neurons. J Neurosci Res 1996; 46:138-151.

70. de Lecea L, Criado JR, Prospero-Garcia O, et al. A cortical neuropeptide with neuronal depressant and sleep-modulating properties. Nature 1996; 381:242-245.

71. Cirelli C, Tononi G. Differences in gene expression between sleep and waking as revealed by mRNA differential display. Brain Res Mol Brain Res 1998; 56:293-305.

72. Cirelli C, Tononi G. Gene expression in the brain across the sleep-waking cycle (1). Brain Res 2000; 885:303-321.

73. Terao A, Steininger TL, Hyder K, et al. Differential increase in the expression of heat shock protein family members during sleep deprivation and during sleep. Neuroscience 2003; 116:187-200.

74. Porkka-Heiskanen T, Smith SE, Taira T, et al. Noradrenergic activity in rat brain during rapid eye movement sleep deprivation and rebound sleep. Am J Physiol 1995; 268:R1456-1463.

75. Toppila J, Stenberg D, Alanko L, et al. REM sleep deprivation induces galanin gene expression in the rat brain. Neurosci Lett 1995; 183:171-174.

76. Kushida CA, Zoltoski RK, Gillin JC. The expression of m1-m3 muscarinic receptor mRNAs in rat brain following REM sleep deprivation. Neuroreport 1995; 6:1705-1708.

77. Maloney KJ, Mainville L, Jones BE. c-Fos expression in dopaminergic and GABAergic neurons of the ventral mesencephalic tegmentum after paradoxical sleep deprivation and recovery. Eur J Neurosci 2002; 15:774-778.

78. Maloney KJ, Mainville L, Jones BE. c-Fos expression in GABAergic, serotonergic, and other neurons of the pontomedullary reticular formation and raphe after paradoxical sleep deprivation and recovery. J Neurosci 2000; 20:4669-4679.

79. Maloney KJ, Mainville L, Jones BE. Differential c-Fos expression in cholinergic, monoaminergic, and GABAergic cell groups of the pontomesencephalic tegmentum after paradoxical sleep deprivation and recovery. J Neurosci 1999; 19:3057-3072.

# 25

## Sleep Length

**MICHAEL H. BONNET**

**Dayton Department of Veterans Affairs Medical Center, Wright State University, Kettering Medical Center, and the Wallace Kettering Neuroscience Institute, Dayton, Ohio, U.S.A.**

### I. Introduction

A good deal is known about the behavioral effects of sleep deprivation and the lawful status of recovery after sleep loss. The data are consistent, persuasive, and extensive. Unfortunately, the data have not clearly identified the need for sleep or exactly what is being recovered. A few have suggested that sleep is not an appetitive drive (like eating) but rather an instinct that allows humans to conserve energy during the dark, when activity would have decreased survival value (1,2). Proponents of sleep as an instinctual behavior present documented cases of several individuals who consistently sleep less than 3 hr each night with no residual sleepiness or performance deficit and suggest that sleep is not an appetitive behavior but rather a genetically determined instinct. This is important to our view of the effects of sleep deprivation because it means that the carefully described lawful effects may not apply in the general case. For example, almost 30% of young adults report normally sleeping 6.5 hr or less on weeknights (3,4). Other studies have shown decreased objective alertness after as little as 1 night of 6 hr of sleep (5) and accumulation of such deficits over consecutive nights (6). Declines in psychomotor performance have been found after as few as 3 nights of 7 hr of sleep (7). Based on these data, one might conclude that almost one third of normal young adults accumulate sufficient sleep deficits across a normal work-week to precipitate significantly impaired alertness and performance. Such data have been used to estimate significant societal costs associated with sleepiness (8,9) and may be used to help form public policy.

However, the alternate viewpoint suggests that this sort of statistical summary is an oversimplification. Almost all partial and total sleep deprivation studies limit their subject populations to healthy young adults who additionally spend 7.5–8.5 hours in bed each night. This is done in part because studies are traditionally planned for 8-hr sleep periods with unitary dose reductions in sleep (i.e., to 6 hr or 4 hr). Individuals who report consistently spending 6 hr in bed are viewed with some suspicion because they may in fact be 8-hr sleepers who are chronically sleep-deprived or because they may not fit into the protocol (i.e., might not be able to maintain sleep for 8 hr). However, it is known that there is a wide variation in usual sleep lengths. A typical population estimate is 7.4 hr/night ± 0.9 hr (10). This implies that 67% of young adults sleep between 6.5 and 8.3 hr, and 5% of young adults sleep less than 5.6 or more than 9.2 hr/night. Relatively little is known about the response to sleep deprivation in groups outside of young adults with "normal" sleep habits. For example, it is unknown whether normal adults who characteristically sleep 6 hr each night have a more efficient sleep system or are simply chronically partially sleep-deprived. If these individuals have a more efficient sleep system, then understanding the differential impact of sleep loss and the rate of recovery of function when sleep is allowed in efficient (i.e., short) and inefficient (i.e., long) sleepers can give valuable information about the sleep process and about the interrelationship between the sleep and arousal systems. If these individuals are simply chronically sleep-deprived, then the perception of decreased need for sleep is clearly not accurate and education is a better goal.

This chapter will review current knowledge about individuals with characteristic long and short sleep patterns, identify some limitations of this research, and suggest some additional studies that might help improve the understanding of differences in sleep requirement versus sleep reduction or sleep deprivation.

## II.  Long and Short Sleepers

Many studies of long- and short-sleeping humans were published between 1970 and 1987. The studies fall into two groups: (a) most of the papers were naturalistic comparisons of people with characteristic sleep lengths of more than 9 hr/day with other individuals sleeping 6 or fewer hr/day; (b) a few studies identified a small group of people with extremely short sleep lengths (less than 3 hr/day) in an attempt to document that such individuals did exist and did not develop symptoms of extreme sleepiness.

Many of the initial studies were based on observations that there might be personality differences between long and short sleepers. Some studies have found no differences (11,12). However, Hartman (13) characterized short sleepers as "involved keeping busy and avoiding psychological problems" while long sleepers were often more shy and creative. More recent studies based on Hartman's interviews of college students have reported that short sleepers showed significantly increased test, achievement, and manifest anxiety (14–16); increased likelihood of type A behavior (17); hypomania (18,19); more disturbed eating patterns (20); decreased fluid intelligence and lower levels of divergent thinking (21,22); more adjustment problems (23); and a more external locus of control (24) as compared with long sleepers. Hicks et al. also found that long sleep was more likely to be a consistent pattern that had existed for more than 5 years whereas the short sleep pattern, at least in college students, was more likely to have been established in the late teens (25). The point of establishment may, therefore, have reflected either an acquired pattern in response to the demands of college (26) or changes in underlying physiology (as the latter seems to produce symptoms of narcolepsy in other individuals at about the same time).

Other studies of long and short sleepers initially concentrated on sleep stage differences in the groups. Short sleepers, by virtue of terminating their sleep much earlier, were consistently found to have less rapid-eye-movement (REM) sleep, less stage 2 and less wake plus stage 1 as a part of their decreased total sleep compared to long sleepers (13,27). Differences in minutes of slow-wave sleep (SWS) were not found. One group of studies by Benoit and colleagues (28–31) examined sleep deprivation in groups of long and short sleepers. The studies indicated that both long and short sleepers had increased total sleep time after sleep deprivation. The proportional increase in total sleep was very similar (127% in short sleepers and 124% in long sleepers), and the increase in total sleep minutes was actually greater in the long sleepers than in the short sleepers (31). One study found that long sleepers had fewer minutes of SWS than short sleepers or regular-length sleepers (who had virtually the same minutes of SWS). These data suggest that the short sleepers were not chronically sleep-deprived compared to the normal sleepers prior to the experiment. However, Benoit et al. also found significantly longer sleep onset latency in their long sleepers as compared to regular and short sleepers, who did not differ (respective latencies to stage 2 were 19, 14, and 11 min [28]), and this might indicate that the long sleepers were sleep-satiated. In support of this finding, Fukuda et al. (32) found that their long sleepers had significantly longer latencies to return to sleep after a standard awakening during the night (58 vs. 14 min). There were some other physiological findings of note in the Benoit et al. studies. Body temperature maximum was similar in the two groups (29), but another paper (30) indicated a higher 24-hr mean heart rate in short sleepers (78.1 ± 0.4 bpm) versus long sleepers (73 ± 0.5 bpm). A second study (33) has shown that short sleepers, when measured across a 28-day period, had elevated presleep (measured only at this time) heart rate.

Only one study has carefully looked at characteristic performance or alertness as a function of habitual sleep duration. Taub (34,35) examined performance in groups of 7.5-hr- and 10-hr-sleeping university students. The long sleepers were found to have significantly shorter reaction time, improved vigilance performance and higher body temperature than the normal sleep group. These data, therefore, would be consistent with the interpretation that even normal sleepers may suffer from chronic partial sleep deprivation with resulting decrements in performance as compared to individuals with longer sleep times. One classic study sought to "make" short sleepers by slowly reducing sleep time by 30 min every 2–4 weeks until subjects were unable to reduce their sleep time any further (36). All of the subjects developed signs of chronic partial sleep deprivation when times in bed were in the 6-hr range and nocturnal sleep latency was reduced from baseline levels of 10 min to 2 min by the end of the study (times in bed in the 4.5–5 hr range). Of most interest, a follow-up study found that subjects who had reported requiring 8 hr of sleep prior to the sleep reduction study were sleeping only 6.3 hr 1 year after the study (37). The data seem to indicate that sleepiness did accumulate during sleep reduction based on the sleep latency data. The question is why the subjects remained short sleepers at the end of the experiment. *Did they habituate to the chronic partial sleep deprivation, or did they adjust to the short sleep times so that they had a new shorter sleep requirement?*

More recent studies (38–41) looked at homeostatic sleep regulation and mood in long and short sleepers before and after sleep deprivation. One major conclusion from the studies was that the time constants calculated for process S, based on the SWS distribution, did not differ in long sleepers as compared to short sleepers. This lack of difference in SWS led the authors to conclude that short sleepers "live under a higher NREMS (non-REM sleep) pressure" (38, p. R51), which implies a chronic sleep debt. The mood results indicated that short sleepers had significantly higher "good mood" at baseline and during sleep deprivation as compared to long sleepers. Both groups reported significantly decreased ability to concentrate during sleep deprivation, but the short sleepers continued to report significantly decreased ability to concentrate 24 hr later, after recovery sleep. The short sleepers tended to report more energy at baseline and throughout deprivation as compared to long sleepers. Only the long sleepers had a significant decrease in energy and increase in tiredness during sleep deprivation. The authors concluded that the long sleepers were more impacted by sleep loss than the short sleepers based on their significant decrease in energy and increase in tiredness during sleep deprivation. At the same time, however, the short sleepers also could be seen as more sensitive to the sleep loss as it took them longer to recover based on the concentration mood scale.

In a second study, long and short sleepers participated in a 40-hour constant routine protocol (39,40). A spectral analysis of waking EEG from this experiment showed that the short sleepers had increased power in the 5.25–9-Hz and the 17.25–18-Hz ranges. Increased time awake (i.e., sleep loss) was also associated with an increase in the 5.25–9-Hz range. These findings of increased theta with sleep loss and in short sleepers therefore also indicated that the short sleepers might have a greater sleep debt than the long sleepers. In the same study (40), blood samples were taken every 30 min to measure thyroid-simulating hormone (TSH) concentrations. TSH was significantly elevated in the short sleepers both prior to and during the sleep loss. Body temperature was also lower in the short sleepers. The authors interpret all of these findings as consistent with higher sleep pressure in the short sleepers. However, the effects of sleep deprivation on TSH and body temperature are open to some speculation. Total sleep loss typically results in an increase in TSH (42), usually associated with remaining awake longer. However, one study (43) has shown a decrease in TSH after partial sleep deprivation. Reports of body temperature change associated with total sleep deprivation are also variable.

There are several other interesting findings in this study. During the constant routine, the long sleepers had higher sleepiness ratings than the short sleepers, but the recovery sleep period was the same length in both groups (15 ± 1.2 vs. 16.1 ± 0.8 hr in the short vs. long sleepers). However, after this recovery sleep, short sleepers still had greater power in the 5.25–9-Hz range.

These findings support the existence of some degree of chronic partial sleep deprivation in the short sleep group. However, many issues remain. In general, these subject groups were selected to demonstrate a habitual difference in sleep length of greater than 3 hr. Unfortunately, as the data have been presented, there is no clear way to understand whether the effects are related to chronic partial sleep deprivation in the short sleepers, sleep satiation in the long sleepers, or a partial effect (i.e., a trait difference, or nondifference between short and long sleepers overlaid by a smaller partial sleep deprivation effect). Parametric studies at fixed sleep lengths including groups of "normal" sleepers could address these issues.

Despite evidence consistent with partial sleep deprivation in the study (38), the authors speculate that their reported differences could be genetic. However, it is also possible that a factor other than pure sleep drive (such as trait level of central nervous system arousal) might act in concert with the sleep system to control total sleep time in these individuals. For example, Freedman (44) found that insomnia patients had increased spectral electroencephalographic (EEG) power at 18–30 Hz in stage 1 and REM sleep, and Bonnet and Arand (45) found that physiological arousal produced by standing or walking prior to data collection caused a significant increase in spectral EEG power at 17 Hz in normal young adults. These data would suggest that the short sleepers in the Aeschbach et al. study (39) were both partially sleep-deprived (hence their decrease in the 5.25–9 Hz range) and at a higher level of central nervous system (CNS) arousal (hence their increase in the 17–18 Hz range). The implication is that increased CNS arousal could decrease sleep length and result in either insomnia (for those who try to stay in bed for 8 hr) or a "decreased sleep requirement" for those who compensate by sleep restriction.

A more recent publication reports melatonin and cortisol in long and short sleepers during the 40-hr constant routine (41). In this study, it was found that the maxima in cortisol and sleepiness were closely related to habitual wake-up time (during the constant routine), which was 2.5 hr later in the long sleepers corresponding to their longer habitual sleep length. In addition, the long sleepers had a longer nocturnal release of melatonin and a longer period of nocturnal low temperature. The authors concluded that these biological markers themselves (i.e., extended periods of low temperature and melatonin excretion) might drive the long sleep in these individuals. Obviously, however, it cannot be determined whether these rhythms determine the long sleep behavior or whether the long sleep behavior results in the establishment of corresponding rhythms. However, the authors also make the interesting observation that the continuing expression of the biological markers of the long and short sleep pattern during the constant routine suggests that long-term exposure to controllers of biological rhythms such as the short and long photoperiods of summer and winter could predispose to longer sleep periods in the winter, for example. Exposure to artificial light in habitual patterns might also help maintain the short sleep pattern.

## III.  Studies of Extreme Short Sleepers

Three groups have studied EEG recordings from individuals demonstrating consistent sleep times of 3 hr or less per night (18,46,47). Jones and Oswald (46) recorded two short sleepers for 3 or 4 consecutive nights to document that both individuals indeed did sleep less than 3 hr/night without appearance of excessive sleepiness or other dysfunction. The other studies came to similar conclusions. One study (18) involved partial sleep deprivation and sleep extension in one subject (who had a normal sleep length of 96 min, a partial sleep deprivation sleep length of 42 min and an extended sleep length of 152 min). Performance tests included a 1-hr vigilance test. Despite characteristic sleep of 1.5 hr, test performance was not consistent with sleep deprivation. In fact, the only unusual conclusion from this case study was that the subject felt groggy (but did not have a decrease in vigilance sensitivity) after the "extended" sleep night.

The results of these studies were used by Meddis to theorize that sleep was not really a restorative process at all (2). Irrespective of theories of sleep, such results imply that there may be a broad range of sleep requirements. Generalizations from groups that have a 7–8 hr sleep requirement may not apply to all individuals.

## IV.  Summary

In individuals without sleep pathology, a pattern of long sleep seems to be a fairly enduring trait. Hicks et al. report that 9% of their college sample slept for more than 9 hr each night and two thirds of those students had had that consistent pattern for more than 5 years (25). Short sleepers were more likely to have developed that pattern more recently. Less than 2% of the total sample had a short sleep pattern for more than 5 years. In general, short sleepers seem to be task-oriented and under some stress to succeed. It is not clear whether this change is in response to natural or inherited changes in underlying physiology (increased sympathetic nervous system activity, for example), which produces a sense of stress and also reduces ability to maintain sleep; or in response to behaviorally mandated changes in sleep (short sleep times reduce REM sleep, for example) that produce mild hypomania that then maintains the short sleep behavior pattern. It is also possible that there are at least two groups of short sleepers: those with a genetic predisposition for short sleep and those with a behavioral imposition. Finally, short sleepers may have a tendency to have some degree of self-imposed chronic partial sleep deprivation in addition to their decreased need for sleep.

## V. Limitations of Previous Research

The normal long sleep pattern seems to be relatively fixed and stable. With the exception of the few documented very short sleepers, the short sleep pattern seems to develop in relationship to periods of increased demand or stress. As such, it is important to differentiate whether this short sleep pattern really is a form of chronic sleep deprivation, which may result in the development of significant residual effects, or whether this pattern reflects a true physiological change. Such a differentiation is currently difficult to make because there are almost no comparative performance data from matched groups of short sleepers, long sleepers, and controls. One sleep deprivation study in long and short sleepers reported mood data, but there are no comprehensible objective alertness or performance data from baseline or sleep deprivation periods in the groups. Data from Taub (34,35) indicated that long sleepers had improved performance compared to normal sleepers, and this implies that even normal sleepers might be chronically sleep-deprived in comparison to long sleepers. However, Aeschbach et al. (38), based on mood data, concluded that long sleepers were more sensitive to sleep deprivation than were short sleepers. Non-EEG physiological data comparing these groups are sparse. Two studies have implied that short sleepers may have higher heart rates than long sleepers, but at least one study found no difference in heart rate. Taub (34,35) found higher body temperature in long sleepers compared to normal sleepers.

## VI. Future Research

As the public health consequences of partial sleep deprivation become clear, recommendations may be made for appropriate sleep hygiene. If recommendations are based on the subset of young adults who normally sleep between 6.5 and 8.3 hr/night (67% of the young adult population), the needs of many individuals (33% of the young adult population, all children, many patients with insomnia, and all older individuals) will not be met. For example, individuals with longer sleep requirements and children may still develop chronic sleep-deprivation-related deficits while following sleep time guidelines established for 7.4-hr sleeping young adults. Even the "normal" 7.4-hr sleeping young adults may be chronically sleep-deprived in comparison with longer sleepers. Previous research supports both the contention that some short sleepers have a reduced sleep need and the contention that short sleepers suffer from chronic partial sleep deprivation. Studies need to differentiate these hypotheses. This is easier to request than to accomplish because there is no accepted standard to judge whether individuals with any reported habitual sleep length obtain adequate sleep or are chronically partially sleep-deprived. Multiple Sleep Latency Tests (MSLTs) have not been done in these groups, perhaps because there are large circadian effects on the MSLT and it would be difficult to determine comparable administration times in subjects with time in bed differences of greater than 3 hr. Use of "usual sleep length" is not informative because it ignores possibly different underlying sleep requirements. Sleep length consistency (i.e., not requiring periodic long sleep periods to recover from partial sleep deprivation) verified by small "oversleep" in a laboratory setting with no externally mandated awakening time could be a better measure of underlying sleep need.

Identification of sleep requirement in a more objective manner could help verify long or short sleep requirement status and allow formation of more homogeneous extreme groups. If it is possible to actually identify groups of individuals on this basis, it will provide evidence that some really do have a reduced sleep requirement. This will then justify exploration of the extreme groups.

At a more theoretical level, it is important to understand the development of sleep deprivation-related impairment as a function of habitually different sleep requirements and sleep stage distributions. Performance and alertness data from sleep deprivation could tell us whether either group is more susceptible to sleep loss. Psychomotor performance data recorded during recovery sleep can tell us whether short sleepers are simply more efficient at recovery of alertness (i.e., if the slope of their return to baseline alertness during recovery sleep is greater than that in long sleepers). One hypothesis of the development of a short sleep pattern is that individuals become short sleepers when circumstances reduce their available sleep time. Reduction of sleep results in loss of REM sleep, and this REM deprivation could make the individual become more hypomanic (which in turn could maintain the short sleep behavior). If this is the case, placing short sleepers in a longer sleep situation would produce REM rebounds, a reduction in hypomania, and a different response to sleep loss. Similarly, placing long sleepers in a shorter sleep situation might reduce REM and produce a hypomania cycle with reduced sensitivity to partial sleep loss. Either response would have significant implications for our understanding of sleep and sleep associated deficits.

Studies of long sleepers and short sleepers all essentially start from different baselines—the individually different baselines of the sleep groups. It has traditionally been believed that these self-selected sleep lengths are based on individual differences in sleep need rather than behaviorally maintained habits. *If conditions change (for example, a new baseline sleep duration of 7.5 hr is required for both habitual 6-hr sleepers and habitual 9-hr sleepers), what would happen?* If sleep duration is based on underlying sleep need, the long sleepers would be partially sleep-deprived for several nights when sleeping 7.5 hr/night and would develop decrements that would be magnified by total sleep loss and would not recover during a 7.5-hr recovery night. On the other hand, short sleepers would be sleep-satiated after sleeping for 7.5 hr, would be less sensitive to sleep deprivation, and would have a more rapid recovery during a 7.5-hr recovery sleep. All of these conditions could maximize differences between long sleepers and short sleepers if their sleep duration is based on their underlying sleep need. Conversely, if habitual sleep duration is maintained from habit, pattern of activity or light exposure, personality, or perceived benefit rather than from biological need, the groups would equalize during the 7.5-hr baseline period and the response to sleep deprivation and the recovery sleep rate would be exactly the same in both groups.

Very little work has addressed the topic of individual differences in response to sleep deprivation. It is clear that such differences exist: total sleep deprivation produces remission of symptoms in depressed patients but does not have such large impact on mood in normals; patients with chronic insomnia should suffer from significant partial sleep deprivation but actually seem less sleepy than normals when tested with the MSLT (48,49). It is certainly possible that individual differences in response to sleep deprivation are related to individual differences in sleep requirement. However, these individual differences may also be related to other intrinsic factors (such as level of central nervous system arousal, biological rhythms, or personality) or extrinsic factors (such as characteristic activity or light exposure patterns).

## Acknowledgments

This work was supported by the Dayton Department of Veterans Affairs Medical Center, Wright State University School of Medicine, and the Sleep-Wake Disorders Research Institute

## References

1.  Webb WB. Sleep the Gentle Tyrant. Boston: Anker, 1992:179.
2.  Meddis R. The Sleep Instinct. London: Routledge & Kegan Paul, 1977:148.
3.  Bonnet MH, Arand DL. We are chronically sleep deprived. Sleep 1995; 18:908–911.
4.  Browman CP, Gordon GC, Tepas DI, Walsh JK. Reported sleep and drug use of workers: a preliminary report. Sleep Res 1977; 6:111.
5.  Rosenthal L, Roehrs TA, Rosen A, Roth T. Level of sleepiness and total sleep time following various time in bed conditions. Sleep 1993; 16:226-232.
6.  Dinges DF, Pack F, Williams K, Gillen KA, Powell JW, Ott GE, Aptowicz C, Pack AI. Cumulative sleepiness, mood disturbance, and psychomotor vigilance performance decrements during a week of sleep restricted to 4–5 hours per night. Sleep 1997; 20:267–277.
7.  Johnson D, Thorne D, Rowland L, Balkin T, Sing H, Thomas M, Wesensten N, Redmond D, Russo M, Welsh A, Aladdin R, Cephus R, Hall S, Powel J, Dinges D,

Belenky G. The effects of partial sleep deprivation on psychomotor vigilance. Sleep 1998; 21(suppl):236.

8.  Leger H. The cost of sleep related accidents: a report for the National Commission on Sleep Disorders Research. Sleep 1994; 17:84–93.

9.  Webb WB. The cost of sleep-related accidents: a reanalysis. Sleep 1995; 18:276-280.

10. White RM. Sleep length and variability: measurement and interrelationships: Unpublished dissertation, University of Florida, 1975.

11. Webb WB, Friel J. Characteristics of "natural" long and short sleepers: a preliminary report. Psychol Rep 1970; 27:63–66.

12. Webb WB, Friel J. Sleep stage and personality characteristics of "natural" long and short sleepers. Science 1971; 171:587–588.

13. Hartman E. Sleep requirement: long sleepers, short sleepers, variable sleepers, and insomniacs. Psychosomatics 1973; 14:95–103.

14. Hicks RA, Pellegrini RJ, Hawkins J. Test anxiety levels of short and long sleeping college students. Psychol Rep 1979; 44:712–714.

15. Hicks RA, Pellegrini RJ. Anxiety levels of short and long sleepers. Psychol Rep 1977; 41: 569–570.

16. Kumar A, Vaidya AK. Anxiety as a personality dimension of short and long sleepers. J Clin Psychol 1984; 40:197–198.

17. Hicks RA, Pellegrini RJ, Martin S, Garbesi L, Elliott D, Hawkins J. Type A behavior and normal habitual sleep duration. Bull Psychonom Soc 1979; 14:185–186.

18. Stuss D, Broughton R. Extreme short sleep: personality profiles and a case study of sleep requirement. Waking Sleeping 1978; 2:101–105.

19. Monk T, Buysse D, Welsh D, Kennedy K, Rose L. A sleep diary and questionnaire study of naturally short sleepers. J Sleep Res 2001; 10:173–179.

20. Hicks RA, Rozette E. Habitual sleep duration and eating disorders in college students. Percept Mot Skills 1986; 62:209–210.

21. Hicks RA, Pellegrini RJ, Cavanaugh A, Sahatjian M, Sandham L. Fluid intelligence levels of short- and long-sleeping college students. Psychol Rep 1978; 43:1325–1326.

22. Hicks RA, Guista M, Schretlen D. Habitual duration of sleep and divergent thinking. Psych Rep 1980; 46:426.

23. Sexton-Radek K. Clinical aspects associated with adjustment in unusual sleepers. Percept Mot Skills 1998; 87:261–262.

24. Hicks RA, Pellegrini RJ. Locus of control in short and long sleepers. Percept Mot Skills 1978; 47:1337–1338.

25. Hicks RA, Pellegrini RJ, Hawkins J, Moore JD. Self-reported consistency of normal habitual sleep durations of college students. Percept Mot Skills 1978; 47:457–458.

26. Bonnet MH, Carswell M. The effect of an environmental shift on sleep. Sleep Res 1977; 6:109.

27. Webb WB, Agnew HWJ. Sleep stage characteristics of long and short sleepers. Science 1970; 168:146–147.

28. Benoit O, Foret J, Bouard G, Merle B, Landau J, Marc ME. Habitual sleep length and patterns of recovery sleep after 24 hour and 36 hour sleep deprivation. Electroencephalogr Clin Neurophysiol 1980; 50:477–485.

29. Benoit O, Foret J, Merle B, Bouard G. Diurnal rhythm of axillary temperature in long and short sleepers: effects of sleep deprivation and sleep displacement. Sleep 1981; 4:359–365.

30. Benoit O, Foret J, Merle B, Reinberg A. Circadian rhythms (temperature, heart rate, vigilance, mood) of short and long sleepers: effects of sleep deprivation. Chronobiologia 1981; 8:341–350.

31. Benoit O, Foret J, Bouard G. The time course of slow wave sleep and REM sleep in habitual long and short sleepers: effect of prior wakefulness. Hum Neurobiol 1983; 2:91–96.

32. Fukuda K, Miyasita A, Inugami M. Sleep onset REM periods observed after sleep interruption in normal short and normal long sleeping subjects. Electroencephalogr Clin Neurophysiol 1987; 67:508–513.

33. Sexton-Radek. Presleep autonomic arousal as a distinguishing factor in type of sleep pattern. Percept Mot Skills 1998; 87:433–434.

34. Taub JM, Berger RJ. Effects of acute sleep pattern alteration depend upon sleep duration. Physiol Psychol 1976; 4:412–420.

35. Taub JM. Behavioral and psychological correlates of a difference in chronic sleep duration. Biol Psychol 1977; 5:29–45.

36. Friedmann J, Globus G, Huntley A, Mullaney D, Naitoh P, Johnson L. Performance and mood during and after gradual sleep reduction. Psychophysiology 1977; 14:245–250.

37. Mullaney DJ, Johnson LC, Naitoh JP, Friedmann JK, Globus GG. Sleep during and after gradual sleep reduction. Psychophysiology 1977; 14:237–244.

38. Aeschbach D, Cajochen C, Landolt H, Borbely AA. Homeostatic sleep regulation in habitual short sleepers and long sleepers. Am J Physiol 1996; 270:R41–R53.

39. Aeschbach D, Postolache TT, Sher L, Matthews JR, Jackson MA, Wehr TA. Evidence from the waking electroencephalogram that short sleepers live under higher homeostatic sleep pressure than long sleepers. Neuroscience 2001; 102:493–502.

40. Aeschbach D, Sher L, Postolache TT, Matthews JR, Jackson MA, Wehr TA. Thyrotropic status as a marker of chronic sleep pressure in habitual short sleepers and long sleepers (abst). J Sleep Res 2002; 11(suppl 1):1–2.

41. Aeschbach D, Sher L, Postolache TT, Matthews JR, Jackson MA, Wehr TA. A longer biological night in long sleepers than in short sleepers. J Clin Endrocrinol Metab 2003; 88:26–30.

42. Gary KA, Winokur A, Douglas SD, Kapoor S, Zaugg L, Dinges DF. Total sleep deprivation and the thyroid axis: effects of sleep and waking activity. Aviat Space Environ Med 1996; 67:513–519.

43. Spiegel K, Leproult R, Van Cauter E. Impact of sleep debt on metabolic and endocrine function. Lancet 1999; 354:1435–1439.

44. Freedman RR. EEG power spectra in sleep-onset insomnia. Electroencephal Clin Neurophysiol 1986; 63:408–413.

45. Bonnet MH, Arand DL. The impact of activity upon spectral EEG parameters. Physiol Behav 2001; 74:291–298.

46. Jones HS, Oswald I. Two cases of healthy insomnia. Electroencephalogr Clin Neurophysiol 1968; 24:378–380.

47. Meddis R, Pearson AJD, Langford G. An extreme case of healthy insomnia. Electroencephaplogr Clin Neurophysiol 1973; 35:213–214.

48. Bonnet MH, Arand DL. 24-Hour metabolic rate in insomniacs and matched normal sleepers. Sleep 1995; 18:581–588.

49. Schneider-Helmert D. Twenty-four-hour sleep-wake function and personality patterns in chronic insomniacs and healthy controls. Sleep 1987; 10:452–462.

# 26

# The Role of Endogenous Sleep-promoting Substances

**FERENC OBAL, JR.**

University of Szeged, Szeged, Hungary

**FABIO GARCIA-GARCIA AND JAMES M. KRUEGER**

Washington State University, Pullman, Washington, U.S.A.

## I. Introduction: The Discovery of Sleep-Regulating Substances

The idea of humoral regulation of sleep dates back to the development of the concept of hormonal regulation by Bayliss and Starling in 1902 (1). In the subsequent years putative hormones regulating various homeostatic functions have been demonstrated by means of transfer experiments. Thus, after appropriate stimulation of a donor animal, tissue fluids were transferred to recipient animals, and these animals produced the anticipated response to the stimulus. Applying this strategy to sleep, Ishimori (see Ref. 2), and Legendre and Piéron (3) reported that brain extracts and cerebrospinal fluid (CSF) samples obtained from sleep-deprived dogs elicited sleep in recipient dogs.

About 60 years after these initial descriptions of endogenous sleep-promoting substances, two theoretically fundamentally different approaches were used to collect tissue fluid samples containing high concentrations of the sleep-promoting substance. One approach assumed that the sleep substance is released during sleep; i.e., the function of this substance is to mediate sleep from the "sleep center" to other areas of the brain. The samples, dialysates of the blood leaving the brain, were collected during sleep after electrical stimulation of the thalamus (4). These experiments resulted in the discovery of the delta-sleep-inducing peptide (DSIP) (5). The other approach, which was also used in the experiments by Ishimori and Legendre and Piéron, assumed that the need for sleep builds up during wakefulness and is expressed by the secretion of a sleep-promoting substance. Since the production of this substance is stimulated by prolongation of wakefulness, the animals were sleep-deprived before collection of the tissue fluids (6,7). This approach led to the identification of muramyl peptides (8), uridine (9), and oxidized glutathione (10) as sleep-promoting substances.

The significance of these identified factors in physiological sleep regulation remains to be elucidated. Meanwhile a significant number of observations implicate six other molecules in sleep regulation. These substances, i.e., adenosine, growth-hormone-releasing hormone (GHRH), interleukin-1β/tumor necrosis factor-α (IL1β/TNF-α), prostaglandin D2 (PGD2), prolactin (PRL), and vasoactive intestinal polypeptide (VIP), are discussed in this review.

## II. Molecules Involved in Sleep Regulation

### A. Adenosine

The cyclic purine nucleoside, adenosine, or the base, adenine, is a component of various molecules that have fundamental roles in cell functions, such as deoxynucleic acid (DNA), coenzymes (e.g., nicotinamide adenine dinucleotide [NAD], nicotinamide adenine dinucleotide phosphate [NADP], flavin-adenine dinucleotide [FAD]), second-messengers cyclic adenosine monophosphate (cAMP), and the compound that stores and provides energy for biochemical processes, adenosine triphosphate (ATP). When intracellular adenosine concentration is high, excess adenosine is released into the extracellular space. This occurs in conditions associated with intense catabolism of ATP. In addition to basic biochemical processes, neurons use large amounts of ATP for the maintenance and recovery of resting ion balance after action potentials, and therefore, prolonged activity may be associated with adenosine release. ATP is also secreted; for example, neurotransmitter vesicles in some neurons (e.g., cholinergic and catecholaminergic neurons) contain ATP. When released into the extracellular space ATP is hydrolyzed by ectoenzymes and adenosine is produced. Wakefulness-associated rises in extracellular adenosine occur in several brain areas, but sustained increases of adenosine persisting during sleep deprivation were found only in the basal forebrain, in an area that corresponds to the location of the cell bodies of wake-active cholinergic neurons (11,12) . Extracellular adenosine elicits hyperpolarization and inhibits neuronal firing via postsynaptic type A1 receptors, inhibits neurotransmitter release via A1 presynaptic receptors, and stimulates neuronal activity by acting on A2 receptors. It seems that adenosine inhibits wake-active neurons in the basal forebrain and may stimulate sleep-active neurons in the preoptic area (13) and in the ventrolateral preoptic nucleus (VLPO) (14). Stimulation is due, in part, to disinhibition of sleep-active neurons via presynaptic A1 receptors, and, in part, to direct stimulation of sleepneurons via A2 receptors.

A number of studies demonstrate that systemic or intracerebroventricular injection of adenosine or locally infused adenosine into the basal forebrain increases the time spent in rapid-eye-movement (REM) and non-REM (NREM) sleep, and electroencephalographic (EEG) slow-wave activity during NREM sleep. In contrast, A1 antagonists decrease sleep (reviewed in Ref. 13). Interestingly, adenosine stimulates and caffeine (an adenosine receptor antagonist) or selective A1 antagonists inhibit rest in Drosophila, although adenosine receptors are not known in this insect (15). Less sleep time and decreases in the EEG slow-wave response to sleep deprivation were reported in A1 receptor knockout mice (16). However, other experiments suggested that sleep deficits did not occur in A1 knockout mice thoroughly adapted to the recording conditions (17). Chronic loss of adenosine action, therefore, might be compensated by other means of sleep regulation.

A1 receptors inhibit whereas A2 receptors stimulate the production of cAMP. Hyperpolarization via A1 receptors is attributed to opening of potassium channels. A1 receptors also elicit metabolic responses (18). Thus, these receptors stimulate translocation of the transcription factor, nuclear factor kappa B (NFκB), into the nucleus of neurons in the basal forebrain via the inositol triphosphate-$Ca^{2+}$ pathway, and may stimulate further synthesis of A1 receptors. Adenosine also elicits c-*fos* expression in noncholinergic basal forebrain neurons (19).

### B. Growth-Hormone-Releasing Hormone

Growth-hormone-releasing hormone (GHRH) is a peptide hypothalamic neurohormone, which is secreted into the pituitary portal circulation from terminals projecting to the median eminence. GHRH delivered to the somatotroph cells in the anterior pituitary stimulates synthesis and secretion of growth hormone (GH). GHRH-containing neurons reside predominantly in the arcuate nucleus, and a smaller number of GHRH-containing neurons are found around the ventromedial nucleus and in the paraventricular nucleus (20). In addition to the median eminence, GHRHergic neurons also send axons to various hypothalamic nuclei, predominantly to the anterior hypothalamus-medial preoptic region (AH/MPO). A major surge of GH secretion is associated with NREM sleep, particularly with deep NREM sleep, in various species (21). Stimulation of GH secretion and NREM sleep are regarded as synchronized but parallel and independent outputs of GHRHergic neurons mediated via projections to the median eminence and the AH/MPO, respectively (22). Hence, microinjection of GHRH directly into the AH/MPO promotes NREM sleep (23), hypophysectomy does not abolish the NREM-sleep-promoting activity of GHRH (24), and a cut in front of the arcuate nucleus decreases NREM sleep (25), yet the pituitary of these rats receives GHRH and continuously secretes GH (26). In vitro studies demonstrate that GHRH elicits calcium signal in GABA (gamma-aminobutyric acid)-ergic neurons in the AH/MPO, and thus, GABAergic neurons may mediate the NREM-sleep-promoting activity of GHRH (27).

Enhancements in NREM sleep (increases in NREM sleep time and intensity) as assessed by EEG slow-wave activity occur in response to GHRH administered via various routes (intracerebroventricular, intravenous, intranasal) in several species (rat, mouse, rabbit, human) (reviewed in Refs. 21,28,29). NREM sleep is suppressed when GHRH actions are acutely inhibited by means of antagonists, immunoneutralization, or stimulation of negative feedbacks in the somatotropic axis [e.g., administration of somatostatin agonists, high doses of GH or insulin-like growth factor-1 (IGF-1)] (29). NREM sleep time is permanently reduced by approximately 10% in animals with chronic GHRH deficiency (mutant *lit/lit* mice and *dw/dw* rats with nonfunctional GHRH receptors, and transgenic mice producing less GHRH) (29). However, NREM sleep responses to sleep deprivation in various models of GHRH deficiencies are inconsistent. Thus, an acute withdrawal of GHRH abolished enhancements in NREM sleep after short-term sleep deprivation in rats (25). Sleep-deprivation-induced stimulation of EEG slow-wave activity was greatly reduced in *dw/dw* rats (30). In contrast, the NREM sleep response to sleep deprivation was not altered in mice with decreased GHRH production or with a defect in GHRH receptors (31,32).

Hypothalamic GHRH synthesis and release, assessed by measuring GHRH messenger ribonucleic acid (mRNA) levels and GHRH contents, respectively, correlate with the diurnal rhythm of NREM sleep in the rat. It seems that both sleep deprivation and subsequent recovery sleep are associated with significant GHRH releases, and that GHRH synthesis is also stimulated during recovery sleep (reviewed in Refs. 25,29). Determination of GHRH receptor mRNA and GHRH binding in the pituitary and hypothalamus suggests that GHRH release is selectively stimulated in the hypothalamus and GHRH might not be secreted into the pituitary blood during sleep deprivation (33). This finding corroborates the observation that GH secretion is generally suppressed during sleep deprivation (34).

Although GHRH has a predominant role in sleep regulation, other members of the somatotropic axis may also modulate sleep. Thus, several lines of evidence indicate that GH may stimulate REM sleep (35), and under chronic conditions, it may also stimulate NREM sleep, particularly the intensity of NREM sleep (36). The latter action might be mediated via IGF-1, which has a modest NREM-sleep-promoting activity (29). Finally, stimulation of somatostatin-2 receptors by somatostatin acutely inhibits NREM sleep (37). This action is attributed to an inhibition of GHRHergic neurons. In addition, somatostatin has been implicated in the promotion of REM sleep (38).

### C.    Interleukin-1 (IL-1) and Tumor Necrosis Factor-$\alpha$ (TNF-$\alpha$)

Cytokines are proteins involved in intercellular communication and are produced by many cell types. Cytokines are best known as mediators of the acute-phase response to microbial challenge and to tissue damage. For instance, cytokines are responsible for somnolence and sleep (as well as fever, anorexia, social withdrawal, and other symptoms of the acute-phase response) during infectious diseases. However, cytokines in much smaller concentrations may also have a role in physiological processes (39). Thus, several lines of evidence suggest that cytokines are also involved in the regulation of spontaneous sleep (40). Several cytokines have NREM-sleep-promoting activity (IL-1β, IL-1α, IL-2, IL-15, IL-18, TNF-α, TNF-β, acidic fibroblast growth factor) whereas other cytokines (e.g., IL-4, IL-10, IL-13, transforming growth factor beta) decrease NREM sleep (40). With regard to their structure, receptors, and signaling pathways, cytokines are related to various growth factors and some hormones (e.g., GH, PRL). Many of these growth factors, such as nerve growth factor (NGF) and brain-derived neurotrophic growth factor (BDNF), are also considered cytokines and exert sleep-promoting activity. There is a strong possibility that some of them are involved in sleep regulation (41).

IL-1β and TNF-α are the best-documented sleep-promoting cytokines. Both glial cells and neurons contain IL-1β and TNF-α (42,43), and these cells, including neurons, also express IL-1 and TNF receptors. The IL type 1 receptor mediates IL-1β actions (the type 2 receptor is a decoy receptor). The type 1 receptor can activate several signaling pathways, but stimulation of NFκB might have particular significance for sleep regulation because translocation of NFκB into the nucleus of cortical (44) and basal forebrain neurons (18) is stimulated by sleep deprivation, and an inhibitor of NFκB translocation suppresses sleep (45). In addition, NFκB may enhance production of IL-1β, TNF-α, NGF, adenosine A1 receptors, and PGD2 (reviewed in Ref. 46). There are two TNF receptors (TNFR), the 55-kD TNFR and the 75-kD TNFR. The sleep-promoting activity of TNF is attributed to the 55-kD TNFR (47). When TNF binds to its receptor, the internal domain of the receptor recruits various adaptor proteins, and the resulting receptor complexes signal via several pathways, including NFκB (48). TNF-α-activated signaling pathways can induce both cell death and activate genes which inhibit apoptosis. The latter occurs more frequently, and NFκB is involved in this mechanism. The extracellular domain of both TNFRs can be shed to form soluble receptors. The 55 kD soluble TNFR is a normal constituent of the CSF (49).

IL-1β and TNF-α promote NREM sleep through multiple brain sites. IL-1 excites sleep-active neurons and inhibits wake-active neurons in the AH/MPO (50). Some hypothalamic neurons are receptive for both IL-1β and GHRH and these neurons are GABAergic (27). IL-1β upregulates hypothalamic GHRH receptors and may also stimulate GHRH synthesis (51). IL-1β injected into the locus ceruleus (52) and dorsal raphe (53) also enhances sleep. Promotion of NREM sleep occurs after microinjection of TNF-α into the AH/MPO (54) or the locus ceruleus (52).

Intracerebral or systemic administration of IL-1β enhances NREM sleep in mice, rats, rabbits, cats, monkeys, and humans (reviewed in Refs. 40,46), and TNF-α promotes NREM sleep in rabbits, mice, rats, and sheep (reviewed in Refs. 40,46). Both NREM sleep time and intensity (EEG slow-wave activity) increase after IL-1β or TNF-α. In rats and cats, only low doses of IL-1 stimulate NREM sleep. In contrast, higher doses decrease NREM sleep, perhaps owing to IL-1β-induced stimulation of corticotropin-releasing hormone (CRH), which is known to suppress NREM sleep (55,56). A correlation is observed between plasma TNF-α concentrations and sleepiness or fatigue in a number of clinical conditions. Thus, TNF-α is elevated in patients with chronic fatigue (57), chronic insomnia (58), and sleep apnea (59). Postdialysis fatigue is associated with higher TNF-α levels (60,61), and cancer patients receiving TNF report fatigue (62). In contrast, administration of the soluble 75-kD TNFR, which binds and decreases TNF levels, reduces fatigue in patients with rheumatoid arthritis (63). There are several routes through which systemic IL-1 or TNF can exert intracerebral actions: they may enter the brain through the circumventricular organs where the blood-brain barrier is deficient, they may be transported into the brain, they may elicit transcription of IL-1 or other signaling molecules in endothelial cells, and they may act via sensory neurons in the nervus vagus. For instance, the sleep-promoting activity of systemic TNF-α is attenuated after vagotomy (64). Systemic IL-1β induces IL-1β mRNA in the hypothalamus and this action is blocked after subdiaphragmatic vagotomy (65). Interestingly, excessive food intake, which enhances NREM sleep, also stimulates IL-1 mRNA expression in the brain, and this action is also blocked by vagotomy (66).

Acute inhibition of IL-1β by means of the IL-1 receptor antagonist (which is also an endogenous ligand of the IL-1 receptors), the soluble IL-1 receptor, or substances that inhibit IL-1 production is followed by decreases in spontaneous sleep (reviewed in Refs. 40,46). TNF-α can also be inhibited by administering anti-TNF-α antibodies or soluble TNFRs, and these substances decrease spontaneous sleep (reviewed in Refs. 40,46). Inhibition of either IL-1β or TNF-α also attenuates sleep rebound after sleep deprivation (40,46). Further, suppression of TNF also blocks enhancements in NREM sleep in response to a mild increase in ambient temperature (67). NREM sleep is permanently reduced in mutant mice lacking type 1 IL-1 receptors, but interestingly, the decreases in NREM sleep occur during the active period of the day (68). Decreases in NREM sleep were found in mice with deficient 55-kD TNF receptor in one study (47) but sleep was normal in mice with the same defect in another experiment (69).

Hypothalamic content and mRNA levels of TNF-α peak during the early light period, when NREM sleep is maximal, in the rat (70,71). IL-1-like activity varies with the sleep-wake cycle in the cerebrospinal fluid of cats (72). IL-1β protein levels in plasma (73) and hypothalamic IL-1β mRNA levels (74) are highest during the sleep period in rats. Sleep deprivation increases IL-1β and TNF-α mRNA levels in the hypothalamus (75–77) and expression of the 55-kD TNFR is also stimulated in the brain (77). In humans, peak levels of IL-1 occur at sleep onset in the blood (78) and IL-1 blood levels also increase during sleep deprivation (79). Blood levels of TNF-α correlate with EEG slow-wave activity (80), and concentrations of circulating TNF-α and the soluble 55-kD TNFR increase after sleep deprivation in humans (81).

Low doses of IL-1β or TNF-α have little effects on REM sleep but higher doses generally suppress this state of vigilance. Inhibition of REM sleep might be related to fever. However, the febrile response to exogenously administered cytokines can be selectively suppressed without blocking the sleep-promoting activity (82).

Downstream biochemical events involved in IL-1β- or TNFα-induced NREM sleep likely involve adenosine, PGD2, nitric oxide, NFκB, and GHRH (reviewed in Ref. 46).

### D. Prostaglandin D2

PGD2 is an unsaturated fatty acid containing a cyclopentane ring. It is produced from arachidonic acid through the cyclooxygenase (COX1 and COX2) pathway. PGH2, the immediate precursor of prostaglandins, is converted into PGD2 by a specific enzyme, the lipocalin-type glutathione-independent PGD synthase in the central nervous system (83).

Brain PGD synthase is expressed predominantly in the epithelial cells of the choroid plexus and in the leptomeninges. Weak expression of PGD synthase is found in some oligodendrocytes but not in neurons (84). The enzyme is secreted into the CSF where it appears as β-trace protein (85). The CSF is the suggested vehicle for PGD2 that carries the molecule to the action site. The prostanoid receptors mediating PGD2 actions also reside in the leptomeninges (86). However, the PGD receptors responsible for sleep promotion are located in the arachnoid cells in a circumscribed area on the surface of the basal forebrain just ventral from the VLPO area (87). PGD2 is assumed to elicit adenosine release from these cells; adenosine diffuses to the VLPO to stimulate the sleep-active neurons in this area. PGD2 also inhibits wake-active neurons perhaps via adenosine. Although the leptomeninges produce PGD2 the stimuli for production must come from the brain. The leptomeninges-CSF should be regarded as amplifier- and humoral-conveying machines through which distant parts of the brain can express their need for sleep to the basal forebrain.

Intracerebroventricular infusion of PGD2 increases NREM and REM sleep in rats and monkeys (88). Single injection of PGD2 into the cerebral ventricles failed to alter sleep in rabbits (89). A tail pinch elicits robust rises in brain PGD2 contents and NREM sleep time in transgenic mice expressing human PGD synthase (90). Intracerebral injection of PGD2 may cause fever but this action is not related to promotion of sleep. Acute inhibition of PGD2 production by means of cyclooxygenase inhibitors or inorganic selenium compounds, which block PGD synthase, elicits decreases in sleep (88). Acute inhibition of COX2 decreases spontaneous NREM sleep in rabbits as well as TNFα-induced NREM sleep (91). Inhibition of PGD synthase also increases the incidence of arousal-like behavior in fetal sheep, and this effect can be reversed by administering PGD2 (92).

PGD2 concentrations in the CSF are higher during the rest period than in the active period, and PGD2 tends to increase in the cerebrospinal fluid and the cortex during NREM sleep compared to values during wakefulness in rats (93,94). Finally, sleep deprivation increases PGD2 levels in the cerebrospinal fluid of rats (93).

### E.  Prolactin

Prolactin (PRL) is a 23-kD polypeptide that is synthesized predominantly in the anterior pituitary. Small amounts of PRL are also produced in other tissues, including the brain, where it may act as a neurotransmitter. In addition to its lactogenic action, PRL has many biological activities (reviewed in Ref. 95), such as regulation of proliferation of various cell types, e.g., astrocytes, anterior pituitary cells, and T lymphocytes (96). Circulating PRL is released from the pituitary. Secretion of PRL is sleep-dependent and is enhanced during NREM sleep (97).

Jouvet et al. suggested that systemic administration of PRL increased REM sleep in cats in which the brainstem is transected at the midpontine level and the pituitary is removed (98). Administration of exogenous PRL stimulates REM sleep in both rabbits and rats (99–102). However, PRL enhances REM sleep only when injected during the diurnal rest period in rats, and PRL increases wakefulness when administered at night (100). Systemic injection of VIP elicits PRL secretion and stimulates REM sleep in rats, and the effects are blocked by immunoneutralization of PRL, suggesting that systemic VIP acts via PRL release on REM sleep (103). Large increases in REM sleep and small, albeit significant, increases in NREM sleep time occur during the rest period in rats rendered hyperprolactinemic by pituitary grafts transplanted under the capsule of the kidney (104). However, increases in REM sleep were not observed in patients with PRL-producing pituitary tumors, instead these patients displayed enhancements in NREM sleep (105). Duration of REM sleep decreases and the circadian rhythm of REM sleep are abolished in hypoprolactinemic rats, though NREM sleep is unaltered in these animals (106). Interestingly, the time spent in REM sleep increased and REM sleep rhythm normalized in the hypoprolactinemic rats kept in constant light or dark (107). Immunoneutralization of systemic PRL causes minor decreases in REM sleep in rats (108).

It is assumed that PRL modulates sleep, predominantly REM sleep, via a central action site, though the mechanism is not known. PRL injection into the central nucleus of the amygdala, an area where microinjections of a cholinergic agonist induces REM sleep (109) and which also contains high concentrations of PRL immunoreactive fibers and receptors (110,111), does not promote REM sleep and decreases NREM sleep (112). In contrast, intrahypothalamic administrations of PRL or antibodies to PRL elicit REM sleep responses (102). PRL may modulate circadian regulation of REM sleep (113), or may directly act in brainstem structures involved in the generation of REM sleep (104). Thus, the firing rate of mesopontine tegmental neurons, which are involved in REM sleep generation (114), increases after PRL injection (115).

PRL has been implicated in the mechanism of sleep enhancement associated with pregnancy in rats (116), and in the stress-induced increases in REM sleep. Stress stimulates PRL release (117). There are some differences in the sleep responses to various stressors (118). Immobilization stress is followed by increases in REM sleep (119) or in both REM and NREM sleep in rats (120). Ether exposure used as a stressor elicits PRL secretion and selective increments in REM sleep, and antibodies to PRL or hypophysectomy block the stress-induced increases in REM sleep (121). In mice, the magnitude of PRL secretion correlates with the immobilization stress-induced REM sleep response (122). PRL release in stress may be elicited by corticotropin-releasing hormone (CRH) (123), and a CRH antagonist, injected prior to stress, inhibits subsequent increases in REM sleep (124). Enhancements in REM sleep were also observed after intracerebroventricular injection of the prolactin-releasing peptide (PrRP) (125,126). PrRP may also stimulate PRL secretion via CRH (127,128). Other observations, however, do not support modulation of REM sleep by CRH (129).

### F.  Vasoactive Intestinal Polypeptide (VIP)

VIP was initially isolated from the duodenum in 1970 (130), and its name is derived from its profound and long-lasting gastrointestinal smooth-muscle-relaxation actions. VIP, like GHRH, is a member of the secretin-glucagon peptide family, and it exhibits high homology with the pituitary-adenylate-cyclase-activating polypeptide (PACAP). The amino acid sequence of VIP is identical in the rat, human and other mammalian species.

VIP is a neurotransmitter in the cerebral cortex, the hypothalamus, amygdala, hippocampus, corpus striatum, and the vagal nuclei of the medulla oblongata (131,132). VIP receptors are widely distributed in cerebral cortex, amygdaloid nuclei, hippocampus, olfactory lobes, thalamus, and the suprachiasmatic nucleus, and are present in lower concentrations in the hippocampus, brainstem, spinal cord, and dorsal root ganglia. VIP is also involved in the release of other hormones such as CRH, PRL, oxytocin, and vasopressin.

VIP promotes REM sleep in normal rats, cats, and rabbits (133–136). Intracerebroventricular administrations of antibodies to VIP or a VIP antagonist selectively decrease REM sleep (133,137). VIP might be identical with the REM sleep-promoting substance accumulating in the CSF of REM-sleep-deprived animals. Thus, CSF obtained from REM-sleep-deprived cats is capable of restoring REM sleep if it is injected intraventricularly in parachlorophenylalanine (PCPA) insomniac cats (138). Furthermore, treatment of these CSF samples with VIP antibodies blocks the REM-sleep-promoting activity (139), thereby suggesting that the CSF of REM-sleep-deprived cats contains a VIP-like sleep factor involved in triggering REM sleep. Further, VIP accumulates in the CSF during REM sleep deprivation and decreases when REM sleep is allowed following REM-sleep deprivation (140).

In the suprachiasmatic and paraventricular nuclei VIP immunoreactivity increases during the dark period, when rodents are mostly awake, and decreases during the subsequent light period, when most of the time is spent in sleep (141,142). In addition, VIP immunoreactivity exhibits diurnal variations in the locus ceruleus nucleus and the periaqueductal gray matter. REM sleep deprivation upregulates VIP receptors in the brainstem areas that are involved in the generation and maintenance of REM sleep (143). The injection of VIP into areas of the brain involved with REM sleep generation induces prolonged increases in REM sleep (144). Thus, the oral pontine reticular nucleus (PnO) may be a target for the induction of REM sleep by VIP. VIP often colocalizes with acetylcholine (145,146). The injection of VIP into the PnO in combination with atropine, a cholinergic muscarinic antagonist, prevents VIP-induced REM-sleep increases (147). Injection of VIP into the medial pontine reticular formation (mPRF) of rats also induces REM sleep (148). Microinjection of cholinergic agonists within the mPRF produces a state that is behaviorally indistinguishable from natural REM sleep (114). These findings suggest that VIP promotes REM sleep via brainstem cholinergic mechanisms. However, VIP administered in combination with atropine in PCPA-treated insomniac cats induces an increase in total-time REM sleep (149), suggesting that the effects of VIP on REM sleep are not dependent on cholinergic mechanisms. Intrahypothalamic VIP is a physiological PRL-releasing hormone (150) and may also stimulate intrahypothalamic PRL synthesis (151).

### G.  Other Molecules

A few additional substances are implicated in sleep regulation, although the evidence for their sleep role is substantially less than that of the molecules discussed above. Oleamide is an unsaturated fatty acid that was isolated from the CSF of a sleep-deprived cat (152). Oleamide is structurally related to the endogenous cannabinoid anandamide, and it is possible that oleamide promotes NREM sleep via cannabinoid receptors directly or indirectly by inhibiting anandamide metabolism (153). Cortistatin is a peptide displaying strong homology with somatostatin. It is an inhibitory neurotransmitter in the cerebral cortex and in the hippocampus (154). Cortistatin seems to promote NREM sleep, but the sleep responses have not been thoroughly studied. Cholecystokinin (CCK) is a peptide hormone released from the duodenum in response to fats and proteins, and might be involved in the mediation of postprandial sleep. CCK promotes NREM sleep (155). The action is peripheral and might be mediated by vagal sensory neurons. Insulin is a peptide hormone released from the pancreas that stimulates glucose uptake by skeletal muscle and adipocytes and has a fundamental role in the regulation of metabolism of sugar, lipid, and protein, and in tissue growth. Promotion of NREM sleep was reported after intracerebroventricular administration of insulin in rats (156). However, the evidence is scarce implicating insulin in sleep regulation, and the sleep-promoting activity of intracerebral insulin might be mediated by IGF-1 receptors (157). Nitric oxide (NO) is also implicated in sleep regulation (158). The findings linking NO to regulation of NREM sleep are controversial (159), whereas the results are consistent that suggest that NO stimulates REM sleep by acting in the pedunculopontine tegmentum in the brainstem (160). Interestingly, neural NO synthase knockout mice have less REM sleep whereas inducible NO synthase knockout mice have more REM sleep (161).

## III. The Role of Sleep-promoting Substances in Sleep Regulation

Several lines of evidence published from various laboratories suggest that the molecules discussed above have a physiological sleep-promoting function. Although it seems likely that additional sleep-regulatory substances will be described in the future, a key question is where the six substances described herein can be placed in a model of sleep regulation. In our theory (162), the need for sleep arises within neuronal groups dispersed throughout the brain. These groups signal to a sleep regulatory network, and when the input to the sleep network is high enough, the sleep network inhibits the wake-promoting networks and synchronizes the sleep mode of the various neuronal groups. The sleep-regulating network resides in the basal forebrain-AH/MPO and the thalamus. This model is inclusive of sleep-promoting molecules that mediate activity-dependent sleep need in the individual neuronal groups, that signal to the sleep network, that signal inside the sleep network, that signal from the sleep network back to the neuronal groups, and those neurotransmitters found in the neural networks involved.

The intracerebral distribution of GHRH determines its function in sleep regulation. A substance, which is strictly localized to the hypothalamus, cannot act as a molecule released use-dependently in various neuronal groups, and cannot be used as a signal molecule between the neuronal groups and the sleep network. Several lines of evidence suggest that the basal forebrain-hypothalamus has a fundamental role in sleep-wake regulation: it contains neuronal networks that promote wakefulness and sleep (163,164). Transmitters in the wake-promoting network include acetylcholine, histamine, and orexin/hypocretin, and perhaps GABA. (GABA in neurons projecting from the basal forebrain to the cortex is assumed to inhibit cortical inhibitory neurons, thereby enhancing cortical activity [165]). Transmitters in the sleep-promoting network are less known. GABA and galanine are likely included (166,167). Neuropeptide Y was identified as the neurotransmitter in a neuron in the basal forebrain that fired during cortical EEG slow-wave activity, and it may correspond to a sleep-active neuron (168). It is suggested that GHRH is also a neurotransmitter in the sleep-promoting network in the hypothalamus. GHRHergic neurons may simultaneously promote NREM sleep and the secretion of a major anabolic hormone of the body, GH. We propose that one function of GHRH is to adjust tissue anabolism to a period when the body is in rest owing to sleep. It is also possible that GHRH conveys need for sleep from other parts of the brain, need for rest from the body, or circadian inputs to sleep regulation. However, currently the stimuli regulating GHRHergic neurons are not clear.

Molecules that express use-dependent sleep need arising in neuronal groups also seem to be involved in the direct maintenance of a synaptic super-structure via expression of molecules regulating neuronal connectivity. These substances, therefore, need to be produced throughout the brain in response to neural use, and, of course, promote sleep. IL-1, TNF, and related growth factors such as NGF and BDNF display these features. It is also characteristic of these molecules that in addition to stimulating the sleep-promoting network in the basal forebrain-hypothalamus, they are capable of enhancing sleep (or inhibiting wakefulness) by acting at other sites, e.g., inhibiting neurons in the locus ceruleus, modulating serotonergic activity, and stimulating other sleep-promoting substances such as NO, PGD2, adenosine, and GHRH. Considering the activity-dependent release of adenosine, this molecule is ideally suited to mediate sleep need as the function of use. In addition, adenosine also stimulates glial synthesis of glycogen (169), a function proposed to be associated with sleep (170,171). Other observations, however, suggest that replenishment of glycogen stores also occurs in wakefulness during sleep deprivation (172). Adenosine is an activity-dependent, locally released sleep-promoting molecule in the basal forebrain where extracellular concentrations of adenosine might be determined by the use of wake-active neurons. Increases and decreases in extracellular adenosine during wakefulness and sleep also occur in the cerebral cortex, thalamus, and brainstem (12). The significance of these variations in extracellular adenosine for sleep remained unclear because, after an initial rise, extracellular adenosine declined during sustained wakefulness, and because perfusion of adenosine into the thalamus failed to promote sleep. However, perfusion of adenosine into the laterodorsal tegmentum does enhance sleep (13). In our model, sleep occurs when a significant number of the neuronal groups signal their need for sleep to the basal forebrain sleep-regulating network, and therefore adenosine application into a limited number of neuronal groups may not elicit sleep. Also theoretically, extracellular adenosine does not have to continuously rise in individual neuronal groups during wakefulness because the activity of the various neuronal groups during sleep deprivation might vary enormously, and some nonstimulated neuronal groups may actually switch to a resting mode. It is possible, therefore, that adenosine contributes to the expression of use-dependent sleep need outside of the basal forebrain. That A1 receptor knockout mice sleep normally and have normal responses to sleep deprivation (17) is strong evidence against a major importance of this molecule. However, this finding may only indicate that multiple molecules are involved in signaling sleep need and that the loss of adenosine action is compensated. As a matter of fact, chronic deficiencies in other sleep-promoting molecules implicated in signaling of sleep need, e.g., IL-1 and TNF, also result in only modest decreases in sleep. Similarly, when lesions are made to sleep-regulating networks, initially, more or less sleep may occur, although as the animal recuperates, sleep tends to return toward control values.

In our model, when the activity of a neuronal group changes in response to use-dependent release of sleep-promoting substances, this neuronal group signals to the sleep-regulating network in the basal forebrain. The sleep-regulating network integrates information received through afferents and the integrated sleep-promoting activity is distributed among the various neuronal groups through efferent projections. However, signaling from the neuronal groups to the sleep-regulating network can be humoral if there is an appropriate medium delivering the sleep-promoting molecules to the basal forebrain. The CSF can act as a vehicle; in fact, accumulation of sleep-promoting materials in the CSF has been repeatedly demonstrated in sleep-deprived animals and VIP may be one of these substances for REM sleep. The humoral mediation also allows integration of sleep need: concentration of the sleep-promoting substance in the CSF should be proportional to the sum of sleep needs arising from the various neuronal groups. PGD2 seems to act as a signal molecule between the neuronal groups and the basal forebrain. There are, however, some issues that are to be addressed in further studies with PGD2. Release of PGD2 from the arachnoid cells has to be regulated by sleep factors produced locally in the neuronal groups. Although IL-1, TNF, and perhaps other growth factors are capable of stimulating PGD2 synthesis, it has to be demonstrated that these substances in fact diffuse to the arachnoid cells and stimulate PGD2 secretion. Currently, it is difficult to envision how the brain tissue could influence PGD2 production in the epithelial cells of the choroid plexus and thus the choroid plexus might not be involved in homeostatic sleep regulation. The dynamics of the changes in PGD2 concentrations in the CSF are not known. PGD2 level increases during sleep deprivation (93) but it is unclear whether it decreases during recovery sleep. For example, PGD2 concentrations in the CSF tend to be higher during spontaneous NREM sleep than during wakefulness (93), and this is not consistent with signaling sleep need to the basal forebrain. Finally, the REM-sleep-promoting activity of circulating PRL may also be mediated via CSF as PRL is transported from blood into the CSF via a choroid plexus transport mechanism.

While GHRH, adenosine, IL-1/TNF, and PGD2 act predominantly on NREM sleep, VIP and PRL stimulate REM sleep. VIP-containing neurons in the brainstem are the most likely source of VIP in the CSF, and thus VIP might be a neurotransmitter in the REM-sleep-regulating network. The physiological role of PRL in REM-sleep regulation is currently not clear but PRL does not seem to have a REM-sleep-triggering function. REM-sleep promotion by PRL might be associated with some metabolic activities of PRL.

## IV. Conclusions

Over the past half century, our understanding of the humoral regulation of sleep has greatly improved. It seems likely that additional sleep-regulatory molecules will be described. Nevertheless, current data strongly support the hypothesis that sleep is regulated by a complex biochemical network, within which no single molecule is necessary for sleep. These substances interact at various levels with sleep-regulatory circuits, none of which also seem to be necessary for sleep to occur. These conclusions speak strongly to the robust nature of sleep and to the likelihood that sleep is a fundamental property of small groups of highly interconnected neurons.

## Acknowledgments

This work was supported by the National Institutes of Health, grant numbers NS25378, NS27250, NS31453, and HD36520 to Dr. James Krueger, and by the Hungarian National Science Foundation (OTKA 043156 ) and Ministry of Health (ETT P-04/033/2000) to Dr. Ferenc Obal, Jr.

## References

1. Bayliss WM, Starling EH. Mechanisms of pancreatic secretion. J Physiol 1902; 28:325–353.
2. Inoué S. Biology of sleep substances. Boca Raton, FL: CRC Press, 1989.
3. Legendre R, Piéron H. Recherches sur le besoin de sommeil consécutif á une veille prlongée. Z Allg Physiol 1913; 14:235–262.
4. Monnier M, Hösli L. Dialysis of sleep and waking factor in blood of the rabbit. Science 1964; 146:796–798.
5. Schoenenberger GA, Maier PF, Tobler HJ, Wilson K, Monnier M. The delta (EEG) sleep inducing peptide (DSIP). XI. Amino acid analysis, sequence, synthesis and activity of the nonapeptide. Pflügers Arch 1978; 376:119–129.
6. Miller TB, Goodrich CA, Pappenheimer JR. Sleep-promoting effects of cerebrospinal fluid from sleep deprived goats. Proc Natl Acad Scii USA 1967; 58:513–517.
7. Uchizono K, Higashi A, Iriki M, et al. Sleep-promoting fractions obtained from the brainstem of sleep-deprived rats. In: Ito M, Kubota K, Tsukahara N, Yagi K, eds. Intergative Control Functions of the Brain, Vol. I. Amsterdam, New York, Oxford: Elsevier/North-Holland Biomedical Press, 392–396.
8. Krueger JM, Pappenheimer JR, Karnovsky ML. The composition of sleep-promoting factor isolated from human urine. J Biol Chem 1982; 257:1664–1669.
9. Komoda Y, Ishikawa M, Nagasaki, H et al. Uridine, a sleep-promoting substance from brainstem of sleep- deprived rats. Biomed Res 1983; 4:223–227.
10. Komoda Y, Honda K, Inoué S. SPS-B, a physiological sleep regulator from the brainstems of sleep-deprived rats, identified as oxidized glutathione. Chem Pharm Bull 1990; 28:2057–2059.
11. Porkka-Heiskanen T, Strecker RE, Thakkar M, Bjorkum AA, Greene RW, McCarley RW. Adenosine: a mediator of the sleep-inducing effects of prolonged wakefulness. Science 1997; 276:1265–1268.

12. Porkka-Heiskanen T, Stecker RE, McCarley RW. Brain site-specificity of extracellular adenosine concentration changes during sleep deprivation and spontaneous sleep: an in vivo microdialysis study. Neuroscience 2000; 99:507–517.

13. Strecker RE, Morairty S, Thakkar MM, et al. Adenosinergic modulation of basal forebrain and preoptic/anterior hypothalamic neuronal activity in the control of behavioral state. Behav Brain Res 2000; 115:183–204.

14. Scammel TE, Gerashchenko DY, Mochizuki T, et al. An adenosine A2a agonist increases sleep and induces Fos in ventrolateral preoptic neurons. Neuroscience 2001; 107:653–663.

15. Hendricks JC, Finn SM, Panckeri KA et al. Rest in Drosophila is a sleep-like state. Neuron 2000; 25:129–138.

16. Kaushal N, Johansson B, Halldner L, Fredholm B, Greene RW. Reduced slow wave activity in the adenosine A1 receptor knockout mice. Soc Neurosci Abstr 2002; 27:2378.

17. Stenberg D, Litonius E, Halldner L, Johansson B, Fredholm B, Porkka-Heiskanen T. Sleep and its homeostatic regulation in adenosine A1–receptor knockout mice. Soc Neurosci Abst 2002; 474.7.

18. Basheer R, Rainnie DG, Porkka-Heiskanen T, Ramesh V, McCarley RW. Adenosine, prolonged wakefulness, and A1–activated NF-kB DNA binding in the basal forebrain of the rat. Neuroscience 2001; 104:731–739.

19. Basheer R, Porkka-Heiskanen T, Stenberg D, McCarley RW. Adenosine and behavioral state control: adenosine increases c-Fos protein and AP1 binding in basal forebrain of rats. Mol Brain Res 1999; 73:1–10.

20. Sawchenko PE, Swanson LW, Rivier J, Vale WW. The distribution of growth-hormone-releasing factor (GRF) immunoreactivity in the central nervous system of the rat: an immunohistochemical study using antisera directed against rat hypothalamic GRF. J Comp Neurol 1985; 237:100–115.

21. Van Cauter E, Plat L. Interrelations between sleep and the somatotropic axis. Sleep 1998; 21:553–565.

22. Obal F, Jr., Alföldi P, Cady AB, Johannsen L, Sáry G, Krueger JM. Growth hormone-releasing factor enhances sleep in rats and rabbits. Am J Physiol 1988; 255:R310–R316.

23. Zhang J, Obal F, Jr., Zheng T, Fang J, Taishi P, Krueger JM. Intrapreoptic microinjection of GHRH or its antagonist alters sleep in rats. J Neurosci 1999; 19:2187–2194.

24. Obal F, Jr., Floyd R, Kapas L, Bodosi B, Krueger JM. Effects of systemic GHRH on sleep in intact and hypophysectomized rats. Am J Physiol 1996; 270:E230–E237.

25. Obal F, Jr. The role of growth hormone-releasing hormone in sleep regulation. In: Borbély AA, Hayaishi O, Sejnowski TJ, Altman JS, eds. The Regulation of Sleep. Strasbourg: HFSP, 2000:112–121.

26. Karteszi M, Fiok J, Makara GB. Lack of episodic growth hormone secretion in rats with anterolateral deafferentation of the medial-basal hypothalamus. J Endocrinol 1983; 94:77–81.

27. De A, Churchill L, Obal F, Jr., Simasko S, Krueger JM. GHRH and IL1( increase cytoplasmic $Ca^{2+}$ levels in cultured hypothalamic GABAergic neurons. Brain Res 2002; 949:209–212.

28.  Steiger A, Antonijevic IA, Bohlhalter S, Frieboes RM, Friess E, Murck H. Effects of hormones on sleep. Horm Res 1998; 49:125–130.

29.  Obal F, Jr., Krueger JM. The somatotropic axis and sleep. Rev Neurol (Paris) 2001; 157:5S12–5S15.

30.  Obal F, Jr., Fang J, Taishi P, Kacsóh B, Gardi J, Krueger JM. Deficiency of growth hormone-releasing hormone signaling is associated with sleep alterations in the dwarf rat. J Neurosci 2001; 21:2912–2918.

31.  Obal F, Jr., Alt J, Taishi P, Gardi J, Krueger JM. Sleep in mice with non-functional growth hormone releasing hormone receptors. Am J Physiol 2003; 284:R131–R139.

32.  Hajdu I, Obal F, Jr., Fang J, Krueger JM, Rollo CD. Sleep of transgenic mice producing excess rat growth hormone. Am J Physiol 2002; 282:R70–R76.

33.  Gardi J, Taishi P, Speth R, Obal F, Jr., Krueger JM. Sleep loss alters hypothalamic growth hormone-releasing hormone receptors in rats. Neurosci Lett 2002; 329:69–72.

34.  Sassin JF, Parker DC, Mace JW, Gotlin RW, Johnson LC, Rossman LG. Human growth hormone release: relation to slow-wave sleep and sleep-waking cycles. Science 1969; 165:513–515.

35.  Drucker-Colin RR, Spanis CW, Hunyadi J, Sassin JF, McGaugh JL. Growth hormone effects on sleep and wakefulness in the rat. Neuroendocrinology 1975; 18:1–8.

36.  Aström C. Interaction between sleep and growth hormone. Acta Neurol Scand 1997; 92:281–296.

37.  Beranek L, Hajdu I, Gardi J, Taishi P, Obal F, Jr., Krueger JM. Central administration of the somatostatin analog octreotide induces captopril-insensitive sleep responses. Am J Physiol 1999; 277:R1297–R1304.

38.  Danguir J. Intracerebroventricular infusion of somatostatin selectively increases paradoxical sleep in rats. Brain Res 1986; 367:26–30.

39.  Vitkovic L, Bockaert J, Jacque C. Inflammatory cytokines: neuromodulators in normal brain? J Neurochem 2000; 74:457–471.

40.  Krueger JM, Obal F, Jr., Fang J, Kubota T, Taishi P. The role of cytokines in physiological sleep regulation. Ann NY Acad Sci 2001; 933:211–221.

41.  Krueger JM. Cytokines and growth factors in sleep regulation. In: Borbély AA, Hayaishi O, Sejnowski TJ, Altman JS, eds. The Regulation of Sleep. Strasbourg: HFSP, 2000:122–131.

42.  Breder CD, Dinarello CA, Saper CB. Interleukin-1 immunoreactive innervation of the human hypothalamus. Science 1988; 240:321–324.

43.  Breder CD, Tsujimoto M, Terano Y, Scott DW, Saper CB. Distribution and characterization of tumor necrosis factor-alpha-like immunoreactivity in the murine central nervous system. J Comp Neurol 1993; 337:543–567.

44.  Chen Z, Gardi J, Kushikata T, Fang J, Krueger JM. Nuclear factor-kappaB-like activity increases in murine cerebral cortex after sleep deprivation. Am J Physiol 1999; 276:R1812–R1818.

45.  Kubota T, Kushikata T, Fang J, Krueger JM. Nuclear factor-kappaB inhibitor peptide inhibits spontaneous and interleukin-1beta-induced sleep. Am J Physiol Regul Integr Comp Physiol 2000; 279:R404–R413.

46. Majde JA, Krueger JM. Neuroimmunology of sleep. In: D'haenen H, DeBoer JA, Westernberg H, Willner P, eds. Textbook of Biological Psychiatry. London: Wiley, 2002.

47. Fang J, Wang Y, Krueger JM. Mice lacking the TNF 55 kD receptor fail to sleep more after TNF alpha treatment. J Neurosci 1997; 17:5949–5955.

48. Wang CY, Majo MW, Korneluk RG, Goeddel DV, Baldwin AS Jr. NFkB antiapoptosis: induction of TRAF1 and TRAF2 and c-IAP2 to suppress caspase-8 activation. Science 1998; 281:1680–1683.

49. Puccioni-Sohler M, Rieckmann P, Kitze B, Lange P, Albrecht M, Flegenhauer K. A soluble form of tumor necrosis factor receptor in cerebrospinal fluid and serum of HTVLV-1–associated hyelopathy and other neurological diseases. Neurology 1995; 242:239–242.

50. Alam N, McGinty D, Imeri L, Opp M, Szymusiak R. Effects of interleukin-1 beta on sleep- and wake-related preoptic anterior hypothalamic neurons in unrestrained rats. Sleep 2001; 24:A59.

51. Taishi P, De A, Teodecki L, Obal F, Jr., Krueger JM. Interleukin-1 beta induces expression of GHRH receptor mRNA on neurons. J Sleep Res 2002; 11 (S1):221–222.

52. De Sarro G, Gareri P, Sinopoli VA, David E, Rotiroti D. Comparative, behavioural and electrocotical effects of tumor necrosis factor-alpha and interleukin-1 microinjected into the locus ceruleus of rat. Life Sci 1997; 60:555–564.

53. Imeri L, Bianchi S, Mariotti M, Opp MR. Interleukin-1 microinjected into the dorsal raphe nucleus enhances NREM sleep in rats. J Sleep Res 2002; 11:107.

54. Kubota T, Li N, Guan Z, Bom RA, Krueger JM. Intrapreoptic microinjection of TNF-alpha enhances non-REMS in rats. Brain Res 2002; 932:37–44.

55. Opp MR, Imeri L. Rat strains that differ in corticotropin-releasing hormone production exhibit different sleep-wake responses to interleukin 1. 2001; 73:272–284.

56. Chang FC, Opp MR. IL-1 is a mediator of increases in slow-wave sleep induced by CRH receptor blockade. Am J Physiol 2000; 279:R793–R802.

57. Moss RB, Mercandetti A, Vohdani A. TNF-alpha and chronic fatigue syndrome. J Clin Immunol 1999; 19:314–316.

58. Vgontzas AN, Zoumakis M, Papanicolaou DA, Bixler EO, Prolo P, Lin HM, Vela-Bueno A, Kales A, Chrousos GP. Chronic insomnia is associated with a shift of interleukin-6 and tumor necrosis factor secretion from nighttime to daytime. Metabolism 2002; 51:887–892.

59. Liu H, Kiu J, Xiong S, Sgen G, Zhang Z, Xu Y. The change in interleukin-6 and tumor necrosis factor in patients with obstructive sleep apnea syndrome. J Tongji Med Univ 2000; 20:200–202.

60. Dreisbach AW, Hendrickson T, Beezhold D, Riesenberg LA, Sklar AH. Elevated levels of tumor necrosis factor alpha in postdialysis fatigue. Int J Artif Organs 1998; 21:83–86.

61. Sklar AH, Beezhold D, Newman N, Hendrickson T, Dreisbach AW. Postdialysis fatigue: lack of effect of a biochmpatible membrane. Am J Kidney Dis 1998; 31:1007–1010.

62. Eskander ED, Harvey HA, Givant E, Lipton A. Phase I study combining tumor necrosis factor with interferon-alpha and interleukin-2. Am J Clin Oncol 1997; 20:511–514.

63. Franklin CM. Clinical experience with soluble TNF p75 receptor in rheumantoid arthritis. Semin Arthitis Rheum 1999; 29:171–181.

64. Kubota T, Fang J, Guan Z, Brundege JM, Krueger JM. Vagotomy attenuates tumor necrosis factor-alpha-induced sleep and EEG delta-activity in rats. Am J Physiol 2001; 280:R1213–R1220.

65. Hansen MK, Taishi P, Chen Z, Krueger JM. Vagotomy blocks the induction of interleukin-2 beta mRNA in the brain of rats in response to systemic interleukin-1 beta. J Neurosci 1998; 18:2247–2253.

66. Hansen M, Kapas L, Fang J, Krueger JM. Cafeteria diet-induced sleep is blocked by subdiaphragmatic vagotomy. Am J Physiol 1998; 274:R168–R174.

67. Takahashi S, Krueger JM. Inhibition of tumor necrosis factor prevents warming-induced sleep responses in rabbits. Am J Physiol 1997; 272:R1325–R1329.

68. Fang J, Wang Y, Krueger JM. The effects of interleukin-1 beta on sleep are mediated by the type I receptor. Am J Physiol 1998; 274:R655–R660.

69. Deboer T, Fontana A, Tobler I. Tumor necrosis factor (TNF) ligand and TNF receptor deficiency affects sleep and the sleep EEG. J Neurosci 2001; 88:839–846.

70. Floyd RA, Krueger JM. Diurnal variations of TNF alpha in the rat brain. Neuroreport 1997; 8:915–918.

71. Bredow S, Taishi P, Guha-Thakurta N, Obal F Jr, Krueger JM. Diurnal variations of tumor necrosis factor-alpha mRNA and alpha-tubulin mRNA in rat brain. J Neuroimmunomod 1997; 4:84–90.

72. Lue FA, Bail FA, Jephtha-Ocholo J, Carayanniotis K, Gorczynski R, Moldofsky H. Sleep and cerebrospinal fluid interleukin-1 like activity in the cat. Int J Neurosci 1998; 42:179–183.

73. Nguyen KT, Deak T, Owens SM, Kohno T, Fleshner M, Watkins LR, Maier SF. Exposure to acute stress induces brain interleukin-1 beta protein in the rat. J Neurosci 1998; 18:2239–2246.

74. Taishi P, Bredow S, Guha-Thakurta N, Obal F Jr, Krueger JM. Diurnal variations of interleukin-1 beta mRNA and beta-actin mRNA in rat brain. J Neuroimmunol 1997; 75:69–74.

75. Mackiewicz M, Sollars PJ, Ogilvie MD, Pack AI. Modulation of IL-1 beta gene expression in the rat CNS during sleep deprivation. Neuroreport 1996; 7:529–533.

76. Veasey SC, Mackiewicz M, Fenik P, Ro M, Ogilvie MD, Pack AL. IL1 beta knockout mice lack the TNF alpha response to sleep deprivation but have normal sleep and sleep recovery. Soc Neurosci Abstr 1997; 23:792.

77. Taishi P, Gardi J, Chen Z, Fang J, Krueger JM. Sleep deprivation increases the expression of TNF alpha mRNA and TNF 55kD receptor mRNA in rat brain. Physiologist 1999; 42:A4.

78. Moldofsky H. Lue FA, Eisen J, Keystone E. Gorcznski RM. The relationship of interleukin-1 and immune functions to sleep in humans. Psychosom Med 1986; 48:309–318.

79. Hohagen F, Timmer J, Weyerbrock A, Fritsch-Montero R, Ganter U, Krieger S, Berger M, Bauer J. Cytokine production during sleep and wakefulness and its relationship to cortisol in healthy humans. Neuropsychobiology 1993; 28:9–16.

80. Darko DF, Miller JC, Gallen C, White J, Koziol J, Brown SJ, Hayduk, Atkinson JH, Assmus J, Munnel DT, Naitotl P, McCutchen A, Mitler MM. Sleep electroencephalogram delta-frequency amplitude, night plasma levels of tumor necrosis fac-

tor alpha, and human immunodeficiency virus infection. Proc Natl Acad Sci USA 2002; 92:12080–12084.

81. Shearer WT, Reuben JM, Mullington JM, Price NJ, Lee BN, Smith EO, Szuba MP, Van Dongen HP, Dinges DF. Soluble TNF-alpha receptor 1 and IL-6 plasma levels in human subjected to the sleep deprivation model of spaceflight. J Allergy Clin Immunol 2001; 107:165–170.

82. Krueger JM, Walter J, Dinarello CA, Wolff SM, Chedid L. Sleep-promoting effects of endogenous pyrogen (interleukin-1). Am J Physiol 1984; 246:R994–R999.

83. Urade Y, Hayaishi O. Prostaglandin D2 and sleep regulation. Bichim Biophys Acta 1999; 1436:606–615.

84. Urade Y, Kitahama K, Ohishi H, Keneko T, Mizuno N, Hayaishi O. Dominant expression of mRNA for prostaglandin D synthase in leptomeninges, choroid plexus and oligodendrocytes of the adult rat brain. Proc Natl Acad Sci USA 1993; 90:9070–9074.

85. Blödorn B, Mäder M, Urade Y, Hayaishi O, Felgenhauer K, Bruck W. Choroid plexus: the major site of mRNA expression for the beta-trace protein (prostaglandin D synthase) in human brain. Neurosci Lett 1996; 209:117–120.

86. Mizoguchi A, Eguchi N, Kimura K et al. Dominant localization of prostaglandin D receptors on arachnoid trabecular cells in mouse basal forebrain and their involvement in the regulation of non-rapid eye movement sleep. Proc Natl Acad Sci USA 2001; 98:11674–11679.

87. Hayaishi O. Regulation of sleep by prostaglandin D2 and adenosine. In: Borbély AA, Hayaishi O, Sejnowski TJ, Altman JS, eds. The Regulation of Sleep. Strasbourg: HFSP, 2000:97–103.

88. Hayaishi O. Molecular mechanisms of sleep-wake regulation: roles of prostaglandins D2 and E2. FASEB J 1991; 5:2575–2581.

89. Krueger JM, Kapas L, Opp MR, Obal F Jr. Prostaglandins E2 and D2 have little effect on rabbit sleep. Physiol Behav 1992; 51:481–485.

90. Pinzar E, Kanaoka Y, Inui T, Eguchi N, Urade Y, Hayaishi O. Prostaglandin D synthase gene is involved in the regulation of non-rapid eye movement sleep. Proc Natl Acad Sci USA 2000; 97:4903–4907.

91. Yoshida H, Kubota T, Krueger JM. A cyclooxygenase-2 inhibitor attenuates spontaneous and TNF(-induced non-rapid eye movement sleep. Submitted.

92. Lee B, Hirst JJ, Walker DW. Prostaglandin D synthase in the prenatal ovine brain and effects of its inhibition with selenium chloride on fetal sleep/wake activity in utero. J Neurosci 2002; 22:5679–5686.

93. Ram A, Pandey HP, Matsumura H. CSF levels of prostaglandins, especially the level of prostaglandin D2, are correlated with increasing propensity towards sleep in rats. Brain Res 1997; 751:81–89.

94. Nicolaidis S, Gerozissis K, Orosco M. Variations des prostaglandines et des monoamines hypothalamiques et corticales révélatrices de la transition entre états de vigilance: étude en microdialyse chez le rat. Rev Neurol (Paris) 2001; 11:5S26–5S33.

95. Goffin V, Binart N, Touraine P, Kelly PA. Prolactin: the new biology of an old hormone. Annu Rev Physiol 2002; 64:47–67.

96. Li-Yuan YL. Prolactin modulation of immune and inflammatory responses. Recent Prog Horm Res 2002; 57:435–455.

97.  Spiegel K, Luthringer R, Follenius M, Schaltenbrand N, Macher JP, Muzet A, Brandenberger G. Temporal relationship between prolactin secretion and slow-wave electroencephalic activity during sleep. Sleep 1995; 18:543–548.

98.  Jouvet M, Buda C, Cespuglio R, Chastrette R, Denoyer M, Sallanon M, Sastre JP. 1986; Hypnogenic effects of some hypothalamo-pituitary peptides. Clin Neuropharmacol 9:S465–S467.

99.  Obal F Jr, Opp M, Cady AB, Johannsen L, Krueger JM. Prolactin, vasoactive intestinal peptide, and peptide histidine methionine elicit selective increases in REM sleep in rabbits. Brain Res 1989; 490:292–300.

100. Roky R, Valatx JL, Jouvet M. Effect of prolactin on the sleep-wake cycle in the rat. Neurosci Lett 1993; 156:117–120.

101. Zhang SQ, Kimura M, Inoue S. Effects of prolactin on sleep in cyclic rats. Psychiatry Clin Neurosci 1999; 53:101–103.

102. Roky R, Valatx JL, Paut-Pagano L, Jouvet M. Hypothalamic injection of prolactin or its antibody alters the rat sleep-wake cycle. Physiol Behav 1994; 55:1015–1019.

103. Obal Jr F, Payne L, Kacsoh B, Opp M, Kapas L, Grosvenor CE, Krueger JM. . Involvement of prolactin in the REM sleep-promoting activity of systemic vasoactive intestinal peptide (VIP). Brain Res 1994; 645:143–149.

104. Obal F Jr, Kacsoh B, Bredow S, Guha-Thakurta N, Krueger JM. Sleep in rats rendered chronically hyperprolactinemic with anterior pituitary grafts. Brain Res 1997; 755:130–136.

105. Frieboes RM, Murck H, Stalla GK, Antonijevic IA, Steiger A. Enhanced slow wave sleep in patients with prolactinoma. J Clin Endocrinol Metab 1998; 83:2706–2710.

106. Valatx JL, Jouvet M. Circadian rhythms of slow-wave sleep and paradoxical sleep are in opposite phase in genetically hypoprolactinemic rats. CR Acad Sci III 1988; 307:789–794.

107. Lobo-Leite L, Claustrant B, Debilly G, Paut-Pagano L, Jouvet M, Valatx JL. Hypoprolactinemic rats under conditions of constant darkness or constant light: effects on the sleep-wake cycle, cerebral temperature and sulfatoxymelatonin levels. Brain Res 1999; 835:282–289.

108. Obal F Jr, Kacsoh B, Alfoldi P, Payne L, Markovic O, Grosvenor C, Krueger JM. Antiserum to prolactin decreases rapid eye movement sleep (REM sleep) in the male rat. Physiol Behav 1992; 52:1063–1068.

109. Calvo JM, Simon-Arceo K, Fernandez-Mas R. Prolonged enhancement of REM sleep produced by carbachol microinjection into the amygdala. Neuroreport 1996; 7:577–80.

110. Siaud P, Manzoni O, Balmefrezol M, Barbanel G, Assenmacher I, Alonso G. The organization of prolactin-like-immunoreactive neurons in the rat central nervous system. light- and electron-microscopic immunocytochemical studies. Cell Tissue Res 1989; 255:107–115.

111. Roky R, Paut-Pagano L, Goffin V, Kitahama K, Valatx JL, Kelly PA, Jouvet M. Distribution of prolactin receptors in the rat forebrain. immunohistochemical study. Neuroendocrinology 1996; 63:422–429.

112. Sanford LD, Nassar P, Ross RJ, Schulkin J, Morrison AR. Prolactin microinjections into the amygdalar central nucleus lead to decreased NREM sleep. Sleep Res Online 1998; 1:109–113.

113. Roky R, Obal F Jr, Valatx JL, Bredow S, Fang J, Pagano LP, Krueger JM. Prolactin and rapid eye movement sleep regulation. Sleep 1995; 18:536–542.
114. Baghdoyan HA, Spotts JL, Snyder SG. Simultaneous pontine and basal forebrain microinjections of carbachol suppress REM sleep. J Neurosci 1993; 13:229–242.
115. Takahashi K, Koyama Y, Kayama Y, Yamamoto M. The effects of prolactin on the mesopontine tegmental neurons. Psychiatry Clin Neurosci 2000; 54:257–258.
116. Zhang S-Q, Kimura M, Inoue S. Bromocriptine-induced blockade of pregnancy affects sleep patterns in rats. Neuroimmunomodulation 1996; 3:219–226.
117. Gala RR. The physiology and mechanisms of the stress-induced changes in prolactin secretion in the rat. Life Sci 1990; 46:1407–1420.
118. García-García F, Beltrán-Parrazal L, Jiménez-Anguiano A, Vega-González A, Drucker-Colín R. Manipulations during forced wakefulness have differential impact on sleep architecture, EEG power spectrum, and Fos induction. Brain Res Bull 1998; 47:317–324.
119. Rampin C, Cespuglio R, Chastrette N, Jouvet M. Immobilization stress induces a paradoxical sleep rebound in rat. Neurosci Lett 1991; 126:113–118.
120. Gonzalez MM, Debilly G, Valatx JL, Jouvet M. Sleep increase after immobilization stress: role of the noradrenergic locus coeruleus system in the rat. Neurosci Lett 1995; 202:5–8.
121. Bodosi B, Obal F Jr, Gardi J, Komlodi J, Fang J, Krueger JM. An ether stressor increases REM sleep in rats: possible role of prolactin. Am J Physiol 2000; 279:R1590–R1598.
122. Meerlo P, Easton A, Bergmann BM, Turek FW. Restraint increases prolactin and REM sleep in C57BL/6J mice but not in BALB/cJ mice. Am J Physiol 2001; 281:R846–R854.
123. Morel G, Enjalbert A, Proulx L, Pelletier G, Barden N, Grossard F, Dubois PM. Effect of corticotropin-releasing factor on the release and synthesis of prolactin. Neuroendocrinology 1989; 49:669–675.
124. Gonzalez MM, Valatx JL. Effect of intracerebroventricular administration of alpha-helical CRH (9–41) on the sleep/waking cycle in rats under normal conditions or after subjection to an acute stressful stimulus. J Sleep Res 1997; 6:164–70.
125. Zhang SQ, Kimura M, Inoue S. Effects of prolactin-releasing peptide (PrRP) on sleep regulation in rats. Psychiatry Clin Neurosci 2000; 54:262–264.
126. Zhang SQ, Inoue S, Kimura M. Sleep-promoting activity of prolactin-releasing peptide (PrRP) in the rat. Neuroreport 2001; 12:3173–3176.
127. Maruyama M, Hirokazu M, Fujiwara K, Noguchi J, Kitada C, Fujino M, Inoue K. Prolactin-releasing peptide as a novel stress mediator in the central nervous system. Endocrinology 2001; 142:2032–2038.
128. Matsumoto H, Maruyama M, Noguchi J, Horikoshi Y, Fujiwara K, Kitada C, Hinuma S, Onda H, Nishimura O, Inoue K, Fujino M. Stimulation of corticotropin-releasing hormone-mediated adrenocorticotropin secretion by central administration of prolactin-releasing peptide in rats. Neurosci Lett 2000; 285:234–238.
129. Chang F-C, Opp MR. Role of corticotropin-releasing hormone in stressor-induced alterations of sleep in rat. 2002. Am J Physiol 283: R400–R407.
130. Said SI, Mutt V. Polypeptide with broad biological activity: isolation from small intestine. Science 1970; 169:1217–1278.

131. Wei Y, Mojsov S. Tissue specific expression of different human receptor types for pituitary adenylate cyclase activating polypeptide and vasoactive intestinal polypeptide: implications for their role in human physiology. J Neuroendocrinol 1996; 8:811–817.

132. Usdin TB, Bonner TI, Mezey E. Two receptors for vasoactive intestinal polypeptide with similar specificity and complementary distributions. Endocrinology 1994; 135:2662–2680.

133. Riou F, Cespuglio R, Jouvet M. Hypnogenic properties of the vasoactive intestinal polypeptide in rats. CR Acad Sci III 1981; 293:679–682.

134. Drucker-Colín R, Bernal-Pedraza J, Fernandez-Cancino F, Oksenberg A. Is vasoactive intestinal polypeptide (VIP) a sleep factor? Peptides 1984; 5:837–840.

135. Drucker-Colin R, Aguilar-Roblero R, Arankowsky-Sandoval G. Sleep factors released from brain of unrestrained cats: a critical appraisal. Ann NY Acad Sci 1986; 473:449–460.

136. Obal F Jr, Sary G, Alfoldi P, Rubicsek G, Obal F. Vasoactive intestinal polypeptide promotes sleep without effects on brain temperature in rats at night. Neurosci Lett 1986; 64:236–240.

137. Mirmiran M, Kruisbrink J, Bos NP, Van der Werf D, Boer GJ. Decrease of rapid-eye-movement sleep in the light by intraventricular application of a VIP-antagonist in the rat. Brain Res 1988; 458:192–194.

138. Prospero-García O, Morales M, Arankowsky-Sandoval G, Drucker-Colin R. Vasoactive intestinal polypeptide (VIP) and cerebrospinal fluid (CSF) of sleep-deprived cats restores REM sleep in insomniac recipients. Brain Res 1986; 385:169–173.

139. Drucker-Colin R, Prospero-Garcia O, Arankowsky-Sandoval G, perez-Monfort R. 1988. Gastropancreatic peptides and sensory stimuli as REM factors. In: Inoué S, Schneider-Helmert D, eds. Sleep peptides: basixc and Clinical Approaches. Berlin:Springer, 1988:73–94.

140. Jimenez-Anguiano A, Baez-Saldana A, Drucker-Colin R. Cerebrospinal fluid (CSF) extracted immediately after REM sleep deprivation prevents REM rebound and contains vasoactive intestinal peptide (VIP). Brain Res 1993; 63:345–348.

141. Morin AJ, Denoroy L, Jouvet M. Daily variations in concentration of vasoactive intestinal peptide immunoreactivity in hypothalamic nuclei of rats rendered diurnal by restricted-schedule feeding. Neurosci Lett 1993; 152:121–124.

142. Schilling J, Nurnberger F. Dynamic changes in the immunoreactivity of neuropeptide systems of the suprachiasmatic nuclei in golden hamsters during the sleep-wake cycle. Cell Tissue Res 1998; 294:233–241.

143. Jimenez-Anguiano A, Garcia-Garcia F, Mendoza-Ramirez JL, Duran-Vazquez A, Drucker-Colin R. Brain distribution of vasoactive intestinal peptide receptors following REM sleep deprivation. Brain Res 1996; 728:37–46.

144. Bourgin P, Lebrand C, Escourrou P, Gaultier C, Franc B, Hamon M, Adrien J. Vasoactive intestinal polypeptide microinjections into the oral pontine tegmentum enhance rapid eye movement sleep in the rat. Neuroscience 1997; 77:351–60.

145. Magistretti PJ. VIP neurons in the cerebral cortex. Trends Pharmacol Sci 1990; 11:250–254.

146. Whittaker VP. Vasoactive intestinal polypeptide (VIP) as a cholinergic co-transmitter: some recent results. Cell Biol Int Rep 1989; 13:1039–1051.

147. Bourgin P, Ahnaou A, Laporte AM, Hamon M, Adrien J. Rapid eye movement sleep induction by vasoactive intestinal peptide infused into the oral pontine tegmentum of the rat may involve muscarinic receptors. Neuroscience 1999;89:291–302.
148. Kohlmeier KA, Reiner PB. Vasoactive intestinal polypeptide excites medial pontine reticular formation neurons in the brainstem rapid eye movement sleep-induction zone. J Neurosci 1999; 19:4073–81.
149. Prospero-Garcia O, Jimenez-Anguiano A, Drucker-Colin R. The combination of VIP and atropine induces REM sleep in cats rendered insomniac by PCPA. Neuropsychopharmacology 1993; 8:387–390.
150. Abe H, Engler D, Molitch ME, Bollinguer-Gruber J, Reinchlin S. Vasoactive intestinal peptide is a physiological mediator of prolactin release in the rat. Endocrinology 1985; 1116:1383–1390.
151. Bredow S, Kacsoh B, Obal F Jr, Fang J, Krueger JM. Increase of prolactin mRNA in the rat hypothalamus after intracerebroventricular injection of VIP or PACAP. Brain Res 1994; 660:301–308.
152. Cravatt BF, Prospero-Garcia O, Siuzdak G, et al. Chemical characterization of a family of brain lipids that induce sleep. Science 1995; 268:1506–1509.
153. Cravatt BF, Giang DK, Mayfield SP, Boger DL, Lerner RA, Gilula NB. Molecular characterization of an enzyme that degrades neuromodulatory fatty-acid amides. Nature 1996; 384:83–87.
154. Spier AD, De Lecea L. Cortistatin: a member of the somatostatin neuropeptide family with distinct physiological functions. Brain Res Rev 2000; 33:228–241.
155. Kapas L, Obal F, Jr., Alföldi P, Rubicsek G, Penke B, Obal F. Effects of nocturnal intraperitoneal administration of cholecystokinin in rats: simultaneous increase in sleep, increase in EEG slow-wave activity, reduction of motor activity, suppression of eating, and decrease in brain temperature. Brain Res 1988; 438:155–164.
156. Danguir J, Nicolaidis S. Chronic intracerebroventricular infusion of insulin causes selective increase of slow wave sleep in rats. Brain Res 1984; 306:97–103.
157. Obal F, Jr., Kapas L, Bodosi B, Krueger JM. Changes in sleep in response to intracerebral injection of insulin-like growth factor-1 (IGF-1) in the rat. Sleep Res Online 1998; 1:87–91.
158. Ribeiro AC, Gilligan JG, Kapas L. Systemic injection of a nitric oxide synthase inhibitor suppresses sleep responses to sleep deprivation in rats. Am J Physiol 2000; 278:R1048–R1056.
159. Burlet.S., Leger L, Cespuglio R. Nitric oxide and sleep in the rat: a puzzling relationship. Neuroscience 1999; 92:627–639.
160. Leonard TO, Lydic R. Pontine nitric oxide modulates acetylcholine release, rapid eye movement sleep generation, and respiratory rate. J Neurosci 1997; 17:774–785.
161. Chen L, Majde JA, Krueger JM. Spontaneous sleep in mice with targeted disruptions of neuronal or inducible nitric oxide synthase genes. Submitted.
162. Krueger JM, Obal F Jr. Sleep function. Frontiers Biosci 2003; 8:511–519.
163. Szymusiak R. Magnocellular nuclei of the basal forebrain: substrates of sleep and arousal regulation. Sleep 1995; 18:478–500.
164. Saper CB, Chou TC, Scammell TE. The sleep switch: hypothalamic control of sleep and wakefulness. Trends Neurosci 2001; 24:726–731.
165. Zaborszky L, Pang K, Somogyi J, Nadasdy Z, Kallo I. The basal forebrain corticopetal system revisited. Ann NY Acad Sci 1999; 877:339–367.

166. Sherin JE, Elmquist JK, Torrealba F, Saper CB. Innervation of histaminergic tuberomammillary neurons by GABAergic and galaninergic neurons in the ventro-lateral preoptic nucleus of the rat. J Neurosci 1998; 18:4705–4721.

167. Chou TC, Bjorkum AA, Gaus SE, Lu J, Scammell TE, Saper CB. Afferents to the ventrolateral preoptic nucleus. J Neurosci 2002; 22:977–990.

168. Duque A, Balatoni B, Detari L, Zaborszky L. EEG correlation of the discharge properties of identified neurons in the basal forebrain. J Neurophysiol 2000; 84:1627–1635.

169. Petit JM, Allaman I, Baudaut J, Tobler I, Borbély AA. Transcriptional regulation of genes related to glycogen metabolism by adenosine: possible involvement in the sleep-wake cycle. J Sleep Res 2002; 11(S1):175.

170. Benington JH, Heller HC. Restoration of brain energy metabolism as the function of sleep. Prog Neurobiol 1995; 45:347–360.

171. Kong J, Shepel N, Holden CP, Mackiewicz M, Pack AI, Geiger JD. Brain glycogen decreases with increased periods of wakefulness: implications for homeostatic drive to sleep. J Neurosci 2002; 22:5581–5587.

172. Gip P, Hagiwara G, Ruby NF, Heller HC. Sleep deprivation decreases glycogen in the cerebellum but not in the cortex of young rats. Am J Physiol 2002; 283:R54–R59.

# 27

# The Role of Pharmacological Interventions for Sleep Deprivation

**JAMES K. WALSH**

St. John's Mercy Medical Center, St. Luke's Hospital, and Saint Louis University, St. Louis, Missouri, U.S.A.

**THOMAS ROTH**

Henry Ford Health System, and University of Michigan, Detroit, Michigan, U.S.A.

## I. Introduction

Human sleep occurs involuntarily. That is, with rare possible exceptions, humans cannot volitionally change their brain state from wakefulness to sleep. The environment and behavior can be manipulated to increase the likelihood of sleep, but the neural activity that brings about sleep is essentially involuntary. Similarly, the maintenance of sleep (i.e., sleep length) and the termination of sleep (awakening) are endogenous processes, rather than under voluntary control. In fact, when individuals wish to impact the awakening process, they rely on external stimuli (e.g., alarm clock). In sum, endogenous neural processes control:

1. conversion of a waking brain to a sleeping brain,
2. sustaining the sleep state,
3. conversion of a sleeping brain to a waking brain.

On the other hand, wakefulness can be volitionally maintained for long periods of time (with the possible exception of infants and young children). This is the only brain state under volitional control of virtually all adult humans. In fact, 21st-century humans seem intent on exploiting this ability to convert extra waking hours and minutes into dollars and cents, as well as to fulfill desires for recreation and enjoyment. Employers encourage shift work and overtime; ambitious individuals work long hours, some holding two full-time jobs. These lifestyle options exist because humans have the capacity to forestall sleep. Self-imposed sleep restriction for social purposes, like poor nutritional habits and lack of adequate exercise, can be viewed as part of a pattern of self-indulgence by a society no longer deferential to its own biology, but rather intent on overriding homeostatic systems.

The lack of voluntary control over sleep generation, and the large degree of voluntary control over sustaining wakefulness (albeit with declining functional ability), underlie the considerations of this chapter. In short, this chapter considers expansion of control over (a) production of sleep and (b) maintenance of high-quality, functional wakefulness with pharmaceuticals. An increase in control over sleep and wakefulness may be unacceptable for some individuals holding an opinion that helping people "feel better" or function more effectively is not a justifiable reason for the use of psychotropic medication without convincing evidence that the health and safety benefits outweigh the risks. The term "pharmacological Calvinism" was used by Klerman (1) to describe this position or attitude. Even John Calvin himself, however, would recognize that modern, industrialized society brings an increase in the number of sleepy people in society (many unavoidably) and, with that, great risk to the sleepy and to those around them. Reduction of danger and misery through pharmacological intervention, when other means are not readily available, seems clearly justifiable, and rather easily distinguishable from recreational drug use. Certainly informed physicians and institutions are essential to define appropriate use, and one could convincingly argue that sleep medicine specialists are best positioned to undertake a strong leadership role in the development of guidelines in this area.

## II.  The Health and Safety Risks of Sleep Deprivation

The consequences and correlates of sleep deprivation in its various forms are extensively reviewed in a number of other chapters (e.g., Chaps. 10–19), and will not be reviewed here. Briefly, there is growing evidence that sleep deprivation and sleep disruption are associated with negative mood, decreased productivity, occupational and transportation accidents, reduced quality of life, poor school attendance, impairment of performance, learning, memory, and physiological changes that theoretically increase the risk of major illnesses, such as diabetes, hypertension, and obesity.

Sleep deprivation not only occurs because of reduced time allotted for sleep (either voluntary or imposed), but also results from inability to obtain adequate duration or quality of sleep. Worldwide, millions of people experience disrupted sleep each day, either on a relatively isolated night or nights or as part of a persistent pattern of inadequate sleep. If the sleep disturbance is of sufficient magnitude, either on a single night or over many nights, negative impact upon waking function becomes likely.

The duration of the problem determines whether transient or chronic insomnia underlies sleep loss. Transient insomnia refers to no more than a few nights of poor sleep, which generally results from challenges such as: (a) acute illness, (b) stress, (c) suboptimal circadian time for sleep, or (d) a disruptive sleep environment. In the absence of these challenges the individuals typically sleep normally. That is, they judge their sleep to be satisfactory. It is reasonable to conclude, therefore, that the impact of transient insomnia on waking function can be extrapolated from partial sleep deprivation research conducted in normal sleepers. Such studies limit the amount of sleep obtained, on one or more nights, just as in the case of transient insomnia.

One possible exception to the parallel between the impact of transient insomnia and the impact of partial sleep deprivation may be stress-related transient insomnia. One could hypothesize that an individual under extreme stress (e.g., a death of a loved one) might experience a pronounced physiological stress response during the day, as well as at night, which might mitigate at least some of the impact of sleep disruption. However, for most transient insomnias, the parallel with sleep deprivation research would appear to be quite appropriate.

Lack of population-based, longitudinal research, combined with diversity in etiology and severity of chronic insomnia, currently precludes a clear understanding of the consequences of chronic insomnia. Available evidence indicates the consequences are not likely to be uniform across diagnostic entities, and in the case of chronic primary insomnia, any presumption of similarity to the impact of sleep deprivation is misguided. Bonnet and Arand (2) and others (3) have documented that primary insomniacs are diurnally hyperaroused, in contrast to the reduction in arousal seen with any form of sleep deprivation, and performance measures fail to consistently demonstrate impairment. On the other hand, occasional studies suggest that chronic insomnia secondary to medical conditions, including some primary sleep disorders (e.g., sleep-disordered breathing, periodic limb movement disorder), has outcomes similar to those seen in sleep deprivation and sleep fragmentation studies (4,5).

## III. Pharmacological Prevention of Sleep Deprivation

The focus of this section will be the prevention of sleep loss through the use of sleep-promoting medications. Choice of sleep medications will not be considered, as others have thoroughly discussed this issue (6). Short-acting benzodiazepine receptor agonists are generally the type of medication recommended for the treatment of transient insomnia and chronic primary insomnia, and as adjunctive therapy for secondary chronic insomnias.

### A. Transient Insomnia

The frequent predictability of transient insomnia provides opportunity for prevention. Perhaps the most straightforward example would involve transient insomnia related to jet lag. Consider the situation of a Californian traveling to the Eastern time zone, needing to rise at 7 A.M. the next day for work. His or her usual bedtime is 11 P.M.; however, 11 P.M. Eastern time corresponds to a Pacific Coast time of 8 P.M., a time of very low physiological sleep tendency. The typical West coast traveler who tries to sleep at 11 P.M. Eastern time will experience significant sleep difficulty because of the mismatch between the desired bedtime and circadian physiology. If bedtime is delayed until 2 A.M. Eastern (11 P.M. Pacific) only a few hours of sleep will be obtained before morning rise time. If the traveler's obligations the next day include important business activities or driving a vehicle, the loss of sleep could produce highly undesirable, even tragic, results. Use of a hypnotic medication to avoid sleep deprivation associated with jet lag seems medically and socially advisable.

Other instances of transient insomnia can also be anticipated, usually based on prior experience. The night before an examination or public presentation is a trigger for many people. A night in a hotel or other strange sleeping environment is often disruptive of sleep. Most of these transient sleep disturbances can be prevented with hypnotic use. Moreover, the availability of extremely short-acting drugs, such as zaleplon, allows pro re nata use without residual morning sedation (7). That is, the decision to take the medication does not have to be prophylactic, but rather the choice can be made when the sleep difficulty occurs, provided 4 or 5 hr remain before the patient must arise.

For many years experts have concluded that transient insomnia is the clearest indication for the use of hypnotic medications (8). Because systematic study of a transient phenomenon is difficult, models of transient insomnia have been developed, particularly to test hypnotic efficacy. Sleep is predictably disrupted by either phase shifts in the timing of sleep (9), sleep in an unfamiliar environment (10), or both factors (11).

The moderate degree of sleep disturbance observed when individuals undergo polysomnographic sleep recordings in a laboratory environment has been termed the "first night effect." Research with this model typically shows that hypnotics reliably increase total sleep time, and reduce sleep latency, as compared to placebo (12).

In circadian-phase–shift research, total sleep time with placebo is reduced by as much as 3 hr as compared to sleep at usual circadian times. As a result, subsequent wake time is characterized by increased sleepiness and performance is often impaired. For example, triazolam was used (13) to counteract the sleep disruptive effects of a 180-degree phase reversal. Total sleep time with triazolam was significantly higher than with placebo, and physiological and performance measures throughout the waking period revealed heightened alertness and performance. That is, the hypnotic treatment significantly improved sleep and promoted alertness during the subsequent "day". Seidel et al. (14) demonstrated very similar effects on sleep and alertness in a 180-degree change in the timing of sleep and wakefulness. Moreover, several studies have demonstrated the efficacy of hypnotics in simulated (15,16) and actual jet lag situations (17,18). In these studies hypnotics maintained sleep-wake function at precircadian challenge levels whereas placebo was associated with curtailed sleep time and consequent impaired waking function.

To date, virtually all published hypnotic-transient insomnia studies indicate that hypnotics are effective when used for 1 to a few nights. A few studies document that the improvement in sleep is accompanied by a higher level of alertness and performance during waking hours, as compared to placebo. Evidence that treatment of transient insomnia reduces or eliminates the sequelae of acute sleep deprivation outside of a laboratory environment is lacking. However, it seems logical that impairment risk will decrease proportionally to the reduction in sleep loss. Moreover, the risk associated with the occasional use of short-acting hypnotics, at recommended doses, is exceedingly low (6,19).

## B. Chronic Insomnia

The consequences of chronic primary insomnia cannot be considered similar to those of sleep deprivation, as stated above. Discussion of the pathophysiology and treatment of this condition is beyond the scope of this chapter. However, many insomnias secondary to medical illness and primary sleep disorders appear to have physiological and behavioral effects similar to those of sleep deprivation. For example, rheumatoid arthritis patients complaining of insomnia and fatigue have moderate levels of physiological sleepiness during the day, and the sleepiness declines after 6 nights of treatment with a short-acting hypnotic (4). Insomnia secondary to periodic limb movement disorder has also been shown to be associated with increased daytime sleepiness, which improves with hypnotic therapy (5). Daytime alertness of elderly insomniacs (of mixed diagnostic categories) also has been shown to improve with 3 nights' use of a short-acting hypnotic (20). It must be cautioned that these studies only evaluated the benefit of short-term hypnotic therapy. Thus, the few data available indicate that acute use of short-acting hypnotics for some chronic insomniacs appears to increase sleep duration and continuity, and improve daytime alertness. Clearly, long-term studies are needed.

## IV. Pharmacological Promotion of Alertness

Sleepiness is an inevitable result of sleep deprivation, and when the magnitude of sleepiness is high, the risk of inattention, poor performance, negative mood, and accidents is great. The majority of individuals affected by sleepiness fall into one of three causal categories: circadian-mediated sleepiness, medical conditions (including sleep disorders), or inadequate time allotted for sleep. Prior chapters review the link between medical (Chap. 6) and sleep (Chap. 5) disorders leading to sleep deprivation and sleepiness. This chapter focuses on pharmacological intervention to promote alertness in each of these types of conditions.

### A.  Circadian-mediated Sleepiness

Two facets of modern society that produce circadian-based sleepiness in significant numbers of people are rapid transmeridian travel (jet lag) and shift work, particularly night shift work. Jet lag was discussed under transient insomnia (above) as sleep disruptive. However, it is the circadian-mediated sleepiness during desired or required waking hours that is often the most problematic component of the jet lag syndrome. When humans remain awake during the endogenous circadian night, whether because of rapid transmeridian travel or because of night shift work, marked sleepiness will be present regardless of the amount of prior sleep, although reduced sleep time will increase sleepiness even further. Clearly, sleep loss and the circadian factor are additive in terms of daytime function. In the jet lag situation the severity of the sleep-wake disruption varies according to the number of time zones crossed, and the duration of sleep-wake symptoms is limited by adjustment of circadian phase in the presence of the light-dark schedule at the destination time zone. Experts estimate that humans' circadian rhythms adapt to the new time zone, depending on light exposure, at the rate of roughly 1 hr/day. Thus, an individual traversing over seven time zones will require about 1 week for his or her endogenous rhythms to synchronize with the new time zone. On the other hand, sleep-wake disruption associated with shift work is not time-limited as the sleep-wake schedule usually remains out of phase with the natural light-dark cycle, and the timing of sleep and wakefulness typically changes from workdays to off days. Only a minimal shift in the phase of the endogenous rhythms occurs in most shift workers within the usual work week (3–5 consecutive night shifts) and, as a result, the sleep-wake disturbance typically is present whenever the timing of sleep is governed by the shift work schedule (21,22)

Nicholson and colleagues (17) have demonstrated significantly increased physiological sleep tendency throughout the day at the destination site after eastward travel over five time zones. This effect persists over several days although the magnitude becomes more moderate. Following westward travel across five time zones, sleepiness is increased predominantly late in the day at the destination site. After 3 days, values close to baseline are found. For the vacationer, sleepiness associated with jet lag may be only a minor nuisance (unless he/she is operating a motor vehicle, in which case major problems may result); but for certain occupations [e.g., airline or military personnel (see Chaps. 12, 15, and 16)], the sleepiness may be disastrous.

Evidence suggests that moderate to severe sleepiness is virtually omnipresent for night shift workers. A recent assessment of 363 shift workers with symptoms of shift work sleep disorder (23) found their nocturnal sleepiness level, studied the night after 3–5 consecutive night shifts, to approximate sleepiness levels after a night of total sleep deprivation (24). The shift workers' mean score on the Multiple Sleep Latency Test (MSLT) at night was 2.75 min. Further, the MSLT score for 90.1% of the shift workers was ≤ 6 min, a level most experts believe to be associated with behavioral impairment and increased accident risk.

## B. Sleepiness Associated with Medical Conditions

The prevalence of sleepiness associated with medical conditions has not been systematically investigated. Included in this category are various renal (25), respiratory (26), gastrointestinal (27), neurological (28), cardiovascular (29), and rheumatological (30) disorders. At least in part, the absence of investigation in this area is because of the common assumption that daytime sleepiness associated with these disorders is thought to be secondary to sleep disturbance and fragmentation. Thus the patients as well as the clinicians focus on the disturbed sleep rather than the daytime sequelae. A patient will more likely tell the doctor that the heartburn is disturbing his/her sleep. The daytime sleepiness associated with the sleep disturbance is likely to be discussed only if specifically asked. One of the challenges in this area is the differentiation of sleepiness and fatigue. Patients, clinicians, and contributors to the literature confuse these terms. Nowhere is this more evident than in the area of sleepiness associated with medical disorders. For example, multiple-sclerosis patients often complain of marked fatigue and their problem seems to be associated only with mild levels of sleepiness (31). In contrast, when Parkinson's patients complain of fatigue it is often significant daytime sleepiness that leads to this complaint (32).

The lack of research in this area is problematic as typically there are four potential sources of daytime sleepiness in medically ill patients reporting daytime sleepiness. First, as mentioned earlier many of these disorders fragment sleep, which in turn negatively impacts daytime alertness. Gastrointentinal reflux and various pain disorders fall into this category. A second potential cause is the increased prevalence of primary sleep disorders associated with several medical conditions. For example, some neurological and cardiovascular disorders are associated with an increased prevalence of sleep-related breathing disorders (33). Similarly, patients with kidney disease have an elevated risk for restless legs syndrome (34). A third cause for the daytime sleepiness is pharmacological. Many of the drugs used to treat these disorders produce daytime sleepiness (35). Included in this category would be tricyclic antidepressants used to manage some rheumatological disorders and dopamine agonists used for the treatment of Parkinson's disease. In another therapeutic context, there is now information about the increased prevalence of sleepiness in cancer patients undergoing chemotherapy. Finally, least investigated is the possibility that sleepiness is a direct result of the disease process itself. This is rarely investigated as the sleepiness is typically attributed to one of the other causes listed above. An example of this is Parkinson's disease. Originally it was felt that the sleepiness in these patients was due to disturbed sleep and increased prevalence of sleep disorders. More recently it was attributed to the dopamine agonists as well as other medications. Although both sleep disruption and drug effects likely contribute to sleepiness, there is reason to believe that sleepiness is an inherent part of Parkinson's. This position is supported by the finding that sleepiness correlates with disease progression, and does not correlate with any aspect of nocturnal sleep (32).

The question as to whether to treat the sleepiness in patients with chronic medical illnesses is complex and important. The treatment of sleepiness is similar to the treatment of pain in these patients, with expected improvements in overall well-being and functionality. In addition, there are reasons to suggest that treating daytime sleepiness may improve the primary condition itself. For example, sleep disruption and the consequent sleepiness is related to increased pain sensitivity (36) and blunts some respiratory reflexes (37). Given the prevalence of fatigue and sleepiness in patients with medical disorders, it is regrettable that no clear guidelines exist as to the use of wake-enhancing drugs in these patients. Clearly the potential benefits exist, but for which patients with what therapeutic benefit remains to be determined.

### C.  Sleepiness Resulting from Inadequate Sleep

Interview or survey studies of populations in other countries suggest daytime sleepiness prevalence rates of about 10–20% (38–41). A preliminary report (42) of an ongoing study with a physiological measure of sleepiness (and using a conservative criterion of excessive daytime sleepiness [EDS]) estimates the prevalence of "excessive daytime sleepiness" in the United States to be 13.4%. The fact that the more sleepy individuals slept better at night, and reported shorter habitual nightly time in bed, suggests that much of the sleepiness is secondary to voluntary or imposed restriction of nightly time in bed.

Estimates of typical nightly sleep amounts, based on large and somewhat representative samples, suggest that in the United States, sleep durations have been declining over the past few decades. In 1960, approximately 86% of adults reported usually getting 7 or more hr of sleep, and 64% reported getting 8 or more hr (43). Annual surveys conducted from 1998 to 2002 indicate that sleep durations of 7 or more or 8 or more hr are reported by about 65% and 35% of adults, respectively (National Sleep Foundation, personal communication, 2003). From a population standpoint, one might infer that tens of millions of people are sleeping significantly less in recent years.

*What underlies the widespread volitional component of sleep restriction, and resultant sleepiness?* Perhaps individuals in industrialized society in the 21st century simply have the desire to experience more, achieve more than is compatible with biological sleep requirements. Certainly 24-hr services, round-the-clock television, the Internet, and other options provide us with the opportunity to experience more by limiting our sleep time. Perhaps trends away from tradition, and a greater emphasis on technology, encourage us to be less deferential to biology—adhering to a regular 8-hr nightly sleep schedule because prior generations did so, because our parents encourage it, or even because our bodies and minds indicate the value of such behavior may not be consistent with a modern mind-set or attitude about the use of technology to increase productivity and entertainment. Self-indulgence is the norm. People measure satisfaction with life in hours and minutes (often translated into currency) or the number of activities in which they participate, rather than actual experienced pleasure or the quality of their work. Staying awake beyond the late-night news, which may be seen only partially between bouts of dozing on the couch, is valued because "we earned it" or because "we just want to relax." Perhaps if we were less sleepy and fatigued, routine life would be more enjoyable, would not take such effort, and the need to extend waking hours just to experience enjoyable wakefulness would not be necessary.

On the other hand, in many cases, work schedules, family obligations, and other factors combine to impose insufficient sleep on us. In addition to night shift workers as previously discussed, early day shift workers, single working parents, caregivers for the elderly, "on-call" personnel, emergency crews, and others find it very difficult to regularly obtain adequate sleep. Mitler et al. (44) found over-the-road truck drivers, for example, averaged only 4.78 hr of sleep per day during 4–5 consecutive days of driving. Although individual differences in biological requirement for sleep almost certainly exist, most sleep scientists and clinicians agree these individual differences are minor and that large segments of our population (e.g., students, shift workers) are sleep deprived. For perspective, it is important to note that when allowed to sleep as needed, young adults average approximately 8.25 hr of sleep per 24 hr (45). Roehrs et al. (46) have shown that increasing sleep duration results in a steady improvement in daytime alertness even among individuals reporting adequate sleep and daytime alertness. Finally, surveys conducted by the National Sleep Foundation demonstrate that average nightly reported sleep time actually is greater in those aged ≥ 65 years, as compared to those aged 18–64, suggesting that when time pressure slackens owing to retirement, more time is allotted to sleep (National Sleep Foundation, personal communication, 2003).

Whatever the reason for insufficient sleep, the sleepiness and neurobehavioral consequences seem inevitable. Prevention of sleep deprivation through lifestyle management, and perhaps with hypnotics, would be first- and second-line recommendations for most situations. However, there are instances in which sleepiness cannot be managed with those approaches. Wake-promoting agents would seem very appropriate for use in some of these situations. It should be noted that the use of medications to modulate the effects of lifestyle is not unique to sleep medicine. The use of artificial sweeteners or lipid-lowering agents, often to correct the effect of inappropriate nutritional choices, has become an acceptable part of daily food selection as well as medical practice.

## V. Wake-Promoting Substances (See Also Chap. 20)

Caffeine is probably the most widely used psychoactive substance in the world and is commonly used to combat sleepiness. A variety of studies have shown it to be effective in reducing sleepiness and enhancing performance, at least when used acutely (47–48). These studies have demonstrated dose-dependent enhanced alertness and daytime function in both people sleeping on their usual schedule and individuals undergoing sleep deprivation (49).

A number of issues, however, prove to be problematic with the use of caffeine. First, tolerance appears to rapidly develop with repeated doses (50). Second, there is substantial interindividual variability in the rate of metabolism and in the frequency of undesired effects such as tremor, jitteriness, and insomnia. Interestingly, despite the widespread use of caffeine, and the strong reluctance of many users to forgo consumption and their inclination to typically escalate dose (i.e., number of servings of coffee or cola), routine caffeine consumption is usually not viewed as drug use, much less drug abuse.

Amphetamines and similar central nervous system stimulants have been available for many years, but the substantial abuse liability and potential cardiovascular adverse effects have largely limited their use to the treatment of narcolepsy and attention-deficit-hyperactivity disorder. There has also been some utilization of amphetamines to combat sleepiness during military operations.

Within the last few years, the role of wake-promoting medication has received renewed and increasing attention with development of modafinil. Although the mechanism through which modafinil works remains to be determined, the low abuse potential (51) and absence of cardiovascular effects (52,53), combined with its clear wake-promoting properties, increase the potential uses for this drug. Studies have shown consistent increases in alertness for narcolepsy (54), in sleep apnea patients (treated with CPAP) with residual sleepiness (55), for shift work sleep disorder (56), and for sleep deprivation (57).

## VI.  Tinkering with Mother Nature: Where Should Society Draw the Line?

Having safe and effective pharmacological tools to choose when we need to sleep and when we need to remain awake presents new and potentially contentious issues for the medical community, various industries, and society as a whole. The use of hypnotics, particularly long-term use, for the treatment of insomnia has been controversial for years. Nevertheless, the pattern of hypnotic use considered for the prevention of sleep deprivation is most likely to be short-term (i.e., less than 1 week) nightly use or potentially longer-term intermittent use. Both of these patterns of use are consistent with most recommendations/guidelines. Thus, little new or additional philosophical concerns are likely to emerge from the concept of preventing sleep deprivation (as opposed to treating transient insomnia) with hypnotics.

On the other hand, pharmacological wake promotion is a new concept brought about by modafinil. Use of modafinil for medical conditions other than narcolepsy has begun to receive the attention of both basic and applied researchers and physicians caring for these patients. Moreover, modafinil consumption is envisioned by some as logical for some critical occupational situations, such as military pilots flying halfway around the world without an opportunity for sleep. *But where does one draw the line? Should over-the-road truck drivers have access to wake-promoting drugs? What about a surgeon performing an emergency operation beginning at 01:00 hr? Or the same surgeon doing the operation at 01:00 hr after being on-call the previous 36 hr because no one else is available?*

Compared to human cloning and other ethical or philosophical concerns emanating from biomedical progress, extending wakefulness/promoting alertness for a few hours, or perhaps even a day or 2 would seem trivial, at least at first glance. *But what if individuals taking modafinil gained a significant advantage in their career or in school because of increased work capacity? Is that consistent with the concept of better living through chemistry? Could the production of a manufacturing plant, or the economy of an impoverished country, be substantially improved with organized pharmacological wake promotion? Moreover, if modafinil is used over the long term, and sleep is insufficient over the long term, will significant medical consequences result (58)?*

## VII. Conclusions

Many aspect of modern society necessitate our dealing with issues relating to perturbations of sleep-wake function. On a clinical level, the increased longevity of our population has resulted in a parallel increase in age-related sleep disorders. From progressive neurological disorders to sleep-related movement and respiratory disorders, a variety of medical conditions leave our aging population with disturbed sleep and impaired wakefulness. The lifestyle of our younger population seems intent on doing away with the difference between night and day, and economic pressures increasingly push toward producing a 24-hr workplace. Finally, safety related to hours of service, whether in the context of medical training, the transportation industry or other areas, has become a major topic for both researchers and regulators. In parallel to these developments, medical research has led to the development of safer sleep- and wake-enhancing pharmaceuticals. *With increased demand for and availability of safe medications the question arises in what context do we accept their use? Moreover, when should the use of these agents be encouraged and by whom? Should sleep-wake disorders be symptomatically managed with these medications on a long term-basis? If not, how do we deal with them?* An argument might be made that widespread use and acceptance of sleep-wake pharmaceuticals would facilitate the evolution to an around-the-clock society. On the other hand, it seems clear that, in most cases, personal and public safety improvements would result from pharmacological sleep promotion or wake enhancement. Certainly no one would question the use of dopamine agonists in restless legs syndrome or the use of wake-enhancing drugs in narcolepsy. *What about drug treatment for sleepiness related to a transmeridian flight or prior to performance of high-risk activities (e.g.,*

*long-haul trucking, performing surgery) after being awake for 24 hr? Does pre-*
*venting an accident perpetuate our taxing the sleep/wake system?* Today we can
essentially initiate and sustain sleep when desired and maintain wakefulness
when desired. Less clear is how to use these tools in the best interest of individuals and society.

## References

1.  Klerman GL. Psychotropic hedonism vs. pharmacological Calvinism. Hastings Cent
    Rep 1972; 2(4):1–3.
2.  Bonnet MH, Arand D. Hyperarousal and insomnia. Sleep Med Rev 1997; 1:97–108.
3.  Vgontzas AN, Bixler EO, Lin H-M, Prolo P, Mastorakos G, Vela-Bueno A, Kales A,
    Chrousos GP. Chronic insomnia is associated with nyctohemeral activation of the
    hypothalamic-pituitary-adrenal axis: clinical implications. J Clin Endocrinol Metab
    2001; 86:3787–3794.
4.  Walsh JK, Muehlbach MJ, Lauter SA, Hilliker NA, Schweitzer PK. Effects of tria-
    zolam on sleep, daytime sleepiness, and morning stiffness in patients with rheuma-
    toid arthritis. J Rheumatol 1996; 23:245–252.
5.  Doghramji K, Browman CP, Gaddy JR, Walsh JK. Triazolam diminishes daytime
    sleepiness and sleep fragmentation in patients with periodic leg movements in sleep.
    J Clin Psychopharmacol 1991; 11:284–290.
6.  Roehrs T, Roth T. Hypnotics: efficacy and adverse effects. In: Kryger M, Roth T,
    Dement WC, eds. Principles and Practice of Sleep Medicine. Philadelphia: Saunders,
    2000:414–418.
7.  Walsh JK, Pollak CP, Scharf MB, Schweitzer PK, and Vogel GW. Lack of residual
    sedation following middle-of-the-night zaleplon administration in sleep maintenance
    insomnia. Clin Neuropharmacol, 2000; 23(1):17–21.
8.  Consensus Conference: Drugs and insomnia. JAMA 1984; 251:2410–2414.
9.  Walsh JK, Schweitzer PK, Sugerman JL, Muehlbach MJ. Transient insomnia associ-
    ated with a three-hour phase advance of sleep time and treatment with zolpidem. J
    Clin Psychopharmacol 1990; 10:184–189.
10. Edinger JD, Fins AL, Sullivan RJ, Marsh GR, Dailey DS, Hope TV, Young M, Shaw
    E, Carlson D, Vasilas D. Sleep in the laboratory and sleep at home: comparisons of
    older insomniacs and normal sleepers. Sleep 1997; 20:1119–1126.
11. Erman MK, Erwin CW, Gengo FM, Jamieson AO, Lemmi H, Mahowald MW,
    Regestein QR, Roth T, Roth-Schecter B, Scharf MB, Vogel GW, Walsh JK, Ware JC.
    Comparative efficacy of zolpidem and temazepam in transient insomnia. Hum
    Psychopharmacol Clin Exp 2001; 16:169–176.
12. Roehrs T, Vogel G, Sterling W, Roth T. Dose effects of temazepam in transient
    insomnia. Arzneimittelforschung 1990; 40:859–862.
13. Bonnet MH, Mitler MM, Gillin JC, James SP, Kripke D, Mendelson W, Mitler M.
    The use of triazolam in phase-advanced sleep. Neuropsychopharmacology 1988;
    1:225–234.
14. Seidel WF, Cohen SA, Bliwise NG, Roth T, Dement WC. Dose-related effects of tri-
    azolam and flurazepam on a circadian rhythm insomnia. Clin Pharmacol Ther 1986;
    40:314–320.

15. Seidel WF, Roth T, Roehrs T, Zorick F, Dement WC. Treatment of a 12–hour shift of sleep schedule with benzodiazepines. Science 1984; 224:1262–1264.

16. Schweitzer PK, Koshorek G, Muehlbach MJ, Morris DD, Roehrs T, Walsh JK, Roth T. Effects of estazolam and triazolam on transient insomnia associated with phase-shifted sleep. Hum Psychopharmacol 1991; 6:99–107.

17. Nicholson AN, Pascoe PA, Spencer MB, Stone BM, Roehrs T, Roth T. Sleep after transmeridian flights. Lancet 1986; 2:1205–1208.

18. Jamieson AO, Zammit GK, Rosenberg RS, Davis JR, Walsh JK. Zolpidem reduces the sleep disturbance of jet lag. Sleep Med 2001; 2:423–430.

19. McCall WV. Pharmacologic treatment of insomnia. In: Lee-Chiong TL, Sateia MJ, Carskadon MA, eds. Sleep Medicine. Philadelphia: Hanley & Belfus, 2002:169–176.

20. Carskadon MA, Seidel WF, Greenblatt DJ, Dement WC. Daytime carryover of triazolam and flurazepam in elderly insomniacs. Sleep 1982; 5(4):361–371.

21. Tepas DI, Walsh JK, Armstrong DA. Comprehensive study of the sleep of shift workers. In: Johnson LC, Tepas DI, Colquhoun WP, Colligan MJ, eds. Biological Rhythms, Sleep and Shift Work. New York: Spectrum, 1981:347–356.

22. Walsh JK, Tepas DI, Moss PD. The EEG sleep of night and rotating shiftworkers. In: Johnson LC, Tepas DI, Colquhoun WP, Colligan MJ, eds. The 24–Hour Workday: A Symposium on Variations in Work-Sleep Schedules. Cincinnati, National Institute for Occupational Safety and Health, 1981:451–466.

23. Walsh JK, Hughes R, Czeisler C, Dinges DF, Niebler G, Roth T. Sleepiness on the night shift in shift work sleep disorder. Sleep 2003; 26(suppl):A110.

24. Rosenthal L, Roehrs TA, Rosen A, Roth T. Level of sleepiness and total sleep time following various time in bed conditions. Sleep 1993; 16:226–232.

25. Walker S, Fine A, Kryger MH. Sleep complaints are common in a dialysis unit. Am J Kidney Dis 1995; 26:751–756.

26. Fleetham J, West P, Mezon B, Conway W, Roth T, Kryger M. Sleep, arousals and oxygen desaturation in chronic obstructive pulmonary disease. Am Rev Respir Dis 1982; 126:429–433.

27. Orr WC. Gastrointestinal functioning during sleep. In: Lee-Chiong TL Jr, Sateia MJ, Carskadon MA, eds. Sleep Medicine. Philadelphia: Hanley & Belfus, 2002:463–469.

28. Henning WA, Walters AS, Chokroverty S. Motor functions and disorders of sleep. In: Chokroverty S, ed. Sleep Disorders Medicine: Basic Science, Technical Considerations, and Clinical Aspects. Boston: Butterworth-Heinemann, 1994:255–294.

29. Verrier RL, Mittleman MA. Sleep-related cardiac risk. In: Kryger MH, Roth T, Dement WC, eds, Principles and Practice of Sleep Medicine. Philadelphia: Saunders, 2000:997–1013.

30. Moldofsky H. Rheumatologic disorders and sleep. In: Lee-Chiong TL Jr, Sateia MJ, Carskadon MA, eds. Sleep Medicine. Philadelphia: Hanley & Belfus 2002:471–476.

31. Rammohan KW, Rosenberg JH, Lynn DJ, Blumenfeld AM, Pollak CP, Nagaraja HN. Efficacy and safety of modafinil (Provigil) for the treatment of fatigue in multiple sclerosis: a two centre phase 2 study. J Neurol Neurosurg Psychiatry 2002; 72(2):179–83.

32. Rye DB, Bliwise DL, Dihenia B, Gurecki P. Daytime sleepiness in Parkinson's disease. J Sleep Res 2000; 9:63–69.

33. George CFP. Hypertension, ischemic heart disease, and stroke. In: Kryger MH, Roth T, Dement WC, eds, Principles and Practice of Sleep Medicine. Philadelphia: Saunders, 2000:1030–1039.

34. Roger SD, Harris DCH, Stewart JH. Possible relation between restless legs and anemia in renal dialysis patients. Lancet 1991; 337:1551.

35. Schweitzer PK. Drugs that disturb sleep and wakefulness. In: Kryger MH, Roth T, Dement WC, eds, Principles and Practice of Sleep Medicine. Philadelphia: Saunders, 2000:441–461.

36. Pascualy R, Buchwald D. Chronic fatigue syndrome and fibromyalgia. In: Kryger MH, Roth T, Dement WC, eds, Principles and Practice of Sleep Medicine. Philadelphia: Saunders, 2000:1040–1049.

37. Leiter JC, Knuth SL, Bartlett D Jr. The effect of sleep deprivation on activity of the genioglossus muscle. Am Rev Respir Dis 1985; 32(6):1242–1245.

38. Souza JC, Magna LA, Reimao R. Excessive daytime sleepiness in Campo Grande general population, Brazil. Arq Neuropsiquiatr 2002; 60(3–A):558–562.

39. Hublin C, Kaprio J. Partinen M, Heikkila K, Koskenvuo M. Daytime sleepiness in an adult Finnish population. J Intern Med 1996; 26:417–423.

40. Hyppa M, Kronholm E. How does Finland sleep? Sleeping habits of the Finnish adult population and the rehabilitation of sleep disturbances [in Finnish]. Finland: Publ Soc Ins Inst; 1987; ML:68:1–110.

41. Ohayon MM, Caulet M, Philip P, Guilleminault C, Priest RG. How sleep and mental disorders are related to complaints of daytime sleepiness. Arch Intern Med 1997; 157:2645–2652.

42. Drake CL, Roehrs TA, Richardson GS, Roth T. Epidemiology and morbidity of excessive daytime sleepiness. Sleep 2002; 25(abstr suppl):A91.

43. Kripke DF, Simons RN, Garfinkel L, Hammond EC. Short and long sleep and sleeping pills. Arch Gen Psychiatry 1979; 36:103–116.

44. Mitler MM, Miller JC, Lipsitz JL, Walsh JK, Wylie CD. The sleep of long-haul truck drivers. N Engl J Med 1997; 337:755–761.

45. Wehr TA, Moul DE, Barbato G, Giesen HA, Seidel J, Baker C, Bender C. Conservation of photoperiod-responsive mechanisms in humans. Am J Physiol 1993; 265:R846–R857.

46. Roehrs T, Shore E, Papineau K, Rosenthal L, Roth T. A two-week sleep extension in sleepy normals. Sleep 1996; 19:576–582.

47. Walsh JK, Muehlbach MJ, Humm TM, Dickins QS, Sugerman JL, Schweitzer PK. Effect of caffeine on physiological sleep tendency and ability to sustain wakefulness at night. Psychopharmacology 1990; *101*:271–273.

48. Muehlbach MJ, Walsh JK. The effects of caffeine on simulated night shift work and subsequent daytime sleep. Sleep 1995; 18:22–29.

49. Zwyghuizen-Doorenbos A, Roehrs T, Lipschultz L, Timms V, Roth T. Effects of caffeine on alertness. Psychopharmacology 1990; 100:36–39.

50. Griffiths RR, Woodson PP. Caffeine physical dependence: a review of human and laboratory animal studies. Psychopharmacology (Berl) 1988; 94(4):437–451.

51. Jasinski DR. An evaluation of the abuse potential of modafinil using methylphenidate as a reference. J Psychopharmacol 2000; 14:53–60.

52. Billiard M, Besset A, Montplaisir J, Laffont F, Goldenberg F, Weill JS, Lubin S. Modafinil: a double-blind multicentric study. Sleep 1994; 17:S107–S112.

53. Simpson LL. The effects of behavioral stimulant doses of amphetamine on blood pressure. Arch Gen Psychiatry 1976; 33:691–695.

54. US Modafinil in Narcolepsy Multicenter Study Group. Randomized trial of modafinil as a treatment for the excessive daytime somnolence of narcolepsy. Neurology 2000; 54:1166–1175.

55. Pack AL, Black JE, Schwartz JR, Matheson JK. Modafinil as adjunct therapy for daytime sleepiness in obstructive sleep apnea. Am J Respir Crit Care Med. 2001; 164(9):1675–1681.

56. Czeisler CA, Dinges DF, Walsh JK, Roth T, Niebler G. Modafinil for the treatment of excessive sleepiness in chronic shift work sleep disorder. Sleep 2003; 26(suppl):A115.

57. Wesensten NJ, Belenky G, Kautz MA, Thorne DR, Reichardt RM, Balkin TJ. Maintaining alertness and performance during sleep deprivation: modafinil versus caffeine. Psychopharmacology (Berl) 2002; 159(3):238–247.

58. Spiegel K, Leproult R, Van Cauter E. Impact of sleep debt on metabolic and endocrine function. Lancet 1999; 354:1435–1439.

# 28

# Eliminating Cumulative Sleep Debt and Sleep Satiation

**MATTHIAS K. LEE**

Virginia Mason Sleep Disorders Center, Seattle, Washington, U.S.A.

**WILLIAM C. DEMENT**

Stanford University, Stanford, California, U.S.A.

## I. Introduction

It is widely accepted that when individuals undergo partial sleep deprivation on a night-after-night basis, they will become progressively more impaired. In recent years, the term "sleep debt" has been used to describe the total accumulation of lost sleep from such partial deprivation. By contrast, when a person obtains substantial extra sleep over and above the daily amount needed, the process has been called sleep satiation. A number of partial sleep deprivation studies have been carried out to study the effect of accumulated sleep loss, but there have been relatively few sleep satiation studies. To address issues involving sleep satiation, it will be necessary to clarify what is meant by chronic partial sleep loss, sleep debt, and sleep need, as well as extra sleep and sleep satiation. *What is the best way to avoid the accumulation and consequences of sleep debt? How can we determine an individual's daily sleep need and therefore establish what constitutes extra sleep? Is it possible to sleep beyond the point of satiety?* These and others are important questions especially in the context of defining proper guidelines for sleep management in our 24 hrs/day-7 days-a-week society.

## II. The Concept and Definition of Sleepiness

In the early days of sleep research, sleep and wakefulness were considered as entirely separate entities and were studied in isolation from one another. All-night sleep was examined in its entirety and minutely dissected with total disregard for either the prior or following hours of wakefulness. Sleep researchers later began to consider these two complementary phases of the daily cycle of existence as mutually interactive. The most obvious interaction between sleep and wakefulness, other than their sequential occurrence in each succeeding 24-hr period, is the predictable fluctuation in daytime alertness as a function of the amount of nocturnal sleep. In other words, the more we sleep, the more we are alert; and the less we sleep, the more we are sleepy in the daytime.

Given that there is a fairly consistent relationship between amount of sleep and daytime alertness, a systematic attempt was made to measure daytime sleepiness quantitatively by means of the Stanford Sleepiness Scale (1). However, the incongruence of individuals often denying subjective daytime sleepiness or choosing flagrantly inappropriate ratings during studies of total sleep deprivation undermined the overall validity of this subjective assessment. It was clear that an objective measure of daytime sleepiness would be a significant advance. This need led directly to the development of the Multiple Sleep Latency Test (MSLT) (2). From the perspective of this test, the simplest definition of sleepiness is that it is an awake condition associated with an increased tendency for a person or an animal to fall asleep.

The MSLT (see also Chap. 2) assesses daytime sleep tendency by measuring the speed of falling asleep. This is defined as sleep latency. In the standard version of the MSLT, the sleep latency is measured every 2 hr. The fundamental concept is that if all competing stimuli are eliminated and the individuals being tested do not attempt to remain awake, then the sleep latency is a valid representation of the underlying physiological sleep tendency.

## III. Primary Factors Affecting Sleep and Wakefulness

As is well known, the sleep tendency at any moment is the net effect of the dynamic interplay of several factors. The main factors include homeostatic sleep drive, circadian influences on sleep propensity, and environmental and situational elements. Some investigators, e.g., Dinges and Kribbs (3), have categorized these factors as describing the "state" of sleepiness, adding that individual differences may also be important.

### A. Homeostatic Factors

The homeostatic mechanism in the human brain responds to sleep reduction by increasing the tendency to fall asleep and, presumably, decreases the tendency to fall asleep in response to an increase in the amount of sleep. Studies measuring MSLT scores during a variety of sleep schedules in human beings have found a very lawful, almost linear, relationship between the mean daytime sleep tendency, or sleep latency profile, and nocturnal amounts of sleep (4). Such results have been routinely obtained with total sleep deprivation. However, it is the accumulation of lost sleep over time in situations entailing chronic partial sleep loss (sleep restriction) that is of the greatest scientific interest and probably has the most important implications for understanding the homeostatic sleep regulatory system.

In the first 24-hr quantitative study of partial sleep loss, Carskadon and Dement (5) restricted subjects to 5 hr of sleep per night for 7 consecutive nights. The mean daily MSLTs decreased from an average of about 16 min at baseline to about 7 min on the 7th day, showing that daytime sleep tendency increased over the 7 days in a cumulative fashion. Dinges et al. (6) performed a similar study with sleep restriction to 4.98 hr/night for 7 consecutive nights and obtained frequent measurements of reaction time using the Psychomotor Vigilance Test (PVT). In the latter study, progressive decrement, measured in the form of increased lapses on the PVT, was observed over the 7 days. Analysis of the temporal profile of the changes in MSLT from the Carskadon paper were compared with the PVT data resulting in an extremely close correlation ($r = -.95$). The close similarity of these curves attests to the precise quantitative nature of the homeostatic process.

The effects of chronic partial sleep deprivation on neurobehavioral functions were further explored in a very comprehensive study by Van Dongen et al. (7). In this study, 48 volunteers were sleep-restricted for a period of 14 days. The subjects were maintained in the laboratory environment for the entire duration of the study and were carefully monitored to ensure that no additional sleep or alerting substances (e.g., caffeine) were taken. The PVT and other tests, including polysomnography and the Stanford Sleepiness Scale, were used to assess changes. Subjects were allowed to sleep 8 hr/night, 6 hr/night, or 4 hr/night for each of the 14 nights. Some subjects were totally sleep-deprived for 3 nights to serve as comparison against the subjects who were partially sleep-deprived.

The results showed that 14 nights of 4 hr of time in bed resulted in PVT lapses in the range seen for subjects who had been completely sleep-deprived for 2 nights. The 6-hr/night group showed PVT lapse results comparable to the 1 night of the total sleep deprivation group. The 8-hr/night group showed no statistically significant changes after 14 days when compared to baseline, and they were certainly nowhere near the level of impairment seen with any of the other sleep deprivation groups. Perhaps the most significant result from this study is the relationship of the PVT lapses with cumulative sleep loss. The PVT lapses increased in near-linear fashion with the accumulation of sleep loss across each day of the experiment. There was no indication of a tendency for a plateau to occur in the progressive changes.

## B.   Circadian Factors

Individuals often do not feel subjectively sleepy and have difficulty falling asleep even when they have accumulated a large amount of sleep loss. It is as if they have become invulnerable to their strong underlying tendency to fall asleep and the associated impairment of performance. As sleep propensity increases progressively as a function of the duration of wakefulness, it is obvious that the ability of human beings to remain effectively awake and alert for long periods of time implies that there are a number of alerting influences that oppose the sleep tendency. External and environmental alerting influences are obvious; these include noise, motion, jostling, internal pain, excitement, anger, muscle activity, and so forth. In addition, a very important internal alerting influence, called clock-dependent alerting, arises periodically from the suprachiasmatic nucleus (SCN) (site of the biological clock).

The SCN is the generator and mediator of circadian rhythms. Forced desynchrony studies have shown a characteristic profile of sleep propensity that varies with a circadian periodicity (8). The role of the biological clock was clarified in the studies of Edgar et al. (9). After continuously recording sleep and wakefulness in squirrel monkeys under constant conditions for several circadian periods, these investigators ablated the suprachiasmatic nucleus and, after suitable recovery, repeated the continuous recordings under the same constant conditions. During baseline, there was a 15–16-hr period of prolonged wakefulness with occasional napping followed by a long period of 8–9 hr of nearly continuous sleep. This typical circadian pattern occurred with no external stimulation whatsoever. After elimination of the biological clock, sleep and wakefulness were completely dispersed throughout the circadian period in very short episodes and there was actually an increase in total sleep time. Edgar et al. concluded that the major role of the biological clock was to alert the brain and to maintain wakefulness for a prolonged period of time, opposing the tendency to fall asleep.

Applying these results to human patterns suggests that relatively high levels of alerting exist in the early morning, followed by lower levels of alerting in the late afternoon. By the middle of the evening, alerting is again high. This has the advantage of offsetting the high levels of homeostatic sleep drive that have accumulated through the day. As clock-dependent alerting subsides again, the homeostatic sleep drive is relatively unopposed and sleep is obtained. As can be inferred from this model, depending on total alerting influence related to circadian time, one can actually have a relatively low propensity to sleep even though the homeostatic sleep drive is fairly high.

## C. Environmental and Situational Elements

It is commonly known from experience that it is easier to fall asleep and maintain sleep while lying down in a dark, quiet, comfortable setting than in a bright, loud, uncomfortable setting. Bonnet and Arand (10) showed that activity that precedes an opportunity to sleep in a modified MSLT markedly influences the latency to sleep. In general, the overall effect of various environmental and situational elements on sleep propensity has not been extensively studied. However, the effects of the homeostatic sleep drive and clock-dependent alerting are fairly well understood.

The two-process model of sleep proposed by Borbely (11) was one of the first characterizations of the independent effects of circadian and homeostatic factors on sleep. In this model, sleep was assumed to be "gated" by the circadian system. As noted, this formulation was modified by Edgar et al. (9). Investigators have utilized the forced desynchronization technique to factor out the relative contributions of these two processes on fatigue and sleepiness (8). The strength of the homeostatic sleep drive is related to the duration of time that a person has been awake. As the day goes on, the homeostatic sleep drive builds until it is reduced by sleep. The studies of partial nightly sleep loss reviewed above have allowed experts to define sleep debt as the sum total of all lost sleep, that is, the nightly amount less than the putative amount needed.

## IV. The Concepts and Definitions of Sleep Need, Sleep Debt, and Extra Sleep

*So what is the daily homeostatic need for sleep?* Strictly speaking, if the function of sleep was known, it could be said that we need the amount of sleep that is required to fulfill this function. If there is more than one function, which seems likely, then it might be that a certain amount of sleep may be needed for one function but that different amounts may be needed for others. Additionally, all mammals exist in two entirely different organismic sleep states, rapid-eye movement (REM) sleep and non-REM (NREM) sleep. One study (12) investigated the effects of selective REM-sleep deprivation with yoked controls simultaneously awakened usually out of NREM sleep together with MSLT assessments on the following days. REM-sleep deprivation for 2 nights had no effect on MSLT scores, but the yoked controls had significantly lower MSLT scores. As REM-sleep loss did not lead to increased sleep tendency, it is suggested that daily sleep need to maintain alertness may not be based simply on number of hours but may also be a frustration of other factors, such as sleep stage and sleep depth. Until all the functions of sleep are known, the most useful and heuristic definition of homeostatic need for sleep is the amount of sleep that, if obtained on a daily basis, does not result in a progressive increase in daytime sleep tendency and sleepiness or a progressive increase in daytime alertness.

Two similar experiments carried out 30 years apart dramatically confirm the concept that human beings can unknowingly carry a large sleep debt. Neither experiment was designed by the researchers primarily to study sleep. In both experiments, brain waves were continuously recorded as one of many measurements of the effects of the experimental protocol on the volunteers.

The first experiment was carried out around 1960 at the U.S. Naval Hospital in Bethesda, Maryland. It was intended to be a test of the role of sensory deprivation on cognitive function. At that time, it was believed that a substantial reduction in sensory input could dramatically impair normal mental processes, and that disorientation, hallucinations, and even psychosis might be the consequence. The study required adult subjects to lie on a comfortable cot in a cubicle where they were completely isolated from light, sound, and interactions with the outside world. The temperature was held constant, neither perceptibly cool nor perceptively warm, and the subjects wore thick gloves to minimize tactile sensations. Brain waves were continuously recorded 24 hr/day by means of very thin wires that were looped through the subject's scalp so they did not have to be replaced. The subjects were required to remain in this situation for seven consecutive 24-hr periods. Having absolutely nothing to do, they generally slept a great deal throughout the first 24-hr period. The mean total sleep time for the group was above 16 hr on the first day. However, the mean total sleep time declined on each successive day, and throughout the last 24-hr period the group mean was just under 8 hr.

The subjects in this experiment were young naval personnel. As we now believe that nearly all young adults are chronically sleep-deprived, it may be assumed that even if the subjects had maintained reasonably normal schedules prior to the experiment, they would have begun the sensory deprivation protocol carrying a substantial sleep debt. We may assume that this sleep debt caused the enormous increase in total sleep time when there was essentially nothing else to do throughout the entire 24 hr. We may further assume that, as the sleep debt was progressively reduced, the associated sleep drive progressively weakened and the total amount of sleep accordingly decreased on each subsequent day. Even with absolutely nothing to do all day long, the subjects were eventually unable to sleep more than 8 hr.

This experiment can also be viewed as a test of the old theory that sensory bombardment of the brain is necessary to maintain wakefulness. As support for this theory, it is an extremely negative result. Although the tremendous reduction in sensory input was maintained for the entire week, there was a very large progressive increase in the amount of time awake. The foregoing U.S. Navy Hospital study was never published. However, one of us (WCD) was acquainted with the investigator and thoroughly familiar with the data contained in the technical report.

The second experiment, carried out more recently by Thomas Wehr and his colleagues at the National Institutes of Health (13), was intended to examine the effect of different photoperiods (duration of time spent in the light each 24-hr day) on the human mood and emotion. The nocturnal portion of the experiment was carried out in a laboratory setting. Sleep parameters were recorded while subjects continuously remained in bed in the dark. When they were out of bed in the light, they were allowed to go about their daily routines. The sleep of each subject was monitored 7 nights a week for 42 consecutive nights. (It should be pointed out that these types of long-term human experimentation require a tremendous organizational effort and cost a great deal of money.)

During the first 7 baseline days, the daily photoperiod during which subjects were out of bed in the light was the conventional 16 hr, and each night they were in bed in the dark from 11 P.M. to 7 A.M. (a total of 8 hr). After 1 week, the 16-hr photoperiod was decreased to 10 hr during which the subjects were out of bed in the light. They were consequently in bed in the dark for 14 hr every night (9 P.M.–11 A.M.) for 35 consecutive nights. During the 6-week period, daily mood scales and a variety of other tests were administered to the subjects.

The subjects' mean nightly baseline sleep time was 7 hr and 36 min. This means they were awake only 24 min during the 8 hr they were in bed in the dark. Such a result also describes an unusually high sleep efficiency (time asleep divided by time in bed) of 95%. It should be pointed out that a low sleep efficiency is reversed by sleep deprivation. When the subjects were switched to the 10-hr photoperiod followed by 14 hr in bed in the dark, their total daily sleep times jumped to amounts greater than 12 hr on the first night and then gradually declined. By the fourth week of the 10-hr photoperiod schedule, total sleep time for the group had leveled off at a nightly average of 8 hr and 15 min. This value was stable even though they continued to lie in bed in the dark for 14 hr every night during which they were awake for a total of 5 hr and 45 min.

The interpretation of these results is that the subjects entered the protocol carrying sizable individual sleep debts, defined as the accumulated loss of sleep. Of course, neither the subjects nor the researchers were aware of such a possibility. The baseline period probably did little to reduce the subjects' sleep debts and may even have resulted in a small increase. As in the Navy Hospital experiment, when the opportunity to sleep was greatly increased, the subjects' large sleep debts caused a very large increase in total daily sleep time. As the subjects' sleep debts decreased, total sleep time per day declined proportionally.

If we assume that the "steady state" value in the last week of the 10-hr-photoperiod (14 hr in bed) schedule represented the real daily sleep need for this group of subjects, we may conclude that all amounts of sleep above these values represented "extra" or "makeup" sleep. Accordingly, the mean "payback" of sleep debt for the group averaged about 30 hr. For purposes of comparison, individuals who were not at all sleep-deprived would have to spend more than 3 consecutive days with no sleep at all to accumulate a sleep debt of similar magnitude.

It is generally felt that sleep debt can only be reduced by obtaining extra sleep; i.e., it does not disappear by other means. In a large U.S. Department of Transportation report titled "Effects of Sleep Schedules on Commercial Motor Vehicle Driver Performance" (14), a study of 66 truck drivers was described. The truck drivers were allowed "baseline" sleep of 3 consecutive nights of 8 hr in bed. A modified MSLT, which utilized only two sleep latency measures, one at 09:40 hr and the other at 15:40 hr, was performed at the end of the 3-night baseline period. The results showed that the drivers were still very sleepy even after 8 hr in bed for 3 consecutive nights. Twenty-four drivers (36%) averaged sleep latencies (fell asleep) in 0–5 min and 31 drivers (47%) averaged sleep latencies in 5–10 min. Only eight drivers (12%) averaged sleep latencies in 10–15 min and only three drivers (5%) fell asleep in 15–20 min. Whatever sleep debt they had before baseline was apparently not substantially reduced even after 3 consecutive nights of 8 hr in bed. We may assume that the drivers needed much more extra sleep beyond their constitutional sleep requirement to clear their sleep debt and to show MSLT scores that would document improved alertness.

*How much sleep is needed to repay sleep debt?* It seems unlikely that exactly 1 extra hr of recovery sleep is needed to repay each hour of accumulated sleep debt (15), although the recovery process needs much more study. Some have suggested that the rate of recovery depends on the age level, with older adults showing improvement in reaction time tests more rapidly than younger adults (16). One experiment showed that older adults had returned to baseline levels on the MSLT after 1 night of recovery sleep, whereas younger adults continued to have shorter MSLT scores (17).

Whether we measure the underlying homeostatic sleep drive by means of the MSLT or by repeated ratings of subjective sleepiness, it should be clear that an individual's need for sleep at night (or the daily quota) may be defined in terms of a standard level of sleepiness or physiological sleep tendency in the daytime in the same manner as we might define the need for fluids. A human being must drink a certain amount of water each day to avoid dehydration. By the same token, a human being must sleep a certain amount each day to maintain a nominal level of alertness and to avoid accumulating a sleep debt. Accordingly, once a sleep debt has been accumulated, it is obvious that repayment would require sleeping amounts beyond the daily sleep need, i.e., obtaining extra sleep.

## V. Potential Benefits of Sleep Debt Reduction and the Way We Feel

In describing the effects of sleep debt reduction, it is desirable to distinguish subjective sleepiness from objective sleepiness, though both are caused by the underlying homeostatic sleep drive. Such a distinction again is analogous to maintaining hydration, in which the feeling or conscious component is experienced as being thirsty and the objective behavior motivated by the biological drive is seeking or drinking water or other suitable fluid to relieve dehydration. Dehydration would correspond to the state of being sleep-deprived. Thus, a moderately dehydrated person might not feel thirsty at any particular moment, in the same way a sleep-deprived person might not feel sleepy at any particular moment. More recently we have attempted to apply the word "sleepy" only to the subjective side of the coin, i.e., the subjective feeling of sleepiness, and to use the phrase "sleep tendency" for the objective side of the coin.

For many years, we have asked Stanford University undergraduates, *"How do you know whether or not you are feeling sleepy?"* We have learned that "sleepiness" appears to refer mostly to the feeling just before sleep onset, for example, the moment that the eyelids start to close involuntarily. In other words, student respondents do not subjectively experience the varying levels of increased sleep tendency as "sleepiness" until the physiological sleep tendency is overtaking them. Thus, until that point arrives, the sensations associated with increased sleep tendency are often characterized as something other than sleepiness. Usually, they are described as tiredness or fatigue. A study by Dement et al. (18) explored the relationship between "tiredness" versus "sleepiness" and "poor sleep." In a survey of 1,010 adults aged 18 years and older, subjects were asked a number of questions about their sleep behaviors as well as a number of other health and lifestyle questions. The percentage of respondents who indicated that they were "tired" on a typical day increased significantly as the usual number of hours of sleep decreased. Furthermore, the percentage of respondents who indicated "fair" or "poor" sleep quality was about three times more likely than those with "good," "very good," or "excellent" sleep to report that they were tired on a typical day. Finally, a much higher percentage of respondents who had sleepiness at least "a few days per week" or "a few days per month" reported always being tired on a typical day as compared to those stating that they were "rarely" or "never" sleepy during the day. These data clearly show that the sensation or expression of "tiredness" is a manifestation of poor sleep and presumably increased sleep drive.

Another study by Dement et al. (19) has shown a correlation between "tiredness" and sleep debt as well as clear benefits of sleep satiation. Fifteen healthy adults were studied by means of MSLT, PVT, and other paper-and-pencil tests. Daily sleep times were monitored by actigraphy and sleep logs. In addition, subjects were given a subjective scale to complete every half hour while awake: 1 (unambiguously alert with no tiredness), 2 (not fully alert, slightly tired), 3 (unambiguously tired), 4 (very tired, but definitely not sleepy, no conscious effort required to maintain attentiveness), and 5 (unambiguously sleepy, conscious effort required to remain attentive). Almost all the ratings were levels 2, 3, and 4 during the baseline week of typical sleep, indicating that people described themselves as tired to some degree much of the time, but rarely sleepy. These results were consistent even though MSLT scores were generally very low. The subjects then obtained as much extra sleep as possible to reduce the sleep debt. MSLT was performed once during baseline and twice during the period of extended sleep.

Each subject who showed clear-cut improvement on the MSLT (usually to an optimal score of 20) had obtained substantial extra sleep. Furthermore, almost all of the ratings for these subjects were 1 or 2, with a remarkable increase in the ratings of peak alertness (level 1) over baseline. There was also a notable disappearance of tiredness and sleepiness after lunch. Another very important result of obtaining extra sleep was the dramatic improvement in satiated subjects' mood, energy levels, and sense of well-being as indicated by daily checklists and questionnaires. On the other hand, with little or no MSLT improvement, subjective tiredness throughout the day was *not* reduced, nor were any of the other benefits observed.

A study by Roehrs et al. (20) supports the assertion that many people who consider their levels of tiredness and sleepiness as "normal" have high levels of sleep propensity. These investigators studied subjects who had no sleep complaints, but had MSLT scores below 6 min. These scores improved when subjects were given the opportunity to extend their sleep. Other MSLT-based reports have found improvement in daytime alertness after extension of sleep. In one study on "oversleeping," time in bed was increased to 11 hr/night for 1 night following either 8.5 hr or 6.5 hr in bed on the previous night (21). In both groups, the MSLT scores and performance measures showed improvement after the night of extra sleep.

One reason that studies of sleep satiation are relatively sparse may be a societal belief that impairment can be caused by "too much sleep." For example, polls of a very large number of Stanford University undergraduates have shown that over 90% believe it is possible to sleep too much. This was called the "Rip Van Winkle effect" by Globus (22), who, some years ago, described a syndrome associated with sleeping late, usually just 1 night. In this study, which was based on questionnaires, Globus reported that a significant number of people have experienced a "worn-out syndrome" after extra sleep. This syndrome was described on the questionnaire as feeling "worn-out, tired, lethargic, in an irritable mood, thinking is fuzzy, and it is difficult to get going on starting the activities of the day." The percentage of respondents who reported experiencing this syndrome at least once was as high as 87%. Taub and Berger (23) showed differences on the Wilkinson vigilance task after subjects slept 11 versus 8 hr, with decrement in the 11-hr group.

The notion that impairment follows "too much sleep" may be rejected for the following reasons. In the first place, the ability to sleep 12 or more hr or into the late afternoon means that an individual has a very large sleep debt. Most nights of prolonged sleep among the population usually follow bouts of severe sleep loss. This is frequently illustrated by the prolonged sleep periods observed in students after "all-nighters" in preparation for final exams. Several hours of extra sleep is almost certainly a negligible reduction of a very large sleep debt. Second, feeling groggy and unrested when waking up after prolonged sleep is discordant with what is expected by the naïve individual. Such individuals do not know that feeling unrested simply reflects a continuing strong physiological sleep tendency. Third, when sleep is markedly extended, individuals are likely to awaken close to the midday dip in alertness. Fourth, and finally, it is likely that muscular aches, discomfort, and/or stiffness are the result of the unusually protracted period of immobility, not specifically the result of too much sleep.

In addition to the foregoing, none of the recent studies of Dement et al. (18,19) and Wehr et al. (13) or any anecdotal reports by individuals after they had obtained extra sleep support the notion of impairment after too much sleep. It should also be pointed out that the subjects in the 14-hr-in-bed study reported feeling much more alert and energetic with a greater sense of well-being toward the end of the study after their total sleep debt reduction had been reduced.

## VI. Summary and Conclusions

Although large-scale controlled studies on chronic partial sleep deprivation and sleep extension are difficult to execute, we have been able to acquire a great deal of knowledge from the well-conducted investigations that have been carried out to date. Chronic partial sleep deprivation unquestionably leads to accumulation of impairment and progressively increased sleep tendency, the sum of which have been referred to as "sleep debt." Once sleep debt has accrued, it can only be paid back by extra sleep.

The process of obtaining extra sleep on a nightly basis for as many nights as possible is called sleep satiation. Compared to sleep deprivation, there are very few studies of sleep satiation in the scientific literature. It seems likely that most people are chronically sleep-deprived, i.e., are carrying a sleep debt. Given the opportunity, they are able to obtain a large quantity of extra sleep. As the sleep debt is "repaid," it is more and more difficult to obtain the same amount of extra sleep. In the studies described in this chapter, a point was reached after which obtaining extra sleep became very difficult, if not impossible.

In spite of the widespread belief that too much sleep (extra sleep) is bad, sleep satiation studies suggest that there are true and substantial benefits that accrue by reducing the sleep debt. These include the disappearance of daytime tiredness, fatigue, and sleepiness; mood elevation; and improvements in performance. Given the pervasive occurrence of chronic sleep loss and observations that sleep satiation is beneficial, we would strongly recommend mounting a sustained and serious scientific effort to investigate sleep satiation much more comprehensively.

## References

1. Hoddes E, Zarcone V, Smythe H, Phillips R, Dement W. Quantification of sleepiness: a new approach. Psychophsiology 1973; 10:431–436.
2. Richardson G, Carskadon M, Flagg W, van den Hoed J, Dement W, Mitler M. Excessive daytime sleepiness in man: multiple sleep latency measurement in narcoleptic and control subjects. Electroencephalogr Clin Neurophysiol 1978; 62:48–67.
3. Dinges D, Kribbs N. Performing while sleepy: effects of experimentally-induced sleepiness. Sleep Sleepiness Perform 1991; 97–128.
4. Carskadon M, Dement W. Daytime sleepiness: quantification of a behavioral state. Neurosci Biobehav Rev 1987; 11:307–317.
5. Carskadon MA, Dement WC. Cumulative effects of sleep restriction on daytime sleepiness. Psychophysiology 1981; 18:107–113.
6. Dinges DF, Pack F, Williams K, Gillen KA, et al. Cumulative sleepiness, mood disturbance, and psychomotor vigilance performance decrements during a week of sleep restricted to 4–5 hours per Night. Sleep 1997; 20:267–277.
7. Van Dongen HPA, Maislin G, Mullington JM, Dinges DF. The cumulative cost of additional wakefulness: dose-response effects on neurobehavioral functions and

sleep physiology from chronic sleep restriction and total sleep deprivation. Sleep 2003; 26:117–126.

8. Dijk D, Duffy J, Riel E, Shanahan T, Czeisler C. Ageing and the circadian and homeostatic regulation of human sleep during forced desynchrony of rest, melatonin and temperature rhythms. Physiol 1999; 516(2):611–627.

9. Edgar D, Dement W, Fuller C. Effect of SCN lesions on sleep in squirrel monkeys: evidence for opponent processes in sleep-wake regulation. J Neurosci 1993; 13(3):1065–1079.

10. Bonnet M, Arand D. Sleepiness as measured by modified multiple sleep latency testing as a function of preceding activity. Sleep 1998; 21:477–483.

11. Borbely A. A two process model of sleep regulation. Hum Neurobiol 1982; 1:195–204.

12. Kykamp K, Rosenthal L, Folkerts M, Roehrs T, Guido P, Roth T. The effects of REM sleep deprivation on the level of sleepiness/alertness. Sleep 1998; 21:609–614.

13. Wehr TA, Moul DE, Barbato G, et al. Conservation of photoperiod-responsive mechanism in humans. Am J Physiol 1993; 265:R846-R857.

14. Federal Motor Carrier Safety Administration. Effects of Sleep Schedules on Commercial Motor Vehicle Driver Performance. Report No. DOT-MC-00-133. 2000.

15. Jewett ME, Dijk D, Kronauer RE, Dinges DF. Dose-response relationship between sleep duration and human psychomotor vigilance and subjective alertness. Sleep 1999; 22:171–180.

16. Bonnet MH. Sleep deprivation. In: Kryger MH, Roth T, Dement WC, eds. Principles and Practice of Sleep Medicine. 3rd ed. Philadelphia: Saunders, 2000:65.

17. Carskadon MA, Dement WC. Sleep loss in elderly volunteers. Sleep 1985; 8:207–221.

18. Dement WC, Hall J, Walsh JK. Tiredness versus sleepiness: semantics or a target for public education? Sleep 2003; 26:485–486

19. Dement WC, Kaplan K, Mah K, Kamdar B. Sleep satiation. I. Effect on subjective feelings of tiredness. Sleep 2003; 26:A207–A208.

20. Roehrs T, Timms V, Zwyghuizen-Doorenbos A, Roth T. Sleep extension in sleepy and alert normals. Sleep 1989; 12:449–457.

21. Carskadon MA, Mancuso J, Keenan S, Littell W, Dement W. Sleepiness following oversleeping. Sleep Res 1986; 15:70.

22. Globus GG. A syndrome associated with sleeping late. Psychosom Med 1969; 31:528–535.

23. Taub JM, Berger RJ. Extended sleep and performance: the Rip Van Winkle effect. Psychon Sci 1969; 16:204–205.

# 29

## A Concluding Note on Sleep Deprivation and Sleep Mechanisms

**ALLAN RECHTSCHAFFEN**

Chicago, Illinois, U.S.A.

Lesion, stimulation, and neuronal activation studies have implicated a plethora of structures and substances in the control of sleep and wakefulness. References to the examples cited below can be found in Barbara Jones' superb review on "Basic Mechanisms of Sleep-Wake States" (1).

Structures implicated in the production or maintenance of sleep include the nucleus of the solitary tract, dorsal medullary reticular formation, raphe nuclei, thalamus, anterior hypothalamus, preoptic area, basal forebrain, orbitofrontal cortex, caudate nucleus, basal ganglia, and cerebral cortex. None of these structures are individually necessary for sleep. No lesion has produced a long lasting total insomnia. After some sleep-reducing lesions, sleep returns toward normal if sufficient time is allowed for recovery.

Structures implicated in the production of wakefulness and/or cortical arousal include the ventral medullary reticular formation, oral pontine reticular formation, midbrain reticular formation, posterior hypothalamus, subthalamus, certain areas of the basal forebrain, and the cortical mantle. None of these brain areas are individually necessary for the production or maintenance of wakefulness or arousal. Normal or near-normal wakefulness-arousal results when lesions are produced gradually or when sufficient time is allowed for recovery.

Although some of these structures exert their effects on sleep and wakefulness via integrated systems, it is clear from the effects of lesions and stimulation that parts of the system can, in the short run, independently increase or reduce the total system outputs. Several different structures seem to be involved, none of which are essential for sleep or wakefulness. Judging from the recovery of sleep and wakefulness after state-reducing lesions, it also appears that sleep and wakefulness may result from different mixtures of mechanistic action at different times. Thus we are left with the impression of a rather diverse, shifting, fluid mechanistic control of sleep and wakefulness.

The fluid picture of sleep-wake control is not improved by an appeal to neurohumoral regulation. Substances implicated in the production or maintenance of sleep include serotonin, GABA, opiate peptides (e.g., endorphin), somatostatin, insulin, bombesin, muramyl peptides, and uridine. One review (2) listed published support for 23 different sleep factors; the list is likely to be substantially longer now. *(Will we better understand how sleep is regulated when we reach 100 sleep factors?)* Chemicals implicated in the production or maintenance of wakefulness include catecholamines, dopamine, acetylcholine, glutamate, histamine, and various peptides. Jones has summarized: ". . . no single chemical transmitter, neuromodulator, or neurohormone has been identified that is necessary or sufficient for the generation and maintenance of sleep or waking. Instead, multiple factors and systems are involved in the onset and maintenance of these states" (1, p.149). This fact is usually ignored when researchers tout their results on individual structures or substances that can affect sleep and/or wakefulness.

This seemingly variable mixture of several different sleep and wake mechanisms seems at odds with the relative stability of total sleep amounts. (This report focuses entirely on *total sleep* rather than specific sleep stages like REM and slow-wave sleep, which depend on more specific mechanisms and appear to be more reactive to presleep experience.)

(a) Although we are fond of social exchanges about having had a good or poor night of sleep, percentage-wise our sleep totals tend to stay relatively stable from night to night, except perhaps for weekends in some age groups. The one study we have located with the greatest number of consecutive, uninterrupted, recorded nights reported on 15 young adults who spent 1 week on a 16/8 hr light/dark schedule, followed 2 weeks later by 4 weeks on a 10/14 hr light/dark schedule (3). Although the variance of individual sleep totals across nights was not described quantitatively, raster plots showed great night-to-night stability on both schedules. We know of no hard data on the matter, but impressionistically it seems that total sleep per 24 hr may be much more stable from day to day than total food intake or physical activity. In rats maintained in constant light, total sleep showed incredibly little variation across rats and across 6 hr blocks of the day (4). Species differences in sleep totals are also stable, as they vary widely (from about 4 hr/day in the elephant to about 20 hr/day in the bat) and the variations are significantly correlated with other variables such as life span, body weight, and metabolic rate (5).

(b) Experimental studies have shown several effects of presleep stimulation on amounts of REM sleep or high-voltage, slow-wave EEG activity, but few effects on total sleep. A review of stimulation effects showed that "In humans, total sleep has not been substantially affected by exercise, prolonged bed rest, increased visual load, or stimulating daytime activities; profound perceptual deprivation produced initial increases in total sleep, but no substantial continuing effect" [Rechtschaffen (6), p. 368]. More extreme experimental manipulations in animals have also had little effect on total sleep. In rats, total sleep was not significantly changed by a presleep array of intense sound, light, and olfactory stimuli (7). The administration to rats of enough thyroxine to produce a large increase in food intake coupled with a significant reduction in weight gain did not change total sleep time by as much as 2% across experimental conditions (8). In cats, 3 hr of electrical stimulation of the brainstem reticular formation did not significantly affect subsequent total sleep (9).

(c) The return to near-normal levels of sleep and wakefulness after experimental brain lesions also indicates a thrust toward baseline sleep levels.

(d) Sleep also shows a certain stability in the way it is expressed. Given the variety of neuronal groups and neurochemicals that can promote sleep or wakefulness, one would think there was ample opportunity for both to be expressed simultaneously—as they seem to be following sleep deprivation. Yet, for the most part, we are normally awake or asleep.

Thus, in spite of the many structures and substances that might potentially participate in the production and maintenance of sleep and wakefulness, and in spite of how they might be variously affected by daily variations in behavior and experience, total daily sleep tends toward a stable amount and stable expression. *How does that happen? With at least 30 different sleep and wake factors variously impinging on nearly 20 sleep-wake brain sites, why do most of us (according to self reports) usually get about 7–8 hr of sleep a night?*

*Does a yet-unidentified master controller, e.g., a specific brain center, balance the outputs of the various sleep and wake mechanisms to produce a stable total output?* If such a center does exist, one would guess that given the many experimental lesions made throughout the brain, it would have been discovered.

*Are the various sleep and wake mechanisms constitutionally fixed to produce a given, fixed, optimal, daily sleep output?* This is unlikely given the apparent compensations for destroyed components of sleep-wake mechanisms and the apparently homeostatic compensations for lost sleep.

The compensations for lost sleep suggest that the master control of *total sleep* may not reside in specific, localizable sleep effectors or neuromodulators, but in a stimulus generated by the need for sleep. Presumably, this need-stimulus activates several sleep centers and substances and deactivates wake centers and substances, which then contribute to the production of sleep to the extent that they are affected. (Conceivably, a need for wakefulness might conversely activate wake mechanisms and deactivate sleep mechanisms.) If one sleep or wake effector were destroyed or blocked by experimental or natural intervention, the need-generated stimulus would opportunistically recruit whatever systems were available to answer the need. When the need was satisfied, the effector systems would remain inactive no matter how prepared they were to function.

Accordingly, insofar as the sleep or wake need was not grossly perturbed by biological or environmental upheaval, sleep and wake amounts would remain stable even though the mix of effector contributions might vary in response to other factors.

The regulation of multiple and often independent mechanisms by—and in the service of—a single functional demand is well established in biology, especially in the protection of vital functions. For example, the maintenance of adequate body heat can be served by increased metabolism, vasoconstriction, piloerection, shivering, brown-fat activation, heat-conserving postures, increased locomotion, and behavioral adjustments like adding clothing. Any or all of these mechanisms may be activated in response to the need for body heat, but may remain inactive when the need is satisfied. In a similar fashion, the existence of multiple sleep-wake effector mechanisms would be insurance for sleep-wake homeostasis rather than a cause for physiological chaos.

Specific sleep-wake effector mechanisms are necessary for responding to sleep-wake needs, and our understanding of sleep-wake regulation would be incomplete without identifying and dissecting the specific mechanisms. Also, pathologically activated or inhibited mechanisms may produce sleep totals that are obviously outside the range of commonsense conceptions of sleep need, e.g., as in idiopathic hypersomnia or fatal familial insomnia. (To follow through with the temperature regulation analogy, malignant hyperthermia can result from a genetically determined excessive contraction of muscle and consequent heat production.) (A daunting challenge for sleep clinicians is to distinguish which sleep disorders result from faulty homeostatic systems and which from pathological mechanisms.) The experimental destruction or stimulation of a contributing mechanism might, especially in the short run, overwhelm the capacity to maintain optimal homeostasis. Nevertheless, according to the perspective now being considered, under ordinary circumstances, in the absence of severe pathology or strong experimental intervention, the regulation of *total* sleep-wake output would be primarily by the need-stimulus, not by the properties of the effector mechanisms.

Although this perspective parsimoniously encompasses the multiplicity of wake-sleep mechanisms, their plasticity and redundancy, the relative stability of total sleep, and rebounds following sleep deprivation, it suffers from a lack of critical, direct evidence. We have no better idea of what the major need-generated stimulus might be than we have of whether there is a master control mechanism. Only further, successful research can resolve these issues.

Prospects for finding a powerful need-stimulus are not-simply rhetorical. From time to time, reasonable candidates emerge. For example, Bennington and Heller (10) have proposed that the depletion of cerebral glycogen (the principal stored energy in the brain) during the elevated cerebral metabolism of wakefulness activates the release of adenosine, which in turn stimulates non-rapid-eye-movement (NREM) sleep (a state of reduced cerebral metabolism), during which glycogen stores are replenished. The theory is attractive because it sets an important, reasonable functional goal for sleep (cerebral energy homeostasis), utilizes a widely distributed need-stimulus (depleted glycogen) that could stimulate widely distributed sleep mechanisms, and specifies a mediator (adenosine) that activates the corrective process (NREM sleep). The theory is well conceived and mechanistic throughout. However, evidence for the theory is mixed. Twenty years ago, Karnovsky et al. (11) showed increases in rat brain glycogen levels during the early minutes of sleep, but little change thereafter—thereby leaving open the question of what function the remainder of sleep might serve. Kong et al. (12) showed theory-consistent results of a decrease in brain glycogen during sleep deprivation, which was reversed with recovery sleep. Gip et al. (13) found that 6 hr of sleep deprivation induced decreases of glycogen level in the cerebellum, but 12 hr of deprivation did not. Glycogen levels were not decreased in the cortex. In fact, in the oldest rats studied (~59 days), cortical glycogen levels were *increased* by sleep deprivation. The authors suggested that prolonged sleep deprivation might result in compensatory changes in glycogen homeostasis even in the absence of undisturbed sleep, *but then why would sleep be necessary?* In a study of three mouse strains (14), sleep deprivation lowered glycogen in the cerebellum and brainstem of two strains, but the third strain showed only an *increase* in cortical glycogen level. The two groups with similar glycogen levels differed most in their compensatory response to sleep loss. The authors took these results to mean that glycogen content is the unlikely endpoint of sleep's role in brain energy homeostasis. Apart from the recent experimental evidence, there is reason to question why electrical brain stimulation (9) or very prolonged sleep deprivation did not increase subsequent slow-wave sleep (4,15), as the glycogen hypothesis would have predicted. Altogether, it seems unlikely that brain glycogen level is the need-stimulus with major control of total sleep, but it does provide an example of the kind of basic, widely distributed biological parameter that might some day provide the answer. New approaches, such as the identification of changes in gene expression during sleep, wakefulness, and sleep deprivation (e.g.,Tononi and Cirelli [16]), offer new promise.

If the control of total sleep depends primarily on a need-stimulus, then sleep deprivation is an essential tool for understanding the activation of sleep mechanisms. We need to identify the brain changes that result from sleep deprivation and, in turn, control the specific sleep effectors. Sleep deprivation studies have had two major bifurcating conceptual trajectories. One examines the disruptive and pathological consequences of sleep loss, which in turn suggest the functional targets of sleep. The other trajectory is to identify the physiological consequences of sleep loss, which then serve as regulators of sleep production. This trajectory is embodied in classic experiments, dating back to Pieron (17), on the search for sleep-producing substances in sleep-deprived animals. Currently, there seems to be much greater interest in pathological consequences. But in the long run, we will need discoveries about the mechanistic controls and how they are homeostatically regulated to provide therapies for sleep disorders and give us a satisfying comprehension of sleep.

## References

1. Jones, BE. Basic mechanisms of sleep-wake states. In: Kryger MH, Roth T, Dement WC, eds. Principles and Practice of Sleep Medicine. Philadelphia: Saunders, 2000:134–54.
2. Garcia-Garcia F, Drucker-Colin R. Endogenous and exogenous factors on sleep-wake cycle regulation. Prog in Neurobiol 1999; 58:297–314.
3. Wehr TA, Moul DE, Barbato G, Giesen HA, Seidel JA, Barker C. Bender C. Conservation of photo-responsive mechanisms in humans. Am J Physiol 1993; 25(Regul Integr Comp Physiol 34):R846–R857.
4. Rechtschaffen A, Bergmann BM, Gilliland MA, Bauer K. Effects of method, duration, and sleep stage on rebounds from sleep deprivation in the rat. Sleep 1999; 22:11–31.
5. Zepelin H, Rechtschaffen A. Mammalian sleep, longevity, and energy metabolism. Brain, Behav, and Evol 1974; 10:425–470.
6. Rechtschaffen A. Current perspectives on the function of sleep. Perspect Biol Med 1998; 43:359–390.
7. Frederickson CJ, Madansky DL, Rechtschaffen A. Sensory stimulation and subsequent sleep. Commun Behav Biol 1969; 4:109–113.
8. Eastman CI, Rechtschaffen A. The effect of thyroxine on sleep in the rat. Sleep 1979; 2:215–32.
9. Frederickson CJ, Hobson JA. Electrical stimulation of the brain stem and subsequent sleep. Arch Ital Biol 1970; 108:564–76.
10. Benington JH, Heller, HC, Restoration of brain energy metabolisms a function of sleep. Prog Neurobiol 1995; 45:347–60.
11. Karnovsky ML, Reich P, Anchors JM, Burrows BL. Changes in brain glycogen during slow-wave sleep in the rat. J Neurochem 1983; 41:1498–1501.
12. Kong J, Shepel PN, Holden CP, Mackiewicz, Pack AI, Geiger JD. Brain glycogen decreases with increased periods of wakefulness: implications for homeostatic drive to sleep. J Neurosci 2002; 22:5581–5587.
13. Gip P, Hagiwara G, Ruby NF, Heller HC. Sleep deprivation decreases glycogen in the cerebellum but not in the cortex of young rats. Am J Physiol Regul Integr Comp Physiol 2002; 283:R54–419.
14. Franken P, Gip P, Hagiwara G. Ruby NF, Heller HC. Changes in brain glycogen after sleep deprivation vary with genotype. American Journal of Physiology Regulatory Integrative and Comparative Physiology 2003;285:R413–9.
15. Everson CA, Gilliland MA, Kushida CA, Pilcher JJ, Fang VS, Refetoff S, Bergmann BM, Rechtschaffen A. Sleep deprivation in the rat. IX. Recovery. Sleep 1989; 12:60–67.
16. Tononi G, Cirelli C. Modulation of brain gene expression during sleep and wakefulness: a review of recent findings. Neuropsychopharmacology 2001; 25(suppl)1:S28–35.
17. Pieron H. Le probleme physiologique du sommeil. Paris, France: Masson, 1913.

# Index

573